ENT

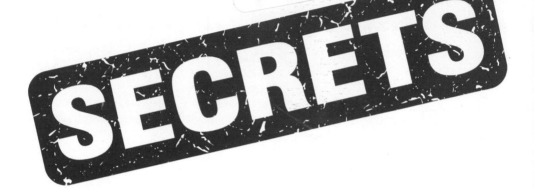

ENT

MELISSA A. SCHOLES, MD
Assistant Professor
Otolaryngology
University of Colorado, Aurora
Colorado
United States

VIJAY R. RAMAKRISHNAN, MD
Professor
Otolaryngology – Head and Neck Surgery
Indiana University School of Medicine,
Indianapolis
Indiana
United States

ELSEVIER

Elsevier
1600 John F. Kennedy Blvd.
Ste 1800
Philadelphia, PA 19103-2899

ENT SECRETS, FIFTH EDITION

ISBN: 978-0-323-73357-1

Previous editions copyrighted 2016, 2005, 2001 and 1996

Content Strategist: Marybeth Thiel
Content Development Specialist: Shweta Pant
Publishing Services Manager: Shereen Jameel
Project Manager: Gayathri S
Design Direction: Bridget Hoette

Printed in India

Last digit is the print number: 9 8 7 6 5 4 3 2 1

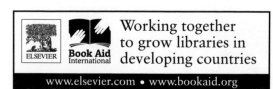

CONTRIBUTORS

Gregory C. Allen, MD, FACS, FAAP
Associate Professor
Department of Otolaryngology – Head and Neck Surgery
University of Colorado School of Medicine, Denver
Colorado
United States;
Associate Profoooor
Department of Pediatrics
University of Colorado School of Medicine, Denver
Colorado
United States;
Faculty Physician
Pediatric Otolaryngology
Children's Hospital Colorado, Aurora
Colorado
United States

Jeremiah A. Alt, MD, PhD
Sinus and Skull Base Surgery Program
Division of Otolaryngology
University of Utah,
Salt Lake City
Utah
United States

Henry P. Barham, MD
Rhinology/Skull Base Surgery
Sinus and Nasal Specialists, Baton Rouge
Louisiana
United States

Ethan Bassett, MD
Assistant Professor
Division of Pediatric Otolaryngology
Nationwide Children's Hospital
The Ohio State University
Columbus, Ohio
United States

Nancy Bauman, MD
Professor
Otolaryngology Head and Neck Surgery
Children's National Health System, George Washington
    University, Washington
District of Columbia
United States

Daniel M. Beswick, MD
Assistant Professor
Otolaryngology – Head and Neck Surgery
University of California Los Angeles,
Los Angeles
California
United States

Lorelei Bourla, MD, MS
Instructor
Department of Medicine
University of Colorado, Aurora
Colorado
United States

Daniel W. Bowles, MD
Associate Professor
Medical Oncology
University of Colorado, Aurora
Colorado
United States

Mariah Brown, MD
Associate Professor
Dermatology
University of Colorado School of Medicine, Aurora
Colorado
United States

Erin J. Buczek, MD, FACS
Assistant Professor
Department of Otolaryngology – Head and Neck Surgery
University of Alabama at Birmingham,
Birmingham
Alabama

Cristina Cabrera-Muffly, MD, FACS
Associate Professor
Otolaryngology
University of Colorado, Englewood
Colorado
United States

Thomas L. Carroll, MD
Assistant Professor
Otolaryngology Head and Neck Surgery
Harvard University School of Medicine, Boston
Massachusetts
United States

Nathan D. Cass, MD
Neurotology Fellow
The Otology Group of Vanderbilt
Vanderbilt University Department of Otolaryngology,
    Nashville
Tennessee
United States

Stephen P. Cass, MD
Professor
Otolaryngology Head and Neck Surgery
University of Colorado Anschutz Medical Campus, Aurora
Colorado
United States

Jeffrey Chain, MD
Private Practice
Comprehensive ENT, Head and Neck Surgery
Denver
Colorado
United States

Kenny H. Chan, MD
Chief
Department of Pediatric Otolaryngology
Children's Hospital Colorado, Aurora
Colorado
United States

Tendy Chiang, MD
Pediatric Otolaryngologist
Department of Otolaryngology
Nationwide Children's Hospital, Columbus
Ohio
United States;
Assistant Professor
Department of Otolaryngology
The Ohio State University College of Medicine, Columbus
Ohio
United States

Farshad Chowdhury, MD
Department of Otolaryngology – Head and Neck Surgery
University of Colorado School of Medicine, Aurora
Colorado
United States

Matthew S. Clary, MD
Associate Professor
Department of Otolaryngology – Head and Neck Surgery
University of Colorado, Aurora
Colorado
United States

Stacy Claycomb, AuD (Doctor of Audiology)
Pediatric Audiologist
Audiology
University of Colorado Hospital, Aurora
Colorado
United States

Luke A. Corsten, MD
Staff Physician
Neurosurgery
The NeuroMedical Center, Baton Rouge
Louisiana
United States

Elizabeth Cuadrado, MS, CCC-SLP, BCS-S
Senior Instructor
Otolaryngology
University of Colorado Anschutz Medical Campus, Aurora
Colorado
United States

Owen A. Darr, MD
Assistant Professor
Otolaryngology – Head and Neck Surgery
University of Colorado, Aurora
Colorado
United States

Elliana Kirsh Devore, MD
Surgical Resident
Department of Otolaryngology – Head and Neck Surgery
Harvard Medical School, Boston
Massachusetts
United States

Allison M. Dobbie, MD
Assistant Professor
Department of Otolaryngology, Division of Pediatric
    Otolaryngology
University of Colorado School of Medicine, Colorado
    Springs
Colorado
United States

Yadrano Ducic, MD, FACS
Staff Physician
Head and Neck Oncologic, Reconstructive and Skull Base
    Surgery, Dallas
Texas
United States

Marcia Eustaquio, MD
Surgeon
Department of Otolaryngology
Denver Health Medical Center, Denver
Colorado
United States;
Associate Professor
Department of Otolaryngology
University of Colorado, Denver
Colorado
United States

Vincent Eusterman, MD, DDS
Associate Professor
Otolaryngology-Head & Neck Surgery
University of Colorado School of Medicine, Aurora
Colorado
United States;
Director
Otolaryngology-Head and Neck Surgery
Denver Health Medical Center, Denver
Colorado
United States

Isabel Fairmont, MD, MS
Resident Physician
Otolaryngology – Head and Neck Surgery
University of Colorado, Aurora
Colorado
United States

Geoffrey Ferril, MD
Assistant Professor
Otolaryngology – Head and Neck Surgery
University of Colorado School of Medicine, Aurora
Colorado
United States

Daniel S. Fink, MD
Assistant Professor, Laryngology
Otolaryngology – Head and Neck Surgery
University of Colorado School of Medicine, Aurora
Colorado
United States

Carol A. Foster, MD
Associate Professor
Otolaryngology
University of Colorado, Aurora
Colorado
United States

Christian R. Francom, MD
Assistant Professor of Pediatric Otolaryngology – Head
    and Neck Surgery
University of Colorado School of Medicine/Children's
    Hospital Colorado
Aurora, Colorado
United States

Norman R. Friedman, MD
Professor
Pediatric Otolaryngology
Children's Hospital Colorado, Aurora
Colorado
United States;
Professor
Otolaryngology
University of Colorado School of Medicine, Aurora
Colorado
United States

Sandra Abbott Gabbard, PhD
President/CEO
Marion Downs Center, Denver
Colorado
United States;
Associate Professor
Pediatrics
University of Colorado, Aurora
Colorado
United States

Anne E. Getz, MD
Department of Otolaryngology – Head and Neck Surgery
University of Colorado, Denver
Colorado
United States

Saied Ghadersohi, MD
Fellow
Pediatric Otolaryngology Head and Neck Surgery
Children's Hospital Colorado, Aurora
Colorado
United States

Sarah A. Gitomer, MD
Assistant Professor
Otolaryngology – Head and Neck Surgery
University of Colorado, Aurora
Colorado
United States

Julie A. Goddard, MD, FACS
Department of Otolaryngology – Head and Neck Surgery
University of California, Irvine
Orange
California
United States

Katherine K. Green, MD, MS
Medical Director, Sleep Center
Otolaryngology
University of Colorado School of Medicine, Aurora
Colorado
United States

Samuel P. Gubbels, MD, FACS
Medical Director, UCHealth Otolaryngology
Director, UCHealth Hearing and Balance Clinics
Associate Professor, Otolaryngology and Neurosurgery
University of Colorado School of Medicine,
Aurora
Colorado
United States

Tamar Hajar, MD
Fellow Physician
Dermatology
University of Colorado School of Medicine, Aurora
Colorado
United States

Erin Hamersley, DO, LCDR, MC, USN
Pediatric Otolaryngologist
Department of Otolaryngology
Naval Medical Center Portsmouth, Virginia
United States;
Assistant Professor
Department of Surgery
Uniformed Services University of the Health Sciences,
    Bethesda
Maryland
United States

Steven Hamilton, MD
Assistant Professor
Otolaryngology – Head and Neck Surgery
University of Colorado School of Medicine, Aurora
Colorado
United States;
Assistant Professor
Pediatric Otolaryngology
Children's Hospital Colorado, Colorado Springs
Colorado
United States

Renee Banakis Hartl, MD, AuD
Resident Physician
Department of Otolaryngology
University of Colorado, Aurora
Colorado
United States

Gabriela Heslop, MD
Resident Physician
Otolaryngology – Head and Neck Surgery
University of Colorado School of Medicine, Aurora
Colorado
United States

Scott Hirsch, MD
Resident-Physician
Otolaryngology
University of Colorado, Anschutz Medical Campus
Aurora
Colorado
United States

Douglas E. Holt, MD
Resident Physician
Radiation Oncology
University of Colorado, Aurora
Colorado
United States

Herman Jenkins, MD
Department of Otolaryngology
University of Colorado School of Medicine
Aurora
Colorado
United States

Marie Jetté, PhD, CCC-SLP
Assistant Professor
Otolaryngology
University of Colorado, Aurora
Colorado
United States

Anjeli Prabhu Kalra, MD
Assistant Professor of Medicine
Allergy and Clinical Immunology
University of Colorado Hospital, Aurora
Colorado
United States

Sana D. Karam, MD, PhD
Department of Radiation Oncology
University of Denver Colorado,
Colorado
United States

Ryota Kashiwazaki, MD
Fellow
Pediatric Otolaryngology
Children's Hospital Colorado, Denver
Colorado
United States

Peggy E. Kelley, MD
Associate Professor
Otolaryngology
University of Colorado, Denver, Aurora
Colorado
United States

Todd T. Kingdom, MD
Professor and Vice Chair Clinical Affairs
Otolaryngology – Head and Neck Surgery
University of Colorado School of Medicine, Aurora
Colorado
United States

Ryan LaRochelle, MD
Resident Physician (Ophthalmology)
Department of Ophthalmology
University of Colorado School of Medicine
United States

Steven Leoniak, MD
Assistant Professor
Otolaryngology – Head and Neck Surgery
University of Colorado, Colorado Springs
Colorado
United States

Alexandra Levitt, MD, MPH
Instructor/Fellow
Department of Ophthalmology
University of Colorado School of Medicine, Aurora
Colorado
United States

Sophie Liao, MD
Assistant Professor
Oculoplastic & Orbital Surgery, Ophthalmology
University of Colorado School of Medicine, Aurora
Colorado
United States;
Medical Director
Sue Anschutz – Rodgers Eye Centers
University of Colorado Hospitals, Aurora
Colorado
United States

Juliana Litts, MA CCC-SLP, Certified Vocologist
Assistant Professor
Otolaryngology – Head and Neck Surgery
University of Colorado, Aurora
Colorado
United States

Scott E. Mann, MD
Assistant Professor
Department of Otolaryngology – Head and Neck Surgery
University of Colorado School of Medicine, Aurora
Colorado
United States

Conner J. Massey, MD
Resident Physician
Otolaryngology – Head and Neck Surgery
University of Colorado School of Medicine, Aurora
Colorado
United States

Jameson K. Mattingly, MD
Assistant Professor
Department of Otolaryngology – Head and Neck Surgery
The Ohio State University Wexner Medical Center
Columbus
Ohio
United States

Brook K. McConnell, MD
Department of Otolaryngology
University of Colorado School of Medicine
Department of Pediatric Otolaryngology
Children's Hospital Colorado, Aurora
Colorado
United States

Jessica D. McDermott, MD
Fellow
Division of Medical Oncology
University of Colorado School of Medicine
Aurora
Colorado
United States

David M. Mirsky, MD
Pediatric Neuroradiologist
Radiology
Children's Hospital Colorado, Aurora
Colorado
United States;
Assistant Professor
Radiology
University of Colorado, Aurora
Colorado
United States

Emily S. Misch, MD, MPH
Resident
Otolaryngology – Head and Neck Surgery
University of Colorado, Aurora
Colorado
United States

Paul Montero, MD
Associate Professor
Surgery
University of Colorado, Aurora
Colorado
United States

Pamela A. Mudd, MD, MBA
Assistant Professor
Pediatric Otolaryngology
Children's National Medical Center, Washington, DC
United States

Matthew Naunheim, MD, MBA
Assistant Professor of Otolaryngology-Head and
    Neck Surgery, Harvard Medical SchoolDivision of
    Laryngology, Massachusetts Eye and Ear
Massachusetts
United States

Stephen S. Newton, MD
Assistant Professor
Otolaryngology
University of Colorado and Children's Hospital of Colorado,
    Colorado Springs
Colorado
United States;
Assistant Professor
Radiology
University of Colorado and Children's Hospital of Colorado,
    Aurora
Colorado
United States

Richard R. Orlandi, MD
Sinus and Skull Base Surgery Program
Division of Otolaryngology
University of Utah,
Salt Lake City
Utah
United States

Erik Peltz, DO
Assistant Professor of Surgery
Surgery
University of Colorado Anschutz Medical Campus, Aurora
Colorado
United States

Cory Portnuff, AuD PhD
UCHealth Hearing and Balance Clinic
University of Colorado Hospital
Department of Otolaryngology – Head and Neck Surgery
University of Colorado School of Medicine
Aurora, Colorado
United States

Jeremy D. Prager, MD, MBA
Associate Professor
Otolaryngology
University of Colorado School of Medicine, Aurora
Colorado
United States;
Associate Professor
Pediatric Otolaryngology
Children's Hospital Colorado, Aurora
Colorado
United States

Allison Ramakrishnan, AuD, MS
Department of Audiology
University of Colorado Hospital
Aurora
Colorado
United States

Vijay R. Ramakrishnan, MD
Professor
Otolaryngology-Head and Neck Surgery
Indiana University School of Medicine
Indianapolis, Indiana
United States

Laylaa Ramos Arriaza, MD, MS
Research Scholar
Otolaryngology – Head and Neck Surgery
University of Colorado, Aurora
Colorado
United States

John Richards, MD
Department of Otolaryngology – Head and Neck Surgery
University of Arizona, Tucson
Arizona
United States

Sanya Richardson, AuD, CCC-A, PASC
Pediatric Audiologist
Audiology, Speech Pathology and Learning Services
Children's Hospital Colorado, Aurora
Colorado
United States

Kenny D. Rodriguez, MD
Resident Physician
Otolaryngology – Head and Neck Surgery
University of Colorado, Aurora
Colorado
United States

Brianne Barnett Roby, MD
Pediatric Otolaryngologist
Pediatric ENT and Facial Plastic Surgery
Children's Hospitals and Clinics of Minnesota, St. Paul
Minnesota
United States;
Assistant Professor
Department of Otolaryngology
University of Minnesota, Minneapolis
Minnesota
United States

Benjamin J. Rubinstein, MD
Assistant Professor
Department of Otolaryngology – Head and Neck Surgery
Eastern Virginia Medical School
Norfolk, Virginia
United States

Melissa A. Scholes, MD
Associate Professor
Otolaryngology
University of Colorado, Aurora
Colorado
United States

Franki Lambert Smith, MD
Associate Professor
Dermatology
University of Rochester Medical Center, Rochester
New York
United States

Fiyin Sokoya, MD
Assistant Professor
Department of Otolaryngology
University of Arizona, Tucson
Arizona
United States

Jeffrey D. Suh, MD
Associate Professor
Division of Head and Neck Surgery
University of California, Los Angeles, Los Angeles
California
United States

Adam M. Terella, MD
Associate Professor
Otolaryngology – Head and Neck Surgery
University of Colorado School of Medicine, Aurora
Colorado
United States

Carissa M. Thomas, MD, PhD, FACS
Assistant Professor
Department of Otolaryngology – Head and Neck Surgery
University of Alabama at Birmingham, Birmingham
Alabama
United States

Kristin Uhler, PhD
Associate Professor
Physical Medicine & Rehabilitation
Children's Hospital Colorado, CU Anschutz, Aurora
Colorado
United States

Thad W. Vickery, MD
Resident Surgeon
Head and Neck Surgery
David Geffen School of Medicine at UCLA, Los Angeles
California
United States

Craig Villari, MD
Bellevue Ear, Nose & Throat,
Bellevue
Washington
United States

Aurora G. Vincent, MD, FACS
Facial Plastic & Reconstructive Surgery
Dwight D. Eisenhower Army Medical Center
Fort Gordon, Georgia
United States

Sean X. Wang, MD
Otolaryngology – Head and Neck Surgery
Sutter Health, Fremont
California
United States

Taylor M. Washburn, MD
Clinical Assistant Professor
Internal Medicine
George E Whalen VA Medical Center, Salt Lake City
Utah
United States

Timothy V. Waxweiler, MD
Associate Professor
Radiation Oncology
University of Colorado, Aurora
Colorado
United States

Todd M. Wine, MD
Physician
Associate Professor
Otolaryngology
University of Colorado Anschutz Medical Campus, Aurora
Colorado
United States;
Pediatric Otolaryngologist
Division of Pediatric Otolaryngology
Children's Hospital of Colorado, Aurora
Colorado
United States

Andrew A. Winkler, MD
Associate Professor
Otolaryngology Head and Neck Surgery
University of Colorado, Denver
Colorado
United States;
Director of Facial Plastic Surgery
Highlands Ranch
United States

William C. Yao, MD
Assistant Professor
Department of Otorhinolaryngology
University of Texas McGovern Medical School at Houston,
  Houston
Texas
United States

Patricia J. Yoon, MD
Associate Professor
Otolaryngology
University of Colorado School of Medicine, Aurora
Colorado
United States;
Faculty
Pediatric Otolaryngology
Children's Hospital Colorado, Aurora
Colorado
United States

PREFACE

Drs. Bruce Jafek and Anne Stark published the first edition of *ENT Secrets* as a communal effort from the University of Colorado Department of Otolaryngology faculty, residents, trainees, and alumni. As the field of otolaryngology has expanded and grown, so has the scope of the contributions from experts in the field across the country. In order to give the most up to date and thorough knowledge, we have come up with this latest edition of *ENT Secrets*. We are indebted to the hard work of all our contributors and thank them for providing excellent content.

CONTENTS

3   ALLERGY AND RHINOLOGY

4   OTOLOGY AND AUDIOLOGY

5   PEDIATRIC OTOLARYNGOLOGY

6   FACIAL PLASTIC SURGERY, RECONSTRUCTION, AND TRAUMA

7   LARYNGOLOGY AND SWALLOWING DISORDERS

TOP 100 EXAMINATION PEARLS

1. If a trachea-innominate bleed occurs in a patient with a cuffed endotracheal or tracheostomy tube, the first step is to overinflate the cuff to tamponade bleeding.
2. A cricothyroidotomy should be converted to a formal tracheotomy within 24 hours, if possible, to minimize the risk of subglottic stenosis.
3. The classic presentation of peritonsillar abscess includes trismus, uvular deviation, muffled voice, and soft palatal edema.
4. In patients with a penicillin allergy, assessing the type of previous reaction in conjunction with penicillin skin testing and oral amoxicillin can determine if penicillin or cephalosporin antibiotics are safe to use.
5. Elevated risk factors for obstructive sleep apnea:
   a. Age greater than 65 years
   b. Body mass index (BMI) greater than 30 kg/m²
   c. Postmenopausal female
   d. African American or Asian race
   e. Male sex
   f. Neck circumference greater than 17 inches in men and 16 inches in women
6. The supraglottis is the most common laryngeal site affected by sarcoidosis. The epiglottis and arytenoids become pale and extremely swollen, giving a "turban-like" appearance.
7. Tension-type headache is the most common type of headache/facial pain.
8. Pediatric autoimmune neuropsychiatric disorder associated with streptococcal infection (PANDAS) is a self-limited condition associated with increased tics and obsessive mannerisms that correlate with elevated anti-streptolysin O titers.
9. Periodic fever, aphthous stomatitis, pharyngitis, cervical adenitis (PFAPA) is a condition defined by high fevers that last 3 to 7 days and recur every 3 to 6 weeks. The cause of PFAPA is unknown but is thought to be either immune-related or infectious.
10. The second branchial cleft is the most common branchial cleft to develop an anomaly.
11. Breslow depth is the most important prognostic factor in melanoma.
12. Cervical lymph node metastasis is a key driver of prognosis in oral cavity cancers and non-HPV-related oropharynx cancers, but less so in HPV-related oropharynx cancers.
13. Smoking through treatment for laryngeal cancer increases the chance for treatment failure and recurrence.
14. HPV-positive and HPV-negative head and neck squamous cell cancers have different drivers of carcinogenesis.
15. Hypopharyngeal cancer is notable for frequent submucosal spread and carries a worse prognosis than laryngeal cancer.
16. Gene sequencing classifier testing tests for RNA expression of several different genes for benign and malignant thyroid nodules. It has a >95% negative predictive value and essentially "rules out" cancer.
17. HIV workup is important in a patient who presents with cystic parotid masses.
18. Carotid body paragangliomas present as a pulsatile neck mass with characteristic CT, MRI, and angiographic findings, including characteristic flow voids and splaying of the external and internal carotid arteries (lyre sign).
19. Excisional lymph node biopsy is the gold standard for diagnosis of lymphoma and subtyping, but core needle biopsy may obtain enough tissue for diagnosis and can be used to direct further workup.
20. The use of ice chips in the mouth during chemotherapy can prevent mucositis by causing vasoconstriction, and rinsing the mouth with buffered saline can treat mucositis.
21. The paranasal sinuses form as evaginations from the nasal cavity. The ethmoid and maxillary sinuses are present at birth, and all sinuses continue to develop postnatally with the sphenoid and frontal sinuses developing last.
22. A patient who requires posterior nasal packing should be admitted to the hospital and placed on telemetry and continuous pulse oximetry.
23. A teenage male presenting with unilateral nasal obstruction and epistaxis should raise suspicion for juvenile nasopharyngeal angiofibroma (JNA). Diagnosis is made by classic history and radiology (widening of the pterygopalatine fossa and anterior bowing of the posterior maxillary sinus wall, or Holman-Miller sign).
24. Occupational exposures are the main risk factors for sinonasal malignancies. Risk factors for adenocarcinoma are wood dust exposure and leather working.

25. Cranial nerve VI is the most medial nerve in the cavernous sinus and is the most commonly injured or affected from sinus pathology.
26. Acute rhinosinusitis is more commonly viral than bacterial, especially within the first 10 days of symptoms.
27. Rhinitis medicamentosa is associated with use of over-the-counter intranasal decongestants that contain α-adrenergic compounds for more than 3 to 5 days.
28. There is an important association between the presence of asthma, chronic rhinosinusitis, airway inflammation, and nasal polyposis, especially in the case of aspirin-exacerbated respiratory disease.
29. The classic nasal deformity in patients with cleft lip and palate includes inferior, posterior, and lateral displacement of the ipsilateral lower lateral cartilage; displacement of the nasal tip, caudal septum, and columella toward the noncleft side; and deviation of the bony septum toward the cleft side.
30. Conservative management is often the first step in managing cerebrospinal fluid leaks resulting from acute nonsurgical trauma.
31. Thyroid eye disease results from autoimmune inflammation of muscle and fat, where the thyroid-stimulating hormone receptor is the autoantigen.
32. Abnormalities of the external ear, including preauricular pits or tags, as well as malformations of the pinnae or ear canal, can be associated with inner ear abnormalities and congenital syndromes and may indicate the need for additional otologic and genetic workup.
33. The severity of cochlear deformities depends significantly on the gestational age of growth arrest or disruption.
34. CT is better for looking at temporal bone masses and lesions, but MRI (of the internal auditory canal with contrast) is the best test for evaluation of acoustic neuromas.
35. Treatment for sudden sensorineural hearing loss (SNHL):
Confirm with audiogram
High-dose oral steroid burst and taper or transtympanic steroid injection
MRI of internal auditory canals to evaluate for acoustic neuroma
36. Multisensory imbalance can be improved using walking aids. Trekking poles are helpful early in the disorder, but as the disease progresses, a rolling walker with handbrakes is the most effective treatment.
37. Patients with headaches and vertigo should be questioned about snoring. Sleep apnea is associated with morning headaches, worsens migraine, and can be associated with recurrent brief dizziness and progressive inner ear disorders such as Ménière's disease.
38. Acoustic feedback occurs when amplified sound leaks out of the receiver back into the microphone and usually occurs with poorly fitting hearing aids or cerumen impaction.
39. MRI is contraindicated for many implanted hearing devices as they have implanted magnets.
40. Bacterial meningitis is slightly more likely after cochlear implantation and all implantees should undergo pneumococcal vaccination prior to implantation per CDC guidelines.
41. For a diagnosis of acute otitis externa, there must be a rapid onset (usually within 48 hours) of symptoms and signs of ear canal inflammation.
42. Amoxicillin remains the first-line therapy for acute otitis media because approximately 80% of bacterial isolates remain susceptible. Pain is an important symptom of otitis externa and otitis media and needs to be treated appropriately.
43. A canal wall-down mastoidectomy is indicated when there is a semicircular canal fistula or posterior canal wall damage due to cholesteatoma, a sclerotic mastoid prevents adequate visualization with a wall-up mastoidectomy, or the patient is unable to attend follow-up or undergo additional surgeries for proper monitoring of recurrent cholesteatoma.
44. Medical therapies for otosclerosis, including sodium fluoride and bisphosphonates, are controversial in their clinical effectiveness.
45. CT is the most used imaging modality to evaluate cholesteatomas.
46. Passive upper eyelid closure can occur by relaxation of the levator palpebrae muscle (innervated by the oculomotor nerve), so upper eyelid motion is not always indicative of an intact facial nerve.
47. The first branch of the facial nerve is the greater superficial petrosal nerve that contains parasympathetic fibers to the lacrimal gland that exits from the anterior margin of the geniculate ganglion.
48. The marginal mandibular and temporal branches of the facial nerve are the branches most at risk during parotidectomy, rhytidectomy, and repair of mandibular fracture.
49. Benign paroxysmal positional vertigo commonly follows an episode of vestibular neuritis. In this situation, vestibular physical therapy (in addition to canalith repositioning) is often helpful to promote full recovery.
50. The key finding that distinguishes conductive hearing loss due to superior semicircular canal dehiscence from that caused by otosclerosis is an intact ipsilateral stapedial reflex.
51. In jugulotympanic paragangliomas, examination of the ear may display a vascular middle ear mass pulsating against the tympanic membrane which blanches upon pneumatic otoscopy. This is known as Brown's sign and seen in approximately 50% of cases.
52. Clinical diagnosis of temporal bone fracture can be made with the presence of three physical findings: hemotympanum, postauricular ecchymosis (Battle's sign), and periorbital ecchymosis (raccoon sign).

53. The most common site of injury to the facial nerve is in the perigeniculate region in 80% to 93% of patients.
54. The pediatric airway is significantly smaller than the adult airway; inflammation and narrowing of the airway can be far more clinically significant in an infant than a similar degree of edema in an adult.
55. Respiratory distress with inspiratory or biphasic stridor in the setting of a strong cry raises suspicion for bilateral true vocal cord paralysis.
56. Urgent intervention is necessary for suspicion of button battery ingestion.
57. Laryngomalacia is the most common cause of stridor in the infant. In most cases, it resolves by age 2 years without surgical intervention.
58. The most common cause of subglottic stenosis is iatrogenic scarring related to endotracheal intubation.
59. Infantile hemangiomas are the most common tumors of infancy.
60. The classic rash associated with scarlet fever appears on the neck and face and then spreads and looks like a sunburn with tiny bumps. The rash will blanch when one presses on it.
61. If mononucleosis is suspected, amoxicillin should be avoided because it may cause a salmon-colored rash.
62. A submucous cleft palate is associated with a higher incidence of post adenoidectomy velopharyngeal insufficiency.
63. Branchial cleft anomalies track deep to the structures of their own arch and superficial to the structures of the subsequent arch.
64. Always evaluate for a normal thyroid gland prior to removing a thyroglossal duct cyst.
65. Pseudotumor of infancy (sternocleidomastoid tumor) responds to conservative treatment by 1 year of age in 80% of cases.
66. A stridulous child with a concomitant hemangioma, particularly in the "beard distribution" of the face, should raise suspicion for a subglottic hemangioma.
67. A higher frequency of cleft lip and palate occurs in Native Americans, those of Asian descent, and those of Latin American descent (1:400). The lowest frequency is reported in African Americans (1:1500 to 2000). Cleft palate alone is fairly consistent among ethnic groups at 1:2000. There is a male predominance in cleft lip and palate, and a female predominance in cleft palate alone.
68. In developed countries, the most common environmental, nongenetic cause of congenital hearing loss is cytomegalovirus infection.
69. Most nonsyndromic genetic hearing loss is caused by mutations in connexins 26 and 30, encoded by *GJB2* and *GJB6*.
70. Patients with an enlarged vestibular aqueduct or Mondini dysplasia should be tested for mutations in *SLC26A4*, which is associated with Pendred syndrome.
71. Alport syndrome is characterized by glomerulonephritis and progressive SNHL. It has a variable inheritance pattern but 85% of cases are X-linked and 15% are autosomal recessive.
72. In children with congenital severe to profound hearing loss in whom *GJB2* and *GJB6* testing is normal, Usher syndrome should be considered.
73. GLUT-1 positivity distinguishes infantile hemangioma (IH) from vascular malformations and other vascular tumors.
74. Propranolol is the first-line treatment for IH unless contraindications for its use exist.
75. The most common mass in the neck in children is a reactive lymph node. Lymphomas are the most common malignancy seen in the neck in children.
76. The key to a Sistrunk procedure is not just resecting the central portion of the hyoid bone, but resecting tongue musculature between the hyoid bone and foramen cecum.
77. Most facial mimetic muscles are superficially situated and receive facial nerve innervation from their deep surface.
78. Most scars improve in appearance without revision 1 to 3 years after the inciting event. Patients should be counseled to wait at least 6 to 12 months before undergoing a scar revision surgery, unless there are obvious scar characteristics that are not expected to improve.
79. The Frankfort horizontal line allows for standardization in photographs and is a cornerstone for facial analysis.
80. A "pollybeak" deformity is a complication of rhinoplasty whereby supratip fullness results in the appearance of a parrot's beak; this can be the result of loss of tip support or supratip scar tissue.
81. From anterior to posterior, the layers of the upper eyelid above the lid crease are as follows: skin, orbicularis oculi, orbital septum, preaponeurotic fat, levator aponeurosis, Müller's muscle, and conjunctiva.
82. Phenol chemical peels are associated with cardiac toxicity and should be applied to individual facial subunits in 15-minute intervals to limit systemic absorption.
83. Facelift is a cosmetic procedure that involves elevating the tissues of the lower face and neck into a more youthful position.
84. The most common complication from facelift surgery is hematoma. It occurs in up to 10% of cases and is more common in men.
85. Botulinum toxin cleaves SNAP-25 at the presynaptic neuromuscular junction, inhibiting acetylcholine release. This leads to temporary muscle paralysis.

86. In the setting of denervation of the facial nerve, there is nerve and motor endplate fibrosis that leads to muscle atrophy. Thus, reinnervation procedures must be completed by 12 to 18 months postinjury before atrophic changes are permanent.

87. Utilization of a full-thickness skin graft, when possible, will limit graft contraction and usually result in an improved texture and color match.

88. When choosing a flap, consider donor-site morbidity, tissue type the flap provides and tissue type being reconstructed, bulk of the flap, and pedicle length.

89. A secured airway must always be verified by observation of equal chest rise/fall, bilateral breath sounds on auscultation, and CO_2 return. A chest radiograph can demonstrate the position of the endotracheal tube above the carina but does not necessarily rule out the possibility of esophageal intubation.

90. What all Le Fort fractures have in common is that they traverse the pterygomaxillary fissure, interrupting the pterygoid plates and resulting in a mobile palate.

91. A "white-eye blowout fracture" is considered a surgical emergency.

92. The hyoid bone is not ossified at birth, but it is the first component of the laryngeal framework to ossify, followed by the thyroid cartilage and the cricoid cartilage.

93. Correct direct laryngoscopy technique greatly enhances visualization of the vocal cords. Always ensure that there are no contraindications to proper neck flexion and head extension (i.e., unstable cervical spine, Down syndrome).

94. Recurrent respiratory papillomatosis is primarily caused by HPV types 6 and 11.

95. There are no targeted treatments for unexplained or neuropathic chronic cough but limited clinical trial data support benefit from treatment with neuromodulators and speech-language therapy.

96. Keeping a cuff inflated on a tracheostomy tube does not mechanically prevent aspiration. It merely contains aspirated material at the level of the cuff, which will leak farther into the airway upon cuff deflation unless subglottic suction is in place.

97. The primary management of vocal fold nodules is voice therapy.

98. The position of the affected true vocal fold does not correlate with the level or extent of the injury to the Vagus nerve or recurrent laryngeal nerve branch. Not all branches of the nerve may recover, and the position of the paralyzed or immobile vocal fold may vary over time.

99. What are the steps in the management of an airway fire?
    a. Turn off the flow of oxygen
    b. Douse fire with saline
    c. Remove damaged tube
    d. Reintubate as atraumatically as possible
    e. Administer IV steroids and antibiotics
    f. Perform bronchoscopy before leaving the operating room to remove any charred tissue or other debris, and evaluate extent of airway injury
    g. Delayed extubation with repeat endoscopic airway examinations

100. Choosing the smallest endotracheal tube that will provide adequate ventilation will help minimize mucosal trauma.

GENERAL ANATOMY AND EMBRYOLOGY WITH RADIOLOGY CORRELATES

Cristina Cabrera-Muffly, MD, FACS

CHAPTER 1

KEY POINTS

1. Eight branches of the external carotid artery:
   - Superior thyroid
   - Ascending pharyngeal
   - Lingual
   - Facial
   - Occipital
   - Posterior auricular
   - Maxillary
   - Superficial temporal
2. Layers of fascia in the neck:
   - Superficial cervical fascia
   - Superficial layer of deep cervical fascia
   - Middle layer of deep cervical fascia
   - Deep layer of deep cervical fascia
3. Characteristics of malignant lymph nodes on neck CT with contrast:
   - Size >1.5 centimeters
   - Round shape
   - Necrotic center
   - Ill-defined margins
4. Facial nerve landmarks:
   - Tragal pointer
   - Tympanomastoid suture line
   - Insertion of the posterior belly of digastric muscle onto the mastoid
5. Best imaging study by region:
   - Cerebellopontine angle – MRI with contrast
   - Neck and salivary glands – CT with contrast or MRI with contrast
   - Sinus – CT without contrast
   - Temporal bone – CT without contrast
   - Thyroid – Ultrasound

Pearls

1. CT scan is best for visualizing temporal bone masses and lesions, but MRI (of the internal auditory canal with contrast) is best for evaluating acoustic neuromas.
2. When a temporal bone fracture is suspected, the best test is a fine cuts CT of temporal bones without contrast.
3. If the nasal turbinates light up on T1 MRI, imaging was performed with contrast.
4. MRI scans commonly over diagnose sinus disease and do not provide detail on outflow obstruction. The most appropriate method to determine chronic sinus disease is CT without contrast (Fig. 1.1).
5. The best imaging method for evaluating thyroid nodules is ultrasound.

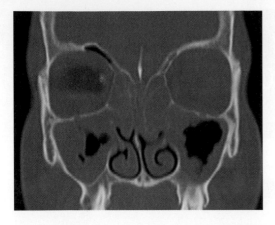

Fig. 1.1 Chronic sinusitis with nasal polyposis on CT scan.

QUESTIONS

1. **When do the sinuses develop?**
   The maxillary sinus is the first to develop in utero. After birth, this sinus enlarges in two stages, once at the age of 3 years and then again between the ages of 7 and 12 years. Neonates have three to four ethmoid cells at birth, which multiply to become 10 to 15 cells by the age of 12 years. The sphenoid sinus begins pneumatization at 3 years of age, and the frontal sinus is the last to develop at approximately 5 years of age. The sphenoid and frontal sinuses do not reach adult size until the teenage years.

2. **What is the difference between agger nasi, Onodi, and Haller ethmoid cells?**
   The agger nasi cell is the most anterior of the ethmoid cells. It is found anterior and superior to the attachment of the middle turbinate to the lateral wall. The Onodi cell is an ethmoid cell that pneumatizes laterally or posteriorly to the anterior wall of the sphenoid. This cell can be adjacent to the optic nerve or carotid artery, so it is important to recognize this variation during sinus surgery. A Haller cell forms when the ethmoid pneumatizes into the medial and inferior orbital walls. If this cell is large, it can cause obstruction of the maxillary ostium.

3. **Name the branches of the internal carotid artery in the neck.**
   Trick question! The internal carotid artery does not branch in the neck.

4. **Name the eight branches of the external carotid artery in the neck.**
   From proximal to distal, the branches are: the superior thyroid, ascending pharyngeal, lingual, facial, occipital, posterior auricular, maxillary, and superficial temporal arteries.

5. **Name the four types of tongue papillae. Where are they located?**
   The four types are circumvallate, fungiform, foliate, and filiform papillae. The circumvallate are located at the junction of the anterior two thirds and posterior one third of the tongue in a "V" shape. Fungiform papillae are found at the tip and lateral edges of the anterior two thirds of the tongue. Foliate papillae are found at the postero-lateral base of tongue. Filiform papillae are found all over the tongue and do not participate in taste sensation.

6. **Describe the landmarks used to locate the facial nerve during parotid surgery.**
   Typical landmarks include the tragal pointer, tympanomastoid suture line, and posterior digastric muscle. The tra-gal pointer refers to the tragus cartilage, which "points" to the location of the nerve 1 centimeter anterior, inferior, and deep to the cartilage. Another method of identification is to follow the tympanomastoid suture line inferiorly to its drop-off point. Six to eight millimeters medial to this point, the facial nerve can be found passing through the stylomastoid foramen. Finally, the nerve can be located just medial to the insertion of the posterior belly of the digastric on the mastoid.

7. **Name each of the major salivary glands and describe the types of saliva produced by each.**
   There are three paired major salivary glands: the parotid, submandibular, and sublingual glands. Each gland has acinar cells that produce either serous or mucinous solution. The parotid glands produce mostly serous saliva. The sublingual glands produce mostly mucinous saliva, and the submandibular glands produce a mixture of the two.

8. **How do the salivary glands develop embryologically?**
   The major salivary glands develop from the first pharyngeal pouch. The glands form during gestational weeks 4 to 9. The parotids form by an ectodermal outpouching into the surrounding mesenchyme. The submandibular

and sublingual glands form from endoderm growing either into the submandibular triangle or floor of the mouth (sublingual).

9. **Describe the embryology of the parathyroid glands.**
The superior parathyroid glands develop from the fourth dorsal branchial pouch, whereas the inferior parathyroid glands develop from the third dorsal branchial pouch. This apparent inversion occurs because the fourth branchial pouch does not migrate during development, but the third branchial pouch descends with the thymus to lie inferior to the fourth pouch. Ectopic parathyroid tissue is present in up to 20% of patients.

10. **Describe the fascial planes of the neck.**
The neck fascia has two main layers: the superficial and deep cervical fascia. The superficial cervical fascia envelops the platysma, facial expression muscles, and the superficial muscular aponeurotic system (SMAS). The deep cervical fascia splits into three parts: the superficial, middle, and deep layers. The superficial layer of the deep cervical fascia envelops the trapezius, sternocleidomastoid, and masseter muscles as well as the parotid and submandibular glands. The middle layer of the deep cervical fascia contains the strap muscles as well as the trachea, esophagus, thyroid, pharynx, and larynx. The deep layer of the deep cervical fascia envelops the cervical vertebrae and paraspinal muscles. All three layers of the deep cervical fascia together form the carotid sheath, enveloping the carotid artery, jugular vein, and vagus nerve (Fig. 1.2).

11. **Describe the lymph node levels of the neck used for staging head and neck cancer.**
The location of the primary tumor determines the likelihood of spread to each particular area. Level I includes the submandibular and submental triangles. Levels II through IV lie along the carotid sheath, superiorly to inferiorly. The boundary between levels II and III is the hyoid bone. The boundary between levels III and IV is the cricoid cartilage. Level V encompasses the posterior triangle, whereas level VI is the central compartment (Fig. 1.3).

12. **Describe the branchial arch derivatives as they relate to the ear.**
The first branchial arch contributes to Meckel's cartilage, which includes the malleus head and neck, incus body and short process, and anterior malleal ligament. It also contributes to the tensor tympani and the first three hillocks of His. The second branchial arch contributes to Reichert's cartilage, which includes the manubrium of the malleus, the long process and lenticular process of the incus, and most of the stapes. It also contributes to the last three hillocks of His. The first branchial pouch contributes to the eustachian tube, mastoid air cells, and inner layer of the tympanic membrane. The first branchial cleft contributes to the external auditory canal and outer layer of the tympanic membrane.

13. **Describe the branchial arch derivatives as they relate to the larynx.**
The third branchial arch contributes to the stylopharyngeus muscle, which elevates the larynx. The fourth branchial arch contributes to thyroid and cuneiform cartilage, the superior laryngeal nerve, and cricothyroid muscle.

FASCIAL LAYERS OF NECK

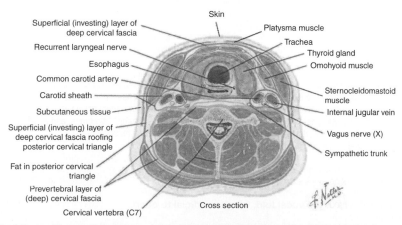

Fig. 1.2 Fascial layers of the neck. (From Goldstone J: *Netter's Surgical Anatomy and Approaches*, Philadelphia: Saunders; 2014:389–398.)

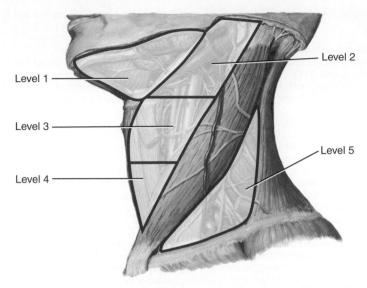

Fig. 1.3 Lymph node levels of the neck commonly used during head and neck cancer staging. (From Goldstone J: Netter's Surgical Anatomy and Approaches, Philadelphia: Saunders; 2014:389–398.)

The fifth and sixth branchial arches contribute to the cricoid, arytenoid, and corniculate cartilages; recurrent laryngeal nerve; and all of the intrinsic laryngeal muscles (except the cricothyroid).

14. **Name the 12 cranial nerves and their functions.**
    I: Olfactory – olfaction
    II: Optic – vision
    III: Oculomotor – motor to all eye muscles except the superior oblique and lateral rectus muscles; parasympathetic to the ciliary muscle (accommodation) and sphincter pupillae muscle (pupil constriction)
    IV: Trochlear – motor to the superior oblique muscle
    V: Trigeminal – sensation from the face; motor to the mastication, tensor tympani, tensor veli palatini, mylohyoid, and anterior digastric muscles
    VI: Abducens – motor to the lateral rectus muscle
    VII: Facial – motor to the facial expression, stapedial, external auricular, occipitofrontalis, stylohyoid, and posterior digastric muscles; parasympathetics to the lacrimal gland (lacrimation) and submandibular and sublingual glands (salivation); taste to the anterior two thirds of the tongue; sensation from the concha, postauricular skin, wall of the external auditory canal, and part of the tympanic membrane
    VIII: Vestibulocochlear – balance and hearing
    IX: Glossopharyngeal – taste; motor to the stylopharyngeus muscle; sensation from the posterior one third of the tongue, tympanic membrane, and external auditory canal; visceral sensation from the carotid body; parasympathetics to the parotid gland (salivation)
    X: Vagus – motor to the pharyngeal muscles (except stylopharyngeal), levator veli palatini, uvulae, palatopharyngeus, palatoglossus, salpingopharyngeus, cricothyroid and pharyngeal constrictors (via superior laryngeal nerve), and all intrinsic muscles of the larynx (via the recurrent laryngeal nerve) except the cricothyroid; parasympathetic innervation to and sensation from the thoracic and abdominal viscera; sensation from the laryngeal mucosa, postauricular skin, external auditory canal, tympanic membrane, and pharynx
    XI: Spinal accessory – motor to the sternocleidomastoid and trapezius muscles
    XII: Hypoglossal – motor to the tongue except the palatoglossus muscle

15. **What muscle is the only vocal fold abductor?**
    The posterior cricoarytenoid is the only abductor of the larynx.

16. **Name the layers of the vocal fold, from superficial to deep.**
    Squamous epithelium
    Lamina propria (three layers: superficial, intermediate, and deep)
    Thyroarytenoid muscle and vocalis muscle (vocal fold body)

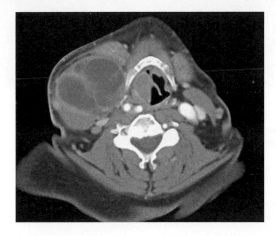

Fig. 1.4 Malignant lymph node on CT scan. Note the large size, necrotic center, and round shape. (Courtesy of Ted Leem, MD, Department of Otolaryngology, University of Colorado.)

17. **Which layers of the vocal fold form the cover? Which form the ligament?**
The cover is formed by the epithelium and superficial lamina propria. The intermediate and deep lamina propria form the vocal ligament.

18. **What is the best type of imaging for the temporal bone?**
CT scan without contrast is best for evaluation of the cortical bone and soft tissue lesions due to its ability to show bony detail.

19. **What is the best type of imaging to evaluate the cerebellopontine angle?**
MRI, with its superior ability to show soft tissue contrast, is best for evaluating tumors and lesions of the cerebellopontine angle. MRI of the internal auditory canals is usually performed with contrast.

20. **What is the best type of imaging to evaluate the thyroid?**
The best type of initial imaging for evaluation of the thyroid is ultrasound.

21. **If you suspect a peritonsillar abscess is present, do you need to obtain imaging?**
No imaging is needed to work up a peritonsillar abscess. If an abscess is suspected in the retropharyngeal or parapharyngeal space, imaging can be helpful in establishing the diagnosis.

22. **How does a PET (positron emission tomography) scan work?**
A radioactive tracer called fludeoxyglucose (very similar to glucose) is given via IV injection. The patient then waits 1 hour to allow for absorption of the tracer. The areas of the body that are most metabolically active (take up the most glucose) are detected by the scanner. PET scans are often used to determine whether cancer metastasis is present. Because cancer cells are usually more metabolically active than normal tissue, these areas will "light up" on the scan.

23. **What changes to the appearance of a lymph node make it suspicious for malignancy on a CT scan with contrast?**
Lymph nodes that are greater than 1 centimeter (1.5 centimeters in the jugulodigastric area), have a necrotic center, have ill-defined margins, or are round (instead of the usual oval shape) are suspicious for malignancy. Lymph nodes with these characteristics should undergo either needle or excisional biopsy, depending on the clinical history (Fig. 1.4).

BIBLIOGRAPHY
Ahmad A, Branstetter BF: CT versus MR: still a tough decision, *Otolaryngol Clin North Am* 41(1):1–22, 2008.
Bailey BJ, Calhoun KH, Healy GB, et al: *Head and Neck Surgery – Otolaryngology*, 3rd ed, Lippincott Williams & Wilkins, 2001.
Deschler DG, Day T, editors: *TNM Staging of Head and Neck Cancer and Neck Dissection Classification*, American Academy of Otolaryngology – Head and Neck Surgery Foundation, 2008.
Grevellec A, Tucker AS: The pharyngeal pouches and clefts: development, evolution, structure, and derivatives, *Semin Cell Dev Biol* 21(3):325–332, 2010.
Myers EN: *Operative Otolaryngology*, Saunders Elsevier, 2008.
Netter FH: *Atlas of Human Anatomy*, Novartis, 1997.
Pasha R: *Otolaryngology Head and Neck Surgery: Clinical Reference Guide*, Plural Publishing, 2006.

CHAPTER 2

ENT EMERGENCIES

Henry P. Barham, MD and Scott E. Mann, MD

KEY POINTS

1. Airway management is the otolaryngologist's main role in emergencies.
2. Epiglottitis is an emergency because of the high potential for airway obstruction.
3. Angioedema involves the reticular dermis as well as the subcutaneous and submucosal layers of nondependent areas.
4. Malignant otitis externa most commonly affects immunocompromised or elderly patients.
5. The mylohyoid muscle boundary is crossed in Ludwig's angina.

Pearls
1. In patients with recurrent angioedema, hereditary angioedema must be considered in addition to adverse reaction to medicines such as ACE inhibitors. For hereditary angioedema, C1 esterase inhibitor levels and complement evaluation should be requested (C4).
2. Ludwig's angina is an odontogenic infection that arises in the submental and submandibular area and causes swelling of the floor of the mouth with displacement of the tongue posteriorly. Upper airway obstruction can proceed rapidly, making intubation difficult or impossible.
3. Definitive diagnosis of invasive fungal sinusitis requires histopathologic analysis, which confirms invasion of the fungal elements into the submucosal tissues including vessels, often resulting in necrosis of the involved mucosa and bone. Clinically, the involved tissue often lacks sensation and may appear pale or necrotic.
4. If a tracheo-innominate bleed occurs in a patient with a cuffed endotracheal or tracheostomy tube, the first step is to overinflate the cuff to tamponade bleeding.
5. A cricothyroidotomy should be converted to a formal tracheotomy within 24 hours, if possible, to minimize the risk of subglottic stenosis.

QUESTIONS

1. **What are the ABCDEs of any medical emergency?**
   A = Airway, B = Breathing, C = Circulation, D = Disability/Drugs (what the patient is taking or what should be given), and E = Exposure/Environmental control.

2. **What are the causes of airway obstruction that require emergent treatment?**
   Etiologies may include but are not limited to: (1) inflammatory changes in the upper airway due to infection, angioedema, or caustic substance exposure, etc.; (2) deep neck space infections; (3) a foreign body within the airway or upper esophagus; (4) blunt or penetrating neck trauma with airway involvement; and (5) bleeding complications including hematoma (posttraumatic or postsurgical).

3. **What is acute epiglottitis and why is it an emergency?**
   Epiglottitis is inflammation of the epiglottis, typically due to an infectious etiology resulting in rapid airway obstruction. When the inflammation involves surrounding structures, including the aryepiglottic folds and arytenoid soft tissues, it is referred to as supraglottitis. Mortality rates can reach 20%, making urgent diagnosis and treatment essential. The incidence has rapidly declined since the introduction of *Haemophilus influenzae* type B vaccination. Commonly a childhood disease in the past, it is now more common in adults. The most common bacteria identified include *H. influenzae*, beta-hemolytic *Streptococcus*, *Staphylococcus aureus*, and *Streptococcus pneumoniae*. Current belief is that George Washington likely died from acute bacterial epiglottitis.

4. **How does the presentation of epiglottitis or supraglottitis differ in adults and children?**
   Children often present with dyspnea, drooling, stridor, or fever. Adults may complain of severe sore throat, odynophagia, and hoarseness. Historically, patients presented acutely but now more patients are presenting in a subacute fashion with slower onset of severe symptoms. The "tripod sign" is classically seen on presentation.

5. **How should epiglottitis be diagnosed and treated?**
   The classic radiographic finding is referred to as the "thumb print sign," described as swelling of the epiglottis on lateral soft tissue neck x-ray. In children, direct visualization via laryngoscopy in the operating room is recommended. Indirect laryngoscopy (fiber-optic nasopharyngeal laryngoscopy) can be considered in adults if the patient is stable enough to tolerate the procedure. Once the diagnosis is made, treatment should consist of airway management and prompt antibiotic administration. Patients with respiratory distress should be intubated. Patients with respiratory stability may be observed closely (in the ICU) with medical management including antibiotics with activity against *H. influenza* (second- or third-generation cephalosporin), humidified air, racemic epinephrine, and intravenous steroids. It is important to remember that patients who are being observed should always have equipment for intubation and cricothyroidotomy available at the bedside.

6. **Describe angioedema.**
   Angioedema is the abrupt onset of nonpitting, nonpruritic edema involving the reticular dermis, subcutaneous, and submucosal layers of nondependent areas. This can affect the lips, soft palate, larynx, and pharynx, causing airway obstruction. Duration typically ranges from 24 to 96 hours. Approximately 25% of the U.S. population will have an episode of urticaria and/or angioedema during their lifetime.

7. **What causes angioedema?**
   The most common causes of acute angioedema include medications, foods, infections, insect venom, contact allergens (latex), and radiology contrast material. Acute angioedema is arbitrarily defined as symptom duration of less than 6 weeks. The evaluation of chronic angioedema and/or urticaria can be challenging. In the majority of cases, no etiology is ever found.

8. **What is involved in the workup of angioedema?**
   In addition to medical history and physical examination, fiber-optic laryngoscopy may be used to determine the degree of laryngeal edema. Patients with angioedema who complain of dyspnea, hoarseness, voice changes, or odynophagia or have stridor on physical exam are likely to have laryngeal involvement. All patients with laryngeal edema require admission to the ICU.

9. **How is angioedema treated?**
   For patients with both angioedema and urticaria, treatment may consist of epinephrine, antihistamines, and corticosteroids. For the majority of these patients, H1 antihistamines are the cornerstone of therapy. Although effective, they can also cause sedation, which can exacerbate respiratory distress. For this reason, second-generation H1 antihistamines (loratadine, cetirizine, desloratadine, and fexofenadine) are preferred. H2 blockers, such as ranitidine, are also necessary to completely interrupt the histamine cascade. Corticosteroids are indicated for patients with anaphylaxis, laryngeal edema, and severe symptoms. Isolated angioedema is often caused by medications, most commonly ACE inhibitors. Patients with recurrent episodes should be evaluated for hereditary angioedema, a deficiency in C1 esterase inhibitor, with laboratory assessment of C1 inhibitor protein and C4 complement factor levels. Danazol can be used for prophylaxis, although newer drugs with better side effect profiles are currently in clinical trials. During acute illness, fresh frozen plasma can be given to replace C1 inhibitor levels.

10. **What are the complications of acute otitis media that require emergent treatment?**
    (1) Mastoiditis with radiologic evidence of coalescence (loss of bony septae within the mastoid); (2) formation of subperiosteal or intracranial abscess; (3) dural venous sinus thrombosis; (4) meningitis; (5) facial nerve paresis; and (6) abducens nerve paresis due to petrous apex involvement or "Gradenigo's syndrome," which is a triad of suppurative otitis media, pain in the distribution of the trigeminal nerve, and abducens nerve palsy.

11. **What are the complications of acute bacterial rhinosinusitis that require emergent treatment?**
    (1) Orbital involvement including cellulitis and abscess formation; (2) intracranial complications including meningitis, intracranial abscess formation, and venous thrombosis; and (3) osteomyelitis of the frontal bone ("Pott's puffy tumor").

12. **What is acute invasive fungal sinusitis and why is it considered an emergency?**
    Acute invasive fungal sinusitis (AIFS) is an aggressive and often fatal angioinvasive infection of the nose, paranasal sinuses, and neighboring structures. It is most often diagnosed in immunocompromised patients with hematologic malignancies, immunosuppression, and poorly controlled diabetes mellitus.

13. **What are the typical causes of AIFS?**
    Typical species responsible for sinonasal invasive infections are *Aspergillus* and zygomycetes (*Rhizopus, Mucor, Rhizomucor*).

14. **How do you diagnose AIFS?**
Nasal endoscopy typically demonstrates areas of mucosal ischemia or frank necrosis that lack sensation. Radiologic studies can show nonspecific findings of sinus mucosal thickening, soft tissue reaction, and possibly bony destruction. The diagnostic gold standard is histopathologic evaluation and culture of nasal biopsies. Histopathologic confirmation of the diagnosis requires the presence of invasive fungal elements within submucosal tissues and vessels.

15. **What are the survival rates associated with AIFS?**
Mortality rates are high, varying from 20% to 80% in the literature. Negative prognostic factors include the presence of hematologic malignancy, advanced age, and intracranial or orbital involvement. Survival success is determined by early diagnosis, prompt initiation of culture-directed antifungal therapy, surgical debridement, and reversal of underlying immunosuppression.

16. **Describe Ludwig's angina.**
Named after Karl Friedrich Wilhelm von Ludwig, it is characterized as a rapidly progressive cellulitis of the soft tissues of the neck and floor of the mouth. With progressive swelling of the soft tissues and elevation and posterior displacement of the tongue, airway obstruction is the most emergent concern. Prior to the development of antibiotics, mortality for Ludwig's angina exceeded 50%. With antibiotic therapy and improved imaging modalities and surgical techniques, mortality currently averages <10%.

17. **What causes Ludwig's angina?**
The majority of cases of Ludwig's angina are of odontogenic origin. Once infection develops, it spreads into the sublingual space and can extend to the pharyngomaxillary and retropharyngeal spaces, encircling the airway. Polymicrobial infection occurs in more than 50% of cases. The most commonly cultured organisms include *Staphylococcus* sp., *Streptococcus* sp., and *Bacteroides* sp.

18. **How is Ludwig's angina diagnosed?**
The majority of patients report dental pain or a history of recent dental procedures and neck swelling. Less common complaints include neck pain, dysphonia, dysphagia, and dysarthria. Less than one third of adults will present in respiratory distress with dyspnea, tachypnea, or stridor. On physical examination, more than 95% of patients have bilateral submandibular swelling and an elevated or protruding tongue.

19. **How is Ludwig's angina managed?**
Any patient presenting in respiratory distress may require immediate intubation, either by routine orotracheal intubation or fiber-optic nasotracheal intubation. In nonintubated patients with Ludwig's angina, airway equipment, including tracheostomy and cricothyroidotomy instruments, should be kept at the bedside. Antibiotics should be initiated as soon as possible. Antibiotics should initially be broad spectrum and cover gram-positive, gram-negative, and anaerobic organisms. Combinations of penicillin, clindamycin, and metronidazole are typically used. Corticosteroid administration can be used in some cases to avoid the need for airway management. More than 50% of patients with Ludwig's angina develop a suppurative fluid collection that requires surgical drainage. Physical examination alone is insufficient in determining which patients require a surgical procedure. CT scan with intravenous contrast is recommended to identify patients who have developed suppurative complications.

20. **What is a tracheo-innominate (TI) fistula?**
TI fistula is a rare but life-threatening complication of tracheostomy, long-term mechanical ventilation, neck tumors, and tracheal surgery. It is the formation of a connection between the trachea and innominate artery that leads to rapid bleeding and possible exsanguination. In patients with a tracheostomy, the incidence of TI fistula is less than 1% but mortality approaches 80%. Patients with a TI fistula secondary to tracheostomy typically present between the first and second week following the procedure. Risk factors for TI fistula include tracheal infection, steroid use, and an anomalous innominate artery. The most common site for fistula formation is at the level of the endotracheal cuff. A large percentage of patients report a brief episode of bright red blood from the tracheal stoma, referred to as a "sentinel bleed."

21. **How is a TI fistula treated?**
Definitive treatment of a TI fistula requires ligation of the innominate artery, often via a sternotomy. Because the most common site for hemorrhage is at the level of the endotracheal cuff, the first maneuver is to overinflate the cuff of the tracheostomy tube to help tamponade the bleeding. If there is still hemorrhage, the cuff should be placed distal to the site of bleeding to protect the airway. A final maneuver is simply to place a finger in the airway and compress the innominate artery against the posterior sternum. Patients with a sentinel bleed require urgent thoracic surgery consultation for bronchoscopy and ligation of the innominate artery.

22. **Which facial fractures require emergent surgical management?**
In select cases, emergent management is required in cases of (1) orbital fractures that have evidence of extraocular muscle entrapment or orbital compartment syndrome; (2) bilateral mandible fractures with "flail mandible" and associated posterior displacement of the tongue and airway compromise; and (3) frontal fractures with depressed or open segments involving dura and large volume CSF leakage.

23. **Describe methods of nonsurgical management of the airway.**
Chin lift: The mandible is lifted away from the chest to move the chin anteriorly.
Jaw thrust: Pressure is applied bilaterally behind the angle of the mandible to displace it anteriorly. This is favored in patients with suspected cervical spine injury.
Oropharyngeal airway: The tube is inserted using a tongue blade into the oropharynx.
Nasopharyngeal airway: Well tolerated in conscious patients. Bypasses base of tongue.
Orotracheal intubation: This is the most common type of definitive airway management. Cervical spine immobilization must be maintained in suspected injuries.
Nasotracheal intubation: Useful with a known cervical spine injury as the spine can be maintained in a neutral position. It is contraindicated in patients with extensive midface trauma.

24. **Describe emergent surgical management of the airway.**
Needle cricothyroidotomy: A large-bore intravenous catheter (12- to 14-gauge) is inserted into the cricothyroid membrane. High-flow oxygen or jet insufflation is used to ventilate the patient. The patient can be adequately ventilated for approximately 30 to 45 minutes until a more definitive airway can be obtained (tracheotomy or intubation).
Surgical cricothyroidotomy: A vertical incision is made in the midline of the neck to expose the area of the cricothyroid membrane. A horizontal incision is then made through the cricothyroid membrane. This incision is dilated if needed using a hemostat, and an endotracheal or tracheostomy tube is inserted. A bougie may be placed prior to the tube if available to help prevent false passage placement. A cricothyroidotomy should be converted to a tracheotomy within 24 hours to prevent possible subglottic stenosis. This procedure is not recommended in children under the age of 12 years.
Awake tracheostomy: The patient is maintained in a semi-upright position with minimal sedation to preserve respiratory effort. The anterior neck is infiltrated with local anesthetic and a standard tracheostomy approach is performed. When the tracheal incision is made, the tube is quickly inserted and the position confirmed, followed by induction of general anesthesia. Further management of the airway and wound is then performed while the patient is anesthetized.

BIBLIOGRAPHY

AAO Resident of Trauma to the Face, Head, and Neck. Available at http://www.entnet.org/mktplace/upload/ResidentTraumaFinallowres.pdf.
Amorosa L, Modugno GC, Pirodda A: Malignant external otitis: review and personal experience, *Acta Otolaryngol Suppl* 521:3–16, 1996.
Bansal A, Miskoff J, Lis RJ: Otolaryngologic critical care, *Crit Care Clin* 19:55–72, 2003.
Berrouschot J, Oeken J, Steiniger L, et al: Perioperative complications of percutaneous dilational tracheostomy, *Laryngoscope* 107(Pt 1):1538–1544, 1997.
Carey MJ: Epiglottitis in adults, *Am J Emerg Med* 14:421–424, 1996.
Budenz CL, El-Kashlan HK, Shelton C, Aygun N, Niparko JK: *Complications of Temporal Bone Infections*, 6th ed, Cummings Otolaryngology, 2015, pp 2156–2176.
Dibbern DA Jr, Dreskin SC: Urticaria and angioedema: an overview, *Immunol Allergy Clin North Am* 24:141–162, 2004.
Gillespie MB, Huchton DM, O'Malley BW: Role of middle turbinate biopsy in the diagnosis of fulminant invasive fungal rhinosinusitis, *Laryngoscope* 110:1832–1836, 2000.
Marple BF: Ludwig angina: a review of current airway management, *Arch Otolaryngol Head Neck Surg* 125:596–599, 1999.
Quinn FB Jr: Ludwig angina, *Arch Otolaryngol Head Neck Surg* 125:599, 1999.
Turner JH, Soudry E, Jayakar VN, et al: Survival outcomes in acute invasive fungal sinusitis: a systematic review and quantitative synthesis of published evidence, *Laryngoscope* 123(5):1112–1118, 2013.

CHAPTER 3

DEEP NECK INFECTIONS

Tendy Chiang, MD and Ethan Bassett, MD

KEY POINTS

1. Initial evaluation of deep neck space infections (DNSI) should be directed toward identifying the acuity and medical stability of the patient; hemodynamic and airway instability may require emergent intervention.
2. Trismus, dysphonia, "hot potato" voice, stridor, and stertor are signs of airway compromise and may require urgent evaluation using flexible fiber-optic laryngoscopy. Tachypnea and oxygen desaturations are late manifestations of airway obstruction and should not be relied on to determine clinical stability.
3. Management with intravenous antibiotics is indicated in stable, antibiotic-naïve patients without any clinical or radiographic features of abscess formation.
4. Infections of the parapharyngeal, prevertebral, and retropharyngeal space can extend into the "danger space," allowing for unrestricted spread of infection into the mediastinum.

Pearls
1. Deep neck space infections most commonly originate from odontogenic sources in adults, whereas tonsillitis and pharyngitis are the most common etiologies in children.
2. There has been a dramatic increase in the incidence of MRSA since the early 2000s, particularly community-acquired MRSA among children.
3. The classic presentation of peritonsillar abscess includes trismus, uvular deviation, muffled voice, and soft palatal edema.

QUESTIONS

1. **What are deep neck space infections?**
   Deep neck space infections (DNSI) encompass a wide spectrum of infectious disorders of the neck. DNSI are typically classified by the fascial space that the infection occupies.

2. **What risk factors are associated with the development of DNSI?**
   Risk factors of DNSI include a low level of education, living more than 1 hour from a tertiary care center, presence of tonsils, *Streptococcus* infections, substance abuse, and poor dental hygiene.

3. **Describe how the neck is organized in terms of fascial planes.**
   The neck is compartmentalized in two main divisions of fascia: the superficial cervical fascia and the deep cervical fascia.

   The superficial cervical fascia includes subcutaneous tissue and envelops the muscles of facial expression. It is continuous with the superficial musculoaponeurotic system (SMAS) and extends inferiorly to involve the platysma.

   The deep cervical fascia is divided into superficial, middle, and deep layers.
   - The **superficial layer** invests the parotid and submandibular glands, muscles of mastication, trapezius, and sternocleidomastoid and forms the stylomandibular ligament.
   - The **middle layer** is composed of two divisions: the *visceral division* invests the larynx, pharynx, trachea, esophagus, thyroid, and parathyroid; the *muscular division* invests the strap muscles.
   - The **deep layer** is also composed of two divisions: the *prevertebral division* envelops the paraspinal muscles and vertebrae; the *alar division* lies atop the prevertebral layer and covers the sympathetic trunk. The carotid sheath represents the confluence of the deep layers of the deep cervical fascia (Fig. 3.1).

4. **Identify the deep neck spaces and anatomic sites that contribute to the infections within these spaces.**
   Deep neck spaces can be suprahyoid, infrahyoid, or span the entire length of the neck. It is important to understand the boundaries of the deep neck spaces because infections often follow these boundaries (or lack thereof)

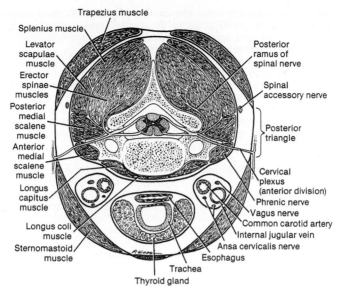

Fig. 3.1 Structures contained by deep cervical fascia: transverse section at the level of CN VII. (From Graney DO: Anatomy. In Cummings CW, et al., eds, Otolaryngology – Head and Neck Surgery, 3rd ed, St. Louis, 1998, Mosby.)

as they spread. DNSI typically are the result of suppuration of lymph nodes from infection at a primary anatomic site.

Suprahyoid:
    Peritonsillar: tonsil
    Parapharyngeal: tonsil, pharynx
    Submandibular: odontogenic, gingiva, submandibular gland
    Sublingual: odontogenic, gingiva, sublingual gland
Infrahyoid: visceral (esophageal perforation)
Spanning the entire length of the neck
    Retropharyngeal: nasal cavity, paranasal sinuses, nasopharynx, vertebral bodies
    Prevertebral: hematogenous spread from vertebrae and intervertebral discs
    "Danger" space: parapharyngeal, retropharyngeal space infections
    Carotid sheath: parapharyngeal, retropharyngeal space infections

5. **What conditions can present in a similar fashion to DNSI?**
   Congenital anomalies can either masquerade as a DNSI or become more clinically apparent when they become infected. Thyroglossal duct cysts, lymphatic malformations, and branchial cleft cysts can rapidly increase in size and present with signs and symptoms identical to DNSI. Prior history of a mass or fullness that waxes and wanes suggests the presence of an underlying congenital lesion.

   Neoplastic processes can also present with rapid neck swelling and features consistent with an infectious process. Fevers, night sweats, and weight loss can be presenting signs of lymphoma. New neck masses in adults are more likely to be malignant when compared to pediatric patients.

6. **What is the "danger space"?**
   The danger space is bound by the alar fascia anteriorly and the prevertebral fascia posteriorly. It extends from the skull base to the thoracic cavity, providing an unrestricted path for the spread of infection into the mediastinum, causing mediastinitis. Infections of the parapharyngeal, retropharyngeal, and prevertebral space can easily extend to this space.

7. **What is the most common major complication of DNSI?**
   Mediastinitis is the most common major complication of DNSI. It typically presents with tachycardia, dyspnea, and pleuritic chest pain. Chest x-ray can demonstrate mediastinal widening. Further evaluation with contrast chest CT is necessary to identify fluid collections that require drainage. Broad-spectrum intravenous antibiotics, early consultation with the thoracic surgery service, and close surveillance in the intensive care unit are recommended.

8. **How are prevertebral space infections different from infections of other deep neck spaces?**
   Prevertebral space infections are generally the result of hematogenous seeding or contiguous spread of infection from discitis or vertebral osteomyelitis. Gram-positive bacteria, especially *Staphylococcus aureus*, are the most common pathogens in these infections; anaerobes are uncommon.

9. **What are the most common etiologies of DNSI?**
   The etiology of DNSI varies with age. Bacterial pharyngitis and tonsillitis with resultant suppuration of parapharyngeal, retropharyngeal, and jugulodigastric lymph nodes are the most common etiologies in children. Odontogenic infections are the most common etiology in adults; bacteria within dental plaque erode tooth enamel to form periapical abscesses that may penetrate the mandible or maxilla to enter the deep spaces of the neck. Other etiologies include cellulitis, trauma, foreign body, intravenous drug use, or congenital lesions such as thyroglossal duct cysts or branchial cleft anomalies.

10. **What are the most common pathogens causing deep neck space infections?**
    Because most of these infections are odontogenic in origin, these infections are usually polymicrobial, involving a large proportion of anaerobic bacteria, especially as the infections spread into deeper neck spaces. Common bacteria include *Streptococcus, Peptostreptococcus, Actinomyces, Fusobacterium,* and *Prevotella* species. *Staphylococcus aureus* (including MRSA), *Pseudomonas aeruginosa*, and other gram-negative rods are more common among immunocompromised hosts, diabetics, and in postoperative infections.

11. **What is the role of methicillin-resistant *Staphylococcus aureus* (MRSA) in deep neck space infections in the USA?**
    Streptococcal species, particularly those of group A *Streptococcus*, remain the most common pathogen responsible for nonpurulent skin and soft tissue infections, such as cellulitis and erysipelas. Purulent skin and soft tissue infections involving the head and neck (abscesses, furuncles, carbuncles, wound infections), on the other hand, are most commonly caused by *S. aureus*. There has been a dramatic increase in the incidence of MRSA since the early 2000s, particularly community-acquired MRSA among children. Up to 70% of pediatric neck abscesses are due to MRSA in some communities. Patients less than 16 months of age with lateral neck abscesses are 10 times more likely to have a *S. aureus* infection than a non–*S. aureus* infection.

12. **What signs and symptoms are common in DNSI?**
    The most common symptoms are neck pain, fever, dysphagia, neck swelling, and odynophagia. Referred pain resulting in otalgia and odynophagia is also common.

13. **What are the key physical exam findings in the evaluation of a patient with DNSI?**
    A complete head and neck exam is essential in all patients with DNSI. Initial interview should devote attention to hoarseness, dyspnea, stridor, stertor, and muffled or "hot potato" voice. Dysphonia should be evaluated with flexible fiber-optic laryngoscopy for possible airway compromise if the patient is stable.
    Inspection and palpation of the head and neck should begin away from the primary site of infection, reserving that portion of the exam for last. Evaluation of the involved area should focus on the size of the area, presence of induration, swelling or fluctuance, and any color change or cellulitic change of the overlying skin. Any cellulitic change should be marked along its periphery to permit accurate surveillance. Presence of crepitus suggests infection with gas-producing organisms.
    Cranial neuropathies can suggest retrograde spread of infection along the valveless venous system of the midface from soft tissue, nasal cavity, or paranasal sinus infection.

14. **What is trismus and why is it significant?**
    Trismus refers to the reduced ability to open the mouth. In the setting of DNSI, it is a sign of inflammation of the parapharyngeal, masseteric, pterygoid, and/or temporal spaces. While seen commonly in odontogenic infections, trismus is also seen with peritonsillar, parapharyngeal, and floor of mouth infections. Severe trismus can lead to difficulty managing secretions and cause airway compromise, presenting challenges for airway intervention should it be needed.

15. **How should suspected deep space neck infections be worked up?**
    Typical diagnostic workup of DNSI includes complete blood count with differential and radiographic evaluations. Atypical presentations (painless, slow growing, association with weight loss and night sweats) should raise suspicion for malignancy. Atypical infectious etiologies should be evaluated with placement of a PPD with chest x-ray, HIV testing, and titers for *Bartonella henselae*.
    Anterior-posterior and lateral neck plain films are useful in evaluation of the retropharyngeal space (Fig. 3.2). Ultrasound and computed tomography are the most common radiographic modalities employed when evaluating DNSI. Ultrasound is effective in differentiating cellulitis from a fluid collection and can also be used for

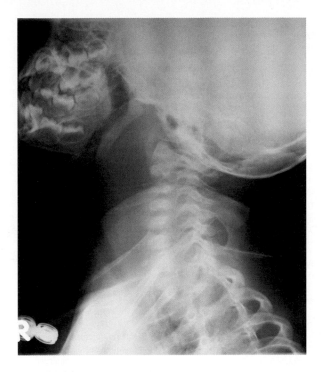

Fig. 3.2 Lateral neck plain film of a pediatric patient with a retropharyngeal abscess showing significant prevertebral thickening.

guidance to localize an abscess cavity. Computed tomography with contrast can demonstrate an abscess in the form of a hypodense focus centrally with peripheral rim enhancement.

16. **How can submandibular space infections be distinguished from sublingual space infections?**
    Submandibular space infections involve the area inferior to the mylohyoid muscle. They are usually the result of apical abscesses of the second or third molars. Sublingual infections, which involve the space superior to the mylohyoid muscle, on the other hand, are usually the result of infections of the mandibular incisors.

17. **Which DNSI pose the greatest risk to the contents of the carotid sheath?**
    The parapharyngeal and retropharyngeal spaces are adjacent to the carotid sheath. Infections of the carotid sheath may lead to complications such as Horner's syndrome (ptosis, miosis, anhydrosis from involvement of the cervical sympathetic chain), cranial nerve palsies, carotid artery rupture, and septic phlebitis of the jugular vein. This can present with neck fullness, a pulsatile neck mass with ecchymosis, and bright red bleeding from the nose, mouth, or external auditory canal.

18. **What are the classic signs of peritonsillar abscess?**
    Peritonsillar abscess is a clinical diagnosis and does not typically require additional diagnostic and radiographic testing. Patients typically present with trismus, muffled voice, uvular deviation, and fullness of the soft palate.
    Management of peritonsillar abscess involves surgical incision and drainage. This procedure is generally tolerated with local anesthesia alone in the clinic or emergency department in cooperative patients, typically the adolescent and adult population. Pediatric patients typically require general anesthesia for management.
    Isolated peritonsillar abscess requires completion of a course of oral antibiotics following drainage. Tonsillectomy is indicated in the setting of recurrent peritonsillar abscess.

19. **What are the indications for surgical intervention for DNSI?**
    Indications for surgical intervention depend on the medical stability of the patient. Patients who are antibiotic-naïve, do not have any airway compromise, and do not have any radiographic features of abscess formation can be managed initially with systemic antibiotic therapy. Any signs of airway compromise, lack of marked improvement after 24 to 72 hours of intravenous antibiotic therapy, or clinical or radiographic signs of abscess formation should undergo incision and drainage.

The goal of incision and drainage should include collection of culture specimens, blunt dissection into the abscess cavity, and disruption of loculations within the abscess cavity to promote drainage. Packing is placed and removed gradually during the postoperative period to prevent re-accumulation of fluid.

20. **What is Lemierre's syndrome?**

    Lemierre's syndrome is septic thrombophlebitis of the internal jugular vein, which is usually the result of hematogenous extension through tonsillar veins. Typical symptoms of pharyngitis lead to fever, lethargy, neck pain, and swelling. Septic emboli can seed in the lungs, resulting in nodular infiltrates on chest x-ray. Contrast CT of the neck demonstrates occlusion of the internal jugular vein. *Fusobacterium necrophorum* is the pathogen isolated in more than 90% of cultures. Metronidazole is the treatment of choice.

21. **What is the hallmark of *Actinomyces israelii* infections involving the head and neck?**

    Infections caused by this bacteria frequently cross fascial planes, forming sinus tracts that drain grainy material commonly referred to as "sulfur granules." Actinomyces is a gram-positive, branching, facultative anaerobe. Fifty percent of cases involve the head and neck. Infections typically present as a nontender, hard, slowly progressive mass in the perimandibular area ("lumpy jaw"). Treatment is a long-term course of penicillin or amoxicillin.

22. **What is Ludwig's angina and what is its major complication?**

    Ludwig's angina is a rapidly spreading infection of the submandibular and sublingual spaces, typically odontogenic in origin. Infection superior to the mylohyoid muscle places the patient at risk for rapid swelling of the floor of the mouth and tongue, resulting in airway obstruction. Patients typically present with trismus, fever, drooling, dysphonia, and dysphagia. On exam, tense swelling of the floor of the mouth and tongue protrusion are present, which can deteriorate quickly into respiratory distress. Intubation can rapidly become difficult, if not impossible. Emergent tracheostomy may be indicated in addition to antibiotics and surgical drainage.

23. **Which empiric antibiotic regimens are appropriate for DNSI?**

    Empiric antibiotics should be administered parenterally and have activity against *Streptococcus* species and oral anaerobes. Appropriate cultures should be obtained if possible prior to initiation of any antimicrobial therapy. Penicillin G plus metronidazole or ampicillin-sulbactam are good choices. For patients who are allergic to penicillin, clindamycin, moxifloxacin, levofloxacin plus metronidazole, or ciprofloxacin plus metronidazole may be used.

    A complete course of antimicrobial therapy typically lasts 10 to 14 days. Marked clinical improvement should be observed prior to conversion from intravenous to oral therapy.

24. **What is a common cause of chronic unilateral regional lymphadenopathy in children?**

    Cat-scratch disease (CSD) presents as lymphadenopathy from infection by *B. henselae*, typically several weeks after inoculation. A history of cat exposure is present in most patients. Lymphadenopathy typically resolves within 2 months but can last up to a year. Early treatment (within the first 30 days) with azithromycin for 5 days demonstrates a significant decrease in lymph node volume, whereas delayed treatment (after 30 days) demonstrates no change in the rate of resolution. Surgical treatment is reserved for persistent discomfort, suppuration, and diagnostic purposes.

25. **Describe the typical presentation of cervical lymphadenitis caused by atypical mycobacterial infection.**

    Infections caused by atypical, or nontuberculous mycobacteria (NTM) typically present with firm, painless lymphadenopathy in the submandibular or perifacial region that does not respond to traditional antibiotic therapy. Over time, the infectious process usually migrates superficially, resulting in violaceous color change of the overlying skin. Resolution can occur over a period of months to years, but can result in drainage and scarring. Medical management consists of a long-term antibiotic regimen, often dual therapy with rifampin and a macrolide; but the mainstay of treatment is often surgical management with removal of infected nodes and adjacent affected tissue.

26. **What is the most common manifestation of tuberculosis of the head and neck?**

    Scrofula is tuberculous lymphadenitis of the cervical region. It typically presents as a unilateral, painless, firm mass without fever or other systemic symptoms. Diagnosis is via biopsy with culture. Treatment includes complete excision of the lymph node, in addition to antimycobacterial therapy.

27. **Discuss the risk factors and typical presentation of necrotizing fasciitis.**

    Necrotizing fasciitis is a rapidly progressive DNSI of the fascial planes that typically occurs in immunosuppressed patients (diabetes, chronic illness, patients undergoing chemotherapy, malnutrition) and presents with pain disproportionate with physical exam. Gas-forming bacteria can produce crepitus and gas bubbles may be seen on imaging within the soft tissues. Disease progression is rapid; early medical management with broad-spectrum IV antibiotics coupled with aggressive surgical debridement of infected tissue is required.

BIBLIOGRAPHY

Barber BR, Dziegielewski PT, Biron VL, et al: Factors associated with severe deep neck space infections: targeting multiple fronts, *J Otolaryngol Head Neck Surg* 43:35, 2014.

Daramola OO, Flanagan CE, Maisel RH, et al: Diagnosis and treatment of deep neck space abscesses, *J Otolaryngol Head Neck Surg* 141:123–130, 2009.

Duggal P, Naseri I, Sobol SE: The increased risk of community-acquired methicillin-resistant *Staphylococcus aureus* neck abscesses in young children, *Laryngoscope* 121:51–55, 2011.

Fraser L, Moore P, Kubba H: Atypical mycobacterial infection of the head and neck in children: a 5-year retrospective review, *Otolaryngol Head Neck Surg* 138:311–314, 2008.

Hull MW, Chow AW: An approach to oral infections and their management, *Curr Infect Dis Rep* 7:17, 2005.

Mandell GL, Bennett JE, Dolin R, editors: *Mandell, Douglas, and Bennett's Principles and Practice of Infectious Diseases*, 7th ed., Churchill Livingstone Elsevier, 2010.

Marioni G, Rinaldi R, Staffieri C, et al: Deep neck infection with dental origin: analysis of 85 consecutive cases (2000–2006), *Acta Otolaryngol* 128(2):201–206, 2008.

Massei F, Gori L, Macchia P, et al: The expanded spectrum of bartonellosis in children, *Infect Dis Clin North Am* 19:691–711, 2005.

Munson PD, Boyce TG, Salomao DR, et al: Cat-scratch disease of the head and neck in a pediatric population: surgical indications and outcomes, *Otolaryngol Head Neck Surg* 139:358–363, 2008.

Reynolds SC, Chow AW: Severe soft tissue infections of the head and neck: a primer for critical care physicians, *Lung* 187:271, 2009.

Smego RA Jr, Foglia G: Actinomycosis, *CID* 26(6):1255–1261, 1998.

Velargo PA, Burke EL, Kluka EA: Pediatric neck abscesses caused by methicillin-resistant *Staphylococcus aureus*: a retrospective study of incidence and susceptibilities over time, *Ear Nose Throat J* 89(9):459–461, 2010.

CHAPTER 4

ANTIMICROBIALS AND PHARMACOTHERAPY

Taylor M. Washburn, MD

KEY POINTS

1. Knowledge of the most common bacteria causing infection, antibiotic methods of action, and microbial resistance mechanisms and patterns can facilitate appropriate drug selection.
2. The most directed antimicrobial therapy is preferred and may require a sample to be obtained for culture and sensitivity testing.
3. Factors to consider when choosing an antibiotic:
   - The antibiotic must have activity against the organism(s)
   - Consider the local resistance patterns
   - Location of the infection and antibiotic penetration
   - Mechanism of action (bacteriocidal versus bacteriostatic)
   - Host factors: age, drug allergy, renal or hepatic dysfunction, pregnancy, immune status, other medications that may cause drug–drug interactions
4. Can β-lactam antibiotics be used if there is a history of penicillin allergy?
   - The nature of the penicillin allergy is important to consider. If the reaction is anaphylaxis, then penicillin should not be used without allergy consultation and possible desensitization. The rate of penicillin cross-reactivity with cephalosporins is low at 2% and use of penicillin skin testing with oral amoxicillin can help determine if cephalosporins can be used safely.
5. Antibiotics with excellent oral absorption:
   - Fluoroquinolones
   - Clindamycin
   - TMP-SMX
   - Doxycycline
   - Linezolid
6. Antibiotics with activity against *Pseudomonas aeruginosa:*
   - Antipseudomonal penicillins: piperacillin-tazobactam
   - Cephalosporins with pseudomonal activity: ceftazidime +/- avibactam, cefepime, ceftolozane-tazobactam
   - Fluoroquinolones: levofloxacin, ciprofloxacin
   - Carbapenems (all but ertapenem)
   - Aztreonam
   - Aminoglycosides
   - Colistin/polymyxin B
7. Commonly used antibiotics with activity against methicillin-resistant *Staphylococcus aureus:*
   - Vancomycin
   - Daptomycin
   - Ceftaroline
   - Linezolid
   - TMP-SMX
   - Clindamycin
   - Tetracyclines

Pearls
1. Ertapenem is the least broad of the carbapenems due to its lack of activity against *Enterococcus* sp. and *P. aeruginosa*.
2. In general, first-generation cephalosporins have the broadest gram-positive coverage and transition to broad gram-negative coverage by fourth-generation cephalosporins.
3. Antibiotics associated with increased risk of *Clostridioides difficile* colitis are clindamycin, fluoroquinolones, cephalosporins, and carbapenems. Macrolides, penicillins, and sulfonamides are less frequently associated.
4. Tetracyclines should not be used in children or pregnant women due to the effect on developing teeth and bones.

QUESTIONS

1. Describe the key factors that influence antibiotic choice.
   - An antimicrobial active against the organism causing the infection should be used. If this is not known, then the typical organisms known to cause the infection should be considered and treatment directed toward these organisms.
   - The anticipated resistance pattern of the organism must be considered. If the organism has been cultured, resistance testing should be done. If susceptibility testing is not possible, local resistance patterns should be taken into consideration when choosing antibiotics.
   - The location of the infection and delivery and penetration of the antibiotic must be considered.
   - The mechanism of action of the antibiotic is important. If the patient does not have an intact immune system, a bacteriocidal antibiotic should be chosen over a bacteriostatic one, if possible.
   - Host factors such as age, history of drug allergy, renal or hepatic dysfunction, pregnancy, drug–drug interactions due to other medications the patient is taking, and immune status must be taken into consideration. Drug dosage adjustment is required for many antibiotics in the setting of renal or hepatic dysfunction.

2. What facts must the clinician consider when deciding between oral and intravenous antibiotic therapy?
   Severity of infection: Oral antibiotics are typically used in mild infections whereas intravenous (IV) antibiotics are chosen for moderate to severe infections. Intravenous antibiotics should be given to patients who are in shock, because oral absorption can be erratic.
   Degree of systemic absorption: If an oral antibiotic is given, the absorption of the antibiotic must be considered. For example, some antibiotics such as aminoglycosides are not given orally due to poor absorption. On the other hand, some antibiotics have excellent oral bioavailability and can be used almost interchangeably with IV antibiotics.

3. What are some advantages of topical antibiotics?
   Some advantages are optimal delivery to the site, ability to deliver higher drug concentration, ability to overcome resistance mechanisms, and minimized systemic side effects. For example, topical eardrops are routinely used to treat otitis externa.

4. Describe the mechanism of action and spectrum of activity of the penicillin class of antibiotics.
   Penicillins are β-lactam antibiotics and are bactericidal. They kill bacteria by inhibiting cell wall synthesis (Table 4.1).

5. Explain the spectrum of activity of the different classes of cephalosporin antibiotics.
   First-generation cephalosporins (intravenous cefazolin, oral cephalexin) primarily have activity against gram-positive cocci, such as *Staphylococcus* sp. and *Streptococcus* sp.

Table 4.1 Clinically Relevant Penicillin Classes and Spectrum of Activity

Classes of Penicillin and Spectrum of Activity				
NATURAL PENICILLINS	**ANTISTAPHYLOCOCCAL PENICILLINS**	**AMINOPENICILLINS**	**CARBOXYPENICILLINS**	**ACYL UREIDOPENICILLINS**
Penicillin G and V	Oxacillin, nafcillin, dicloxacillin	Ampicillin, amoxicillin	Ticarcillin-clavulanate	Piperacillin-tazobactam
GPC, GNC, and some GNR. Also spirochetes and actinomyces	Methicillin sensitive staphylococci, penicillin-susceptible strains of *Streptococci*, anaerobic GPC	Essentially the same as natural penicillins, including *Haemophilus influenzae*	Increased gram-negative coverage including *Pseudomonas aeruginosa*	Excellent gram-positive and gram-negative coverage, including *Pseudomonas aeruginosa*
Susceptible to all β-lactamases	Not active against gram-negative organisms	Susceptible to β-lactamases	Less active against penicillin-resistant *Streptococcus* sp.	Enhanced activity against some β-lactamases

GPC, gram-positive cocci; GNC, gram-negative cocci; GNR, gram-negative rods.

Second-generation cephalosporins (cefuroxime) have increased activity against gram-negative respiratory pathogens, including *Haemophilus influenzae* and *Moraxella catarrhalis*. However, second-generation cephalosporins have limited activity against many Enterobacteriaceae. Cefuroxime is active against penicillin-sensitive strains of *Streptococcus pneumoniae*.

Third-generation cephalosporins (intravenous ceftriaxone and ceftazidime, oral cefixime and cefditoren) demonstrate increased activity against gram-negative organisms. Some of the drugs in this class, such as ceftriaxone, also have activity against penicillin-resistant *S. pneumoniae*.

Fourth-generation cephalosporins (cefepime is the only drug in this class available in the United States) have the broadest activity against gram-negative organisms, including *P. aeruginosa*.

Fifth-generation or methicillin-resistant *Staphylococcus aureus* (MRSA) active cephalosporins (the only approved agent in this class is ceftaroline) have excellent activity against MRSA and other gram-positive organisms including *S. pneumoniae*. The gram-negative activity of this drug is similar to that of ceftriaxone.

6. **Can β-lactams be safely used in patients who report a history of penicillin allergy?**
   A history of low-risk reaction (i.e., remote reaction that was not anaphylaxis) may be an indication for oral amoxicillin challenge. Higher risk reactions (i.e., features of IgE-mediated reactions) likely need penicillin skin testing prior to oral amoxicillin testing, if negative. Many patients who report a history of penicillin allergy (assumed to be an allergy to any antibiotic in the penicillin class) in fact have negative penicillin skin tests.
   Of patients with a history of penicillin allergy, 2% of patients with a positive skin test to penicillin have allergy to cephalosporins. Therefore, the risk is low but still present. The history of the penicillin reaction, penicillin skin testing, and possible oral amoxicillin challenge can all be used to determine if cephalosporins can be used safely.

7. **In addition to the penicillin and cephalosporin class of antibiotics, the carbapenems are also β-lactam antibiotics. What is their range of antimicrobial activity?**
   There are four carbapenems available for use in the United States: ertapenem, imipenem, doripenem, and meropenem. All have a very broad range of antimicrobial activity, including gram-positive organisms, gram-negative organisms (including drug-resistant gram-negatives), and anaerobic organisms. Ertapenem is the least broad of the carbapenems due to its lack of activity against *Enterococcus* sp. and *P. aeruginosa*.

8. **There are differences in antimicrobial coverage between the various agents of the fluoroquinolone class of antibiotics. Describe the mechanism of action of the fluoroquinolones and the differences in coverage between the drugs in this class.**
   Fluoroquinolones are bactericidal antibiotics that work by inhibiting bacterial DNA synthesis (Table 4.2).

9. **The macrolides are used frequently for infections of the head and neck. How do they work and what is their antimicrobial activity?**
   There are three members of the macrolide class of antibiotics: erythromycin, azithromycin, and clarithromycin. They are bacteriostatic antibiotics that inhibit RNA protein synthesis. Erythromycin has fairly broad antimicrobial activity, with activity against gram-positive and gram-negative organisms. Azithromycin and clarithromycin are the newest agents in the class and were developed with an even broader range of antimicrobial activity. Azithromycin and clarithromycin are more easily absorbed than erythromycin with fewer gastrointestinal side effects.

10. **Describe the spectrum of activity of clindamycin.**
    Clindamycin has good activity against gram-positive organisms, including *Staphylococcus aureus* (including MRSA) and *Streptococcus* sp. including *S. pyogenes*, *S. pneumoniae*, and members of the viridans streptococcus group. The special quality of clindamycin is the anaerobic coverage it provides. The adage is to use clindamycin for "anaerobic infections above the diaphragm" because clindamycin has activity against the anaerobes found in the oral cavity including *Peptostreptococcus* sp. and *Veillonella* sp.

Table 4.2 Antimicrobial Activity of the Fluoroquinolones	
Common coverage	Gram-negative bacilli, including *Enterobacteriaceae* and respiratory pathogens such as *Haemophilus influenzae*. Gram-positive respiratory pathogens such as *Neisseria* sp. and *Moraxella catarrhalis*. Atypical respiratory pathogens that can cause pneumonia, such as *Legionella pneumophilia*, *Mycoplasma pneumoniae*, and *Chlamydophilia pneumoniae*.
Ciprofloxacin	Broadest gram-negative activity, including *Pseudomonas aeruginosa*. Limited activity against *Streptococcus* sp. (not typically used for head and neck infections).
Levofloxacin, moxifloxacin	Best activity against *Streptococcus* sp. Levofloxacin also has activity against *Pseudomonas aeruginosa*.

11. **Which classes of antibiotics are most frequently associated with *Clostridioides difficile* infection?**
Prior antibiotic use is the primary risk factor for development of *C. difficile*–associated diarrhea. The antibiotics associated with increased risk are clindamycin, fluoroquinolones, broad-spectrum penicillins and cephalosporins, and carbapenems. Macrolides and sulfonamides are less frequently associated.

12. **Trimethoprim-sulfamethoxazole (TMP-SMX) is a bactericidal antibiotic that works by inhibiting bacterial production of folic acid. Describe the antimicrobial spectrum of action of the drug and its major side effects.**
TMP-SMZ is a fairly broad-spectrum antibiotic, with activity against a wide range of aerobic gram-positive and gram-negative bacteria. Examples include *S. aureus* (both methicillin-sensitive and methicillin-resistant), *S. pneumoniae*, *M. catarrhalis*, and *H. influenzae* and enteric aerobic gram-negative bacilli.
    The most common side effects of TMP-SMX are gastrointestinal upset and dermatologic reactions such as rash. More severe dermatologic reactions can occur including Stevens-Johnson syndrome and toxic epidermal necrolysis. Nephrotoxicity can also occur.

13. **Describe the mechanism of action of the tetracyclines and their spectrum of activity.**
Tetracyclines (doxycycline, minocycline, tetracycline) are bacteriostatic antibiotics that work by inhibiting bacterial protein synthesis. Tetracyclines are active against a wide range of gram-positive and gram-negative organisms, including respiratory pathogens such as *S. pneumoniae, H. influenzae*, and *Mycoplasma pneumoniae*. Tetracyclines should not be used in children or pregnant women due to the effect on developing teeth and bones.

14. **Name the antibiotics with activity against MRSA.**
The most commonly used IV agent is vancomycin, which is an inhibitor of bacterial cell wall synthesis. Other intravenous agents with MRSA activity include daptomycin, linezolid, and ceftaroline.
    There are also a number of oral agents with activity against MRSA. These include TMP-SMX, clindamycin, tetracyclines, and oral linezolid. The fluoroquinolones do have activity against *S. aureus* including MRSA but should not be used as monotherapy for staphylococcal infections because resistance can rapidly develop.

15. **Fungal infections of the head and neck are uncommon but can be devastating. What are the classes of antifungal medications and what infections do they treat?**
Azoles are the most commonly used antifungal medications. Examples of medications in this class include fluconazole, itraconazole, posaconazole, and voriconazole.
    Micafungin, caspofungin, and anidulafungin are all echinocandins. These are used for invasive candidiasis due to particular species of *Candida* including *Candida krusei* and *Candida glabrata*.
    Polyene amphotericin B is typically reserved for serious fungal infections, including invasive rhinosinusitis due to mucormycosis. The different formulations of the medication are conventional amphotericin B and liposomal amphotericin B. The liposomal form of the drug has less nephrotoxicity, so it is more commonly used (Table 4.3).

16. **Herpes simplex virus (HSV) is a frequent cause of orolabial infections. What are the oral antiviral medications used for this infection?**
Acyclovir is commonly used for orolabial HSV infections. Other oral antiviral medications used for HSV are valacyclovir and famciclovir.

Table 4.3 Overview of Characteristics of Antibiotics Used in Head and Neck Infections

CLASS	ACTIVITY	MECHANISM OF ACTION
Penicillins	Bactericidal	Inhibit cell wall synthesis
Cephalosporins	Bactericidal	Interfere with cell wall synthesis
Carbapenems	Bactericidal	Inhibit cell wall synthesis
Fluoroquinolones	Bactericidal	Inhibit DNA gyrase
Macrolides	Bacteriostatic	Inhibit protein synthesis
Clindamycin	Bacteriostatic	Inhibit protein synthesis
Trimethoprim/sulfamethoxazole	Bacteriostatic	Folate antagonist/inhibit folate synthesis
Vancomycin	Bactericidal	Inhibit cell wall synthesis and RNA synthesis
Tetracyclines	Bacteriostatic	Inhibit protein synthesis
Aminoglycosides	Bactericidal	Inhibit protein synthesis

BIBLIOGRAPHY

Andes DR, Craig WA. Cephalosporins. In Mandell, Douglas, and *Bennett's Principles and Practice of Infectious Diseases (Volume 1)*, 7th ed, Churchill Livingstone, 2009, pp 323–339.

Jorgenson MR, DePestel DD, Carver PL: Ceftaroline fosamil: a novel broad-spectrum cephalosporin with activity against methicillin-resistant *Staphylococcus aureus*, *Ann Pharmacother* 45(11):1384–1398, 2011.

Kachrimanidou M, Malisiovas N: Clostridium difficile infection: a comprehensive review, *Crit Rev Microbiol* 37(3):178–187, 2011.

Nathwani D, Wood MJ: Penicillins: A current review of their clinical pharmacology and therapeutic use, *Drugs* 45(6):866–894, 1993.

Roberts MC: Tetracycline therapy: update, *Clin Infect Dis* 36(4):462–467, 2003.

Shenoy ES, Macy E, Rowe T, et al: Evaluation and management of Penicillin allergy: a review, *JAMA* 321(2):188–199, 2019.

Wolfson JS, Hooper DC: Fluoroquinolone antimicrobial agents, *Clin Microbiol Rev* 2(4):378–424, 1989.

Zhanel GG, Dueck M, Hoban DJ, et al: Review of macrolides and ketolides: focus on respiratory tract infections, *Drugs* 61(4):443–498, 2001.

Zhanel GG, Wiebe R, Dilay L, et al: Comparative review of the carbapenems, *Drugs* 67(7):1027–1052, 2007.

Zinner SH, Mayer KH: Sulfonamides and trimethoprim. In Mandell, Douglas, and *Bennett's Principles and Practice of Infectious Diseases*, 7th ed, *Sulfonamides and trimethoprim* Churchill Livingstone, 2009, pp 475–486.

CHAPTER 5

ADULT SNORING AND OBSTRUCTIVE SLEEP APNEA

Katherine K. Green, MD, MS and Sarah A. Gitomer, MD

KEY POINTS

1. Obstructive sleep apnea (OSA) is a major problem in the United States and is associated with serious health complications. Noninvasive treatment with continuous positive airway pressure (CPAP) therapy remains the gold standard therapy, and it is typically recommended that patients try CPAP before considering alternative treatment options. For patients who are intolerant to CPAP therapy, surgical alternatives may be appropriate.
2. History and physical exam can help differentiate between snoring and sleep apnea. A thorough history and physical, input from a bed partner, and the Epworth Sleepiness Scale can help determine which patients need further diagnostic workup, such as polysomnography.
3. Identification of the site of airway obstruction should be performed prior to any attempted OSA surgery. Drug-induced sleep endoscopy may help to define the site of obstruction. A wide variety of surgical techniques are used for the treatment of OSA. Surgery should be tailored for each patient based on anatomic variations, severity of sleep apnea, and patient preference.

Pearls
1. Elevated risk factors for OSA:
   a. Age greater than 65 years
   b. Body mass index (BMI) greater than 30 kg/m²
   c. Postmenopausal female
   d. African American or Asian race
   e. Male sex
   f. Neck circumference greater than 17 inches in men and 16 inches in women
2. Although obesity is a risk factor for sleep apnea, an underweight patient may also have severe OSA.
3. Patients with OSA most likely to respond best to surgical therapy are those with "kissing" or 4+ tonsils.
4. Tracheotomy remains the most definitive surgical treatment for OSA. It bypasses the upper airway entirely and is effective in almost all patients, including those with severe disease.
5. Patients with craniofacial anomalies may benefit from correction of their skeletal deformity prior to soft tissue surgery for the treatment of OSA.

QUESTIONS

1. **What is the difference between snoring and obstructive sleep apnea (OSA)? What about sleep-disordered breathing (SDB) and upper airway resistance syndrome (UARS)?**
   Snoring is simply noisy breathing during sleep that occurs due to the vibration of lax tissue in the upper airway. SDB is characterized by snoring along with symptoms suggestive of OSA, including daytime somnolence and snoring. Sleep-disordered breathing exists along a continuum of severity. UARS represents the mildest form of SDB and is characterized by a normal apnea-hypopnea index (AHI) with an elevated respiratory disturbance index (RDI), indicative of respiratory events that fragment sleep quality but are not severe enough to cause oxygen desaturation. OSA, the most severe form of SDB, affects quality of life and is potentially life-threatening. In adults, OSA is defined by an AHI of greater than five events per hour during sleep, as revealed by polysomnography. OSA is caused by upper airway tissue collapse resulting in airway obstruction.

2. **How common is snoring? What about sleep apnea?**
   Snoring is very common across the population. Based on self-report questionnaires and questionnaires, 40% of middle-aged men and 28% of middle-aged women snore. This increased to as high as 84% and 73%, respectively, in the seventh decade of life. It is estimated that as many as 3% to 7% of men and 2% to 5% of women have OSA. It has been shown that the prevalence is even higher in obese, senior, postmenopausal,

and minority populations. The risk of OSA is higher when a person has a close relative (parent, child, or sibling) with OSA.

3. What causes snoring and OSA?

Snoring is caused by variations in airflow across dynamic portions of the upper airway, which results in the vibration of soft tissues. Most commonly, it occurs in the areas of the uvula, soft palate, tonsillar pillars, and/or pharyngeal walls. Occasionally, it may also occur at the base of the tongue or the epiglottis. OSA occurs secondary to collapse at the anatomic levels mentioned above, with airway collapse that is significant enough to not only result in vibratory snoring but also affect airflow and disruption in oxygen saturation. Obesity often contributes to snoring and apnea due to increased weight of the neck tissues; increased fat in the parapharyngeal space, which narrows the pharynx; redundancy in the soft palate; and fullness in the tongue base.

4. What is obstructive sleep apnea (OSA)?

OSA refers to a collection of conditions and syndromes that have periods of *apnea*, a temporary cessation of breathing (defined as intermittent cessation of airflow during sleep that lasts 10 seconds or longer), and/or hypopneas (defined as a partial reduction in airflow that results in oxygen desaturation) as key occurrences. It was initially described in the early 1800s. One of the first accounts was written by Charles Dickens in 1837 and titled *The Posthumous Papers of the Pickwick Club*. Subsequently, William Osler coined the term "pickwickian" in 1918 to describe the obese, hypersomnolent patient. The pathogenesis and pathophysiology of OSA have been extensively studied. During sleep, the upper airway is occluded, resulting in an episode of obstructive apnea. As a result, the patient experiences brief arousal from sleep. With the return of breathing, the patient typically returns to sleep quickly. This sequence is repeated many times.

5. What are the subclassifications of sleep apnea?

Over the years, various sleep apnea syndromes have been described and classified into three main types: *central, obstructive,* and *mixed*. Central sleep apnea refers to apneas notable for cessation of airflow due to cessation of *breathing effort*. Obstructive sleep apnea (OSA) refers to apnea due primarily to the collapse of the upper airway during sleep. Mixed apnea refers to apnea with both central and obstructive characteristics. Of the three main types of apneas, OSA is the most common and has received the most scientific interest and study.

6. What are common symptoms of obstructive sleep apnea?

Snoring, restless sleep, witnessed episodes of choking or gasping for air while sleeping, excessive daytime somnolence, morning headaches, nocturia, changes in mood (depression, irritability, anxiety, aggression), poor concentration, memory loss, night sweats, and bruxism.

7. What medical comorbidities can predispose patients to sleep apnea?

- **Obesity:** Obesity is very common in patients with OSA. Although being overweight is not necessary for OSA, truncal obesity predisposes patients to sleep apnea. In patients with a small airway diameter at baseline, even modest weight gain can cause OSA.
- **Hypothyroidism:** There appears to be a link between hypothyroidism and OSA beyond increased BMI alone. It is thought that mucoprotein and hyaluronic acid deposition in the upper airway may be related to increased airway compression. Treating underlying hypothyroidism often improves sleep apnea, independent of weight change or pulmonary function.
- **Acromegaly:** Tongue enlargement and skeletal changes, including increased head size, can also impact the airway and predispose patients to OSA.
- **Gastroesophageal reflux disease (GERD):** GERD is commonly present alongside OSA. Changing intrathoracic pressures and obesity predispose patients to reflux, and the inflammation caused by untreated GERD has been shown to worsen sleep apnea.
- **Polycystic ovarian syndrome:** Hormone dysregulation in PCOS can lead to increased frequency of apneic episodes in women with an anatomic predisposition for pharyngeal collapse. Hormonal changes associated with postmenopausal women have also been shown to cause a higher incidence of OSA.

8. What medical complications can arise if OSA is untreated?

Systemic hypertension, myocardial infarction, vascular accidents, congestive heart failure, cor pulmonale, atherosclerosis, atrial fibrillation, ventricular arrhythmias, pulmonary hypertension, glaucoma, decreased seizure threshold, diminished libido, cognitive impairment, and death.

9. What should an in-office clinical exam of the snoring patient with OSA include?

A complete head and neck examination should be performed. The nose should be examined for signs of obstruction due to a deviated septum, hypertrophic turbinates, or allergic rhinitis. Improving nasal congestion may decrease the intensity and frequency of primary snoring, and in patients with OSA, CPAP therapy may be more comfortable. Examination of the oral cavity may reveal potential obstruction due to large tonsils, redundant soft palate and uvula, redundant lateral pharyngeal walls, and/or a full base of the tongue. Patients may also have a high-arched hard

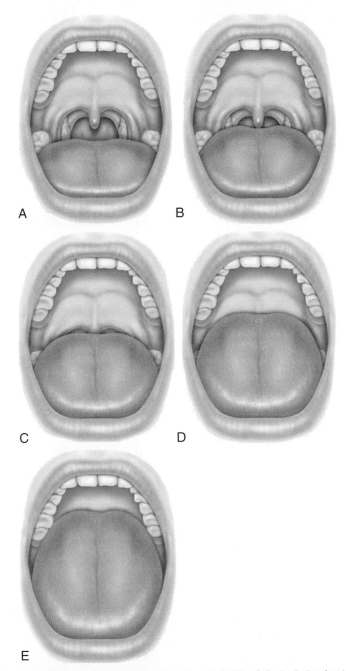

Fig. 5.1 Friedman tongue position. A, I: visualization of the entire uvula and tonsils/pillars. **B,** IIa: visualization of most of the uvula but tonsils/pillars are absent. **C,** IIb: visualization of the entire soft palate to the base of the uvula. **D,** III: visualization of some of the soft palate, but structures distal to this are not seen. **E,** IV: visualization of the hard palate only. (Reprint permission obtained from Dr. Michael Friedman.)

palate, retrognathia, and micrognathia. The Friedman tongue position classification system can be used together with BMI and tonsil size to predict patients' response to palate surgery and/or tonsillectomy (Fig. 5.1). The system grades the view of the uvula and tonsillar pillars while the patient opens his or her mouth with the tongue in a neutral position. Obstruction with a lower Friedman tongue position (1 or 2, as opposed to 3 or 4) is associated with the success of tonsillectomy and/or palate procedures (Fig. 5.2).

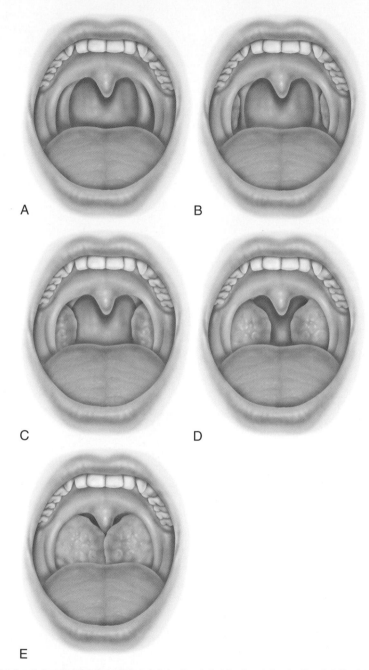

Fig. 5.2 A, Tonsil grade 0, postsurgical; **B,** tonsil grade 1; **C,** tonsil grade 2; **d,** tonsil grade 3; **e,** tonsil grade 4. (Reprint permission obtained from Dr. Michael Friedman.)

10. **How is OSA diagnosed?**

The gold standard for diagnosing OSA is in-lab-monitored polysomnography, but the most common pathway of testing in the United States is home sleep testing. The history and physical, along with supplementary question-naires such as the Epworth Sleepiness Scale (ESS), can help identify patients who would benefit from a sleep study to diagnose sleep apnea. In-lab sleep studies measure brain activity, leg muscle movements, cardiac rhythm, eye movements, oxygen saturation, respiratory effort, and air movement at the nose and mouth. Polysomnography can differentiate between primary snoring, OSA, and central sleep apnea and can characterize the severity of apnea. This test requires the patient to spend the night in a formal sleep laboratory. Portable monitoring devices for home sleep studies vary by manufacturer but in general tend to measure respiratory flow, pulse oximetry, heart rate, and respiratory effort.

11. **What defines obstructive sleep apnea on polysomnography in adults? What is the difference between AHI and RDI?**
    The diagnostic criteria for OSA in adults are an apnea-hypopnea index (AHI) greater than 5 or a respiratory disturbance index (RDI) greater than 5. AHI is defined as the number of apneic or hypopneic episodes per hour. On polysomnography, obstructive apnea is defined as cessation of airflow due to anatomic airway obstruction for 10 seconds, and hypopnea is defined as reduction in ventilation by at least 30% of baseline for 10 seconds associated with at least a 4% oxygen desaturation. RDI is similar to AHI but also includes respiratory effort–related arousals (RERAs). RERAs do not fulfill the criteria of apnea or hypopnea but still result in arousal from sleep. AHI between 5 and 15 is considered mild OSA, 16 to 30 is considered moderate OSA, and any number greater than 30 is considered severe OSA.

12. **Describe the classic sleep pattern seen in OSA.**
    Although sleep quality is highly variable, patients with OSA exhibit a quick onset of sleep and multiple arousals. The patient maintains relatively more stage I and II sleep and less stage III and rapid eye movement (REM) sleep. Sleep fragmentation results in sleep deprivation symptoms.

13. **During which stage of sleep do most obstructive events occur?**
    While sleep-disordered breathing events can occur during all stages of sleep, obstructive events are often worse during REM sleep. During REM sleep muscles are the most relaxed and thus upper airway collapse is most likely. For patients who are relatively deprived of REM sleep due to this fragmentation, a hallmark of successful treatment of OSA is REM rebound, or a significant increase in REM sleep (clinical increase in dreaming) due to correction of previous sleep deprivation.

14. **Should everyone who snores undergo a sleep study?**
    When snoring is accompanied by symptoms of OSA, such as hypersomnolence, morning headache, and restless sleep, a thorough examination and sleep study are indicated. When snoring is socially disruptive but is not accompanied by symptoms of sleep apnea, the picture is not so clear. Symptoms of sleep apnea correlate poorly with the presence and severity of OSA, and even "apneas" witnessed by bed partners may not be predictive of OSA. The only reasonably accurate method for detecting OSA remains a formal sleep study. Therefore current recommendations suggest obtaining a sleep study prior to any surgery for sleep apnea or snoring.

15. **What are some treatments for primary snoring?**
    Weight loss, tonsillectomy (if adenotonsillar hypertrophy is present), positional therapy, and improved nasal breathing are the most common treatments for snoring because they decrease vibrations of the soft palate. Stiffening of the soft palate can also be accomplished using a variety of techniques. Most palate stiffening techniques can be performed in offices under local anesthesia. Options for palate stiffening include submucosal radiofrequency, placement of woven polyester implants, suture techniques, and injection of sclerosing agents. Mandibular advancement devices (oral appliances that hold the jaw forward) can also be effective in improving snoring.

16. **Are there behavioral or lifestyle adjustments that can change the severity of OSA?**
    - Reducing or eliminating alcohol or sedatives because they may cause excess relaxation of tissues, which may exacerbate soft tissue collapse.
    - Treatment of underlying medical conditions: anti-reflux medications, thyroid replacement therapy, and hormone replacement therapy.
    - For many patients, weight loss has been shown to result in improvement in or even resolution of OSA.
    - For some patients, OSA can be dependent on position, with events occurring more frequently during supine sleep. Positional therapy devices prevent patients from rolling onto their back at night, and this strict avoidance of supine sleep can improve OSA severity in some patients.

17. **What is positive airway pressure therapy (PAP therapy), and why is it first-line therapy for OSA?**
    PAP therapy involves the administration of pressurized air through the nose or mouth by wearing a mask attached to a machine while sleeping. The pressure of the airflow stents the airway open, particularly during the inspiratory phase, when negative pressure would otherwise cause the pharyngeal walls to collapse. CPAP provides one fixed pressure throughout the night, and it provides one pressure at a time but can auto-adjust throughout the night across a range of pressures depending on whether the machine is sensing respiratory events. Bi-level positive airway pressure (BiPAP) provides two different pressures, a higher pressure when patients are breathing in and a lower pressure when breathing out.

18. **Why would you recommend surgery over CPAP alone?**

    In general, surgery should only be offered to patients who have tried and failed CPAP therapy, and if a patient is able to wear CPAP comfortably and effectively, then no surgery is necessary. If patients have primary symptoms related to areas that may contribute to airway obstruction (tonsillar hypertrophy causing chronic or recurrent acute tonsillitis, septal deviation causing nasal congestion, etc.), it may be reasonable to consider those procedures in conjunction with recommending CPAP.

19. **If surgery is indicated, how do you select the operation to be performed?**

    The challenge confronting the surgeon is to know what part of the upper airway causes obstruction to airflow. Sleep studies (polysomnography and home sleep testing) do not provide any indication of the site of obstruction. The site of obstruction also does not correlate very well with the severity of sleep apnea. If the surgeon treats the wrong part of the airway, or if there are multiple sites of obstruction, it is less likely that sleep apnea will improve to a degree such that no other treatment is needed. Given the several sites where airway obstruction may exist, a diagnostic procedure called drug-induced sleep endoscopy to identify the site of obstruction while the patient is asleep may be helpful (see more details below).

    Several types of operations are currently being used to treat sleep apnea. The most common surgery performed on adults in the USA is uvulopalatopharyngoplasty (UPPP). The success rate of this operation is approximately 50%.

    - **Nose:** Nasal obstruction can be treated by septoplasty, turbinate reduction, or sinus surgery if appropriate. Nasal surgery is unlikely to improve obstructive sleep apnea but may increase the success and comfort of CPAP therapy.
    - Adenoidectomy is often performed in children. It is 80% to 90% effective, often in conjunction with tonsillectomy, for improving nasal airway, snoring, and apnea in children. This operation is rarely necessary for adults.
    - **Tonsils:** Tonsillectomy for tonsillar hypertrophy. In adults with OSA tonsillectomy is often performed as part of a UPPP.
    - **Palate:** Older procedures for palate intervention include snoreplasty (sclerosants injected into the palate to cause scarring and shrinkage), laser-assisted uvulopalatoplasty (LAUP), submucosal radiofrequency device, or UPPP. These procedures have variable success rates, and minimally invasive procedures such as snoreplasty or LAUP procedures are unlikely to treat sleep apnea but may decrease the intensity of snoring in some patients. Newer surgical techniques include expansion pharyngoplasty and lateral pharyngoplasty, and studies indicate that these palate surgeries may have a higher and more predictable success rate for improving palate obstruction, with a lower risk of complications. Because these techniques are relatively new, they are not yet widely used in practice as UPPPs.
    - **Tongue base:** Transoral robotic surgery, coblation or radiofrequency tongue base reduction, lag screw and suture suspension of the tongue and hyoid, genioglossus advancement, hyoid suspension, distraction osteogenesis, partial midline glossectomy, and maxillomandibular advancement are used to reduce obstruction at the tongue base.
    - After any surgical intervention for sleep apnea, repeat polysomnography should be performed at approximately 3 months to assess the efficacy of the intervention.

20. **What is a drug-induced sleep endoscopy (DISE)?**

    Studies have shown that awake airway examination findings do not correlate with the success of surgical interventions, and this poses a challenge in deciding which of the above procedures may have the highest chance of success. DISE, a relatively new technique, helps to evaluate the airway during sleep to determine which areas of the throat have the most prominent collapse during apneic events. Patients are examined in a lightly sedated sleep that is intended to mimic natural sleep. A flexible fiber-optic scope is passed through the nose to evaluate the upper airway to reveal the site of obstruction. This enables the surgeon to adequately address these sites while preserving areas that are not involved. Data on the validity of this procedure are scant yet promising, but this procedure may not be widely available in all areas.

21. **What is UPPP? What are the complications associated with it?**

    Uvulopalatopharyngoplasty, or "U triple-P," is the most commonly performed surgical procedure for OSA. Under general anesthesia, the tonsils are removed along with a portion of the anterior and posterior pillars and part of the soft palate. The remaining tonsillar pillars are sutured together and the uvula is shortened. The operation decreases the amount of soft tissue in the oropharynx and, as such, it is most successful in patients with isolated palatal collapse. The efficacy of UPPP alone in improving AHI over time ranges from 40% to 70%, depending on patient selection. Bleeding is the most common postoperative complication, occasionally requiring another visit to the operating room for control. Transient velopharyngeal insufficiency with nasal regurgitation occurs in 5% to 10% of patients but is rarely permanent. Nasopharyngeal stenosis is a very rare but devastating complication in which the nasopharynx scars completely. Patients may also complain of dry mouth, tightness in the throat, increased gag reflex, and/or change in taste, and in some studies up to 30% of patients may have persistent symptoms of globus sensation after UPPP.

22. **What is upper airway stimulation (UAS)? Which patients qualify for this therapy?**
    The concept of upper airway stimulation is a newer technique aimed at increasing the tone of the tongue during inspiration while sleeping. With proper patient selection the success rates of this procedure are comparable with those of other surgical interventions for OSA. These devices work to stimulate specific branches of the hypoglossal nerve and protrude and stiffen the tongue when activated to open and stabilize the airway. Inspire therapy is the first FDA-approved hypoglossal nerve stimulator for clinical use. It involves the placement of three components of the device: a stimulation lead with a cuff that gets placed in the neck around the branches of the hypoglossal nerve, a sensing lead that gets placed in the intercostal space to sense inspiration vs expiration, and an IPG generator that gets placed beneath the subcutaneous tissue overlying the pectoralis major muscle.
    Criteria for qualification of Inspire are controlled by the FDA and insurance regulations and may continue to change as we understand who is most likely to benefit from therapy. Currently, the device is approved for:
    1. Patients aged 18 years and older (although clinical trials are currently being conducted on adolescent populations)
    2. Patients who have tried and failed CPAP therapy first and are unable to tolerate CPAP
    3. Patients who have exclusively obstructive sleep apnea ($<25\%$ central sleep apnea on a recent sleep study)
    4. Patients with a body mass index of ≤ 32 kg/m^2 (some insurance companies have increased this cutoff to 35 kg/m^2)

CONTROVERSIES

1. Further research as to whether sleep endoscopy improves surgical outcomes is needed.
2. There currently exist two different but accepted definitions of hypopnea.
    a. Recommended:
        i. Ventilation drop by $\geq 30\%$ of pre-event baseline.
        ii. The duration of the $\geq 30\%$ drop in signal excursion is ≥ 10 seconds.
        iii. There is a $\geq 3\%$ oxygen desaturation from the pre-event baseline and/or the event is associated with arousal.
    b. Alternate version:
        i. Ventilation drops by $\geq 30\%$ of pre-event baseline.
        ii. The duration of the $\geq 30\%$ drop in signal excursion is ≥ 10 seconds.
        iii. There is a $\geq 4\%$ oxygen desaturation from pre-event baseline.

BIBLIOGRAPHY

American Academy of Otolaryngolgy–Head and Neck Surgery. Clinical indicators: palatopharyngoplasty for obstructive sleep apnea. American Available at: http://www.entnet.org/sites/default/files/UPPP-CI%20Updated%208-7-14.pdf. Accessed April 11, 2015.

Friedman M, Ibrahim H, Bass L: Clinical staging for sleep-disordered breathing, *Otolaryngol Head Neck Surg* 127:13–21, 2002.

Hohenhorst W, Ravesloot MJL, Kezirian EJ, et al: Drug-induced sleep endoscopy in adults with sleep-disordered breathing: technique and the VOTE classification system, *Oper Tech Otolaryngol Head Neck Surg* 23(1):11–18, 2012.

Katsantonis GP: Uvulopalatopharyngoplasty for obstructive sleep apnea and snoring, *Oper Tech Otolaryngol Head Neck Surg* 2(2): 100–103, 1991.

Punjabi NM: The epidemiology of adult obstructive sleep apnea, *Proc Am Thorac Soc* 5(2):136–143, 2008.

Strollo PJ Jr, Soose RJ, Maurer JT, et al: Upper-airway stimulation for obstructive sleep apnea, *N Engl J Med* 370(2):139–149, 2014.

Terris DJ: Multilevel pharyngeal surgery for obstructive sleep apnea: indications and techniques, *Oper Tech Otolaryngol Head Neck Surg* 11:12–20, 2000.

Walker RP: Snoring and obstructive sleep apnea. In: Bailey BJ, Johnson JT, Newlands SD, eds: *Head & Neck Surgery: Otolaryngology*, 4th ed, Philadelphia, 2006, Lippincott Williams & Wilkins, pp. 645–665.

Weaver EM, Maynard C, Yueh B: Survival of veterans with sleep apnea: continuous positive airway pressure vs. surgery, *Otolaryngol Head Neck Surg* 130:659–665, 2004.

Young T, Palta M, Dempsey J, et al: The occurrence of sleep-disordered breathing among middle-aged adults, *N Engl J Med* 328: 1230–1235, 1993.

CHAPTER 6

HEAD AND NECK MANIFESTATIONS OF SYSTEMIC DISEASE

Melissa A. Scholes, MD

KEY POINTS

1. Granulomatosis with polyangiitis is the most common vasculitis disease affecting the head and neck.
2. In patients with recurrent inflammation of the cartilages of the nose, ears, or larynx, you must consider a diagnosis of relapsing polychondritis.
3. Sjögren's syndrome (SS) is a systemic autoimmune disorder that is associated with inflammation of the epithelial tissues, including the salivary and lacrimal glands.

Pearls

1. The diagnosis of granulomatosis with polyangiitis requires biopsies of involved sites and testing for antineutrophil cytoplasmic antibodies.
2. Relapsing polychondritis is diagnosed with three of the following signs with positive biopsies from two separate sites and response to steroids: (1) bilateral auricular chondritis, (2) nonerosive seronegative inflammatory polyarthritis, (3) nasal chondritis, (4) ocular inflammation, (5) laryngotracheal chondritis, and (6) audiovestibular damage.
3. The supraglottis is the most common laryngeal site affected by sarcoidosis. The epiglottis and arytenoids become pale and extremely swollen, giving a "turban-like" appearance.
4. Eosinophilia with granulomatosis and polyangiitis is characterized by sinusitis, asthma, and tissue and blood eosinophilia.
5. Inflammatory bowel disease, Crohn's disease, and ulcerative colitis can cause recurrent aphthous ulcers.

QUESTIONS

1. **What's the most common granulomatous disease affecting the head and neck? What are its main otolaryngologic manifestations?**

   Granulomatosis with polyangiitis (GPA) is a systemic disease characterized by necrotizing granulomas of the upper and lower respiratory tract, vasculitis, and glomerulonephritis. It is the most common granulomatous disease of the head and neck. Rhinologic symptoms include rhinitis, congestion, sinusitis, and inflammation that can be severe and progress to nasal septal perforation or nasal stenosis. GPA affects the larynx and trachea and can cause hoarseness, cough, hemoptysis, wheezing, and stridor and can progress to subglottic stenosis. Oral cavity manifestations include gingival hyperplasia and tooth mobility.

2. **How do you diagnose GPA, and what is the differential diagnosis?**

   The diagnosis of GPA is based on clinical symptoms, biopsy, and a positive antineutrophil cytoplasmic antibody (C-ANCA) test. C-ANCA is highly specific and sensitive for GPA, but a negative result does not completely rule out GPA. A liberal biopsy of involved nasal mucosa is recommended to look for the characteristic necrotizing granulomas and vasculitis. Isolated oral or laryngeal/tracheal involvement can occur but is less common, and these areas should be biopsied if diagnosis in unclear. Tissue culture should also be done to rule out bacterial or fungal disease.

3. **What is the treatment for GPA?**

   Since GPA is a systemic disease, it is best treated in a multidisciplinary fashion with specialists from otolaryngology, rheumatology, nephrology, and other fields. Medical treatment includes immunosuppression with cyclophosphamide, methotrexate, or glucocorticoids. In severe cases, the biologic agent rituximab may be indicated. After control of systemic disease, nasal or airway reconstruction may be needed, but care must be taken to control the disease medically to prevent relapse and further damage to airway structures.

4. **What autoimmune disease affects the cartilages of the head and neck in a recurrent fashion?**
Relapsing polychondritis (RP) is a rheumatologic disorder that involves the cartilages of the nose, ears, and airway as well as systemic involvement of the lymph nodes, lungs, and joints. It typically occurs in the fourth decade of life and affects men and women equally. The incidence is three cases per million.

5. **What are some of the symptoms of RP?**
Most cases of RP present with recurrent auricular chondritis and arthropathy. Patients can also have audiovestibular system damage, nasal and laryngotracheal chondritis, cardiovascular vasculitis, and ocular inflammation. Nasal symptoms include crusting, drainage, and epistaxis and are usually brought on by mucosal disruption and cartilage exposure. Chronic inflammation can cause septal perforation and saddle nose deformity. Airway involvement can be severe and lead to stenosis and collapse of the laryngeal cartilages and trachea, causing obstruction, and patients may need tracheostomy.

6. **How do you diagnose RP?**
There is no specific laboratory test for RP, but markers of inflammation are often increased, including erythrocyte sedimentation rate (ESR), C-reactive protein (CRP), and anti nuclear antibodies (ANAs). There are clinical criteria for the diagnosis or RP and include at least three of the following: (1) bilateral auricular chondritis, (2) non erosive seronegative inflammatory polyarthritis, (3) nasal chondritis, (4) ocular inflammation, (5) laryngotracheal chondritis, and (6) audiovestibular damage. Stricter criteria require at least two separate areas of biopsy-proven chondritis with response to steroid. Biopsy specimens show chondritis, chondrolysis, and perichondritis.

7. **How do you treat RP?**
As an autoimmune disease, RP is treated by immunosuppression including corticosteroids and cytotoxic medications. Additional workup may be needed such as imaging, pulmonary function testing, and echocardiography to determine extent of disease. Surgery is directed at the organ system involved and may involve airway and nasal reconstruction.

8. **Describe how T-cell lymphoma affects the head and neck.**
T-cell lymphoma usually starts with nasal obstruction followed by purulent rhinorrhea and bloody discharge. Mucosal ulcerations appear on the lateral nasal mucosa with extension into the palate, sinuses, and upper lip; disease is usually unilateral. Oronasal fistula and nasoseptal destruction with extensive crusting and friable, pale mucosa develop in 40% of cases. Systemic symptoms such as fever, weight loss, and malaise are common. Treatment usually consists of radiation and multiagent chemotherapy and bone marrow transplantation.

9. **Describe the histopathology of T-cell lymphoma.**
T-cell lymphoma is characterized by a polymorphic lymphocyte infiltration that causes angioinvasion with infarction of the blood vessels that leads to tissue destruction. T-cell markers are usually present, including CD2, CD7, CD45RO, CD43, and the natural killer cell marker CD57. Epstein-Barr virus (EBV) is associated with nasal T-cell lymphoma, and EBV DNA and RNA have been detected in tumor cells. However, the exact role of EBV remains to be determined.

10. **What disease presents with eosinophilia, asthma, and sinusitis?**
Eosinophilic granulomatosis with polyangiitis (EGPA) is a rare systemic necrotizing vasculitis associated with sinopulmonary disease and blood and tissue eosinophilia. It was previously known as Churg-Strauss syndrome. Like GPA, it is associated with C-ANCA. Ear, nose, and throat involvement includes middle ear effusion, allergic rhinitis, nasal congestion, recurrent sinusitis, and nasal polyps and occurs in 75% to 80% of patients with this disease.

11. **What systemic granulomatous disease characterized by noncaseating granulomas can first present with nasal symptoms?**
Sarcoidosis is a multisystem granulomatous disease that is characterized by noncaseating granulomas involving multiple sites in the body, most commonly the lungs. Nasal symptoms of inflammation such as obstruction, epistaxis, and anosmia may be the first signs of the disease. Nasal sarcoidosis involves the septum and inferior turbinate, most commonly with dry and friable mucosa. Nodules can occur in the nasal mucosa and are characterized by a yellow appearance and composed of intramucosal granulomas.

12. **What is the most common part of the larynx involved in sarcoidosis?**
The supraglottis is most commonly involved in sarcoidosis, followed by the subglottis. The vocal folds are usually spared. The supraglottis becomes very erythematous and pale and has been described as "turban-like" in appearance (Fig. 6.1). Biopsy shows the characteristic granulomas and diffuse lymphocyte infiltration. The laryngeal manifestations can present with hoarseness, dyspnea, stridor, dysphagia, and cough, but these are usually slow to develop.

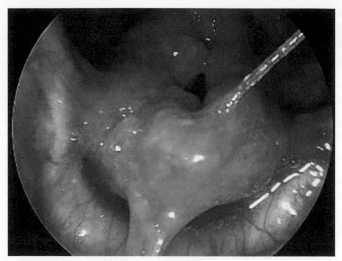

Fig. 16.1 Supraglottic changes of sarcoidosis causing a "turban-like" appearance.

13. **What is Heerfordt syndrome?**

    Heerfordt syndrome is a rare sarcoid variant that presents with fever, parotid gland enlargement, uveitis, and facial nerve palsy. It is also known as uveoparotid fever.

14. **What is pemphigus vulgaris?**

    Pemphigus vulgaris is an idiopathic autoimmune disorder affecting the mucosal membranes and skin where there is formation of intraepithelial blebs secondary to IgG autoantibodies binding to intercellular adhesion molecules. These blebs can occur in the nose, mouth, or larynx. Isolated laryngeal lesions are rare and can present with hoarseness, stridor, and dyspnea. Laryngeal lesions may not have characteristic bleb appearance on scope because the mechanism of swallowing may slough off the lesions, leaving a tan fibrotic lesion with a halo of erythema. The pain associated with mucosal involvement can be severe. Biopsy is recommended for definitive diagnosis. Pemphigus vulgaris is treated with immunosuppressants.

15. **What is the Nikolsky sign?**

    The Nikolsky sign in the induction of blistering via mechanical pressure at the edge of a blister or on normal skin. This can be elicited in pemphigus vulgaris.

16. **How does mucous membrane pemphigoid differ from pemphigus vulgaris?**

    Mucous membrane pemphigoid (MMP) or bullous pemphigoid (BP) is a subepithelial blistering disorder caused by deposition of immunoglobulins and complement within the epidermal or mucosal basement membrane. In bullous pemphigoid, there is formation of firm, fluid-filled blisters on the skin. MMP is characterized by recurrent inflammation and erosion of the mucosa, most commonly in the oral cavity. Many patients have multiple comorbidities, and there is a link between BP and neurologic disorders and malignancy. Biopsy is important to confirm diagnosis. Nikolsky sign is absent.

17. **What is the name of the chronic mucocutaneous autoimmune process that affects the oral cavity?**

    Lichen planus is an autoimmune disorder that can be precipitated by several conditions, including genetic predisposition, drug exposure, stress, and dental material hypersensitivity. It can appear in different patterns and forms such as bullous, plaque-like, atrophic, and reticular (lacy lines also known as Wickham striae).

18. **Where do the lesions of lichen planus occur?**

    The lesions of lichen planus most often occur on the buccal mucosa, gingiva, and tongue but can occur on the lip and hard palate. Some evidence shows that these lesions may have malignant potential. Thus histopathologic samples are required to differentiate this from other oral lesions. Regular follow-up is needed once diagnosed to monitor for change. Treatment is in the form of immunosuppression, either local (topical glucocorticoids) or systemic, depending on the severity of the disease.

19. **What is the most common medical disorder that causes dry mouth and salivary dysfunction?**
Sjögren's syndrome (SS) is a systemic autoimmune disorder that is associated with inflammation of the epithelial tissues, including the salivary and lacrimal glands. It can occur alone as primary disease or can be secondary and related to other autoimmune diseases such as scleroderma, systemic lupus erythematosus, and polyarteritis nodosa. The salivary and lacrimal glands become infiltrated by mononuclear infiltrates and are associated with anti-Ro (SS-A) and anti-La (SS-B) autoantibodies. Symptoms can be severe, including exocrine gland dysfunction with resulting dry mouth developing into cracked tissues that are vulnerable to infections, gingivitis, and dysphagia. People with this disease are at increased risk for dental caries and impaired eating and require routine dental care.

20. **What condition associated with Sjögren's syndrome also includes tightening of the face?**
Scleroderma is a systemic disorder of unknown etiology that mainly affects the skin and oral cavity. Collagen is deposited in the tissues and around nerves and vessels. Head and neck involvement is common. Fibrosis occurs in the muscles of mastication and tongue, resulting in difficulty opening the mouth and impaired eating and speaking. Telangiectasias may form in the nasal cavity and lead to epistaxis.

21. **Which diseases of the gastrointestinal tract cause oral ulcers?**
Inflammatory bowel disease, Crohn's disease, and ulcerative colitis can cause recurrent aphthous ulcers. Oral ulcers in ulcerative colitis are usually associated with arthritis, iritis, and erythema nodosum. Crohn's disease can include additional mucosal involvement, including nodular swellings, cobblestoning of the mucosa, and deep granulomatous-appearing ulcers.

22. **What disorder includes recurrent aphthous oral ulcers, genital ulcers, and ocular inflammation?**
Behçet syndrome is an idiopathic condition that manifests with recurrent oral ulcers along with genital ulcers, arthritis, and inflammation of the gastrointestinal tract and the eyes. Ulcers can also occur in the nasal cavity and cause rhinorrhea, septal ulceration, and pain. Oral ulcers usually precede the other sites of involvement. Treatment is supportive with immunosuppression.

23. **What joints are affected by rheumatoid arthritis?**
Rheumatoid arthritis (RA) can affect the temporomandibular and cricoarytenoid joints. RA is an autoimmune arthritis that affects synovial tissues. Women are two to three times more likely to develop RA than men.

24. **What are the laryngeal manifestations of RA?**
RA affects the larynx in two forms. With active inflammation, the arytenoids will be swollen and erythematous on laryngoscopy. This evolves to the chronic form with destruction of the cricoarytenoid joint and ankylosis of the vocal folds that may be bilateral. In the case of bilateral impairment, urgent medical and surgical management may be needed to avoid airway compromise. Additionally, RA can cause submucosal nodules in the vocal folds that can cause hoarseness. The nodules are treated medically and eventually removed surgically if needed.

BIBLIOGRAPHY

Batra PS, Wrobel BB, Trimarchi M: Systemic Disease of the Nose and Sinuses. In Flint Paul W, editor: *Cummings Otolaryngology Head and Neck Surgery*, 7th ed., Elsevier, 2021, pp 788–794.

Cereceda-Monteoliva N, Rouhani MJ, Maughan EF, Rotman A, Orban N, Al Yaghchi C, Sandhu G: Sarcoidosis of the ear, nose and throat: A review of the literature, *Clin Otolaryngol* 46(5):935–940, 2021 Sep; doi: 10.1111/coa.13814, Epub 2021 Jun 8. PMID: 34051056.

De Virgilio A, Greco A, Magliulo G, Gallo A, Ruoppolo G, Conte M, Martellucci S, de Vincentiis M: Polyarteritis nodosa: A contemporary overview, *Autoimmun Rev* 15(6):564–570, 2016 Jun; doi: 10.1016/j.autrev.2016.02.015, Epub 2016 Feb 13. PMID: 26884100.

Leahy KP: Laryngeal and Tracheal Manifestations of Systemic Disease. In Flint Paul W, editor: *Cummings Otolaryngology Head and Neck Surgery*, 7th ed., Elsevier, 2021, pp 180–184.

Nadol JB, Quesnel AM: Otologic Manifestation of Systemic Disease. In Flint Paul W, editor: *Cummings Otolaryngology Head and Neck Surgery*, 7th ed., Elsevier, 2021, pp 2293–2310.

Taylor SC, Clayburgh DR, Rosenbaum JT, Schindler JS: Clinical manifestations and treatment of idiopathic and Wegener granulomatosis-associated subglottic stenosis, *JAMA Otolaryngol Head Neck Surg* 139(1):76–81, 2013 Jan; doi: 10.1001/jamaoto.2013.1135, PMID: 23329095.

Turner MD: Oral Manifestation of Systemic Diseases. In Flint Paul W, editor: *Cummings Otolaryngology Head and Neck Surgery*, 7th ed., Elsevier, 2021, pp 185–197.

CHAPTER 7

FACIAL PAIN AND HEADACHE

Laylaa Ramos Arriaza, MD, MS and Vijay R. Ramakrishnan, MD

KEY POINTS

1. Headaches can be classified as primary, secondary, or both. Primary headaches occur in the absence of another disorder known to cause headaches (e.g., tension-type or migraine headache). Secondary headaches occur in the presence of another disorder that is known to cause headaches (e.g., headache attributed to rhinosinusitis).
2. The majority of patients with "sinus headaches" will meet International Classification of Headache Disorders (ICHD) criteria for migraine disorder.
3. Cortical spreading depression is the leading theory for the etiology of migraine disorder. It is a slowly propagated wave of depolarization followed by suppression of brain activity and results in the release of neuropeptide transmitters such as substance P, calcitonin gene-related peptide, and neurokinin A.
4. Temporomandibular disorder can be divided into three categories: myofascial disorder, disc displacement, and arthritis/arthrosis/arthralgia.

Pearls
1. Postherpetic neuralgia occurs in approximately 25% of patients previously diagnosed with herpes zoster.
2. Tension-type headache is the most common type of headache/facial pain.
3. First-line treatment of persistent idiopathic facial pain is tricyclic antidepressants.
4. Triptans are the first-line medical abortive therapy for migraine disorder.
5. Substance P is a neuropeptide that has been associated with the sensation of pain during a migraine and is released from trigeminocervical axons promoting plasma protein extravasation.

QUESTIONS

1. **What is the difference between primary and secondary headache?**
   A headache is labeled a primary headache if it occurs in the absence of a disorder that is known to cause headaches. A secondary headache is a new headache that occurs in close temporal relation to another disorder that is known to cause headache. Headaches can also be categorized as having both primary and secondary components, such as a primary headache that becomes chronic or at least two-fold worsened by another headache-causing disorder.

2. **What is the differential diagnosis for facial pain?**
   - Primary headache: Common types include tension-type headache, migraine headache, and trigeminal autonomic cephalalgias.
      Other primary headache disorders: Primary cough headache, primary exercise headache, primary thunderclap headache, cold-stimulus headache, external pressure headache, primary stabbing headache, nummular headache, hypnic headache, and new daily persistent headache.
   - Secondary headache: Trigeminal neuralgia, persistent idiopathic facial pain, temporomandibular disorder, headache attributed to cranial or cervical disorder, substance abuse and/or withdrawal, intracranial infection, headache attributed to disorder of the eyes (acute glaucoma, refractive error, heterophoria, heterotropia), and psychiatric disorder.

3. **What is the prevalence of headache?**
   Worldwide headache prevalence for the adult population is 46% for headache in general, 42% for tension-type headache, 11% for migraine, and 3% for chronic daily headache. Based on years lived with disability, headaches are 1 of the 10 most disabling conditions and 1 of the 5 most disabling for women.

4. **How do you diagnose and treat tension-type headache?**
   Tension-type headaches are episodic and typically bilateral, pressing or tightening in quality, of mild to moderate intensity, and last from minutes to days. The pain does not worsen with routine physical activity and is not associated with nausea. Photophobia or phonophobia may be present. Other International Classification of Headache

Disorders – 3rd edition (ICHD-III) diagnoses should be ruled out. Treatment consists of aspirin or NSAIDs for occasional mild tension-type headache; the addition of caffeine can make treatment more effective. Acetaminophen is preferred in pregnancy. More severe headaches can require a prescription analgesic. Amitriptyline is the most effective prophylactic pharmaceutical for tension-type headaches.

5. **What are the adult diagnostic criteria for migraine headache without aura?**
   For a headache to meet ICHD-III criteria as a migraine without aura, a person must suffer at least five headaches that include the following characteristics: (1) must last between 4 and 72 hours; (2) have at least two of the following: unilateral location, pulsating quality, moderate/severe pain intensity, or aggravation by physical activity; (3) must have either nausea and/or vomiting or photophobia/phonophobia during headache; and (4) must not meet other criteria.

6. **Why do migraine headaches occur?**
   Cortical spreading depression (CSD) is the currently accepted etiology for migraine with aura. CSD is transient neuronal and glial cell excitation followed by long-lasting depression, slowly propagating across the cerebral cortex and gray matter. During CSD, there are significant changes in the levels of extracellular ions and neurotransmitters (such as glutamate, acetylcholine, and substance P), leading to activation of dural nociceptors and central trigeminovascular neurons in the superficial and deep laminae of the trigeminocervical complex, contributing to the clinical manifestation of migraines.

7. **What is the first-line medical option for abortive therapy for migraine headache?**
   Triptans are the main first-line medical option for abortive therapy for migraines. They are synthetic serotonin analogs that activate the 5-HT1B and 5-HT1D serotonin receptors, constricting cranial blood vessels and inhibiting release of proinflammatory neuropeptides.

8. **Is "sinus headache" recognized as a type of headache?**
   The ICHD-III lists "sinus headache" as an outmoded term for a type of secondary headache. This condition is recognized as headache attributed to disorder of the nose or paranasal sinuses and further attributed to acute rhinosinusitis or chronic or recurring rhinosinusitis.

9. **Is imaging necessary to diagnose someone with headache attributed to disorder of the nose or paranasal sinuses?**
   While imaging can help, it is not mandatory. ICHD-III states that headache attributed to rhinosinusitis must demonstrate clinical, endoscopic, and/or imaging evidence of current or past infection or inflammation. In addition, evidence of headache causation is established by at least two of the following: (1) headache with a temporal relation to rhinosinusitis, (2) headache correlates with rhinosinusitis symptoms, (3) headache is exacerbated by pressure over the sinuses, and (4) headache localizes to the side of rhinosinusitis.

10. **What percentage of patients presenting with complaints of sinus headache will meet International Headache Society (IHS) criteria for migraine headache syndrome?**
    Many patients who have a chief complaint of sinus headache actually fulfill IHS criteria for migraine. One large study screened patients with a history of sinus headache and found that 88% actually fulfilled IHS criteria for migraine-type headache.

11. **Describe the diagnostic criteria and initial management of trigeminal neuralgia.**
    Trigeminal neuralgia is characterized by unilateral paroxysmal attacks of severe facial pain that lasts from a fraction of a second to 2 minutes. The pain is described as electric shock-like, shooting, stabbing, or sharp. Diagnosis is established clinically and must include recurrent paroxysm of unilateral facial pain in one or more divisions of the trigeminal nerve precipitated by innocuous stimuli and not described by another ICHD-III diagnosis. First-line pharmacotherapy is carbamazepine.

12. **What is the most common division of the trigeminal nerve to be affected by trigeminal postherpetic neuralgia?**
    The first division of the trigeminal nerve is most commonly affected in trigeminal postherpetic neuralgia. However, the second and third divisions can also be involved. Typically, the pain is burning and may be pruritic. Patients can also have sensory abnormalities and allodynia in the affected territory. Pale or light purple scars may be present as sequelae of the herpetic eruption. Trigeminal postherpetic neuralgia occurs in approximately 10% of patients with herpes zoster ophthalmicus. Tricyclic antidepressants, gabapentin, pregabalin, opioids, and lidocaine patches are medical options with inconsistent efficacy.

13. **What is persistent idiopathic facial pain?**
    Persistent idiopathic facial pain, formerly referred to as atypical facial pain, is a type of secondary headache. It is a type of facial and/or oral pain that occurs in the absence of clinical neurologic deficit or dental etiology. The pain

is poorly localized; does not follow a nerve distribution; and is qualified as dull, aching, or nagging. Additionally, it must recur daily for more than 2 hours per day over 3 months to meet diagnostic criteria. Treatment includes tricyclic antidepressants and/or other medications used to treat neuropathic pain, such as gabapentin.

14. **Describe contact point headaches.**
Contact point headaches are assumed to be associated with an intranasal contact point, where two structures within the nasal cavity meet (most commonly a large septal spur). The contact point can be identified on clinical exam with endoscopy or radiologically. It is believed that stimulation from the mucosal contact point can result in referred pain via the trigeminal nerve. Therefore, there should be a correlation between the headache and contact point regarding time, symptoms, and location. ICHD-III recognizes contact point headaches as a category of secondary headaches.

15. **Is there evidence that patients with headache and contact points may benefit from surgical intervention?**
Level 4 evidence suggests a potential benefit from surgery in these patients. However, interestingly, the majority of people who have mucosal contact points have no associated facial pain. There is also debate whether the improvement in facial pain following removal of contact points in some patients may be due to cognitive dissonance and/or neuroplasticity. A trial of topical anesthesia to the contact point region can be used as a diagnostic test prior to considering surgical intervention.

16. **What are the three groups of temporomandibular disorders?**
Muscle disorders with myofascial pain; disc displacement with or without reduction; and arthralgia, arthritis, arthrosis.

17. **What is the prevalence of temporomandibular disorders?**
In a meta-analysis of TMD patients, 45.3% patients had Group I disorders (myofascial), 41.1% had Group II disorders (disc displacement), and 30.1% had Group III disorders (arthralgia, arthritis, arthrosis). Some patients may have more than one type. Group I and Group II disorders are more common in the general population, each with a prevalence of approximately 10%.

18. **Describe the criteria for the diagnosis of Temporomandibular Joint (TMJ) pain disorders.**
Criteria for temporomandibular pain: Pain relates directly to jaw movements and mastication, tenderness to palpation of the muscles of mastication and/or over the temporomandibular joint, and confirmation of the presence and location of pain source with relief from anesthetic blocking.
Criteria for temporomandibular dysfunction: Interference with mandibular movement, restriction of mandibular movement, and sudden change in occlusional relationships.
First-line treatment for TMJ disorders typically involves conservative management with analgesics, anti-inflammatory agents, application of local heat, and bite appliances.

19. **What is the CSF pressure level used as a cut-off for diagnosing Idiopathic Intracranial Hypertension (IIH)?**
Twenty-five centimeters H_2O is the common pressure limit used as diagnostic criteria for IIH. However, children can have normal opening pressures of up to 28 centimeters H_2O. This is measured by lumbar puncture performed in the lateral decubitus position, without sedative medications or other medications that have the potential to alter intracranial pressure.

CONTROVERSIES

1. **What causes the neurologic symptoms of migraine headache?**
Recent literature supports that the cortical spreading depression that initiates migraines leads to release of proinflammatory mediators, such as substance P, calcitonin gene-related peptide, and neurokinin A. These inflammatory pathways provide a persistent stimulus that sensitizes trigeminal nerve endings. The parenchymal inflammatory response and trigeminal stimulation leads to pain.

2. **Is there a role for empiric triptan therapy in patients with a diagnosis of sinus headache?**
A high percentage of patients with a self-diagnosis or physician diagnosis of sinus headache may have a migraine-type headache. It has been proposed that empiric migraine therapy (triptans) may be employed in patients with sinus headache, with one study demonstrating improvement in 82% of patients.

3. **Is there a role for interventional therapies in patients with facial pain and headache?**
The role of interventional procedures is still being defined, such as the use of neural blockade in the anterior ethmoid and sphenopalatine region using a steroid and local anesthesia mixture or Botox injections. Radiofrequency ablation of the pterygopalatine ganglion has also been anecdotally described, but the efficacy of these treatment options and their possible complications are still poorly understood.

Bibliography

Bendtsen L, Evers S, Linde M, et al: EFNS guideline on the treatment of tension-type headache - report of an EFNS task force, *Eur J Neurol* 17:1318–1325, 2010.

Ferrari MD, Klever RR, Terwindt GM, et al: Migraine pathophysiology: lessons from mouse models and human genetics, *Lancet Neurol* 14:65–80, 2015.

Gonzalez-Quintanilla V, Pascual J: Other primary headaches: an update, *Neurol Clin* 37:871–891, 2019.

Gronseth G, Cruccu G, Alksne J, et al: Practice parameter: the diagnostic evaluation and treatment of trigeminal neuralgia (an evidence-based review): report of the Quality Standards Subcommittee of the American Academy of Neurology and the European Federation of Neurological Societies, *Neurology* 71:1183–1190, 2008.

Headache Classification Committee of the International Headache Society (IHS): The International Classification of Headache Disorders, *Cephalalgia* 38:1–211, 2018.

Texakalidis P, Tora MS, Boulis NM: Neurosurgeons' armamentarium for the management of refractory postherpetic neuralgia: a systematic literature review, *Stereotact Funct Neurosurg* 97:55–65, 2019.

Wall M, Corbett JJ: Revised diagnostic criteria for the pseudotumor cerebri syndrome in adults and children, *Neurology* 83:198–199, 2014.

CHAPTER 8

TASTE AND SMELL

Laylaa Ramos Arriaza, MD, MS and Vijay R. Ramakrishnan, MD

KEY POINTS

1. Chemosensation (the perception of chemicals) relies on three sensory systems: taste, olfaction, and somatosensory.
2. Chemosensory dysfunction can severely influence quality of life, ranging from safety issues such as detection of a gas leak to higher functions such as emotion and memory.
3. Flavor results from the combination of taste, smell, and somatosensory-mediated sensations of temperature, texture, and pungency.

Pearls
1. There are five described tastes: salty, sour, sweet, bitter, and umami. Fat is being considered as a possible sixth taste.
2. Taste receptor cells assembled into taste buds allow for detection of different tastes. These taste buds are distributed across three types of papillae of the tongue: fungiform, foliate, circumvallate. The fourth type of papillae found on the tongue are filiform; they lack taste buds and therefore do not participate in taste.
3. Anosmia is the absence of olfactory function. Hyposmia describes reduced olfactory function. Dysosmia means changes in odor quality, including parosmia (altered perception of an odor) and phantosmia (perception of an odor when that odor is not present).
4. Common causes of olfactory dysfunction include upper respiratory infection, head trauma, sinonasal disease, medication, chemical exposure, and dementia.

QUESTIONS

1. **What is the purpose of the chemosensory system?**
   We detect chemicals through three different sensory systems: taste, olfaction, and somatosensory. Taste refers to the sensation arising from taste receptors and is used to evaluate the nutritious content of food and avoid ingestion of toxic substances. Smell is the detection of volatile odorants though olfactory and somatosensory systems. Olfaction is the perception of odorants through activation of odorant receptors and is mediated by cranial nerve (CN) I. Smell is also important for social interactions and memory. Trigeminal somatosensory fibers detect thermal, mechanical, and chemical stimuli and initiate protective respiratory reflexes.

2. **What are the consequences of taste or smell dysfunction?**
   Chemosensation is an integral aspect of how we interact with the environment and guides our behavior. Loss of these senses can lead to hazardous situations, such as food poisoning and the inability to detect fire or gas. The disruption of appetitive cues can lead to weight changes and nutritional deficiencies. People without taste often lose the desire to eat and may require medical intervention to restore their appetite.

3. **What is the impact of taste or smell dysfunction on quality of life?**
   Olfactory dysfunction negatively impacts quality of life through eating behaviors, social behaviors, environmental hazard exposures, and mental health. There is a well-established relationship between olfaction, emotion, and memory. The loss of chemosensation impairs the ability to feel motivated and engage in pleasurable activities and is associated with lower perception of quality of life, changes in mood, and depression.

   Social chemical cues play a role in determining our social behavior. Odorants are reported to influence mate selection and cause females to synchronize their menstrual cycle, indicating a biological importance for olfactory cues.

4. **What is the relationship between taste, smell, and flavor?**
   The flavor of our food is the combination of taste, smell, and the somatosensory-mediated sensations of temperature, texture, and pungency. Patients presenting with taste complaints may actually suffer from olfactory dysfunction as a result.

5. **Describe the trigeminal (CN V) contribution to smell.**
   The trigeminal system mediates the perception of touch, pressure, temperature, and nociception (pain or irritation) and displays a limited spectrum of sensations compared to olfaction. The ophthalmic and maxillary branches of the trigeminal nerve innervate the nasal cavity. Most odorants can activate the trigeminal system, and individuals with impaired olfaction (CN I) may still be able to detect odors (often strong irritating odors such as gasoline or ammonia) through trigeminal sensations.

6. **What are the five basic tastes?**
   Salty, sour, sweet, bitter, and umami. Umami is the detection of L-amino acids and is also described as savory. Sweet is indicative of energy-rich foods. The detection of salt allows us to control proper dietary electrolytic balance. Sour and bitter are used to warn against noxious/poisonous compounds. Fatty taste may be considered a new, sixth taste.

7. **Where are taste receptors located?**
   Taste receptors are located on taste receptor cells. *Taste buds* are bundles of taste receptor cells. Taste receptors are also found on specialized chemosensory cells, ciliated cells, and smooth muscle cells in the airway and are thought to mediate the perception of irritants. Taste-sensing of food also occurs within the gastrointestinal tract as taste receptors are expressed by enteroendocrine cells.

8. **Where are taste buds located?**
   Taste buds are located on a large portion of the tongue dorsum within small protrusions of epithelium called *papillae.* Taste buds are also found on the soft palate, larynx, pharynx, and epiglottis, and these taste buds are innervated by the vagus nerve (CN X).

9. **Describe the four types of papillae.**
   The anterior two thirds of the tongue contains *fungiform* papillae. Fungiform papillae contain 1 to 15 taste buds each and are innervated by the chorda tympani branch of the facial nerve (CN VII). There are approximately 750 fungiform papillae.
   The posterior aspects of the tongue contain *circumvallate* and *foliate* papillae and are innervated by the glossopharyngeal nerve (CN IX). Humans have 8 to 12 circumvallate papillae arranged in a V-shape on the dorsal tongue and a few foliate papillae on the lateral sides, each housing dozens of taste buds.
   Filiform papillae are distributed throughout the tongue dorsum. They contribute to the mechanical distribution of chemicals on the tongue and do not contain taste buds.

10. **Describe the central processing of taste.**
    Taste receptor cells transmit taste information to neural fibers within the taste bud, which project from neurons located in the sensory ganglia of cranial nerves VII, IX, and X. The cranial nerves enter the central nervous system at the brainstem and converge to form the solitary tract. Afferent information enters the thalamus and proceeds to the gustatory cortex.

11. **Where is olfactory epithelium found?**
    The olfactory epithelium is located in the superior and posterior aspect of the nasal cavity, including parts of the nasal septum and superior and middle turbinates.

12. **Describe the cellular composition of the olfactory epithelium.**
    The olfactory epithelium is a pseudostratified columnar epithelial tissue comprised of several cell types. *Bipolar sensory neurons* extend an apical dendrite to the epithelial surface from which cilia extend to detect odors. The basal pole extends into an axon, which crosses the cribriform plate and enters the olfactory bulb. The axons of the sensory neurons are ensheathed by *olfactory ensheathing cells*, which have received clinical interest for their ability to support axon growth. *Basal cells* produce new olfactory sensory neurons as the old neurons die or are damaged. Supporting or *sustentacular* cells regulate and maintain the mucus layer into which odorants dissolve. Flask-shaped *microvillar* cells have an unclear function but can respond to odorants and may play a role in reception.

13. **Where are olfactory receptors located?**
    We are able to distinguish over 1000 odorants through a large multigene family of receptors that detect specific chemical structures within odorant molecules. Olfactory receptors are located on the cilia of bipolar sensory neurons within the olfactory epithelium. Each sensory neuron expresses only one type of receptor.

14. **Describe the processing of olfactory stimuli.**
    Odorant molecules that enter the nasal cavity and diffuse through the mucus layer bind to specific odorant receptors depending on their chemical structure. Odor-evoked responses are conducted through the sensory neuron axons, which converge with axons expressing the same receptor type into circular structures called *glomeruli* in the olfactory bulb. Information about the odorant is encoded by the pattern of sensory neurons and the glomeruli

they activate, forming a chemotopic map. Second-order neurons (mitral and tufted cells) transmit the response through the olfactory tract to regions in the frontal lobe and dorsomedial temporal lobe. There is a structural overlap of olfactory-responsive regions and those related to emotion, memory, and motivation. These regions include the amygdala, entorhinal cortex, orbital cortex, striatum, hypothalamus, and hippocampus. The structural overlap is thought to contribute to the salience of olfactory memories and emotional responses.

15. What are the terms used to describe olfactory dysfunction?

Olfactory dysfunction is divided into quantitative and qualitative disorders. Quantitative dysfunction is the reduced ability to sense an odor without distorting its quality; hyposmia and functional anosmia are subtypes. *Dysosmias,* or qualitative dysfunction, include *parosmia* (altered perception of an odor) and *phantosmia* (perception of an odor when that odor is not present). *Anosmia* is the absence of olfactory function. *Hyposmia* describes reduced olfactory function. *Hyperosmia* is enhanced perception of smell.

16. What are the terms used to describe taste dysfunction?

Ageusia is the absence of the ability to taste. *Hypogeusia* describes reduced taste perception. *Dysgeusias* are changes in taste quality, including *parageusia* (altered perception of tastant) and *phantogeusia* (taste detection in the absence of stimulus).

17. How are sensory dysfunctions classified?

Disruption of the transmission of sensory information can occur at multiple levels from the peripheral elements to areas within the central nervous system.

- Transport or *conductive losses* refer to conditions that interfere with access to receptor cells. Transport losses in taste can result from infections, oral inflammation, and dry mouth (xerostomia). Transport losses in olfaction can result from mucosal inflammation, structural obstructions, and alterations in nasal mucus.
- *Sensory losses* refer to conditions that disrupt receptor cell function, including the loss of receptor cells due to injury. Olfactory neuron disruption can occur from head injury, sinonasal disease, respiratory tract infections, and chemical exposure. Taste receptor cell loss may be caused by medications, radiation therapy, infection, and endocrine disorders.
- *Neural losses* refer to disruptions in the transmission of information upstream of receptor cells. For olfaction this includes injury to the olfactory bulb and cortex. Neural losses in taste can occur following damage to the chorda tympani, facial, vagus, and glossopharyngeal nerves as well as with brain injury.

18. What are the major causes of taste disorders?

Respiratory infections, head trauma, middle ear surgery, radiation therapy, medication side effects, chemical exposure, endocrine disorders, and poor oral hygiene. Isolated taste dysfunction is very rare, with a prevalence of 0.001% of the population.

19. What are the major causes of olfactory disorders?

Olfactory dysfunction affects up to 20% of the general adult population; two thirds of cases are due to sinonasal disease, infection, and trauma. The prevalence of olfactory dysfunction increases with age, with estimates of 24% to 40% in individuals over 50 years of age. Other causes include normal aging, medication, environmental and chemical exposure, endocrine dysfunction, neurologic disorders, depression.

20. What are key questions to ask during evaluation of the patient with a taste or smell problem?

Inquire about any prior history of dysfunction, including possible precipitating events such as upper respiratory infections, nasal obstruction, sinonasal disease, head trauma, or prior ear surgery. Ask if the onset was gradual of sudden or if it fluctuates. Determine whether the loss is complete or partial and if there are any distortions/hallucinations in taste or olfaction. Inquire about cognition, medication use, appetite, and changes in weight. Medical history and social history, including occupation, should be included.

21. What should you look for on physical examination of a patient with a taste or smell problem?

Examination of the oral cavity should include focusing on the tongue, teeth, gums, lips, and hard and soft palate. The nasal examination should assess for septal deviation, turbinate enlargement, allergic appearance of mucosa, or presence of nasal polyps or purulence. Mucus character and signs of epithelial irritation or inflammation should be assessed in the nasal cavity and oral cavity. Ear examination should assess the middle ear space to rule out disease affecting the chorda tympani.

22. How do you proceed with the workup for taste and/or smell dysfunction?

Formal testing may include threshold and odorant identification tests for olfactory and/or taste loss. MRI may be indicated to rule out central processes and can demonstrate presence of sinus inflammation. If indicated, additional workup may include biopsy, screening for autoimmune conditions, IgE levels, and salivary flow.

23. **How do you assess olfactory function?**

Patients often do not accurately report deficits in olfaction; therefore, it is important to obtain an objective measurement of olfactory function. Validated subjective and psychophysical olfactory assessments along with imaging and electrophysiology may be used for olfactory testing. The two most frequently used standardized tests are the Smell Identification Test (SIT), an odor identification "scratch and sniff" test, and Sniffin' Sticks, an odor identification, discrimination, and threshold assessment using odor-dispensing pens. Odor identification and discrimination tasks are generally thought to assess peripheral and central processing, whereas threshold testing reflects mainly peripheral processing. Direct measures of odor-evoked responses are not often used, but the ability of sensory neurons to respond can be measured using electroolfactograms (EOGs) and cortical responses can be assessed using electroencephalograms (EEGs) or functional imaging.

24. **Will steroid administration help sense of smell?**

Steroid administration is frequently used to reduce inflammation and clear obstruction of the olfactory cleft. Rapid improvement of olfactory function is often observed; however, this is usually transient and permanent restoration of normal function is unlikely. Systemic administration is more effective than topical application, but extended administration of systemic steroids puts the patient at risk of side effects.

25. **Will surgery help sense of smell?**

If the deficit is due to obstruction of the olfactory cleft, then restoring airflow with surgery will aid in recovery of olfactory function. Sinus surgery to decrease infection and/or inflammation often provides some degree of benefit, particularly in patients with nasal polyps. While improvement of olfactory function is possible, it may be transient and/or incomplete.

26. **Will olfactory training therapy help sense of smell?**

Patients with olfactory loss who expose themselves to four intense odors twice a day for 12 weeks demonstrate improvement from olfactory training. Patients scores of Sniffin' Sticks increase as well as their thresholds for the four odors compared to baseline. Given the high prevalence of this disorder, it is a high priority research area that will hopefully yield understanding of the pathophysiology and identify novel treatments.

BIBLIOGRAPHY

Chandrashekar J, Hoon MA, Ryba NJP, et al: The receptors and cells for mammalian taste, *Nature* 444:288–294, 2006.
Doty R: The olfactory system and its disorders, *Semin Neurol* 29:74–81, 2009.
Hummel T, Rissom K, Reden J, et al: Effects of Olfactory Training in Patients with Olfactory Loss, *Laryngoscope* 119:3, 2009.
Hummel T, Whitcroft KL, Andrews P, et al: Position paper on olfactory dysfunction, *Rhinol Suppl* 54:1–30, 2017.
Kinnamon SC: Taste receptor signaling-from tongues to lungs, *Acta Physiol* 204:158–168, 2011.
London B, Nabet B, Fisher AR, et al: Predictors of prognosis in patients with olfactory disturbance, *Ann Neurol* 63:159–166, 2008.
Whitcroft KL, Hummel T: Clinical diagnosis and current management strategies for olfactory dysfunction: a review, *JAMA Otolaryngol Head Neck Surg* 145(9):846–853.
Yang J, Pinto JM: The epidemiology of olfactory disorders, *Curr Otorhinolaryngol Rep* 4(2):130–141, 2016.

CHAPTER 9

PHARYNGITIS AND LARYNGITIS

Steven Hamilton, MD

KEY POINTS

1. Infections are the most common cause of pharyngitis. Viral infections are more common than bacterial, with 50% to 60% of cases caused by common viruses.
2. The AAO-HNS Clinical Practice Guideline for Tonsillectomy in Children from 2018 strongly recommends watchful waiting for recurrent throat infections if there have been <7 episodes in the past year, <5 episodes per year in the past 2 years, or <3 episodes per year in the past 3 years.
3. Group A streptococcal pharyngitis should be treated with antibiotics to prevent potential complications of rheumatic fever. Treatment should be initiated within 10 days of symptoms.
4. Any patient with chronic laryngitis for over 2 weeks, those with worrisome symptoms, or those with a high risk history of cancer should be evaluated by an otolaryngologist to rule out the presence of other causes of symptoms, including malignancy.

Pearls

1. Pediatric autoimmune neuropsychiatric disorder associated with streptococcal infection (PANDAS) is a self-limited condition associated with increased tics and obsessive mannerisms that correlate with elevated ASO titers.
2. Periodic fever, aphthous stomatitis, pharyngitis, and cervical adenitis (PFAPA) is a condition characterized by high fever that lasts 3 to 7 days and recurs every 3 to 6 weeks. The cause of PFAPA is unknown but it is thought to be either immune related or infectious.
3. The majority of patients who receive amoxicillin to treat infectious mononucleosis will develop a diffuse rash due to hypersensitivity. This is often confused with penicillin allergy.

QUESTIONS

1. **What is pharyngitis?**
   Pharyngitis, simply stated, is inflammation of the pharyngeal mucosa and submucosa. Classically, a clinical diagnosis of pharyngitis includes inflammation of the tonsils. This is often referred to as pharyngotonsillitis.

2. **What is laryngitis?**
   Laryngitis is acute or chronic inflammation of the laryngeal mucosa.

3. **Why are these conditions important?**
   "Sore throat" is one of the most common chief complaints seen in the primary care setting. Acute or chronic inflammation of the pharynx, tonsils, and/or larynx leads to difficulty in phonation, swallowing, and breathing. This inflammation is often associated with significant discomfort, and certain conditions can lead to acute upper airway compromise. Pharyngitis and tonsillitis account for over 14 million visits per year to clinics, urgent care centers, and emergency departments. The economic burden of these conditions in the United States has been estimated to be over $1.2 billion. Half of this cost could be saved by adherence to current clinical guidelines and avoidance of overprescribing antibiotics.

4. **What is the most common cause of pharyngitis?**
   Infections are the most common cause of pharyngitis. Viral infections are more common than bacterial infections, with 50% to 60% of cases caused by common viruses. Viral causes include rhinovirus, coronavirus, adenovirus (associated with conjunctivitis), herpes simplex virus, Epstein-Barr virus (EBV), coxsackievirus, HIV, and cytomegalovirus. Typically, viral infections have a less severe course with lower fever and symptoms of an upper respiratory infection (cough, runny nose, and sneezing). The majority of bacterial cases are caused by group A streptococcus (10% of all adult cases of pharyngitis and 30% of cases in children). Other bacterial causes include syphilis, pertussis, gonorrhea, diphtheria, and *Fusobacterium*. Fungal pharyngitis, typically caused by *Candida albicans*, is uncommon, except in select populations such as immunocompetent infants and the immunocomprised.

Other causes of pharyngitis include postnasal drip, irritants (smoking, dust, dry heat, chemicals), laryngo-pharyngeal reflux, chronic mouth breathing, voice abuse, granulomatous diseases, chronic allergies, and connective tissue disorders. Malignancy should be a part of the differential diagnosis of atypical presentations or courses of pharyngitis.

5. **How does one diagnose group A streptococcal (GAS) pharyngitis? What is the treatment of this infection?**
The symptoms of GAS pharyngitis include high fever, headache, palatal/tonsillar petechiae, exudative tonsillitis, and tender cervical lymphadenopathy. Cough and rhinorrhea are not usually observed. However, clinical features alone do not readily distinguish between GAS pharyngitis and viral pharyngitis. Swabbing the throat to test for GAS pharyngitis with a rapid antigen detection test (RADT) and/or culture should be performed for diagnosis. A negative RADT should be followed with a culture in children, given that the sensitivity of the test can be as low as 70%. It is over 95% specific; thus a positive test should not be followed by a culture. It is not recommended that a negative test in adults be followed routinely by a culture due to the low incidence of GAS pharyngitis in adults and the low risk of developing rheumatic fever. Children under the age of 3 years are routinely not tested unless they have an older sibling with GAS pharyngitis because the risk of GAS infection and rheumatic fever is very low in this population.

GAS pharyngitis should be treated with antibiotics to prevent the potential complications of rheumatic fever. Treatment should be initiated within 10 days of symptom onset. Other benefits of treatment include a shorter duration of symptoms and cessation of contagious status after 24 hours of treatment.

Oral penicillin or amoxicillin for 10 days is the recommended treatment for GAS pharyngitis. Alternatively, a single dose of intramuscular benzathine penicillin G may be administered. For patients with a penicillin allergy, treatment with an oral cephalosporin, a macrolide, or clindamycin is indicated. The treatment duration should be 10 days, unless azithromycin is used. The treatment course for azithromycin is only 5 days.

6. **What are the potential serious complications of group A streptococcal pharyngitis?**
   a. Acute rheumatic fever occurs when antibodies produced during a GAS infection react with myocardial tissue and other areas of the body. This can lead to carditis, polyarthritis, chorea, and serpiginous rash. Permanent damage to the heart valves (primarily the mitral valve) can result from rheumatic fever. This usually occurs 10 to 20 years after an episode of acute rheumatic fever, although some children may exhibit symptoms while still acutely ill with GAS pharyngitis. Rheumatic fever is the major cause of GAS pharyngitis infections that are treated with antibiotics.
   b. Poststreptococcal glomerulonephritis (PSGN): An acute nephritic syndrome that occurs 1 to 2 weeks after infection. This is caused by the antigen-antibody deposits in the glomeruli. Up to 50% of cases are subclinical, with only microscopic hematuria. Symptoms can be much worse with gross hematuria (relatively painless), low complement (C3) levels; edema of the extremities; and hypertension. Treatment is usually supportive, and antibiotics have not been proven to be preventative or curative of PSGN.
   c. Scarlet fever – A secondary condition caused by side effects of the exotoxin produced by a GAS pharyngeal infection. Signs and symptoms include skin erythema that usually initiates in the trunk, strawberry tongue, desquamation of the perioral skin, cervical lymphadenopathy, and fever. The patient is treated with antibiotics.
   d. Pediatric autoimmune neuropsychiatric disorder associated with streptococcal infection (PANDAS) is a self-limiting condition associated with increased tics and obsessive mannerisms that correlate with elevated ASO titers. Patients usually have a previous diagnosis of obsessive-compulsive disorder. This diagnosis is controversial and there is no definitive consensus that treatment with tonsillectomy or antibiotics is curative.
   e. Suppurative complications such as peritonsillar or retropharyngeal abscesses may occur following GAS pharyngitis or other causes of pharyngitis. These complications may require surgical incision and drainage.
   f. Necrotizing fasciitis is rarely seen with GAS pharyngitis but can be a life-threatening complication requiring repeated surgical debridement.
   g. Recent dermatology studies have proposed a link between guttate psoriasis and GAS infections. Anecdotal evidence of improvement in psoriasis symptoms with tonsillectomy has been reported.

7. **What are the indications for tonsillectomy as a treatment for recurrent throat infections? What are some of the potential modifying factors to consider when recommending tonsillectomy for recurrent throat infections?**
The AAO-HNS Clinical Practice Guideline for Tonsillectomy in Children from 2018 strongly recommends watchful waiting for recurrent throat infections if there have been <7 episodes in the past year, <5 episodes per year in the past 2 years, or <3 episodes per year in the past 3 years. The guidelines suggest that clinicians may recommend tonsillectomy for patients with recurrent throat infections if they exceed the number of infections listed above.

Modifying factors to the above criteria, which may favor tonsillectomy, include but are not limited to multiple antibiotic allergies/intolerance, PFAPA, or a history of >1 peritonsillar abscess.

8. **What is PFAPA?**
   Periodic **fever**, **aphthous** stomatitis, **pharyngitis**, and cervical **adenitis** (**PFAPA**) is a condition characterized by high fever that lasts 3 to 7 days and recurs every 3 to 6 weeks. Patients always have a fever and will have between one and three of the other symptoms. The cause of PFAPA is unknown but it is thought to be either immune related or infectious. Treatment of fevers with acetaminophen, ibuprofen, or prednisone can be effective, and tonsillectomy has been shown to reduce symptoms or be curative.

9. **What causes mononucleosis and how is it diagnosed?**
   Infectious mononucleosis is a viral pharyngitis caused primarily by the Epstein-Barr virus (EBV) in up to 90% of cases. Cytomegalovirus and other viruses may also be responsible. This disease is spread by oral contact and is commonly known as the "kissing disease." It most often affects children and young adults.

   Infectious mononucleosis typically presents with high fever, malaise, gray/white tonsils that are hypertrophic, odynophagia, dysphagia, hepatosplenomegaly, and posterior cervical chain lymphadenopathy.

   A complete blood count (CBC) with differential, erythrocyte sedimentation rate (ESR), LFTs, heterophile antibody test (monospot), and EBV antibody titers may all assist in diagnosis. Elevated lymphocytes and monocytes are seen on differential CBC. LFT and ESR are likely to be elevated in mononucleosis and not in GAS pharyngitis. The Monospot test is 85% sensitive and nearly 100% specific. During the first 2 weeks of infection, only 60% of the cases have positive tests. This increases to nearly all cases by the sixth week of infection. In a suspected case with an early negative test, the patient may be tested weekly following a negative test. Alternatively, EBV serologies may be checked to confirm a diagnosis and should be checked in children under the age of 5 years, as the Monospot test is often negative in young children with mononucleosis.

10. **How is mononucleosis treated and what special considerations should be taken with this disease?**
    Supportive care is the primary treatment for infectious mononucleosis. IV fluids and bed rest are indicated. Patients should avoid contact sports until they are cleared of hepatosplenomegaly by ultrasound due to an increased risk of splenic rupture in these patients. Upper airway obstruction can occur and may necessitate treatment with steroids, nasopharyngeal airway, intubation, or even tracheotomy in the most severe cases. Antibiotics should only be used if there is an additional secondary bacterial infection. The majority of patients who receive amoxicillin will develop a diffuse rash due to hypersensitivity. This is often confused with penicillin allergy.

11. **What is the concern with prescribing antibiotics for viral pharyngitis?**
    Inappropriate prescription of antibiotics for viral pharyngitis is ineffective, may lead to unwanted side effects or reactions, and can increase antibiotic resistance. It has been estimated that nearly 50% of antibiotic prescriptions for pharyngitis are associated with viral infections. This equates to nearly $3 billion unnecessarily prescribed medications. In addition, prescribing broad-spectrum antibiotics (macrolides and fluoroquinolones) has increased nearly four-fold since the early 2000s.

12. **What is Lemierre's syndrome and what bacteria is responsible for this syndrome?**
    Lemierre's syndrome is a rare but potentially fatal complication of bacterial pharyngitis caused by *Fusobacterium necrophorum* (anaerobic gram-negative rod). CT findings in this disease show internal jugular vein thrombophlebitis with a filling defect. Symptoms include pharyngitis that progresses to spiking "picket fence" fevers with malaise, unilateral neck swelling/tenderness, trismus, and potentially septic emboli to liver, lungs, and joints. Initial treatment is IV antibiotics with beta-lactamase-resistant coverage. The effectiveness of anticoagulation therapy is controversial, but it is often prescribed. Abscess drainage, surgical debridement, and excision of the affected jugular vein have been described. Recent studies have shown that *F. necrophorum* causes up to 10% of endemic bacterial pharyngitis infections in young adults. It is also the most common bacteria isolated from peritonsillar abscesses in this population.

13. **What is diphtheria and why is it not commonly seen in the United States?**
    Diphtheria is an uncommon cause of bacterial pharyngitis in the United States due to the high prevalence of those vaccinated against this disease. There are approximately 200 to 300 cases reported annually in the United States. The disease typically affects unvaccinated children aged >6 years. It is caused by *Corynebacterium diphtheriae* and can be treated with diphtheria antitoxin, penicillin, or erythromycin. Characteristic green-gray plaques or exudates are seen on the tonsils, pharynx, and larynx. An airway compromise can be observed. The breath of patients with this infection has been described as smelling like acetone. Nephritis and neurologic infections are two potential systemic complications.

14. **What is the difference between acute and chronic laryngitis?**
    Laryngitis is often diagnosed clinically by the presence of a hoarse voice, dysphonia, and odynophagia. The presence of symptoms for >2 weeks is typically defined as chronic laryngitis.

15. **What is the common cause of acute laryngitis and how is it treated?**
    Up to 60% of cases of acute laryngitis in adults are caused by viruses that cause the common cold, with *rhinovirus* being the most common. Antibiotics are not typically indicated for episodes of acute laryngitis unless a bacterial cause is identified by culture. Obtaining a culture is not commonly advised unless the symptoms are atypical. Imaging is not indicated unless there is a concern for airway compromise. Laryngoscopy is often not performed for acute laryngitis. Treatment consists of voice rest, use of an air humidifier, hydration, over-the-counter antipyretics/analgesics, and avoidance of decongestants due to their drying effects. Most hospitals now have rapid viral PCR testing, which can be beneficial for diagnosis.

16. **What are some more rare causes of acute laryngitis?**
    History and physical examination can help define the cause of acute laryngitis and direct further workup if necessary. A history of exposure to chemicals or smoke warrants evaluation for inhalational injuries. Unattended young children may need further evaluation for an aerodigestive foreign body or caustic ingestion. High fever, airway compromise, or other abnormal symptoms can indicate a more serious infection. Some common serious infections are listed below:
    a. Laryngotracheobronchitis (croup): Symptoms of croup usually consist of onset of stridor and barky cough that worsens with agitation or overnight after a normal URI prodrome. Croup typically affects patients aged 6 months to 3 years. Over 95% of patients can be managed as outpatients with supportive care and steroids. Patients rarely require hospitalization for oxygen support, high-flow nasal cannula, heliox, or other more invasive ventilatory measures. *Parainfluenza* is the most common cause of infection. The classic "steeple sign" can be seen on an A/P neck x-ray.
    b. Supraglottitis/epiglottitis: This constitutes an airway emergency. Patients typically present with a rapid onset of high fever, dysphagia, drooling, dysphonia, stridor, and toxic appearance. Classically, this is seen in children and is caused by *H. influenzae* type B. Immunizations have decreased this incidence. An increase in polymicrobial infections (most commonly *Staphylococcus* or *Streptococcus*) that affect teenagers or adults has been observed. Lateral neck x-rays often show the "thumb" sign, indicating a swollen epiglottis. Antibiotics are administered and intubation in the operating room or an urgent surgically established airway may be necessary.
    c. Bacterial tracheitis: This condition usually occurs in children with symptoms of croup who show a rapid decline. Methicillin-sensitive *Staphylococcus aureus* is the most common cause of bacterial infections. Pain with palpation of the thyroid cartilage, loss of voice, high fever, and acute decline in respiratory status may indicate bacterial tracheitis. The presence of thick, purulent secretions or pseudomembranes in the subglottis and trachea on rigid endoscopy is diagnostic. Aggressive management of the airway with debridement and intubation is often required. IV antibiotics with vancomycin or oxacillin plus a third-generation cephalosporin are administered empirically until culture-guided therapy can be initiated.

17. **What are the more common causes of chronic laryngitis and how are they treated?**
    Chronic laryngitis is more commonly caused by environmental factors, such as smoking, inhalational exposure, or laryngopharyngeal reflux. In-office laryngoscopy can be used to diagnose fungal laryngitis in immunocompromised patients or those on chronic inhaled steroids. This is most often caused by *Candida* species and is treated with nystatin. Cultures are usually not taken because of the difficulty of obtaining a sample in the office.

18. **What evaluation should be performed in all patients with laryngitis symptoms that persist past 2 weeks?**
    Any patient with chronic laryngitis for over 2 weeks, those with worrisome symptoms, or those with a high risk history of cancer should be evaluated by an otolaryngologist to rule out the presence of other causes of symptoms, including malignancy.

CONTROVERSIES

PANDAS, or its broader iteration, pediatric acute-onset neuropsychiatric syndrome (PANS), as a diagnosis is controversial because its origin, natural history, treatment, and prognosis have not been clearly defined. Definitive proof of an autoimmune marker is lacking, and treatment in terms of medications and surgeries has yielded mixed results. Response rates to psychiatric intervention appear similar to those of non-PANDAS/PANS-associated obsessive-compulsive disorder (OCD). However, cohort studies have shown an association between infection and the emergence of psychiatric symptoms. More work is needed to better understand the disease process and its possible implications.

BIBLIOGRAPHY

Allen CT, Nussenbaum B, Merati AL: Acute and chronic laryngopharyngitis. In: Flint P, et al: eds: *Cummings Otolaryngology: Head and Neck Surgery*, 7th ed, Philadelphia, 2021, Mosby, pp. 897–905.
Carpenter PS, Kendall KA: MRSA chronic bacterial laryngitis: a growing problem, *Laryngoscope* 128:921–925, 2018.
Centor RM, Atkinson TP, Ratliff AE, et al: The clinical presentation of fusobacterium-positive and streptococcal-positive pharyngitis in a university health clinic, *Ann Intern Med* 162:241–247, 2015.

Harris AM, Hicks LA, Qaseem A: Appropriate antibiotic use for acute respiratory tract infection in adults: advice for high-value care from the American College of Physicians and Centers of Disease Control and Prevention, *Ann Intern Med* 164:425–434, 2016.

Hayward GN, Hay AD, Moore MV, et al: Effect of oral dexamethasone without immediate antibiotics vs placebo on acute sore throat in adults, *JAMA* 317(15):1535–1543, 2017.

Li RM, Kiemeney M: Infections of the neck, *Emerg Med Clin North Am* 37:95–107, 2019.

Mitchell RB, Archer SM, Ishman SL, et al: Clinical practice guideline: tonsillectomy in children (update), *Otolaryngol Head Neck Surg* 160(Suppl):S1–S42, 2019.

Shulman ST, Bisno AL, Clegg AW, et al: Clinical practice guideline for the diagnosis and management of group A streptococcal pharyngitis: 2012 update by the Infectious Diseases Society of America, *Clin Infect Dis* 55(10):1279–1282, 2012.

Wilbur C, Bitnun A, Kronenberg S, et al: PANDAS/PANS in childhood: controversies and evidence, *Paediatr Child Health* 24(2):85–91, 2019.

HEAD AND NECK ANATOMY AND EMBRYOLOGY WITH RADIOLOGY CORRELATES

John Richards, MD, Farshad Chowdhury, MD, Carissa M. Thomas, MD, PhD, FACS and Fiyin Sokoya, MD

CHAPTER 10

KEY POINTS

1. The six branchial arches form the skeletal and muscular derivatives of the head and neck and the six pharyngeal pouches form the endothelium and glands. Each arch is associated with a nerve and artery.
2. Aberrant embryologic development can cause first, second, third, and fourth branchial cleft anomalies. Branchial cleft anomalies have associated sinus tracts, which pass deep to their associated aortic arch derivatives.
3. Cervical lymphadenectomy (neck dissection) is based on lymphatic drainage patterns to regional lymph nodes delineated by sublevels of the neck.
4. The upper aerodigestive tract is divided into the nasal cavity, oral cavity, nasopharynx, oropharynx, hypopharynx, and larynx.
5. Deep neck space infections can travel through the neck and into adjacent regions via the retropharyngeal, danger, and prevertebral spaces.

Pearls
1. The second branchial cleft is the most common branchial cleft to develop an anomaly.
2. The soft palate divides the nasopharynx from the oropharynx, and the hyoid bone separates the oropharynx from the hypopharynx.
3. The parapharyngeal space has two compartments: pre-styloid and post-styloid, with different contents.
4. The retropharyngeal space extends from the skull base to the mediastinum, the danger space extends from the skull base to the diaphragm, and the prevertebral space extends from the clivus to the coccyx.
5. The lymphatics in the neck are subdivided into seven different levels with boundaries formed by anatomic landmarks.

QUESTIONS

1. **What are the skeletal derivatives of the six branchial arches?**
   See Table 10.1. The first and second arches have cartilaginous precursors: Meckel's and Reichert's, respectively.

2. **What are the muscular derivatives of the six branchial arches?**
   See Table 10.1.

3. **What do the six pharyngeal pouches form?**
   See Table 10.2. The pharyngeal pouches are composed of endoderm and form glandular structures.

4. **What cranial nerve innervates the derivatives of each branchial arch?**
   See Table 10.1. The cranial nerve associated with each branchial arch innervates the muscles formed by the same branchial arch.

5. **List the aortic arch artery associated with each branchial arch.**
   See Table 10.1.

Table 10.1

BRANCHIAL ARCH	SKELETAL DERIVATIVES	MUSCLE DERIVATIVES	CRANIAL NERVES (CN)	AORTIC ARCH ARTERY
First	Meckel's cartilage: Proximal – Body and ramus of the mandible, sphenomandibular ligament, anterior malleolar ligament, malleus (except for the manubrium), and incus (except for the long process). Distal – Withers; the body of the mandible is formed from intramembranous growth. Maxillary process forms the premaxilla, maxilla, zygoma and part of the temporal bone.	Muscles of mastication: temporalis, masseter, and medial and lateral pterygoid muscles. Tensor tympani, tensor veli palatini, anterior belly of the digastric, and mylohyoid muscles.	Trigeminal nerve (CN V)	Maxillary artery
Second	Reichert's cartilage: Proximal – Styloid process, manubrium of the malleus, long process of the incus, and stapes superstructure. Central – Withers and forms a band, the stylohyoid ligament. Distal – Superior body and lesser cornu of the hyoid bone.	Muscles of facial expression and posterior belly of the digastric, stylohyoid, and stapedius muscles.	Facial nerve (CN VII)	Stapedial artery (degenerates)
Third	Inferior body and greater cornu of the hyoid bone	Stylopharyngeus muscle	Glossopharyngeal nerve (CN IX)	Common and internal carotid arteries
Fourth	Thyroid, cricoid, arytenoid, corniculate, and cuneiform laryngeal cartilages	Pharyngeal muscles (superior, middle, and inferior constrictor muscles), striated muscle of the upper half of the esophagus, and extrinsic and intrinsic muscles of the larynx.	Vagus nerve (CN X)	Aorta (left); proximal subclavian artery (right)
Sixth	Thyroid, cricoid, arytenoid, corniculate, and cuneiform laryngeal cartilages	Pharyngeal muscles (superior, middle, and inferior constrictor muscles), striated muscle of the upper half of the esophagus, and extrinsic and intrinsic muscles of the larynx.	Vagus nerve (CN X)	Ductus arteriosus and pulmonary artery (left); pulmonary artery (right)

Table 10.2	
PHARYNGEAL POUCH	**POUCH DERIVATIVES**
First	Inner layer of the tympanic membrane, middle ear mucosa, and eustachian tube
Second	Epithelial lining of the palatine tonsil
Third	Superior forms the inferior parathyroid glands and inferior forms the thymus
Fourth	Superior parathyroid glands
Fifth, sixth	Parafollicular (C) cells

6. Describe the potential tracts of the branchial cleft sinuses.

   Sinus tracts typically have a pattern of passing deep to the associated aortic arch derivatives. It is important to attempt surgical excision of both the sinus tract along as well as the branchial cleft cyst to prevent recurrence.

   First branchial cleft anomalies are duplications of the membranous part of the external auditory canal and are divided into two types. Type I is of ectodermal origin and is a duplication anomaly of the external auditory canal located antero-inferior to the lobule. Type II is of ectodermal and mesodermal origin, duplicates the cartilage in addition to the external auditory canal, and presents below the angle of the mandible. First branchial cleft tracts may pass medial or lateral to the main trunk of the facial nerve or between branches.

   Second branchial cleft anomalies present below the angle of the mandible, at the anterior border of the sternocleidomastoid muscle (SCM). The tract passes deep to the external carotid artery, stylohyoid, and digastric muscle and superficial to the internal carotid artery, opening in the tonsillar fossa.

   Third branchial cleft anomalies present anterior to the SCM and lower in the neck than second branchial cleft anomalies. The tract passes deep to the glossopharyngeal nerve and the internal carotid artery and superficial to the vagus nerve, opening in the pharynx at the thyrohyoid membrane or piriform sinus.

   Fourth branchial cleft anomalies are predominantly left-sided, presenting as thyroid masses or paratracheal masses in the lateral neck. The tract of this sinus passes deep to the superior laryngeal nerve and superficial to the recurrent laryngeal nerve opening into the hypopharynx.

7. What is the most common branchial cleft anomaly?

   Second branchial cleft anomalies are the most common (approximately 95% of all anomalies). First branchial cleft anomalies are the second most common. Third and fourth branchial cleft anomalies are rare.

8. What are the boundaries and subsites of the oral cavity?
   - Anterior: Vermillion border of the lip
   - Superior: Hard–soft palate junction
   - Lateral: Tonsillar pillars
   - Posterior/inferior: Circumvallate papillae of the tongue
   - Subsites: Lip, oral tongue (anterior two-thirds), buccal mucosa, floor of mouth, hard palate, upper and lower gingiva (alveolar ridges), and retromolar trigone

9. What are the boundaries of the nasopharynx (Figure 10.1)?
   - Anterior: Posterior nasal cavity
   - Superior: Sphenoid sinus
   - Posterior: First and second vertebrae
   - Inferior: Soft palate
   - Lateral: Eustachian tube, torus tubarius, and the fossa of Rosenmüller

10. What are the boundaries and subsites of the oropharynx (Figure 10.1)?
    - Anterior: Oral cavity
    - Superior: Soft palate
    - Posterior: Posterior pharyngeal wall
    - Inferior: Hyoid
    - Subsites: Base of tongue (posterior third), palatine tonsil/lateral pharyngeal wall, soft palate, and posterior pharyngeal wall

11. What are the boundaries and subsites of the hypopharynx (Figure 10.1)?
    - Anterior: Larynx
    - Superior: Hyoid bone and pharyngoepiglottic folds
    - Posterior: Retropharyngeal space
    - Inferior: Esophageal introitus at the cricopharyngeus muscle
    - Subsites: Piriform sinuses, postcricoid area, and posterior pharyngeal wall

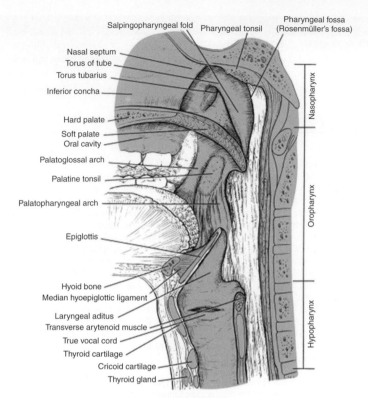

Fig. 10.1 Anatomic subsites and structures of the upper aerodigestive tract.

12. Describe the orientation of the piriform sinuses of the hypopharynx.
    The piriform sinuses are an inverted pyramid with the base at the level of the pharyngoepiglottic fold and the apex extending to just below the cricoid cartilage.

13. Describe the different layers of the deep cervical fascia.
    Deep fascia is divided into three layers: the superficial (investing), middle (pre-tracheal or visceral), and deep layers (prevertebral). The superficial layer is underneath the platysma and invests the superficial neck structures. The middle layer encloses the visceral structures including the trachea and esophagus. The deep layer surrounds the deep muscles of the neck and cervical vertebrae.

14. What layers of deep cervical fascia make up the carotid sheath and what does it contain?
    The carotid sheath is composed of all three layers of deep cervical fascia. The contents of the carotid sheath include the carotid artery, internal jugular vein, vagus nerve, and the sympathetic chain.

15. Where are the retropharyngeal space, danger space, and prevertebral space?
    - Retropharyngeal Space Boundaries
      - Superior: Skull base
      - Inferior: Mediastinum at the tracheal bifurcation
      - Anterior: Buccopharyngeal fascia lining the posterior pharynx and esophagus
      - Posterior: Alar fascia over the danger space
      - Lateral: Carotid sheath
    - Danger Space Boundaries
      - Superior: Skull base
      - Inferior: Diaphragm
      - Anterior: Alar fascia and retropharyngeal space
      - Posterior: Prevertebral fascia and prevertebral space
      - Lateral: Transverse process of the vertebrae

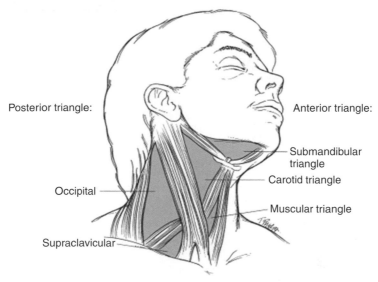

Posterior triangle:

Anterior triangle:

Submandibular triangle

Carotid triangle

Occipital

Muscular triangle

Supraclavicular

Fig. 10.2 Boundaries of the triangles of the neck.

- Prevertebral Space Boundaries
  - Superior: Clivus of the skull base
  - Inferior: Coccyx
  - Anterior: Prevertebral fascia and danger space
  - Posterior: Vertebral bodies
  - Lateral: Transverse process of the vertebrae

16. **Describe the lymphatics of the retropharyngeal space.**
    There are two groups of retropharyngeal lymph nodes (RPLNs): lateral and medial. The lateral RPLNs are also known as Rouvière nodes and are subdivided into the lateral nasopharyngeal and lateral oropharyngeal lymph nodes.

17. **Describe the cervical triangles of the neck (Figure 10.2).**
    - The SCMs divide each side of the neck into two major triangles: anterior and posterior.
      - The anterior triangle is further divided into the submandibular, carotid, and muscular triangles.
      - The submandibular triangle is bordered by the mandible and the posterior and anterior bellies of the digastric muscle.
      - The carotid triangle is bordered by the posterior belly of the digastric, the SCM, and the omohyoid.
      - The muscular triangle is bordered by the midline of the neck, the SCM, and the omohyoid.
      - The posterior triangle is formed by the SCM anteriorly, the clavicle inferiorly, and the anterior border of the trapezius posteriorly.
      - The omohyoid divides the posterior triangle into a small inferior subclavian triangle and a larger posterior occipital triangle.

18. **Describe the contents of the posterior cervical triangle.**
    The cutaneous branches of the cervical plexus, the spinal accessory nerve (cranial nerve XI), and the suprascapular and transverse cervical vessels are found in the posterior cervical triangle.
    It also contains the deep muscles of the neck, including semispinalis capitis, splenius capitis, levator scapulae, and the scalene muscles.

19. **What are the boundaries of the lymphatic levels of the neck?**
    Lymph node levels have boundaries that are identified anatomically during surgical dissection or via radiographic correlates.
    Certain neck level borders have different radiographic and surgical landmarks. The radiographic landmarks are in parentheses:

Level I

Level Ia – Submental
- Superior: Mandible
- Inferior: Hyoid bone
- Lateral: Ipsilateral anterior belly of the digastric muscle
- Medial: Midline of the neck from the mandible to the hyoid

Level Ib – Submandibular
- Superior: Mandible
- Inferior: Digastric attachment to hyoid (inferior edge of hyoid)
- Lateral/posterior: Posterior belly of the digastric muscle
- Medial: Anterior belly of the digastric muscle

Level II

Level IIa – Upper Jugular Region
- Superior: Skull base
- Inferior: Carotid bifurcation (hyoid bone)
- Lateral/posterior: Spinal accessory nerve (posterior border of internal jugular vein)
- Medial: Lateral border of the sternohyoid and stylohyoid muscles

Level IIb – Submuscular recess
- Superior: Skull base
- Inferior: Carotid bifurcation (hyoid bone)
- Lateral/posterior: Lateral border of the SCM
- Medial: Spinal accessory nerve (medial border of internal carotid artery)

Level III – Mid-Jugular
- Superior: Carotid bifurcation (hyoid bone)
- Inferior: Omohyoid muscle (inferior border of cricoid cartilage)
- Lateral/posterior: Sensory branches of cervical plexus (lateral border of the SCM)
- Medial: Lateral border of the sternohyoid muscle (medial border of common carotid artery)

Level IV – Lower Jugular
- Superior: Omohyoid muscle (inferior border of cricoid cartilage)
- Inferior: Clavicle
- Lateral/posterior: Sensory branches of cervical plexus (lateral border of the SCM)
- Medial: Lateral border of the sternohyoid muscle (medial border of common carotid artery)

Level V – Posterior Triangle

Level Va
- Superior: Convergence of SCM and trapezius muscles
- Inferior: Inferior border of cricoid cartilage
- Lateral: Anterior border of the trapezius muscle
- Medial: Sensory branches of cervical plexus (lateral border of the SCM)

Level Vb
- Superior: Inferior border of cricoid cartilage
- Inferior: Clavicle
- Lateral: Anterior border of the trapezius muscle
- Medial: Sensory branches of cervical plexus (lateral border of the SCM)

Level VI – Anterior Compartment
- Superior: Hyoid
- Inferior: Suprasternal notch
- Lateral: Common carotid arteries

Level VII – Superior Mediastinal
- Superior: Superior border of the sternum
- Inferior: Innominate artery
- Lateral: Innominate artery and left common carotid artery

20. Name the cranial nerves and skull base foramina where they exit.
    - Cranial nerve I: Olfactory nerve—Cribriform plate of the ethmoid bone
    - Cranial nerve II: Optic nerve—Optic canal
    - Cranial nerve III: Oculomotor nerve—Superior orbital fissure
    - Cranial nerve IV: Trochlear nerve—Superior orbital fissure
    - Cranial nerve V: Trigeminal nerve
        - V1: Ophthalmic nerve—Superior orbital fissure
        - V2: Maxillary nerve—Foramen rotundum
        - V3: Mandibular nerve—Foramen ovale

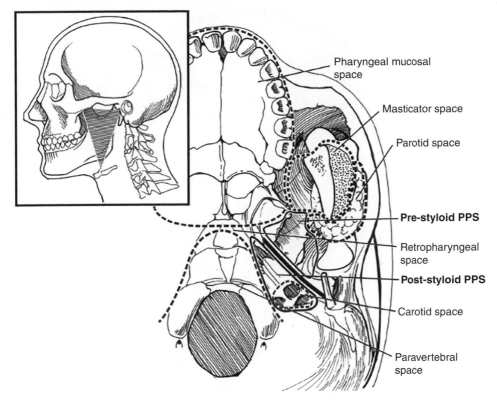

Pharyngeal mucosal space

Masticator space

Parotid space

Pre-styloid PPS

Retropharyngeal space

Post-styloid PPS

Carotid space

Paravertebral space

Fig. 10.3 Boundaries, compartments, and contents of the parapharyngeal space. (From Paz D, Eran A: Imaging of the parapharyngeal space, *Oper Tech Otolaryngol Head Neck Surgl* 25(3):220–226, 2014.)

- Cranial nerve VI: Abducens nerve—Superior orbital fissure
- Cranial nerve VII: Facial nerve
  - Motor division—Stylomastoid foramen
  - Chorda tympani—Petrotympanic fissure
- Cranial nerve VIII: Vestibulocochlear nerve—Internal acoustic meatus
- Cranial nerve IX: Glossopharyngeal nerve—Jugular foramen
- Cranial nerve X: Vagus nerve—Jugular foramen
- Cranial nerve XI: Accessory nerve—Jugular foramen
- Cranial nerve XII: Hypoglossal nerve—Hypoglossal canal

21. Describe the parapharyngeal space and list the contents of each compartment (Figure 10.3).
    The parapharyngeal space is an inverted pyramid with the base at the skull base and the apex at the greater cornu of the hyoid bone.
    Boundaries of the Parapharyngeal Space
    - Anterior: Pterygomandibular raphe and pterygoid muscles
    - Posterior: Vertebral fascia
    - Superior: Skull base
    - Inferior: Hyoid bone
    - Lateral: Mandible, deep parotid gland
    - Medial: Pharynx (superior constrictor muscle, buccopharyngeal fascia)
    Compartments and their contents
    - Pre-styloid compartment: Internal maxillary artery, pterygoid venous plexus, minor salivary gland tissue, and fat
    - Post-styloid compartment: Neurovascular bundle including carotid artery, internal jugular vein, sympathetic chain, and cranial nerves IX, X, XI.

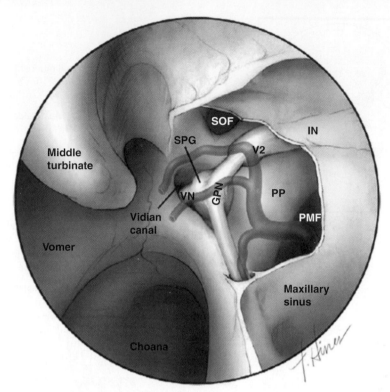

Fig. 10.4 Boundaries, communications, and contents of the pterygopalatine fossa. (From Statham MM, Tami TA: Endoscopic anatomy of the pterygopalatine fossa, *Oper Tech Otolaryngol Head Neck Surg* 17(3):197–200, 2006.) GPN, Greater palatine nerve; IN, Infraorbital nerve; PMF, pterygomaxillary fissure; PP, pterygoid process; SOF, Superior orbtial fissure; SPG, Sphenopalatine ganglion; VN, Vidian nerve

22. **Describe the pterygopalatine fossa (Figure 10.4).**
    The pterygopalatine fossa is the space below the apex of the orbit.
    Boundaries of the Pterygopalatine Fossa
    - Anterior: Maxilla
    - Posterior: Pterygoid plates of the sphenoid bone
    - Superior: Medial half of the inferior orbital fissure
    - Inferior: Upper end of the palatine canal
    - Lateral: Pterygomaxillary fissure
    - Medial: Sphenopalatine foramen and perpendicular plate of the palatine bone
    Communications of the Pterygopalatine Fossa
    - Anterior: Maxillary sinus (no direct communication)
    - Superior: Orbital cavity through the inferior orbital fissure
    - Posterior: Middle cranial fossa through foramen rotundum and the pterygoid canal
    - Inferior: Oral cavity through the palatine canal
    - Lateral: Infratemporal fossa through the pterygomaxillary fissure
    - Medial: Nasal cavity through the sphenopalatine foramen
    Contents of the Pterygopalatine Fossa
    - Fat
    - Maxillary artery
    - Maxillary division of the trigeminal nerve
    - Pterygopalatine ganglion: Parasympathetic ganglion where postganglionic nerves innervate the lacrimal gland and nasal mucosa.

23. **Where is the mental foramen located?**
    The mental nerve exits the mandible through the mental foramen at approximately the second premolar.

24. **Name the muscles of mastication, where they attach, and their primary action.**
    - Masseter muscle – arises from the maxillary process of the zygomatic bone and zygomatic arch and attaches to the angle of the mandible with its primary action to elevate the mandible and bring the teeth into occlusion.
    - Temporalis muscle – arises from the temporal fossa and inserts on the coronoid process and elevates and retracts the mandible.
    - Medial pterygoid muscle – the deep portion arises from the medial surface of the lateral pterygoid plate of the sphenoid bone, the superficial portion arises from the maxillary tuberosity and pyramidal process of the palatine bone, and both attach to the medial surface of the ramus and angle of the mandible. The primary action is to elevate the mandible.
    - Lateral pterygoid muscle – the upper portion arises from the infratemporal surface and crest of the greater wing of the sphenoid bone and the lower portion arises from the lateral surface of the lateral pterygoid plate of the sphenoid bone, and both attach to the coronoid process of the mandible. The primary actions are to depress and protrude the mandible.

25. **How can the internal carotid artery be distinguished from the external carotid artery?**
    The external carotid artery is anterolateral to the internal carotid artery. The internal carotid artery has no branches until it enters the skull base.

26. **What are the branches of the external carotid artery from proximal to distal?**
    - Superior thyroid artery
    - Ascending pharyngeal artery
    - Lingual artery
    - Facial artery
    - Occipital artery
    - Posterior auricular artery
    - Maxillary artery *(terminal branch)*
    - Superficial temporal artery *(terminal branch)*

27. **Name the branches of the thyrocervical trunk.**
    - Suprascapular artery
    - Transverse cervical artery
    - Inferior thyroid artery

BIBLIOGRAPHY

Bailey BJ, Johnson JT, Newlands SD: *Head and Neck Surgery—Otolaryngology*, Philadelphia, 2006, Lippincott Williams & Wilkins.
Cummings CW, Flint PW: *Cummings Otolaryngology: Head & Neck Surgery*, Philadelphia, 2010, Mosby Elsevier.
Coskun HH, Ferlito A, Medina JE, et al: Retropharyngeal lymph node metastases in head and neck malignancies, *Head Neck* 33(10):1520–1529, 2011.
Lalwani AK: *Current Diagnosis & Treatment in Otolaryngology: Head & Neck Surgery*, New York, 2008, McGraw-Hill Medical.
Paz D, Eran A: Imaging of the parapharyngeal space, *Oper Tech Otolaryngol Head Neck Surg* 25(3):220–226, 2014.
Statham MM, Tami TA: Endoscopic anatomy of the pterygopalatine fossa, *Oper Tech Otolaryngol Head Neck Surg* 17(3):197–200, 2006.

CHAPTER 11

TUMOR BIOLOGY

Jessica D. McDermott, MD and Daniel W. Bowles, MD

KEY POINTS

1. Cancer development requires an accumulation of genetic and cellular alterations.
2. The most common risk factors associated with head and neck squamous cell cancer in the United States are tobacco use, alcohol use, and the HPV virus (type 16).
3. HPV-positive and HPV-negative HNSCC have different drivers of carcinogenesis.
4. There are recurring DNA translocations and receptor overexpression patterns in different salivary gland cancers.
5. The key molecular drivers in differentiated thyroid cancer are BRAF mutations and RET translocations.
6. Dysregulation of cell cycle progression, angiogenesis, and immune tolerance are hallmarks of tumorigenesis.
7. Therapies targeting EGFR and immune checkpoint inhibitors are approved in HNSCC, with many more novel targeted therapies under investigation.

QUESTIONS

1. **What is the multi-hit theory of carcinogenesis?**
   This theory postulates that cells must acquire multiple mutations or aberrations in order to develop into cancer. Different types of tumors may result from different cellular changes.

2. **What biological processes contribute to cancer development, growth, and persistence?**
   Aberrant cell signaling controlling mitosis and cell differentiation
   Decreased apoptosis (programmed cell death)
   Angiogenesis (the growth of new blood vessels)
   Immune system dysregulation and evasion

3. **What are some molecular techniques used to analyze causes of head and neck cancer development?**
   Immunohistochemistry (IHC): stains for proteins in tumor specimens
   Fluorescence in situ hybridization (FISH): uses fluorescent probes to analyze for DNA translocations
   Next-generation sequencing: several methods that allow a wide number of genes to be analyzed for mutations and/or fusions simultaneously

4. **What are oncogenes, proto-oncogenes, and tumor suppressor genes?**
   An oncogene is a gene that confers the potential to cause cancer, and a proto-oncogene is a normal gene that can contribute to cancer formation when mutated. A tumor suppressor gene is one that protects a cell from transitioning to cancer. Mutations in tumor suppressor genes that cause loss of function may allow the cell to progress to cancer, especially when combined with overexpression of oncogenes and mutations in proto-oncogenes.

SQUAMOUS CELL CARCINOMAS OF THE HEAD AND NECK

5. **What are the most common risk factors for head and neck squamous cell cancer (HNSCC) worldwide?**
   Tobacco use
   Alcohol consumption
   Human papillomavirus (HPV) infection, especially in oropharyngeal cancer
   Betel nut chewing
   Epstein-Barr virus (EBV) in nasopharyngeal cancer
   Viral infections with hepatitis C (HCV) and human immunodeficiency virus (HIV)
   Immunosuppression

6. **What is the concept of field cancerization?**
Field cancerization refers to epithelium changes adjacent to an invasive cancer showing precancerous alterations such as dysplasia or carcinoma in situ. This is more common in smoking-related cancers, implying that such risk factors may be more broadly impacting the tissues.

7. **Which "high-risk" HPV virus type is most implicated in HNSCC?**
HPV type 16. Less commonly found are HPV types 18, 31, and 33.

8. **How does HPV cause HNSCC?**
HPV is a DNA virus that inserts genes into host DNA, which then act as oncogenes.
E6 protein: an oncoprotein that inactivates p53, a host tumor suppressor protein that blocks apoptosis
E7 protein: an oncoprotein that inactivates the retinoblastoma (Rb) tumor suppressor protein and promotes host DNA synthesis and cell cycle progression

9. **How is HPV detected in patients with HNSCC?**
P16 protein overexpression by immunohistochemistry. P16 is downstream of Rb, and when Rb is destroyed by HPV oncoproteins, P16 protein levels increase.
HPV in situ hybridization and polymerase chain reaction. These detect HPV DNA in cancer cells.
P16 and HPV DNA testing correlate approximately 85% of the time.

10. **What key molecular pathways are important in HNSCC pathogenesis?**
p53, a tumor suppressor gene
Epidermal growth factor receptor (EGFR)
Phosphoinositide 3-kinase (PI3K)
NOTCH-1
The tumor suppressor genes cyclin-dependent kinase inhibitor 2A (CDKN2A) and cyclin D1 (CCND1)

11. **How does the molecular landscape differ between HPV-positive and HPV-negative HNSCCs?**
    1. There is significant heterogeneity in both HPV-positive and HPV-negative cancers. In general, HPV-negative cancers are more likely to have mutations or alterations in the p53, EGFR, CDKN2A, and NOTCH pathways. HPV-positive tumors are more likely to have inactivation of p53 by viral proteins (E6 and E7) and PIK3CA (the gene encoding PI3K) mutations.
    2. HPV-positive tumors tend to have increased T cell infiltrates and markers of immune activation compared with HPV-negative tumors, but the tumoral expression of PD-L1 is similar.

12. **What is the role of EGFR in HNSCC?**
EGFR is a member of a family of tyrosine kinases that is overactivated in HNSCC. This results in increased activation of downstream pathways including Ras/Raf/MAPK and PI3K-Akt and transcription pathways promoting angiogenesis, proliferation, metastasis, and invasion.
EGFR is more frequently upregulated in HPV-negative cancers and is associated with poor prognosis

13. **Which molecular pathway has an FDA-approved targeted drug for treatment of HNSCC?**
Cetuximab, an IgG1 human monoclonal antibody, targets the extracellular domain of EGFR. It is FDA approved to treat HNSCC with radiation or in the metastatic setting. EGFR expression does not predict response to cetuximab. Recent studies suggest it may be less effective than cisplatin with radiation for HPV-related oropharynx cancers.

14. **How does the immune system play a role in the development and progression of HNSCC?**
Changes in immune cell populations, altered regulation of immune checkpoints, and defects in antigen presentation and cytokine release result in immune dysfunction of the tumor microenvironment. This allows tumors to avoid recognition and immune surveillance.

15. **What immune checkpoint pathways has targeted drugs approved for use in HNSCC?**
The programmed death 1 (PD-1) pathway includes PD-1 expression on immune cells and programmed death ligand 1 (PD-L1) expression on immune cells. This pathway is frequently upregulated in HNSCC, allowing adaptive immune resistance.
Pembrolizumab and nivolumab (both PD-1 inhibitors) are approved for use in metastatic HNSCC.

SALIVARY GLAND CANCERS

16. **What receptors are overexpressed in salivary gland tumors and may be exploited as potential biological targets for treatment?**

    Androgen receptor is increased in salivary duct carcinoma (90% to 100%), adenocarcinoma, and carcinoma ex pleomorphic adenoma.

    EGFR is increased in adenoid cystic carcinoma (36% to 85%), mucoepidermoid carcinoma (53% to 100%), adenocarcinoma (60%), salivary duct cancers (9% to 40%), and others.

    HER2/neu receptor is involved in cell growth and differentiation. It is increased mostly in salivary duct cancers (30% to 35%) but can also be found in adenocarcinomas (14% to 21%) and mucoepidermoid carcinoma (0% to 38%). HER2 targeted drugs may be helpful in HER2-expressing tumors.

17. **What recurring translocations commonly occur in salivary gland cancers?**

    t(11;19), producing the fusion protein CRTC1-MAML2, is seen in mucoepidermoid carcinomas (found in approximately 30%).

    t(6;9) MYB-NFIB translocations are seen in adenoid cystic carcinomas. It is estimated that 80% to 90% of adenoid cystic carcinomas have MYB activation by gene fusion.

    t(12;15) ETV-NTRK3 translocations are seen in mammary analogue secretory carcinomas (found in >90%). There are two FDA-approved drugs for treating NTRK fusion salivary gland cancers.

    RET gene fusions may be seen in salivary duct carcinomas.

THYROID CANCERS

18. **What are the different histologic types of thyroid cancer and what cells do they arise from?**

    Papillary: well-differentiated tumor of the thyroid epithelium
    Follicular: well-differentiated tumor of the thyroid epithelium
    Medullary: neuroendocrine tumor of the parafollicular or C cells of the thyroid gland
    Anaplastic: undifferentiated tumors of the thyroid follicular epithelium
    Hürthle cell: follicular epithelium

19. **What genetic mutations and fusions are commonly found in papillary thyroid cancer (PTC)?**

    RET/PTC: RET codes for a glial cell line–derived neurotrophic factor receptor that has tyrosine kinase activity. RET fusions are present in approximately 20% of metastatic PTCs.

    NTRK: NTRK is a nerve growth factor with tyrosine kinase activity. NTRK1 and NTRK3 fusions are present in <5% of PTCs.

    BRAF: Activates the RAF/MEK/MAPK signaling pathway, promoting tumorigenesis, invasion, metastasis, and recurrence. Mutations occur in 40% to 60% of PTC overall but more frequently in advanced PTC.

20. **What genetic mutations are commonly found in follicular thyroid cancers (FTCs)?**

    Translocation t(2;3)(q13:p25): resulting in a fusion protein of PAX8 (a thyroid transcription factor) and PPAR-gamma-1 (a transcription factor that stimulates cell differentiation and inhibits cell growth). Estimated to occur in approximately 40% of FTC.

    HRAS/KRAS/NRAS: proto-oncogenes that affect the MAPK and PI3K-AKT pathways, promoting tumorigenesis, invasion, and metastasis (30% to 45% of FTC).

    PTEN: mutation or deletion inactivates the gene, which activates the PI3K pathway, promoting tumorigenesis and invasiveness (10% to 15% of FTC).

21. **What genetic mutations are commonly found in anaplastic thyroid cancer (ATC)?**

    BRAF: V600E-activating mutations are seen in approximately 40% of ATCs. The combination of dabrafenib/trametinib is approved to treat BRAF-mutated ATC.

    TP53: an inactivating mutation that promotes tumor progression. Seen in 70% to 80% of ATCs.

    PIK3CA: an activating mutation affecting the PI3K-AKT pathway, promoting tumorigenesis and invasiveness (15% to 25% of ATC).

    RAS: activating mutation affecting the MAPK and PI3K-AKT pathways (20% to 30% of ATC).

22. **What is the major gene mutated in medullary thyroid cancer (MTC)?**

    RET: a proto-oncogene that has gain-of-function mutations in medullary thyroid cancer, resulting in tumor pathogenesis
    Sporadic MTC: somatic mutations seen in 20% to 80%, often associated with worse prognosis.
    Familial MTC: >95% have RET mutations. Seen in patients with MEN2A and familial MTC.

BIBLIOGRAPHY

Alsahafi E, Begg K, Amelio I, et al: Clinical update on head and neck cancer: molecular biology and ongoing challenges, *Cell Death Dis* 10:540, 2019.

Chow LQM: Head and neck cancer, *N Engl J Med* 382(1):60–72, 2020.

Guzzo M, Locati LD, Prott FJ, et al: Major and minor salivary gland tumors, *Crit Rev Oncol Hematol* 74(2):134–148, 2010.

Leemans CR, Snijders PJF, Brakenhoff RH: The molecular landscape of head and neck cancer, *Nat Rev Cancer* 18(5):269–282, 2018.

Pozdeyev N, Gay LM, Sokol ES, et al: Genetic analysis of 779 advanced differentiated and anaplastic thyroid cancers, *Clin Cancer Res* 24(13):3059–3068, 2018.

Ross JS, Gay LM, Wang K, et al: Comprehensive genomic profiles of metastatic and relapsed salivary gland carcinomas are associated with tumor type and reveal new routes to targeted therapies, *Ann Oncol* 28(10):2539–2546, 2017.

Solomon B, Young RJ, Rischin D: Head and neck squamous cell carcinoma: genomics and emerging biomarkers for immunomodulatory cancer treatments, *Semin Cancer Biol* 52:228–240, 2018.

Stenman G: Fusion oncogenes in salivary gland tumors: molecular and clinical consequences, *Head Neck Pathol* 7(Suppl 1):S12–S19, 2013.

Xing M: Molecular pathogenesis and mechanisms of thyroid cancer, *Nat Rev Cancer* 13(3):184–199, 2013.

CHAPTER 12

SKIN CANCER

Tamar Hajar, MD, Franki Lambert Smith, MD and Mariah Brown, MD

KEY POINTS

1. Skin cancer incidence
   - Normal population: basal cell carcinoma > squamous cell carcinoma > melanoma > Merkel cell carcinoma
   - Transplant population: squamous cell carcinoma > basal cell carcinoma > melanoma > Merkel cell carcinoma
2. Patients at higher risk for nonmelanoma skin cancer
   - Fair-skinned with light eyes
   - Previous history of significant sun exposure and blistering sunburns
   - Personal or family history of skin cancer
   - History of chemical exposure
   - Genetic syndromes
   - Immunosuppression
   - Male sex
   - Older age
3. Important prognostic factors for melanoma
   - Breslow depth
   - Ulceration
   - Presence of nodal or distant metastases
4. Systemic treatment options for Stage 3 or Stage 4 melanoma
5. Checkpoint inhibitors (anti-programmed cell death 1 [PD-1] antibodies and the anti-cytotoxic T-lymphocyte-associated protein 4 [CTLA-4])
6. Targeted therapy (small-molecule inhibitors of BRAF and MEK)

Pearls
1. Breslow depth is the most important prognostic factor in melanoma.
2. Squamous cell carcinoma is the most common type of skin cancer in transplant recipients.

QUESTIONS

1. **What are the common cutaneous malignancies?**

   Cutaneous malignancies are classified into melanoma and nonmelanoma skin cancers. Nonmelanoma skin cancers include basal cell carcinoma and squamous cell carcinoma, which account for the majority of all skin cancers. Melanoma skin cancers account for only 5% of cutaneous malignancies but result in 90% of the mortality from skin cancer in patients less than 50 years old. Rare nonmelanoma skin cancers include Merkel cell carcinoma, dermatofibrosarcoma protuberans, sebaceous carcinoma, and cutaneous T-cell lymphoma. Overall, there are more skin cancers in the United States than all other malignancies combined, and it is estimated that 20% of the population of the United States will develop a skin cancer during their lifetime.

2. **What is a basal cell carcinoma?**

   Basal cell carcinoma (BCC) is a cutaneous neoplasm that arises from the basal layer of the epidermis. It is the most common cancer in humans and the most common type of skin cancer. BCC is more commonly found in men, although in the last decade the incidence has been increasing in women. It is most diagnosed in middle-aged individuals with a median age of diagnosis of 68 years. BCC accounts for up to 75% of all nonmelanoma skin cancers.

   BCC is classified according to histologic appearance, including *superficial, nodular, micronodular, desmoplastic, pigmented,* and *basosquamous* BCCs. The classic appearance of a BCC is a skin-colored to pink pearly papule or plaque with a rolled border and possibly central ulceration (Fig. 12.1A and 12.1B). Superficial BCCs present as thin, pink, scaly papules or plaques and are most common on the trunk in younger patients (Fig. 12.1C). Desmoplastic BCCs, also known as morpheaform, infiltrating, or sclerosing BCCs, may have a more subtle clinical appearance, presenting as flat, slightly atrophic lesions, similar to a scar (Fig. 12.1D). Desmoplastic and

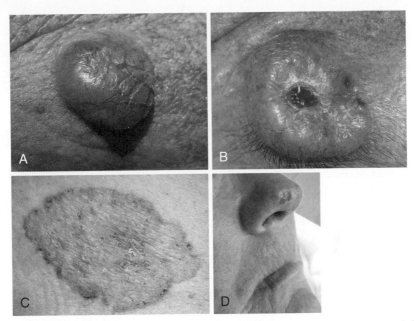

Fig. 12.1 Variants of basal cell carcinoma (BCC). A, Nodular BCC with classic pearly appearance and dilated blood vessels. **B**, Ulcerated nodular BCC. **C**, Superficial BCC demonstrating pink plaque with scale. **D**, Desmoplastic BCC with scarred appearance. (From Fitzsimons Army Medical Center.)

basosquamous BCCs have a more aggressive clinical course and a higher risk of recurrence than other histologic subtypes of BCC. Risk factors for BCC include intermittent rather than cumulative ultraviolet (UV) exposure, fair skin, immunosuppression, indoor tanning, ionizing radiation, exposure to chemicals such as arsenic, coal tar psoralen plus ultraviolet A (UVA) radiation, and rare genetic syndromes, such as basal cell nevus syndrome (Gorlin's syndrome). Although BCCs can be locally aggressive, they almost never metastasize (rate 1/35,000).

3. **What is squamous cell carcinoma?**
   Squamous cell carcinoma (SCC) is the second most common cutaneous malignancy and arises from the keratinocytes within the epidermis. SCC represents approximately 20% of all skin cancers and can have a more aggressive clinical course than BCC. SCC in situ, also known as Bowen's disease, is confined to the epidermis of the skin and presents as a thin, pink, scaly papule or plaque (Fig. 12.2A). Invasive SCC presents as a pink, crusted papule or nodule on sun-damaged skin (Fig. 12.2B). Common locations for SCC are sun-exposed areas such as the face, forearms, and dorsal hands. SCCs associated with human papillomavirus (HPV) can occur on the hands, feet, and genitals. SCCs can also occur in areas of chronic inflammation such as a stasis ulcer or burn site (Marjolin's ulcer).

   Risk factors for SCC include fair skin, UV exposure, male sex, immunosuppression such as in human immunodeficiency virus (HIV) and solid organ transplant, cigarette smoking, HPV infection, indoor tanning, ionizing radiation, exposure to chemicals such as arsenic, coal tar psoralen plus UVA, mineral oil, soot and mechlorethamine, certain medications, chronic nonhealing ulcers and scars, chronic inflammatory skin conditions, and rare genetic syndromes. The risk of metastatic SCC is less than 5% in sun-exposed skin but can be significantly higher for tumors with known risk factors. Metastases from SCC are most often found in regional lymph nodes but can also be distant. The role of sentinel lymph node biopsy (SLNB) in the evaluation and management of high-risk SCC is debated.

4. **What makes an SCC high risk?**
   Although most SCCs can be successfully treated surgically, there is a subset that are associated with higher rates of recurrence, metastasis, and death. It is estimated that approximately 3000 to 9000 Americans die each year from SCC, a rate comparable to deaths from melanoma. SCCs are considered high risk based on several factors, including location, etiology, histologic features, and host immune status. High-risk factors include the following:
   - **Diameter:** A tumor diameter of >2 centimeters, especially those >4 centimeters in their greatest dimension.
   - **Depth:** Tumors that are >2 millimeters deep but especially those >6 millimeters in thickness, extension beyond the subcutaneous fat, and bony invasion.

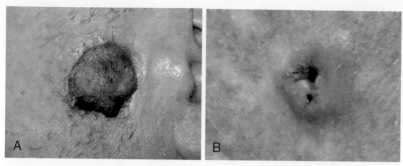

Fig. 12.2 Squamous cell carcinoma (SCC). A, Large SCC composed of fungating hyperkeratotic plaque. **B,** Pink hyperkeratotic papule with central ulceration.

- **Perineural involvement:** Perineural involvement of nerves >0.1 millimeter in diameter (large caliber) or clinical/radiographic evidence of named nerve involvement or tumor cells within the nerve sheath of a nerve lying deeper than the dermis.
- **Histology:** Poorly differentiated tumor on histopathology
- **Previously treated/recurrent SCC**
- **Anatomic site:** Ear, lip, genitals
- **SCC arising in a scar or a site of chronic inflammation**
- **Host immune status**: immunosuppression, chronic lymphocytic leukemia, genetic DNA repair defects such as xeroderma pigmentosum

5. **How is SCC staged?**
   Several staging systems exist for cutaneous SCC. The American Joint Committee on Cancer (AJCC) staging system was most recently revised in October 2016 (eighth edition) to better stratify high-risk SCC (Table 12.7). An alternative staging system, the Brigham and Women's Hospital (BWH) staging system, was proposed in 2013 in order to identify which T2 tumors were higher risk. Patients with high-risk SCCs based on staging may need imaging, adjuvant treatment such as radiation, and closer clinical follow-up.

6. **What are the most common cutaneous malignancies in the transplant population?**
   Transplant recipients are more likely to develop numerous aggressive nonmelanoma skin cancers and should be counseled on the importance of sun-protective measures, regular skin exams, and skin self-checks. SCC is by far the most common cutaneous malignancy in transplant recipients. Transplant recipients are 65 to 250 times more likely to develop SCCs than the general population and 6 to 16 times more likely to develop BCCs. The reported risk of developing an invasive melanoma is two fold higher in the transplant population than in the general population in White people and 17 times greater in Black people. Kaposi's sarcoma and Merkel cell carcinoma are also seen more commonly in transplant recipients. Rates of skin cancer development and skin cancer mortality increase with the length of immunosuppression and level of immunosuppression and in patients with a baseline high risk for skin cancer. Mortality from skin cancer may approach 27% in cardiac transplant recipients.

7. **What is Merkel cell carcinoma?**
   Merkel cell carcinoma (MCC) is a rare and aggressive cutaneous neoplasm that is more common in older immunosuppressed patients. It presents as a rapidly enlarging pink or violaceous nodule on the head and neck or other sun-exposed areas. MCC was suspected to have a neuroendocrine origin for many years; however, in 2008, it was discovered that a polyomavirus was present in the majority of MCCs and the tumor is now considered to be infectious in origin, similar to HPV-induced malignancies. Other risk factors that contribute to the etiology of MCC include UV radiation exposure and immunosuppression (24-fold higher risk). MCCs grow rapidly, and up to 30% are metastatic at presentation. Treatment consists of surgical excision, often with SLNB and lymph node dissection if necessary, followed by adjuvant radiation therapy to the surgical site and nodal basin. Even with therapy, outcomes are poor, with 5-year mortality at 30%.

8. **What is a keratoacanthoma and how is it treated?**
   Keratoacanthoma (KA) is a type of SCC that presents as an enlarging skin-colored or red nodule, often with a central crater that may be filled with keratinous debris (Fig. 12.3). KAs usually develop over a few weeks and then are often reported to spontaneously resolve over months, leaving a scar. KAs are generally solitary but can be multiple in certain genetic syndromes. Given the difficulty in distinguishing a KA from a well-differentiated SCC, both clinically and histologically, these tumors are best considered a variant of well-differentiated SCC and treated as such.

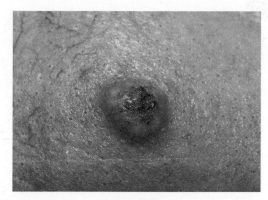

Fig. 12.3 Keratoacanthoma. Dome-shaped nodule with central crater. (From Fitzpatrick JE, Aeling JL: *Dermatology Secrets in Color*, 2nd ed, Philadelphia, 2000, Hanley & Belfus.)

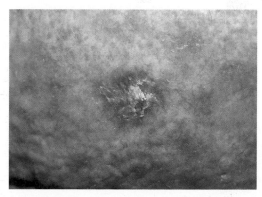

Fig. 12.4 Actinic keratosis. Scaly pink papule on sun-exposed skin. (From Fitzpatrick JE, Aeling JL: *Dermatology Secrets in Color*, 2nd ed, Philadelphia, 2000, Hanley & Belfus.)

9. **What is an actinic keratosis and how is it treated?**
   An actinic keratosis (AK) is a precancerous lesion that presents as a skin-colored to pink rough papule on sun-exposed skin (Fig. 12.4). Often, AKs are more easily felt than seen and patients describe them as areas that develop a crust that later falls off and reforms. If left untreated, AKs can develop into invasive SCC. Although the rate of transformation is thought to be roughly 1/100 per year, up to 60% of SCCs arise from an AK. As a result, it is recommended that AKs be treated in most cases rather than observed. AKs can be treated with destructive mechanisms such as curettage, cryotherapy, dermabrasion, or photodynamic therapy; topical medications such as fluorouracil, imiquimod, Ingenol mebutate, and diclofenac; and field-ablative techniques such as chemical peels and laser resurfacing. Isolated lesions are most often treated with destructive methods such as cryotherapy. Field-directed therapy is generally recommended for patients with a larger number of AKs. AKs are not treated surgically, because they are non malignant, ill-defined, and often diffusely present across sun-damaged skin. The risk factors for AKs are similar to those for SCC.

10. **What is actinic cheilitis?**
    Actinic cheilitis describes the precancerous sun damage changes that typically occur on the lower lip of older adults. It is the mucosal equivalent of an AK but has a higher risk of transformation to SCC. Actinic cheilitis can be treated similar to AKs with cryotherapy, topical agents, or photodynamic therapy.

11. **What is Mohs micrographic surgery?**
    Mohs micrographic surgery (MMS) is a technique for treating skin cancer developed by Dr. Frederic Mohs in 1938. The modern technique of MMS is a single-day procedure performed under local anesthesia designed to provide high cure rates and conserve normal, uninvolved skin. During MMS, a skin cancer is removed in a specific beveled

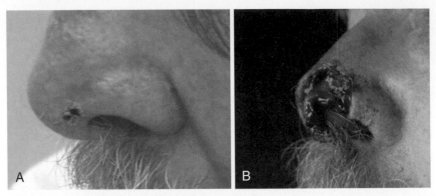

Fig. 12.5 Before and after Mohs microscopic surgery (MMS). A, Pre-MMS. Desmoplastic basal cell carcinoma on the nasal tip. It is difficult to determine extent and depth of tumor. **B,** Post-MMS. Large defect involving cartilage and nasal mucosa after four stages of MMS.

disc shape and the resected tissue is mapped out with ink to provide accurate orientation. This tissue is then processed into frozen sections and stained, using a method of horizontal *en face* sections that allows for visualization of 100% of the peripheral and deep margins (standard tissue processing examines <1% of the surgical margin). The tissue is examined under the microscope by the Mohs surgeon and the areas of tumor are precisely mapped out. If needed, the patient then has additional tissue removed only in the areas that were positive for tumor. Each excision and visualization of tissue is referred to as a Mohs stage. As many stages as necessary are taken to ensure that the entire tumor is completely removed (Fig. 12.5), at which time surgical reconstruction may be performed. Because all margins are examined during MMS, it offers high cure rates while promoting tissue conservation.

12. **What tumors can be treated with MMS?**
    MMS is predominantly used to treat BCC and SCC, as these comprise 95% of all skin cancers. However, more rare cutaneous tumors can also be treated with MMS. Certain types of cutaneous tumors may be treated with MMS using immunohistochemistry tissue stains to help better visualize the tumor cells. Many Mohs surgeons use immunohistochemistry stains such as SOX-10, MART-1, and/or Mel-5 to treat melanoma in situ (particularly the lentigo maligna variant) with MMS.

13. **What are the indications for MMS?**
    MMS is reserved for skin cancers in anatomic locations where tissue conservation is key or for high-risk tumors, due to the cost and time-consuming nature of the procedure. MMS is usually considered appropriate for skin cancers of the face, neck, scalp, hands, feet, and genitalia. Skin cancers in other anatomic locations may be candidates for MMS if they are recurrent, are large, have an aggressive histologic subtype of SCC or BCC, are present in an immunocompromised host, or are a less common skin cancer (see Table 12.1).

Table 12.1 Rare Nonmelanoma Skin Cancers Appropriate for Mohs Microscopic Surgery
Adenocystic carcinoma
Apocrine/eccrine carcinoma
Atypical fibroxanthoma
Dermatofibrosarcoma protuberans
Extramammary Paget's disease
Leiomyosarcoma
Undifferentiated pleomorphic sarcoma
Merkel cell carcinoma
Microcystic adnexal carcinoma
Mucinous carcinoma
Sebaceous carcinoma

14. **What are other treatments for nonmelanoma skin cancer besides MMS?**
Other treatment options for nonmelanoma skin cancer include excision, electrodesiccation and curettage, cryosurgery, topical therapies, or radiation therapy. Excision can be performed for BCCs and SCCs, anticipating margins of 4 to 5 millimeters from clinically visible tumors. Larger margins will be needed for higher-risk tumors, and clear margins should be confirmed with histologic examination. Electrodesiccation and curettage is a destructive technique that allows for localized treatment of low-risk skin cancers without the need for sutures or histologic examination. However, the technique can result in suboptimal scars and lower cure rates than excision or MMS. Cryosurgery or topical treatments, including 5-fluorouracil, imiquimod, and photodynamic therapy, are best limited to treatment of superficial variants of SCC and BCC. Radiation can be used to treat skin cancers but is often reserved for inoperable tumors, patients who cannot tolerate surgery, or adjuvant therapy after complete surgical removal.

15. **What are Hedgehog inhibitors?**
BCC formation is driven by mutations in the Hedgehog signaling pathway. There are two Hedgehog pathway inhibitors that have been U.S. Food an Drug Administration (FDA) approved for the treatment of locally advanced or metastatic BCC – vismodegib and sonidegib. These two agents are small-molecule oral agents that target the mutation present in the majority of sporadic BCCs and in basal cell nevus syndrome. Most BCCs have a mutation in the *PTCH* gene that leads to constitutive activation of the Smoothened receptor, which in turn leads to gene replication and BCC formation. Both vismodegib and sonidegib have similar response rates for locally advanced BCCs – between 55% and 62%. However, vismodegib has been found to be superior when treating metastatic disease. The most common side effects of these medications include nausea, nonscarring alopecia, dysgeusia, muscle cramps, and teratogenicity.

16. **What is melanoma?**
Melanoma is a malignancy that arises from aberrant growth of melanocytes, the pigment-containing cells that exist in the basal cell layer of the epidermis and within moles (nevi). Melanoma is most frequently seen in fair-skinned individuals with histories of intense, intermittent UV exposure. It is the most common cancer in female patients aged 25 to 29 years. Approximately 75% of melanomas arise de novo and the remainder arise from pre-existing nevi. The four main types of melanoma are *superficial spreading* melanoma (70%), *nodular* melanoma (15%–30%), *lentigo maligna* melanoma (up to 15%), and *acral lentiginous* (5%–10%). Less common variations of melanoma are *spitzoid* melanoma, *desmoplastic* melanoma, and *amelanotic* melanoma.

17. **What is the clinical appearance of melanoma?**
Melanomas are usually heavily pigmented, with color variations of brown, black, and blue but may also include red or pink areas, as well as lighter areas that represent tumor regression (Fig. 12.6). Melanomas are often asymmetric with irregular borders and variegated color. Common symptoms are pain, itching, or bleeding, but many tumors are symptomatic. Amelanotic (nonpigmented) melanomas are much more difficult to diagnose clinically and often present as a pink, rapidly enlarging nodule that may ulcerate and bleed.

18. **What are the ABCDEs of melanoma?**
    - Asymmetry (if a lesion is bisected, one half is not identical to the other half)
    - Border irregularities
    - Color variegation (presence of multiple shades of red, blue, black, gray, or white)
    - Diameter ≥6 millimeters
    - Evolution: a lesion that is changing in size, shape, or color

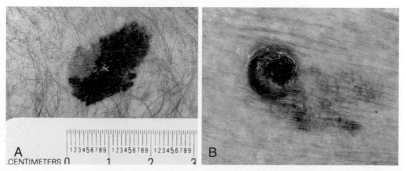

Fig. 12.6 Melanoma. A, Superficial spreading melanoma with asymmetry, irregular borders, and color variegation. **B**, Superficial spreading and nodular melanoma with ulceration. (From Fitzpatrick JE, Aeling JL: *Dermatology Secrets in Color*, 2nd ed, Philadelphia, 2000, Hanley & Belfus.)

Table 12.2	ABCDEs of Melanoma
A	Asymmetry: Melanomas are not uniform in size, shape, or color.
B	Border: Melanomas often have borders that are not smooth or clearly demarcated.
C	Color: Melanomas may contain varying shades of pigment and colors such as red, white, and blue.
D	Diameter: Most melanomas are >6 millimeters (the diameter of a pencil eraser); however, suspicious lesions <6 millimeters should still be biopsied.
E	Evolution: Patients with melanoma often note changes in shape, size, color, or symptomatology. Any new pigmented lesion in a patient >35 years old should be evaluated.

19. **What are lentigo maligna and lentigo maligna melanoma?**

    Lentigo maligna is a variant of melanoma in situ with a characteristic histologic and clinical appearance. Lentigo maligna presents clinically as a slow-growing, irregularly hyperpigmented patch on sun-exposed skin (Fig. 12.7). Lentigo maligna melanoma (LMM) represents lentigo maligna with areas of tumor invasion into the dermis and is the third most common type of melanoma (up to 15%). Lentigo maligna and lentigo maligna melanoma are most often seen in elderly patients on sun-exposed areas.

20. **What are risk factors for melanoma?**

    Risk factors for melanoma consist of genetic, skin type, and environmental factors. Most commonly, genetic susceptibility is related to an inherited phenotype of fair skin. Patients with multiple benign moles (>50) also have an increased risk of melanoma development, and the development of moles is linked with childhood sun exposure. Melanoma risk is also increased in individuals with a first-degree relative with a melanoma. True genetic predisposition (i.e., familial melanoma) is much rarer and is most commonly associated with defects in *CDKN2A*, the gene that encodes the proteins p16 and p14. Patients with multiple atypical moles and a family history of melanoma, described as dysplastic nevus syndrome, have an elevated risk of melanoma. Patients with large congenital nevi (>20 centimeters) also have an elevated risk of developing melanoma. Sun exposure is the most important environmental risk factor for melanoma, and it has been shown that people living at latitudes closer to the equator (i.e., Florida, Australia) have a much higher incidence of melanoma. Times of intense, intermittent sun exposure are associated with the development of superficial spreading and nodular melanoma, while a high cumulative sun exposure is associated with the development of LMM.

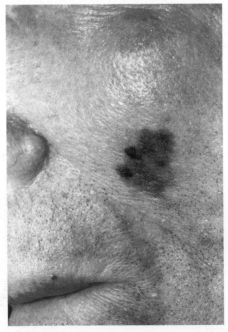

Fig. 12.7 Lentigo maligna. Irregular pigmented patch on sun-exposed skin. (From Fitzpatrick JE, Aeling JL: *Dermatology Secrets in Color*, 2nd ed, Philadelphia, 2000, Hanley & Belfus.)

21. **What is Breslow depth?**
    Breslow depth is a measurement in millimeters of the tumor depth from the granular layer of the epidermis to the base of the melanoma. It is the most important prognostic indicator for melanomas. Clark's level, a measurement of melanoma depth based on skin anatomy, is no longer used for melanoma staging but may still be reported by some pathologists.

22. **How is melanoma staged?**
    Melanoma is staged by the TNM staging system from the American Joint Commission on Cancer (AJCC), most recently updated in 2017 (Table 12.3). Clinical staging includes histologic staging of the primary melanoma and evaluation for metastases. Pathology reports for melanoma have transitioned from a narrative form to a more

Table 12.3 Melanoma TNM Classification

T CLASSIFICATION	THICKNESS	ULCERATION STATUS/MITOSES	5-YEAR % SURVIVAL	10-YEAR % SURVIVAL
TX: Primary tumor thickness cannot be assessed (e.g., diagnosis by curettage)	Not applicable	Not applicable	Not applicable	Not applicable
T0: No evidence of primary tumor (e.g., unknown primary or completely regressed melanoma)	Not applicable	Not applicable	Not applicable	Not applicable
Tis	Not applicable	Not applicable	Not applicable	Not applicable
T1	≤1.0 mm	Unknown or unspecified		
T1a	<0.8 mm	Without ulceration	99%	98%
T1b	<0.8 mm	With ulceration	99%	96%
	0.8 to 1 mm	With or without ulceration		
T2	>1 to 2 mm	Unknown or unspecified		
T2a	>1 to 2 mm	Without ulceration	96%	92%
T2b	>1 to 2 mm	With ulceration	93%	88%
T3	>2 to 4 mm	Unknown or unspecified		
T3a	>2 to 4 mm	Without ulceration	94%	88%
T3b	>2 to 4 mm	With ulceration	86%	81%
T4	>4 mm	Unknown or unspecified		
T4a	>4 mm	Without ulceration	90%	83%
T4b	>4 mm	With ulceration	82%	75%

REGIONAL LYMPH NODES (N)

N CATEGORY	EXTENT OF REGIONAL LYMPH NODE AND/OR LYMPHATIC METASTASIS	
	NUMBER OF TUMOR-INVOLVED REGIONAL LYMPH NODES	PRESENCE OF IN-TRANSIT, SATELLITE, AND/OR MICROSATELLITE METASTASES
NX	Regional nodes not assessed (e.g., SLN biopsy not performed, regional nodes previously removed for another reason). **Exception:** Pathologic N category is not required for T1 melanomas, use cN.	No
N0	No regional metastases detected	No

Table 12.3 Melanoma TNM Classification (*Continued*)

REGIONAL LYMPH NODES (N)

	EXTENT OF REGIONAL LYMPH NODE AND/OR LYMPHATIC METASTASIS	
N CATEGORY	**NUMBER OF TUMOR-INVOLVED REGIONAL LYMPH NODES**	**PRESENCE OF IN-TRANSIT, SATELLITE, AND/OR MICROSATELLITE METASTASES**
N1	One tumor-involved node or in-transit, satellite, and/or microsatellite metastases with no tumor-involved nodes	
N1a	One clinically occult (i.e., detected by SLN biopsy)	No
N1b	One clinically detected	No
N1c	No regional lymph node disease	Yes
N2	Two or three tumor-involved nodes or in-transit, satellite, and/or microsatellite metastases with one tumor-involved node	
N2a	Two or three clinically occult (i.e., detected by SLN biopsy)	No
N2b	Two or three, at least one of which was clinically detected	No
N2c	One clinically occult or clinically detected	Yes
N3	Four or more tumor-involved nodes or in-transit, satellite, and/or microsatellite metastases with two or more tumor-involved nodes or any number of matted nodes without or with in-transit, satellite, and/or microsatellite metastases	
N3a	Four or more clinically occult (i.e., detected by SLN biopsy)	No
N3b	Four or more, at least one of which was clinically detected, or presence of any number of matted nodes	No
N3c	Two or more clinically occult or clinically detected and/or presence of any number of matted nodes	Yes

DISTANT METASTASIS (M)

M CATEGORY	**M CRITERIA**	
	ANATOMIC SITE	**LDH LEVEL**
M0	No evidence of distant metastasis	Not applicable
M1	Evidence of distant metastasis	See below
M1a	Distant metastasis to skin, soft tissue including muscle, and/or non regional lymph node	Not recorded or unspecified
M1a(0)		Not elevated
M1a(1)		Elevated
M1b	Distant metastasis to lung with or without M1a sites of disease	Not recorded or unspecified
M1b(0)		Not elevated
M1b(1)		Elevated
M1c	Distant metastasis to non-CNS visceral sites with or without M1a or M1b sites of disease	Not recorded or unspecified
M1c(0)		Not elevated
M1c(1)		Elevated
M1d	Distant metastasis to CNS with or without M1a, M1b, or M1c sites of disease	Not recorded or unspecified
M1d(0)		Normal
M1d(1)		Elevated

SLN, sentinel lymph node.
Data from the American Joint Committee on Cancer website https://cancerstaging.org/Pages/default.aspx.

structured synoptic reporting system, which helps pathologists ensure that all necessary data elements for staging are included. Pathologic staging includes histologic evaluation of the initial biopsy, including any additional staging information from the wide local excision (surgical), as well as information about the regional lymph nodes after sentinel lymph node biopsy (SLN; required for all >T1 melanomas).

23. **What is an SLNB and how is it performed?**
SLNB is a technique that is performed to determine whether cancer has spread from the skin to the regional draining lymphatics. Sentinel lymph node (SLN) status is an important prognostic indicator used in the staging of melanoma. SLN status is one of the most important prognostic factors for long-term survival. A radioactive tracer and/or a blue dye is injected into the melanoma site and then the lymph node (or sometimes multiple lymph nodes) that most strongly picks up these markers is removed and evaluated. Normally, wide local excision of the melanoma is done at the time of SLNB to prevent disruption of lymphatics, which could alter the normal drainage pattern. SLN status impacts further management, including type and frequency of clinic visits, imaging surveillance type and frequency, complete lymph node dissection, and adjuvant therapy.

24. **When is an SLNB recommended for patients with melanoma?**
SLNB is recommended for patients with clinically negative lymph nodes and a primary melanoma at intermediate or high risk for lymph node metastasis (>5%), which include melanomas that are >1 miillimeter deep. SLNB is not recommended for low-risk melanomas, such as those with a Breslow depth of <0.8 miillimeter without ulceration. Consideration and thorough discussion with patients should be held for those with a melanoma that is <8 miillimeter deep with ulceration or other high-risk features, such as high mitotic rate (particularly in younger individuals) and/or lymphovascular invasion and for those who have melanomas 0.8 to 1 millimeter in depth with or without ulceration. SLNB has a low rate of morbidity, but would not be indicated in patients for whom a positive result would not change management (i.e., patients who are very elderly or who have multiple comorbidities or those with clinical or radiographic metastases).

25. **What is the treatment for localized primary melanoma?**
Surgical excision, with margins based on Breslow depth (Table 12.5). There is some debate as to whether >2 cm margins should be taken on thicker melanomas (Breslow depth >2 millimeters).

26. **What are checkpoint inhibitors and what is their role in the treatment of melanoma?**
In the past decade, melanoma treatment has been advanced by the development of immunotherapy – medications that activate the body's immune system to destroy tumor cells. These immunotherapy medications are called checkpoint inhibitors and include the anti–programmed cell death 1 [PD-1] antibodies (pembrolizumab, nivolumab) and the anti-cytotoxic T-lymphocyte-associated protein 4 [CTLA-4] antibody (ipilimumab). Immunotherapy has been shown to prolong progression-free and overall survival in clinical trials for stage III and stage IV disease. PD1 inhibitors are given as an infusion every 2 to 3 weeks and ipilimumab is given as a series of four infusions 3 weeks apart.

Table 12.4 American Joint Committee on Cancer Eighth Edition Stage Groupings for Cutaneous Melanoma

CLINICAL (CTNM)					
WHEN T IS...	AND N IS...	AND M IS...	THEN THE CLINICAL STAGE GROUP IS...	5-YEAR % SURVIVAL	10-YEAR % SURVIVAL
Tis	N0	M0	0	NA	NA
T1a	N0	M0	IA	99%	98%
T1b	N0	M0	IB	97%	94%
T2a	N0	M0	IB	97%	94%
T2b	N0	M0	IIA	94%	88%
T3a	N0	M0	IIA	94%	88%
T3b	N0	M0	IIB	87%	82%
T4a	N0	M0	IIB	87%	82%
T4b	N0	M0	IIC	82%	75%
Any T, Tis	≥N1	M0	III	NA	NA
Any T	Any N	M1	IV	NA	NA

(*Continued*)

Table 12.4 American Joint Committee on Cancer Eighth Edition Stage Groupings for Cutaneous Melanoma (*Continued*)

PATHOLOGIC (PTNM)

WHEN T IS...	AND N IS...	AND M IS...	THEN THE PATHOLOGIC STAGE GROUP IS...	5-YEAR % SURVIVAL	10-YEAR % SURVIVAL
Tis	N0	M0	0		
T1a	N0	M0	IA	99%	98%
T1b	N0	M0	IA	99%	98%
T2a	N0	M0	IB	97%	94%
T2b	N0	M0	IIA	94%	88%
T3a	N0	M0	IIA	94%	88%
T3b	N0	M0	IIB	87%	82%
T4a	N0	M0	IIB	87%	82%
T4b	N0	M0	IIC	82%	75%
T0	N1b, N1c	M0	IIIB	83%	77%
T0	N2b, N2c, N3b, or N3c	M0	IIIC	69%	60%
T1a/b-T2a	N1a or N2a	M0	IIIA	93%	88%
T1a/b-T2a	N1b/c or N2b	M0	IIIB	83%	77%
T2b/T3a	N1a–N2b	M0	IIIB	83%	77%
T1a-T3a	N2c or N3a/b/c	M0	IIIC	69%	60%
T3b/T4a	Any N ≥N1	M0	IIIC	69%	60%
T4b	N1a–N2c	M0	IIIC	69%	60%
T4b	N3a/b/c	M0	IIID	32%	24%
Any T, Tis	Any N	M1	IV		

Data from the American Joint Committee on Cancer website https://cancerstaging.org/Pages/default.aspx.

Table 12.5 Excisional Margins for Melanoma

MELANOMA BRESLOW DEPTH	MARGIN (CM)
Melanoma in situ (excluding lentigo maligna which may need larger margins)	0.5–1
≤1 mm	1–2
1.01–2.0 mm	1–2
>2 mm	2

Both types of medication can have immune-mediated toxicities, but typically the side effects of ipilimumab therapy are more severe than those seen with PD-1 inhibitors. Double-agent therapy, using both a PD-1 inhibitor and ipilimumab, has shown improved survival for metastatic melanoma when compared with either single agent. However, the combination of these medications is associated with serious (grade >3) adverse events in 23% to 60% of patients.

27. What is targeted therapy for melanoma?

Many melanomas have specific mutations in the mitogen-activated protein kinase (MAPK) pathway. Up to 70% of melanomas have a mutation in the MAPK pathway resulting in oncogenesis – 50% have a V600 mutation in *BRAF* and 15% to 20% have a mutation in *NRAS*. Targeted therapy with BRAF inhibitors (dabrafenib, vemurafenib, and encorafenib) showed dramatic anti tumor activity in initial clinical trials. However, patients later developed disease progression due to reactivation of the MAPK pathway. As a result, agents that inhibit another aspect of the MAPK pathway (MEK enzyme inhibitors – trametinib, cobimetinib, and bimetinib) are used in combination with BRAF inhibitors for patients with metastatic melanoma. Studies have shown that this combination has higher response rates and longer long-term survival rates for patients with metastatic melanoma.

Table 12.6 Ultraviolet Spectrum

ULTRAVIOLET RADIATION TYPE	WAVELENGTH (NM)
UVC	270–290
UVB	290–315
UVA	315–400

28. **What is the treatment for melanoma that has spread to the lymph nodes but has not metastasized distantly (Stage III)?**
For patients with Stage III melanoma (positive SLNB or clinically involved lymph nodes), adjuvant immunotherapy with a PD-1 inhibitor is recommended. In patients with a BRAF V600 mutation, a combination of a BRAF inhibitor plus an MAPK inhibitor can also be considered.

29. **What is the treatment for metastatic melanoma?**
Once melanoma has spread to the lymph nodes or other distant sites, mortality sharply increases, and systemic therapy is commonly indicated. Metastatic melanoma is not very responsive to radiation or traditional chemotherapy but may respond to immunotherapy, as noted above. For some patients, surgical removal or radiation therapy of metastatic lesions may be indicated, but these interventions are unlikely to impact overall mortality and are considered more palliative.

30. **What is the association between UV light and skin cancer?**
UV radiation emitted from the sun consists of ultraviolet C (UVC), ultraviolet B (UVB), and ultraviolet A (UVA). UVC is almost completely blocked by the Earth's atmosphere and UVB is somewhat blocked by the atmosphere; 95% of UV radiation that reaches the Earth's surface is UVA, and the remainder is UVB. Exposure to UV radiation has repeatedly been shown to increase the risk of nonmelanoma and melanoma skin cancers by inducing DNA mutations and causing immunosuppression within the skin, which decreases DNA repair. It was previously thought that UVB is responsible for most skin cancers; however, UVA is now thought to play a larger role. Tanning beds, which predominantly emit UVA light, have been associated with an increased risk of BCC, SCC, and melanoma. UVC is profoundly carcinogenic but does not contribute to skin cancer formation because it is blocked from reaching the ground by the Earth's atmosphere (Table 12.6).

31. **What are important methods of photoprotection?**
Photoprotection should be recommended for all patients, especially those at high risk for skin cancer or with a history of skin cancer. Photoprotection is multifactorial and includes avoidance of sun during peak hours of UV radiation (10:00 am to 2:00 pm), protective clothing, wide-brimmed hats, and sunscreen for exposed areas. Photoprotection is measured in UV protection factor (UPF) for clothing and hats and sun protection factor (SPF) for sunscreens. Sunscreens are composed of organic and inorganic compounds that absorb and scatter UV light. Chemical sunscreens (organic filters) absorb UV radiation and convert it to a small amount of heat. Mineral sunscreens (inorganic filters) form a protective barrier over the skin by reflecting and scattering UV light. Sunscreens should be "broad spectrum," meaning that they block both UVB and UVA for optimal photoprotection. It is important to note that protocols to determine sunscreen SPF include application of 2 mg/cm^2 of sunscreen, but most people apply a much smaller density of sunscreen. As a result, frequent reapplications (every 2 to 4 hours) and use of high SPF products is recommended.

32. **What is dermoscopy?**
Dermoscopy is a noninvasive diagnostic technique performed in the office setting. It is performed with a dermatoscope, a hand held instrument with polarized or nonpolarized light and a magnifier. Dermatoscopes allow for the visualization of certain structures in the epidermis and at the dermatoepidermal junction. Although this practice requires formal training, the utility of dermoscopy to distinguish between benign and malignant lesions has been well-demonstrated in the literature.

CONTROVERSIES

33. **What is the role of immunotherapy in the management of nonmelanoma skin cancers?**
In recent years, PD-1 inhibitors for advanced SCC have been proven to be more effective than other treatment modalities such as chemotherapeutic agents and monoclonal antibodies such as cetuximab. As a result, the PD-1 inhibitor cemiplimab was approved by the FDA in 2018 for the treatment of locally advanced or metastatic SCC. Unfortunately, immunotherapy is not recommended for solid organ transplant recipients with advanced SCC, due to the risk of transplant rejection. Investigation into the possible role for checkpoint inhibitors in the management of advanced BCC is in the early stages.

Table 12.7 American Joint Committee on Cancer (AJCC) Squamous Cell Carcinoma Tumor Staging System and Brigham and Women's Hospital (BWH) Staging System

AJCC Eighth Edition	
T1	<2 cm in greatest diameter
T2	>2 cm, but <4 cm in greatest diameter
T3	Tumor is >4 cm in greatest diameter, minor bone invasion, perineural invasion, or deep invasion
T4a	Tumor with gross cortical bone and/or marrow invasion
T4b	Tumor with skull bone invasion and/or skull base foramen involvement
BWH	
T1	0 High risk factors
T2a	1 High risk factor
T2b	2–3 High risk factors
T4	4 High risk factors or bone invasion

*BWH high-risk factors include tumor diameter >2 centimeters, poorly differentiated histology, perineural invasion of nerve(s) >0.1 millimeter in caliber, or tumor invasion beyond subcutaneous fat (excluding bone).

34. **Should SLNBs be performed for SCC?**
There have been no randomized clinical trials establishing when SLNBs are appropriate in cutaneous SCC. Retrospective studies have not shown that SLN status in SCC impacts relapse-free survival or overall survival. Currently, SLNB is not considered the standard of care for high-risk SCC, but more studies are needed to make definitive recommendations on the role of SLNB in SCC management.

BIBLIOGRAPHY

Amber K, McLeod MP, Nouri K: The Merkel cell polyomavirus and its involvement in Merkel cell carcinoma, *Dermatol Surg* 39(2): 232–238, 2013.
Balch CM, Gershenwald JE, Soong SJ, et al: Final version of 2009 AJCC melanoma staging and classification, *J Clin Oncol* 27(36): 6199–6206, 2009.
Bolognia J, Jorizzo JL, Rapini RP: *Dermatology*, St. Louis, MO, 2008, Mosby/Elsevier.
Chapman PB, Hauschild A, Robert C: Improved survival with vemurafenib in melanoma with BRAF V600E mutation, *N Eng J Med* 364(26):2507–2516, 2011.
Clarke CA, Robbins HA, Tatalovich Z, et al: Risk of Merkel cell carcinoma after solid organ transplantation, *J Natl Cancer Inst* 107(2): 2015, dju382.
Costantino D, Lowe L, Brown DL: Basosquamous carcinoma-an under-recognized, high-risk cutaneous neoplasm: case study and review of the literature, *J Plast Reconstr Aesthet Surg* 59(4):424–428, 2006.
Demer AM, Vance KK, Cheraghi N, et al: Benefit of Mohs micrographic surgery over wide local excision for melanoma of the head and neck: a rational approach to treatment, *Dermatol Surg* 45(3):381–389, 2019.
Hollenbeak CS, Todd MM, Billingsley EM, et al: Increased incidence of melanoma in renal transplantation recipients, *Cancer* 104(9): 1962–1967, 2005.
Jambusaria-Pahlajani A, Kanetsky PA, Kria PS, et al: Evaluation of AJCC tumor staging for cutaneous squamous cell carcinoma and a proposed alternative tumor staging system, *JAMA Dermatol* 149(4):402–410, 2013.
Lhote R, Lambert J, Lejeune J, et al: Sentinel lymph node biopsy in cutaneous squamous cell carcinoma series of 37 cases and systematic review of the literature, *Acta Derm Venereol* 98(7):671–676, 2018.
Migden MR, Rischin D, Schmults CD, et al: PD-1 blockade with cemiplimab in advanced cutaneous squamous-cell carcinoma, *N Engl J Med* 379(4):341–351, 2018.
Mudigonda T, Levender MM, O'Neill JL, et al: Incidence, risk factors, and preventative management of skin cancers in organ transplant recipients: a review of single- and multicenter retrospective studies from 2006 to 2010, *Dermatol Surg* 39(3 Pt 1):345–364, 2013.
Rigel DS, Friedman RJ, Kopf AW: Lifetime risk for development of skin cancer in the U.S. population: current risk is now 1 in 5, *J Am Acad Dermatol* 35(6):1012–1013, 1996.
Robbins HA, Clarke CA, Arron ST, et al: Melanoma risk and survival among organ transplant recipients, *J Invest Dermatol* 135(11):2657–2665, 2015.
Schmitt AR, Brewer JD, Bordeaux JS, et al: Staging for cutaneous squamous cell carcinoma as a predictor of sentinel lymph node biopsy results: meta-analysis of American Joint Committee on Cancer criteria and a proposed alternative system, *JAMA Dermatol* 150(1):19–24, 2014.
Sladden MJ, Balch C, Barzilai DA, et al: Surgical excision margins for primary cutaneous melanoma, *Cochrane Database Syst Rev* 7(4):CD004835, 2009.
Weber JS, Mandala M, Del Vecchio M, et al: Adjuvant therapy with nivolumab versus ipilimumab after complete resection of stage III/IV melanoma: updated results from a phase III trial (CheckMate 238), *J Clin Oncol* 36S, 2018.
Xie P, Lefrançois P: Efficacy, safety, and comparison of sonic hedgehog inhibitors in basal cell carcinomas: a systematic review and meta-analysis, *J Am Acad Dermatol* 79(6): 1089-1100.e17, 2018.
Yélamos O, Braun RP, Liopyris K, et al: Usefulness of dermoscopy to improve the clinical and histopathologic diagnosis of skin cancers, *J Am Acad Dermatol* 80(2):365–367, 2019.

CHAPTER 13

ORAL CAVITY AND OROPHARYNX MALIGNANCY

Julie A. Goddard, MD, FACS

KEY POINTS

1. Despite their proximity, oral cavity and oropharyngeal cancers can behave differently and thus are treated differently.
2. Premalignant lesions of the oral cavity warrant evaluation and follow-up. Biopsies of clinically different lesions show nonspecific dysplasia.
3. Pathologic depth of invasion is the main determinant in treatment decisions and staging for oral cavity cancer.
4. Recent discoveries about human papillomavirus (HPV) have changed the face of oropharynx cancer.

Pearls
1. Oral cavity cancer most commonly spreads to lymph nodes in levels I, II, and III. Oropharynx cancer most commonly spreads to lymph nodes in levels II, III, IV.
2. Tumor (T) staging of oral cavity and oropharynx tumors can generally be remembered by size criteria (T1 = 0–2 centimeters, T2 = 2–4 centimeters, T3 = >4 centimeters, T4 = extension to adjacent structures).
3. Oral cavity cancer is primarily treated with surgery, whereas oropharynx cancer is often treated primarily in a nonsurgical fashion with radiation with or without chemotherapy.
4. Cervical lymph node metastasis is a key driver of prognosis in oral cavity cancers and non-HPV-related oropharynx cancers but less so in HPV-related oropharynx cancers.

QUESTIONS

1. **The oral cavity extends from the lip to the circumvallate papillae inferiorly and the junction of the hard and soft palate superiorly. Name the eight subsites within the oral cavity.**
   1. Mucosal lip
   2. Buccal mucosa
   3. Lower (mandibular) alveolar ridge/gingiva
   4. Upper (maxillary) alveolar ridge/gingiva
   5. Retromolar trigone
   6. Hard palate
   7. Floor of mouth
   8. Oral tongue (anterior two-thirds)

2. **What is the most common type of malignancy within the oral cavity?**
   Squamous cell carcinoma: As in all head and neck sites, squamous cell carcinoma (SCC) is by far the most common type of tumor seen. More than 90% of oral cavity cancers are SCC. Other malignant tumors include minor salivary gland malignancies, Kaposi's sarcoma, other sarcomas, melanoma, and, rarely, lymphoma.

3. **Where in the oral cavity are minor salivary gland malignancies most commonly seen? What is the most common type?**
   Within the oral cavity, minor salivary gland malignancies most commonly occur on the hard palate. Adenoid cystic carcinoma is the most common tumor of the minor salivary glands.

4. **What are the most common subsites for oral cavity SCC?**
   a. Lips: Overall, 15% to 30% of oral cancers arise from mucosal (wet) and external vermilion (dry) lip combined. The lower lip is much more common a site than the upper lip (>90% arise in the lower lip). American Joint Committee on Cancer (AJCC) staging and National Comprehensive Cancer Network (NCCN) guidelines now separate mucosal lip squamous carcinoma (included as oral cavity) and vermilion dry lip carcinoma (included

with cutaneous squamous cell carcinoma). The external vermilion (dry) lip is exposed to external environmental factors, such as ultraviolet radiation from the sun, and thus a tumor in this area behaves more like cutaneous SCC. Current classifications of lip cancers make the true mucosal lip a less common subsite, although much of the historical data are based on all lip cancers being staged within the oral cavity.
  b. Oral tongue: 20% to 30% of oral cavity cancers. The lateral tongue is more common than the dorsal tongue.

5. **Discuss three premalignant clinical lesions or conditions of the oral cavity**
   a. Leukoplakia: Defined as a white keratotic plaque or patch that cannot be rubbed off. Often seen due to chronic trauma or irritation of oral mucosa. Most are benign, but malignant potential/transformation rate is very difficult to predict. Baseline biopsy and follow-up or excision are recommended depending on pathologic findings.
   b. Erythroplakia (red plaque/lesion): Red mucosal plaque not arising from an obvious mechanical or inflammatory cause. Has much higher malignant potential than leukoplakia (estimated to be seven times more malignant potential). Can be seen in conjunction with leukoplakia. More aggressive therapy recommended than that for leukoplakia.
   c. Oral lichen planus: Lacy white lines primarily noted on buccal mucosa, known as Wickham's striae (buccal mucosa is classic location, but changes can be seen throughout the oral cavity). Exact cause is unknown but thought to be immune-mediated (lymphocytic infiltration of epithelial layers seen). Associated with pain and burning, and the clinical course waxes and wanes. Treated with topical steroids, systemic steroids, and sometimes other immunosuppressants. Lifetime malignant transformation risk is 5% to 10%.

   Note: The above are *clinical*, rather than *pathologic*, descriptions of premalignant conditions. Dysplasia, which can be seen in any of these lesions, is the pathologic description of premalignant change describing degrees of cellular change. Dysplasia can be described as mild, moderate, and severe. Severe dysplasia and carcinoma in situ are often utilized interchangeably by pathologists.

6. **Are oral cavity SCCs commonly caused by human papillomavirus (HPV)?**
   No. Whereas *oropharynx* SCC is very commonly driven by HPV, only a small percentage (<3%) of oral cavity cancers are truly HPV-associated.

7. **Where in the neck do regional metastases of oral cavity SCC most commonly appear and how is this clinically significant?**
   Regional nodal disease from oral cavity SCC most commonly presents in the upper cervical lymph nodes – level I (submental and submandibular) and levels II and III (upper and middle jugular nodes). This relatively predictable nodal drainage of oral cavity subsites has led to the use of what is termed supraomohyoid neck dissection (includes levels I, II, and III) being utilized for elective nodal dissection in oral cavity cancers. The finding of microscopic nodal disease in levels III and IV without level I and II disease in more than 15% of patients with *oral tongue* cancer in a 1997 study has led to some recommending inclusion of level IV in elective neck dissections for oral tongue cancer.

8. **How is cancer of the oral cavity staged?**
   SCC of the oral cavity is staged according to the tumor, node, metastasis (TNM) system by the AJCC, currently in its eighth edition, utilized since 2017. Within the oral cavity, size and depth of invasion (DOI) are major factors determining T stage (eighth edition AJCC included DOI in T staging for the first time).
   T staging
   Tx: Primary tumor cannot be assessed
   Tis: Carcinoma in situ
   T1: Tumor ≤ 2 cm with DOI ≤ 5 mm
   T2: Tumor ≤ 2 cm with DOI > 5 mm or tumor > 2 cm and ≤ 4 cm with DOI ≤ 10 mm
   T3: Tumor > 2 cm and ≤ 4 cm with DOI > 10 mm or tumor > 4 cm with DOI ≤ 10 mm
   T4a: Moderately advanced local disease.
   Tumor > 4 cm, with DOI > 10 mm or tumor invades adjacent structures only (e.g., through cortical bone of the mandible or maxilla, or involves the maxillary sinus or skin of the face). Note: Superficial erosion of bone or tooth socket by a gingival primary is not sufficient to classify a tumor as T4.
   T4b: Very advanced local disease.
   Tumor invades masticator space, pterygoid plates, or skull base and/or encases internal carotid artery
   Nodal staging was previously the same for most head and neck squamous cell cancers. However, the eight edition of AJCC staging has changed nodal staging such that it differs between head and neck sites. Clinical (cN) nodal staging for oral cavity cancers now includes a clinical (based upon exam/imaging) assessment of extranodal extension (ENE). cN staging for oral cavity cancers is as follows:
   Clinical N staging
   Nx: Regional lymph nodes cannot be assessed
   N0: No regional lymph node metastasis

N1: Metastasis in a single ipsilateral lymph node, 3 centimeters or smaller in greatest dimension, and ENE(-)

N2a: Metastasis in a single ipsilateral lymph node larger than 3 centimeters but not larger than 6 centimeters in greatest dimension and ENE(-)

N2b: Metastases in multiple ipsilateral lymph nodes, none greater than 6 centimeters in greatest dimension, and ENE(-)

N2c: Metastases in bilateral or contralateral lymph nodes, none larger than 6 centimeters in greatest dimension, and ENE(-)

N3a: Metastasis in a lymph node larger than 6 centimeters in greatest dimension and ENE(-)

N3b: Metastasis in any node(s) and clinically overt ENE(+)

9. **How is depth of invasion (DOI) utilized in treatment of small oral tongue cancers?**
DOI correlates with risk of nodal metastasis, risk of recurrence, and prognosis. DOI and tumor thickness are not technically synonymous, because exophytic tumors can be very thick but have shallow depth of invasion into underlying structures. True DOI is measured from the basement membrane. Especially in oral tongue cancer, DOI has been studied as a deciding factor regarding elective treatment of a clinically node-negative neck. Multiple trials have supported tumor DOI of 4 millimeters as a cutoff point regarding elective treatment of the neck. Tumors with depth of invasion of 4 millimeters or greater are associated with more than 20% incidence of microscopic nodal metastasis and thus elective neck treatment is generally recommended, most commonly with neck dissection at the time of resection. Current investigation into sentinel node biopsy is ongoing, and elective neck irradiation is also considered acceptable oncologically, though less commonly utilized.

10. **What does the initial workup for patients with oral cavity or oropharynx cancer typically include?**
Complete history and physical examination, radiographic imaging (neck computed tomography [CT] with contrast or magnetic resonance imaging with gadolinium), dental evaluation, tissue biopsy, and chest imaging. It is currently more common to utilize chest CT or positron emission tomography (PET)/CT over plain chest x-ray; however, use of PET/CT as the primary staging imaging modality for all patients with head and neck cancer is a subject of ongoing study. Generally, most patients will have laboratory evaluation including liver function tests, although an abnormal liver function test leading to the finding of liver metastases at initial presentation is a rare scenario.

11. **What is the recommended treatment for oral cavity cancer?**
Primary surgery is accepted as first-line therapy for all oral cavity sites. Surgical excision of all involved structures including a margin of normal tissue is performed. The generally accepted *pathologically* negative margin is 5 millimeters. Due to tissue shrinkage, clinical margins measured and excised by the surgeon intraoperatively are 1 to 2 centimeters.

12. **What factors are the indications for postoperative adjuvant radiation therapy after resection of oral SCC to minimize risk of locoregional recurrence?**
Tumor factors
   a. Locally advanced T3 or T4 lesions
   b. High-grade histology
   c. Presence of perineural invasion or lymphovascular invasion on pathology
   d. Infiltrating rather than pushing borders of tumor
   e. Positive or close (<5 millimeters on pathologic specimen) margins of surgical resection
   f. Surgeon concern regarding adequacy of resection regardless of histologic surgical margins
      Nodal factors
   g. N stage higher than N1
   h. Surgical contamination (excisional or incisional nodal biopsy prior to definitive surgery)
   i. Presence of extracapsular extension (extranodal extension or ENE)
      Note: Positive margins and presence of extracapsular extension are even higher-risk features for recurrence and are used as indications to give chemotherapy in addition to radiation therapy postoperatively.

13. **What are the subsites within the oropharynx?**
The oropharynx is bounded by the junction of the hard and soft palate and circumvallate papillae anteriorly, superior surface of the soft palate superiorly, and pharyngoepiglottic fold inferiorly. Subsites include:
   a. Tonsils (palatine)
   b. Base of tongue and vallecula
   c. Soft palate
   d. Tonsillar pillars
   e. Posterior and lateral pharyngeal walls

14. **What is the primary lymphatic drainage of the oropharynx?**
    Lymphatic drainage is primarily to the jugular lymphatics in levels II, III, and IV. Nodal metastases are most often seen in level II. Isolated nodal metastasis to levels I or V is rare from oropharynx tumors. Subsites within the oropharynx known specifically to have rich bilateral lymphatic drainage are the base of the tongue and the soft palate (as well as the posterior pharyngeal wall, which is generally a much less common primary site for SCC). Oropharyngeal structures also drain to retropharyngeal and parapharyngeal lymph nodes.

15. **Which is more common to present as an isolated neck mass: oral cavity or oropharyngeal SCC?**
    Oropharyngeal cancer may commonly present as an isolated neck mass without other symptoms, whereas oral cancer more commonly presents with oral cavity symptoms such as pain, bleeding, ulcer/visible lesion, change in speech, and/or ear pain.

16. **List the common symptoms of oropharyngeal cancer.**
    Oropharyngeal cancer commonly presents with throat pain or fullness, dysphagia, odynophagia, ear pain (referred), neck mass (often painless), change in voice (muffled voice), foul breath or foul taste, and expectorating bloody secretions. With more advanced disease, patients may have trismus, difficulty with tongue mobility due to deep infiltration, or airway obstruction.

17. **How do oral and pharyngeal neoplasms refer pain to the ipsilateral ear?**
    Otalgia is referred from the pharynx by way of the pharyngeal cranial nerves IX and X, which also supply sensory innervation to the ear. The tongue and floor of the mouth are supplied by the lingual branch of V3. V3 also provides sensation to the external auditory canal, tympanic membrane, and temporomandibular joint through the auriculotemporal nerve. In some patients, the sensation of otalgia is much more prominent than oral or throat pain.

18. **Why should one be wary of the diagnosis of "branchial cleft cyst" in a 55-year-old patient?**
    Oropharyngeal SCC very commonly presents with cystic nodal metastases. Since the most common cervical location of these is level II of the neck, these metastases are in the presenting location of a second branchial cleft cyst. These cystic metastases can have a thin wall and be full of clear/serous fluid just like the branchial cleft cyst. We often cannot rely on fine-needle aspiration (FNA) for diagnosis as the fluid obtained from either type of neck mass may look similar under the microscope – degenerated squamous cells and debris can be seen in the fluid of both a malignant nodal metastasis and a branchial cleft cyst. Though it is possible for an adult to have a congenital branchial anomaly present later in life, this is an uncommon scenario, and one must think of a cystic neck mass in an adult as *cancer until proven otherwise.*

19. **The incidence of some head and neck malignancies in the United States has been declining slowly in the recent past (likely due to decreased rates of smoking). However, the rate of oropharyngeal cancer is increasing significantly. To what factor is this attributed?**
    HPV-associated oropharyngeal cancer is increasing dramatically in the United States and some European countries. Since the late 1990s and early 2000s, HPV has risen to the forefront of discussion in oropharyngeal SCC and the incidence of HPV-associated oropharyngeal cancer exceeds that of HPV-negative cancers. Primary sites that are most associated with HPV are the tonsil and the base of tongue. The virus is felt to preferentially affect the lymphoid tissue in these sites (though similar lymphoid tissue in the nasopharynx does not seem to be similarly affected – nasopharyngeal cancer rates have not shown similar increase rates). The overall prognosis associated with HPV-positive SCC is significantly better than that of HPV-negative SCC and thus these two are now staged differently in the eighth edition of AJCC staging (see question 23).

20. **Which subtype of HPV is considered to be the highest risk for association with oropharyngeal malignancy?**
    HPV 16 is by far the most common subtype of HPV associated with oropharyngeal SCC. Types 18, 31, and 33 are also considered high-risk subtypes but are not commonly seen in oropharyngeal cancer. Overexpression of the p16 protein can be evaluated by immunohistochemistry on pathologic specimens and is commonly utilized as a surrogate marker for HPV-positive tumors (designated p16+ vs p16−).

21. **How does HPV cause oropharyngeal cancer?**
    Viral proteins E6 and E7 cause inactivation of the p53 tumor suppressor gene, allowing malignant cells to proceed through normal cell cycle checkpoints and continue to replicate.

22. **How do patients with oropharyngeal cancer diagnosed commonly today differ from those seen more than 30 years ago?**
    We are more commonly seeing HPV-positive oropharyngeal cancer in younger (40s–50s) patients with little to no smoking history. Specifically, the incidence is expanding in the White male population (although the female

incidence is expanding as well). HPV-associated tumors present with early cervical nodal metastases, but these patients are noted to have an overall better prognosis than their HPV-negative counterparts.

23. **How are oropharyngeal cancers staged?**
The AJCC TNM system. The eighth edition of the AJCC TNM system brought significant change to the staging of oropharyngeal SCC as HPV-mediated (p16+) SCC of the oropharynx is a new classification. Though T (tumor) staging is fairly similar between p16+ and p16−, the nodal staging is quite different. Nodal staging for p16− oropharynx cancer is similar to that for oral cavity cancer.

HPV-mediated (p16+) Oropharyngeal Cancer Staging

T staging	*Clinical N staging*
T0: No primary identified	Nx: Regional lymph nodes cannot be assessed
T1: Tumor 2 centimeters or smaller in greatest dimension	N0: No regional lymph node metastases
T2: Tumor larger than 2 centimeters but not larger than 4 centimeters in greatest dimension	N1: One or more ipsilateral lymph nodes, none larger than 6 centimeters
T3: Tumor larger than 4 centimeters in greatest dimension or extension to the lingual surface of the epiglottis	N2: Contralateral or bilateral lymph nodes, none larger than 6 centimeters
T4: Moderately advanced local disease: Tumor invades the larynx, extrinsic muscle of tongue, medial pterygoid, hard palate, or mandible or beyond (*Note: Mucosal extension to lingual surface of epiglottis from primary tumors of the base of tongue and vallecula does not constitute invasion of the larynx.)	N3: Lymph node(s) larger than 6 centimeters

p16− Oropharyngeal Cancer Staging

T staging	*Clinical N staging*
TX: Primary tumor cannot be assessed	Nx: Regional lymph nodes cannot be assessed
Tis: Carcinoma in situ	N0: No regional lymph node metastasis
T1: Tumor 2 centimeters or smaller in greatest dimension	N1: Metastasis in a single ipsilateral lymph node, 3 centimeters or smaller in greatest dimension, and ENE(−)
T2: Tumor larger than 2 centimeters but not larger than 4 centimeters in greatest dimension	N2a: Metastasis in single ipsilateral lymph node larger than 3 centimeters but not larger than 6 centimeters in greatest dimension and ENE(−)
T3: Tumor larger than 4 centimeters in greatest dimension or extension to the lingual surface of the epiglottis	N2b: Metastases in multiple ipsilateral lymph nodes, none greater than 6 centimeters in greatest dimension, and ENE(−)
T4a: Moderately advanced local disease Tumor invades the larynx, extrinsic muscle of tongue, medial pterygoid, hard palate, or mandible or beyond (*Note: Mucosal extension to lingual surface of epiglottis from primary tumors of the base of tongue and vallecula does not constitute invasion of the larynx.)	N2c: Metastases in bilateral or contralateral lymph nodes, none larger than 6 centimeters in greatest dimension, and ENE(−)
T4b: Very advanced local disease Tumor invades lateral pterygoid muscle, pterygoid plates, lateral nasopharynx, and skull base or encases carotid artery	N3a: Metastasis in a lymph node larger than 6 centimeters in greatest dimension and ENE(−) N3b: Metastasis in any node(s) and clinically overt ENE(+)

24. **How does primary treatment of oropharyngeal SCC differ from treatment of oral cavity SCC?**
Whereas the unequivocal recommendation for primary treatment of oral cavity cancer is surgical excision, oropharyngeal cancer is commonly treated primarily with radiation with or without chemotherapy. Based initially on studies from the 1990s and 2000s regarding "organ preservation" therapy for laryngeal cancer showing similar oncologic outcomes between nonsurgical therapy and laryngectomy for larynx cancer, further evidence amassed for nonsurgical treatment of oropharyngeal cancer providing oncologic outcome similar to surgery plus postoperative radiation and significantly less morbidity. Thus, radiation-based therapy became the standard of care for treatment of most oropharyngeal SCCs over the last 30 years. With improved technology to allow for less-invasive access to the oropharynx (TLM and TORS – see below), surgical therapy for oropharyngeal cancer has re-emerged and is offered for early-stage tumors. This is the subject of much ongoing research.

25. **Describe two techniques for a minimally invasive approach to the oropharynx.**
a. Transoral laser CO_2 microsurgery (TLM) – Initially described in the 1970s, this is a technique utilized initially for laryngeal surgery and subsequently applied to tumors of the oropharynx and hypopharynx. It utilizes laryn-

goscopes of various types to provide access to the pharynx and binocular microscopy for magnified view of the tumor. A CO_2 laser is used as the cutting and coagulating instrument. This technique is traditionally limited by line of sight – the structures being visualized are in a straight line with the laryngoscope used and the laser travels in a straight line from the microscope (though use of a CO_2 laser fiber has allowed for some degree of angled application).

   b. Transoral robotic surgery (TORS) – Initially described in 2005, this technique utilizes robotic arms inserted into the mouth held open by a suspended retractor and controlled by the surgeon at a distant console. High-definition binocular magnification angled at 0° or 30° is used for visualization and the robotic arms can be fitted with various grasping, cautery, or cutting instruments (including a laser fiber). This technique has become more widely utilized for access to the oropharynx than TLM.

26. **How does the presence of cervical nodal metastases affect the overall prognosis for oral cavity and oropharyngeal cancer?**
    Prior to p16+ oropharyngeal cancers, cervical nodal metastasis was generally associated with a worse prognosis for all head and neck sites, with survival rates diminished by up to 50% compared with patients lacking cervical nodal disease. While this holds true for oral cavity and p16– oropharyngeal cancer groups where nodal disease is a driver of prognosis, cervical nodal disease is not as strongly associated with overall prognosis in p16+ oropharyngeal cancers.

27. **How will the HPV vaccine impact oropharyngeal SCC?**
    In June 2020, the US FDA approved the GARDASIL 9 vaccine for prevention of oropharyngeal and other head and neck cancers. GARDASIL 9 includes protection against HPV types 6, 11, 16, 18, 31, 33, 45, 52, and 58. Types 6 and 11 are associated with anogenital warts, and the other types have been associated with cervical, anogenital, and head and neck cancers. Prior versions of HPV vaccines have been approved since 2006 for prevention of HPV in association with cervical and anogenital cancers, but the FDA head-and-neck indication has only recently come about. However, with use of the vaccine since the first decade of this century, head and neck oncologists are hopeful that this will change the incidence over time. Based on recent population studies, the overall incidence of HPV-associated oropharyngeal cancer in the United States is projected to drop only modestly by 2045 (14.3 vs 13.8 per 100,000 people). However, the decrease in incidence is more notable in younger patients younger than 55 years of age and use of the vaccine is predicted to prevent 6334 cases of HPV-associated oropharyngeal SCC between 2018 and 2045. Though the clinical benefit of this vaccine in oropharyngeal cancer will take many years to realize, experts remain optimistic about this intervention as an effective preventative measure.

BIBLIOGRAPHY

Bernier J, Domenge C, Ozsahin M, et al: Postoperative irradiation with or without concomitant chemotherapy for locally advanced head and neck cancer, *N Engl J Med* 350(19):1945–1952, 2004.

Byers RM, Weber RS, Andrews T, et al: Frequency and therapeutic implications of "skip metastases" in the neck from squamous cell carcinoma of the oral tongue, *Head Neck* 19(1):14–19, 1997.

Chaturvedi AK, Engels EA, Pfeiffer RM, et al: Human papillomavirus and rising oropharyngeal cancer incidence in the United States, *J Clin Oncol* 29(32):4294–4301, 2011.

Cooper JS, Pajak TF, Forastiere AA, et al: Postoperative concurrent radiotherapy and chemotherapy for high-risk squamous-cell carcinoma of the head and neck, *N Engl J Med* 350(19):1937–1944, 2004.

Edge S, Byrd DR, Compton CC, et al: *AJCC Cancer Staging Manual*, 7th ed, New York, 2010, Springer.

Holsinger FC, Sweeney AD, Jantharapattana K, et al: The emergence of endoscopic head and neck surgery, *Curr Oncol Rep* 12(3):216–222, 2010.

Huang SH, Hwang D, Lockwood G, et al: Predictive value of tumor thickness for cervical lymph node involvement in squamous cell carcinoma of the oral cavity: a meta-analysis of reported studies, *Cancer* 115(7):1489–1497, 2009.

Liang XH, Lewis J, Foote R, et al: Prevalence and significance of human papillomavirus in oral tongue cancer: the Mayo Clinic experience, *J Oral Maxillofac Surg* 66(9):1875–1880, 2008.

Machado J, Reiss PP, Zhang T, et al: Low prevalence of human papillomavirus in oral cavity carcinomas, *Head Neck Oncol* 12(2):6, 2011.

Monroe MM, Gross ND: Management of the clinical node-negative neck in early-stage oral cavity squamous cell carcinoma, *Otolaryngol Clin N Am* 45(5):1181–1193, 2012.

Myers EM, Suen JY, Myers JN, et al: *Cancer of the Head and Neck*, 4th ed, Philadelphia, 2003, Saunders.

NCCN Guidelines Version 3.2021, 04/27/2021. Available at www.nccn.org.

Shah JP, Patel SG, Singh B: *Jatin Shah's Head and Neck Surgery and Oncology*, 4th ed, Philadelphia, 2012, Elsevier Mosby.

Zhang Z, Fakhry C, D'Souza G: Projected association of human papillomavirus vaccination with oropharynx cancer incidence in the US, 2020–2045, *JAMA Oncol* 7(10):e212907, 2021.

CHAPTER 14

CANCER OF THE HYPOPHARYNX, LARYNX, AND ESOPHAGUS

Marcia Eustaquio, MD

KEY POINTS

1. The most affected subsite for laryngeal cancer is the glottis.
2. Smokers are approximately 20 times more likely than nonsmokers to develop laryngeal cancer. Smoking and alcohol intake are synergistic risk factors for the development of laryngeal cancer.
3. Conservation surgery or radiation are treatment options for voice preservation in early laryngeal cancer.
4. The supraglottis has bilateral lymphatic drainage.
5. Hypopharyngeal cancers have a poor prognosis and are usually discovered at a later stage than laryngeal cancers.

Pearls
1. Smoking through out treatment for laryngeal cancer increases the chance for treatment failure and recurrence.
2. Both surgery and radiation therapy have similarly good outcomes for early glottic squamous cell carcinomas.
3. At least one cricoarytenoid joint must be preserved in conservation laryngeal surgery for voicing.
4. Hypopharyngeal cancer is notable for frequent submucosal spread and carries a worse prognosis than cancer of the larynx.

QUESTIONS

1. **Describe the general anatomic divisions of the larynx.**
   Vertically, the larynx is subdivided into three regions: the supraglottis, the glottis, and the subglottis. The division of these three subsites reflects embryologic development and natural barriers to cancer spread.

   The *supraglottis* can be thought of as a three-dimensional box containing a suprahyoid and infrahyoid epiglottis, the aryepiglottic folds, arytenoids, ventricles, and false vocal folds. It extends from the superior surface of the epiglottis and the superior edge of the aryepiglottic folds to a horizontal plane passing through the lateral margin of the ventricle and the superior surface of the true vocal folds. The supraglottis has bilateral lymphatic drainage to the upper and middle jugular lymph nodes.

   The *glottis* begins at the superior surface of the true vocal fold and extends inferiorly 1 centimeter. Laterally, it is bordered by the thyroid cartilage with the lateral ventricle coming to the superior most extent. It contains the anterior and posterior commissures. The vocal folds themselves have sparse lymphatics; therefore deep invasion is needed for unilateral lymphatic spread.

   The *subglottis* begins at the inferior border of the glottis (1 centimeter below the supraglottis) and proceeds to the inferior border of the cricoid cartilage.

2. **Regarding the divisions of the larynx, where does laryngeal cancer commonly occur?**
   Laryngeal cancer most commonly arises in the glottis (60%), followed by the supraglottis (35%) and subglottis (2%); another 3% are transglottic and involve multiple subsites. An overwhelming 95% of glottic cancers arise from the true vocal cords. Because of natural barriers to spread and early presenting symptoms, laryngeal cancer is often confined to the larynx at time of diagnosis (60% of cases).

3. **How common is laryngeal cancer?**
   Laryngeal cancer is the second most common malignancy of the head and neck (after oral cavity/oropharynx). Currently, in the United States, there are over 12,000 new cases of laryngeal cancer annually. One-third of these patients will die from their disease. The number of new cases is declining by roughly 2% to 3% per year due to decreased smoking. Laryngeal cancer is 3.8 times more common in men than women, though the gender disparity has narrowed in recent years due to the increased proportion of female smokers.

4. **What are the risk factors for laryngeal cancer?**
Tobacco and alcohol are the primary risk factors for laryngeal cancer. The risk is thought to be directly proportional to the duration and intensity of exposure. Smoking and alcohol are synergistic in increasing cancer risk rather than merely additive. Risk does decrease slowly after cessation but does not return to baseline for at least 20 years. Patients who continue to smoke through out their treatment are at a higher risk of recurrence and development of a second primary. There are conflicting data as to whether laryngopharyngeal reflux could be a risk factor. One meta-analysis has shown an increased risk in patients with confirmed gastroesophageal reflux disease. Human papillomavirus has not definitively been shown to be a cause of laryngeal cancer.

5. **What types of cancers are found in the larynx?**
Squamous cell carcinoma (SCC) is the most common type of malignancy found in the larynx, accounting for more than 95% of all tumors. Variations of SCC include verrucous carcinoma (2% to 4%) and spindle cell carcinoma. Verrucous carcinoma carries an improved prognosis, while spindle cell variants are more aggressive. Both subtypes are typically treated with surgical excision.
   Less common nonepithelial tumors include adenoid cystic carcinoma, mucoepidermoid carcinoma, sarcoma (e.g., fibrosarcoma, chondrosarcoma, liposarcoma), neuroendocrine tumor (e.g., paragangliomas, carcinoid), contiguous lesions (i.e., thyroid), and metastatic lesions.

6. **How might a patient with laryngeal cancer present?**
Hoarseness, dysphagia, odynophagia, referred otalgia, globus sensation, weight loss, and neck mass can all be presenting symptoms. Glottic cancers tend to present early with hoarseness, whereas airway obstruction and hemoptysis are later findings. Supraglottic cancers often present with dysphagia and odynophagia. Otalgia can occur due to pharyngeal extension. Hoarseness occurs secondary to transglottic extension or arytenoid involvement. Airway obstruction can be gradual with bulky disease or may be acute in onset from a ball–valve type of obstruction. Supraglottic tumors are usually discovered later and have a poorer prognosis as these symptoms arise with progression beyond the supraglottis. Subglottic carcinomas present with signs and symptoms of early airway obstruction such as biphasic stridor.

7. **Discuss the workup of laryngeal cancer.**
History and physical exam should address symptoms such as dyspnea, stridor, dysphagia, odynophagia, otalgia, weight loss, and hoarseness. Special attention should be paid to risk factors for carcinoma, primarily smoking, alcohol, and history of cancer. It is important to determine overall health and functional status as this will play a key role in determining treatment. A complete head and neck exam should be performed with careful visualization and palpation of the oral cavity, oropharynx, and neck. Laryngoscopy should be performed with any lesions characterized by location, size, endophytic or exophytic nature, vocal cord mobility, and patency of the airway.
   In cases other than a T1 glottic primary, additional imaging should be ordered to evaluate extent of disease and metastatic potential. Computed tomography (CT) of the neck with contrast is the most utilized modality. Magnetic resonance imaging (MRI) can also be useful and is more sensitive in differentiating soft tissue and cartilage involvement. Positron emission tomography (PET) may be helpful in advanced stages for metastatic workup. Operative endoscopy should be pursued with direct visualization, palpation, and tissue sampling. In select cases, debulking and/or airway stabilization will also be warranted.

8. **What is the significance of a paralyzed vocal fold?**
A fixed or paralyzed vocal fold is one that appears immobile on examination and can be associated with hoarseness or aspiration. A cord can be rendered immobile in several ways, including mass effect of the tumor, cricoarytenoid joint involvement, or recurrent laryngeal nerve involvement. Vocal cord immobility upstages laryngeal and hypopharyngeal cancers to T3. This is in contrast to a partially immobile or paretic vocal fold. A vocal fold with decreased mobility is characterized as at least a T2 cancer.

9. **What membranous structures help prevent the spread of cancer outside of the larynx?**
There are two fibroelastic membranes that help prevent cancer spread from the larynx. The *conus elasticus* helps support the vocal folds and extends from the cricoid cartilage to the vocal ligaments. It is the lower part of the elastic membrane of the larynx. The *quadrangular membrane* supports the supraglottis and begins superiorly at the lateral margin of the epiglottis and proceeds inferiorly to the false cords. This is the upper part of the elastic membrane of the larynx. This quadrangular membrane and the conus elasticus are separated by the laryngeal ventricle and form the medial boundary of the paraglottic space (Fig. 14.1).

10. **Discuss the routes of local spread and nodal metastasis of SCC for the different laryngeal regions.**
Laryngeal cancer may spread by direct extension or through the lymphatics. Local extension may occur through the paraglottic space, which is a fibrofatty-filled space bounded medially by the conus elasticus and quadrangular membrane, laterally by the thyrohyoid membrane and thyroid cartilage lamina, and posteriorly by the medial mucosa of the piriform sinus. Entry of a mass into this space, commonly from the laryngeal ventricle, allows for

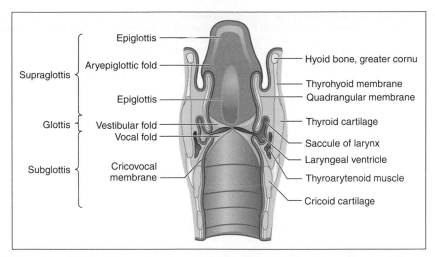

Fig. 14.1 Coronal view of the internal larynx with quadrangular membrane and conus elasticus (cricovocal membrane). (From Bogart BI, Ort V: *Elsevier's Integrated Anatomy and Embryology*, 1st ed, Philadelphia, 2007, Elsevier.)

transglottic extension. Paraglottic space involvement upstages any laryngeal carcinoma to T3. The pre-epiglottic space is a fibrofatty-filled space bounded superiorly by the hyoepiglottic ligament, anteriorly by the thyrohyoid membrane and thyroid cartilage, and posteriorly by the epiglottis and thyroepiglottic membrane. It is continuous laterally with the paraglottic space. Glottic cancer can invade from the anterior commissure along Broyles' ligament into the thyroid cartilage and via lacunae of the epiglottis into the pre-epiglottic space.

Regional lymphatic spread also occurs. The lymphatics of the supraglottis follow the superior laryngeal arteries draining to the upper and middle jugular lymph nodes in levels 2 and 3. Bilateral lymphatics allow cancer to spread to the ipsilateral or contralateral lymph nodes. The incidence of nodal metastasis varies from 0% to 57% depending on the primary tumor stage. The glottis is without notable lymphatic drainage; regional nodal spread for glottic cancer is below 10%. Subglottic carcinoma extends to and through the cricothyroid membrane to involve the lateral paratracheal and cervical lymphatics as well as the medial prelaryngeal (Delphian) node. There is also rich lymphatic drainage from the postcricoid area.

11. **How is laryngeal carcinoma staged?**
Laryngeal cancers are staged based on their site of origin in the supraglottis, glottis, or subglottis, according to the TNM classification system of the American Joint Committee on Cancer (AJCC) (Table 14.1). For a patient to have clinical evidence of extranodal extension, the nodal disease must be fixed to the skin or underlying muscle or cause nerve dysfunction through invasion on clinical exam. On imaging, extranodal extension is present if invasion into adjacent structures and ill-defined borders are observed. If the patient has had a neck dissection, they will be staged pathologically, where extranodal extension is then defined by extension of the tumor outside of the nodal capsule (Table 14.2).

12. **How is laryngeal cancer treated?**
The patient's functional status, location of the cancer, and its stage are critical in determining the appropriate modality. Early cancers are usually addressed with single-modality therapy. Radiation therapy and surgical excision have been shown to be statistically equivalent in terms of disease-free and overall survival. Advanced laryngeal cancers (stages 3–4) should be addressed with multimodal therapy. For high-volume tumors, this may mean conservation surgery in select cases or total laryngectomy, with postoperative radiation with or without chemotherapy. High-level evidence favors combined chemotherapy and radiation over radiation alone as a primary treatment modality for advanced stage cancers.

13. **What are the surgical options for early laryngeal cancer?**
Many early laryngeal cancers may be treated via conservation surgery with excellent local control rates. Traditional surgical resection has included open approaches, but transoral robotic and transoral laser techniques are now more commonly utilized. T1 and T2 lesions are usually amenable to surgery, but other factors such as whether the tumor is exophytic or endophytic and the precise location of the tumor are important. Exophytic tumors located on the central portion of the cord or on the epiglottis are more easily excised than endophytic tumors located near the arytenoid or anterior commissure, for instance. Contraindications to conservation laryngeal surgery include more than 5 millimeters of subglottic extension, extension into the postcricoid space, involvement of the base of tongue

Table 14.1 Tumor Staging

Supraglottis	T1. Limited to one subsite, with normal vocal cord mobility
	T2. Invades mucosa of more than one adjacent subsite of the supraglottis or glottis or a region outside the supraglottis, without fixation of larynx
	T3. Limited to the larynx with vocal cord fixation and/or invasion of the postcricoid area, pre-epiglottic tissues, paraglottic space, and/or erosion of the inner laminae of the thyroid cartilage
	T4a. Invades through the thyroid cartilage and/or tissues beyond the larynx
	T4b. Invades the prevertebral space, encases the carotid artery, or invades the mediastinal structures
Glottis	T1a. Limited to one vocal cord
	T1b. Involves both vocal cords
	T2. Extends to the supraglottis and/or subglottis and/or with impaired cord mobility
	T3. Limited to the larynx with vocal cord fixation or involvement of the inner layer of cartilage
	T4a. Invades through the thyroid cartilage and/or tissues beyond the larynx
	T4b. Invades the prevertebral space, encases the carotid artery, or invades the mediastinal structures
Subglottis	T1. Limited to the subglottis
	T2. Extends to the vocal cord(s) with normal/impaired mobility
	T3. Limited to the larynx with vocal cord fixation
	T4a. Invades the cricoid or thyroid cartilage and/or tissues beyond the larynx
	T4b. Invades the prevertebral space, encases the carotid artery, or invades the mediastinal structures

(Data from American Joint Committee on Cancer: Larynx. In: *AJCC Cancer Staging Manual*, 8th ed, Chicago, 2018, American College of Surgeons, p 149–162.)

Table 14.2 Nodal Staging

CLINICAL NODAL STAGING	
cN0	No reginal lymph node metastasis
cN1	Metastasis in a single ipsilateral lymph node, 3 centimeters or smaller in greatest dimension, and ENE(−)
cN2a	Metastasis in a single ipsilateral node, >3 centimeters but not larger than 6 centimeters in greatest dimension, and ENE(−)
cN2b	Metastasis in multiple ipsilateral nodes, none larger than 6 centimeters in greatest dimension, and ENE(−)
cN2c	Metastasis in bilateral or contralateral lymph nodes, none larger than 6 centimeters in greatest dimension, and ENE(−)
cN3a	Metastasis in a single lymph node, larger than 6 centimeters in greatest dimension, and ENE(−)
cN3b	Metastasis in any lymph node(s) with clinically overt ENE(+)
PATHOLOGIC NODAL STAGING	
pN0	No reginal lymph node metastasis
pN1	Metastasis in a single ipsilateral lymph node, 3 centimeters or smaller in greatest dimension, and ENE(−)
pN2a	Metastasis in a single ipsilateral lymph nodes, 3 centimeters or smaller in greatest dimension, and ENE(+)
	Or metastasis in a single ipsilateral node, more 3 centimeters but not larger than 6cm in greatest dimension, and ENE(−)
pN2b	Metastasis in multiple ipsilateral nodes, none larger than 6 centimeters in greatest dimension, and ENE(−)
pN2c	Metastasis in bilateral or contralateral lymph nodes, none larger than 6 centimeters in greatest dimension, and ENE(−)
pN3a	Metastasis in a single lymph node, larger than 6 centimeters in greatest dimension, and ENE(−)
pN3b	Metastasis in a single ipsilateral node, larger than 3 centimeters in greatest dimension, and ENE(+)
	Or multiple ipsilateral, contralateral, or bilateral lymph nodes, any with ENE(+)
	Or a single contralateral node of any size and ENE(+)

(Data from American Joint Committee on Cancer: Larynx. In: *AJCC Cancer Staging Manual*, 8th ed, Chicago, 2018, American College of Surgeons, pp 149–162.)

or piriform sinus, cartilage invasion, bilateral vocal cord fixation, or bilateral arytenoid involvement. Glottic T1a tumors are treated with cordectomy, while larger T1 or T2 lesions may be amenable to vertical partial laryngectomy through an open or transoral approach. Supraglottic T1 and T2 lesions may be treated with supraglottic (horizontal) laryngectomy or supracricoid partial laryngectomy through an open or transoral approach.

14. **What is the difference between horizontal hemilaryngectomy and vertical partial laryngectomy?**
    In both instances, the resection must be oncologically sound with preservation of at least one cricoarytenoid unit (the cricoid cartilage, one arytenoid cartilage, associated musculature, and superior and recurrent laryngeal nerves). Horizontal hemilaryngectomy, or supraglottic laryngectomy, is indicated for T1, T2, or select T3 supraglottic tumors that do not involve the true vocal fold or associated cartilages. The open procedure removes the bilateral supraglottis but spares the true vocal folds and arytenoids. Voice and swallowing outcomes are typically good. If the tumor involves one vocal fold or cricoarytenoid joint a supracricoid laryngectomy may be performed. This leaves one cricoarytenoid joint intact and removes a portion of the thyroid cartilage. Vertical partial laryngectomy, or hemilaryngectomy, is indicated for T1, T2, and select T3 glottic lesions (not involving commissure or associated cartilages). This procedure removes the ipsilateral vocal fold, false cord, ventricle, and overlying thyroid cartilage. Postoperatively, patients have a functional glottic voice.

15. **What are the subsites of the hypopharynx and their oncologic considerations?**
    1. The *piriform sinus* is the inferior extent of the hypopharynx. It is typically subdivided into anterior, lateral, posterior, and apical walls. The medial limits of the piriform sinus are the larynx, aryepiglottic folds, arytenoids, and cricoid. The piriform sinus is the most common site for hypopharyngeal cancer (65%–75%). Cancer may extend from here into the subglottis, thyroid cartilage, postcricoid region, or cricoarytenoid joint. Three of every four patients presenting with hypopharyngeal cancer within the piriform sinus have regional metastasis, resulting in a poorer prognosis.
    2. The *postcricoid space* spans from the posterior aspect of the arytenoids to the esophageal introitus, anterior to the posterior pharyngeal wall. Cancer here can directly invade the cricoid and can also involve the recurrent laryngeal nerve by spreading laterally into the tracheoesophageal groove.
    3. The *posterior pharyngeal wall* extends from the level of the hyoid bone to the cricopharyngeus muscle, which marks the transition to cervical esophagus. Extension posteriorly through the potential retropharyngeal space can lead to involvement of the prevertebral tissues.

16. **After total laryngectomy, what voice options are available for the patient?**
    Immediately after surgery, all patients should be supplied with a writing board or picture board to assist in communication while in the hospital. For long-term rehabilitation, the most used methods of speech are the electrolarynx, esophageal speech, and a tracheoesophageal prosthesis. The electrolarynx is the most common method of post-laryngectomy speech. This inexpensive device is easier to master than other voicing techniques. It uses patient-induced upper aerodigestive tract vibrations to create a mechanical voice. Drawbacks include the need for an independent power supply, difficultly being understood by others (particularly on the phone), and the need for additional equipment. Esophageal speech is another option with good voice quality for some but is harder to learn. With this method, patients use vibration of the pharyngoesophageal mucosa along with oral air trapping to produce speech. It requires much patience and practice, but no extra equipment is required. Finally, placement of a tracheoesophageal prosthesis is another common method of voice management. This method allows expired air from the tracheal stoma to enter the esophagus via a surgically created tracheoesophageal fistula. This method allows a stronger, more natural voice. Creation of an tracheoesophageal puncture requires a procedure that may be complicated by breakdown of the surrounding tissue or a fistulous tract. This is sometimes done at the time of laryngectomy or as an additional procedure after completion of treatment and healing. Success may be hampered by pharyngeal constrictor spasm and increased risk of aspiration. Proficient use of the tracheoesophageal prosthesis requires practice and training with speech therapy, and the prosthesis itself requires dexterity, can be costly, and must be replaced and cleaned on a regular basis.

17. **What is the prognosis for laryngeal cancer? Has this improved over the last few years?**
    Survival of patients with laryngeal cancer has improved slightly over the past several decades. Only early-stage glottic cancer carries a good prognosis. Unfortunately, most supraglottic cancers present at a later stage and thus have poor survival rates. Prognosis is worse for esophageal cancer compared to laryngeal cancer (Table 14.3).

18. **What are risk factors for esophageal cancer?**
    The predominant risk factors for SCC of the esophagus are smoking and alcohol consumption. Additional risk factors are poor socioeconomic status, low intake of fresh fruits and vegetables, copious consumption of hot tea, and hookah smoking. An increased risk of adenocarcinoma has also been shown in smokers, but alcohol has not been implicated as an independent risk factor. The primary risk factor for adenocarcinoma is thought to be dysplasia (Barrett's esophagus) due to gastroesophageal reflux disease (GERD). It has been postulated that the increasing rate of obesity is responsible for the rising rates of esophageal adenocarcinoma by increasing the severity of GERD as an independent risk factor.

Table 14.3 Five-Year Survival Rates

	LARYNGEAL CANCER	ESOPHAGEAL CANCER
Local	77.4%	46.7%
Reginal metastasis	44.7%	25.1%
Distant metastasis	33.3%	4.8%
All stages	60.3%	19.9%

(Howlader N, Noone AM, Krapcho M, et al, eds: *SEER Cancer Statistics Review, 1975–2016,* Bethesda, MD, National Cancer Institute. Available at https://seer.cancer.gov/csr/1975_2016/, based on November 2018 SEER data submission, posted to the SEER web site, April 2019.)

19. **What is the most common type of esophageal cancer?**
    Esophageal cancer is a relatively uncommon cancer that carries a poor prognosis. Worldwide, SCC is the most common form of esophageal cancer, and this was historically true in the United States. Over the last 40 years, the epidemiology has shifted in the United States, with adenocarcinoma accounting for two-thirds of new cases. The esophagus can be divided into a proximal, middle, and distal third. Adenocarcinoma is found most often in the distal third, while SCC can be found along the entire length of the esophagus with predilection for the upper two-thirds.

CONTROVERSIES

20. **Discuss the treatment options for early glottic cancers.**
    Both radiation therapy and conservation surgery offer excellent and equal cure rates. The decision therefore often falls to the preferences of the patient. Benefits of surgery include a one-time treatment, histopathologic confirmation of free tumor margins, and sparing of radiation therapy for future treatment if needed. Radiation therapy offers a nonsurgical alternative and generally a better voice outcome when compared to open procedures or tumors involving the full thickness of the cord. Drawbacks to radiation include length of treatment, expense, and a decreased chance of laryngeal preservation with recurrence. A key point to remember is that the T1–T2 definition of "early glottic cancers" encompasses a broad range of tumors. Each case should be evaluated, preferably by a multidisciplinary panel, regarding ease of surgical resection and radiation therapy and the risks and benefits of each.

21. **How should the N0 neck be addressed in laryngeal cancer?**
    Treatment options for the N0 neck include observation, elective neck dissection, or radiation therapy. The location of the primary cancer and any previous treatments must be considered. For glottic tumors that have not extended into the supraglottis, elective treatment of the neck may not be necessary because there is poor lymphatic drainage from the glottis. For advanced glottic tumors with supraglottic extension or for primary supraglottic tumors T2 or greater, there is debate on whether to electively treat the neck. There are no randomized controlled trials, and the literature relies heavily on retrospective reviews. Many of these do not show a benefit with treatment; however, some of the larger series support elective treatment of the neck based on improved locoregional control. In the case of recurrent laryngeal cancer after radiation treatment, if there has never been clinical evidence of neck disease, there is not strong evidence to support elective treatment of the neck. Elective neck dissection in such cases may also lead to an increased rate of postoperative complications.

BIBLIOGRAPHY

American Cancer Society: Statistics on laryngeal and hypopharyngeal cancer, 2014. Available at https://www.cancer.org/cancer/laryngealandhypopharyngealcancer/detailedguide.

Armstrong WB, Vokes DE, Maisel RH: Malignant tumors of the larynx In: Flint P, ed: *Cummings Otolaryngology: Head and Neck Surgery,* 5th ed, Philadelphia, 2010, Mosby, pp 1482.

Flint PW: Minimally invasive techniques for management of early glottic cancer, *Otolaryngol Clin North Am* 35(5):1055–1066, 2002.

Forastiere A, Koch W, Trotti A, et al: Head and neck cancer, *N Engl J Med* 345(26):1890–1900, 2001.

Gilbert J, Forastiere AA: Organ preservation trials for laryngeal cancer, *Otolaryngol Clin North Am* 35(5):1035–1054, 2002.

Goudakos JK, Markou K, Nikolaou A, et al: Management of the clinically negative neck (N0) of supraglottic laryngeal carcinoma: a systematic review, *Eur J Surg Oncol* 35(3):223–229, 2008.

Howlader N, Noone AM, Krapcho M, et al: *SEER Cancer Statistics Review, 1975–2016,* Bethesda, MD, April 2019, National Cancer Institute. Available at https://seer.cancer.gov/csr/1975_2016/, based on November 2018 SEER data submission, posted to the SEER web site, April 2019.

Redaelli de Zinis LO, Nicolai P, Tomenzoli D, et al: The distribution of lymph node metastases in supraglottic squamous cell carcinoma: therapeutic implications, *Head Neck* 24(10):913–920, 2002.

Talamini R, Bosetti C, La Vecchia C, et al: Combined effect of tobacco and alcohol on laryngeal cancer risk: a case–control study, *Cancer Causes Control* 13(10):957–964, 2002.

Tufano RP: Organ preservation surgery for laryngeal cancer, *Otolaryngol Clin North Am* 35(5):1067–1080, 2002.

Zhang D, Zhou J, Chen B, et al: Gastroesophageal reflux and carcinoma of the larynx or pharynx: a meta-analysis, *Acta Otolaryngol* 134(10):982–989, 2014.

CHAPTER 15

DISEASES OF THE SALIVARY GLANDS

Farshad Chowdhury, MD and Carissa M. Thomas, MD, PhD, FACS

KEY POINTS

1. It is important to know multiple ways to identify the facial nerve during parotidectomy.
2. Differentiate between infectious, inflammatory, granulomatous, autoimmune, and neoplastic processes based on history, physical examination, laboratory tests, and radiographic imaging.
3. Know the prevalence and malignancy rates of neoplasms in each major salivary gland.

Pearls

1. Mumps and *Staphylococcus aureus* are the most common causes of viral and acute suppurative sialadenitis, respectively.
2. The most common benign salivary gland tumors are pleomorphic adenomas in adults and hemangiomas in children.
3. The most common malignant salivary gland tumor in the parotid is mucoepidermoid carcinoma.
4. HIV workup is important in a patient who presents with cystic parotid masses.

QUESTIONS

1. **Describe the histology of the salivary gland secretory unit.**
   From proximal to distal: Acinar cells –> intercalated duct –> striated duct –> excretory duct. Contractile myoepithelial cells surround the acini and intercalated ducts (Fig. 15.1).

2. **What volume of saliva is produced daily? When is each salivary gland most active?**
   Approximately 1500 mL of saliva is produced daily. At rest, the submandibular glands are the most active (producing two-thirds of all saliva). When stimulated by nausea, food, olfaction, or mastication, the parotid glands become the most active.

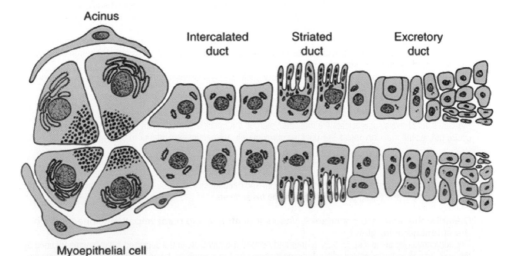

Fig. 15.1 Histology of the salivary gland unit. (From Cummings CW, Flint PW: *Cummings Otolaryngology Head & Neck Surgery*, 5th ed, Philadelphia, 2010, Elsevier-Mosby.)

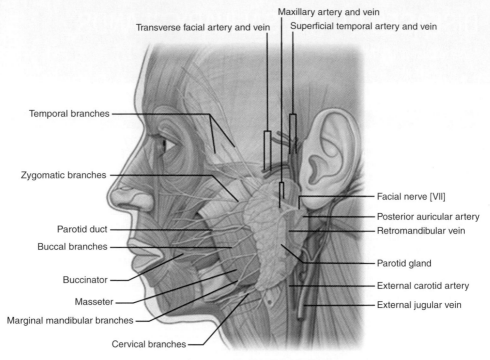

Maxillary artery and vein

Transverse facial artery and vein

Superficial temporal artery and vein

Temporal branches

Zygomatic branches

Parotid duct

Buccal branches

Buccinator

Masseter

Marginal mandibular branches

Cervical branches

Facial nerve [VII]

Posterior auricular artery

Retromandibular vein

Parotid gland

External carotid artery

External jugular vein

© Elsevier Ltd. Drake et al: Gray's Anatomy for Students www.studentconsult.com

Fig. 15.2 Anatomy of the parotid gland and surrounding structures. (From Drake R, Vogl AW, Mitchell AWM: *Gray's Anatomy for Students*, Philadelphia, 2009, Elsevier.)

3. **Describe the anatomic boundaries, vascular anatomy, and parasympathetic innervation of the parotid gland.**
   The parotid gland (Fig. 15.2) is located in the lateral face (parotid space), bordered by the masseter muscle anteriorly/medially, the zygomatic arch superiorly, the tragal cartilage posteriorly, the angle/ramus of the mandible posteriorly/medially, and the sternocleidomastoid muscle (SCM) inferiorly. It is enveloped by the parotidomasseteric fascia, a continuation of the superficial layer of the deep cervical fascia.
   The external carotid artery lies medial to the parotid and branches into the maxillary and superficial temporal arteries. Venous anatomy is variable: the maxillary and superficial temporal veins form the retromandibular vein and join the external jugular vein.
   Parasympathetic innervation: inferior salivatory nucleus –> glossopharyngeal nerve (CN IX) –> Jacobson's nerve –> lesser petrosal nerve –> otic ganglion –> auriculotemporal nerve.

4. **What is the name and course of the parotid duct?**
   Stensen's duct travels superficial to the masseter, pierces the buccinator muscle, and enters the oral cavity opposite the second maxillary molar. The duct is approximately 1.5 centimeters inferior to the zygoma.

5. **What divides the parotid into superficial and deep portions anatomically and radiographically?**
   The facial nerve separates the parotid into superficial and deep lobes (not a true fascial plane). The retromandibular vein is a surrogate radiographic landmark for the facial nerve.

6. **Describe the anatomic boundaries, vascular anatomy, and parasympathetic innervation of the submandibular gland.**
   The submandibular gland (Fig. 15.3) is inferior and deep to the mandible in the submandibular triangle (defined by the anterior and posterior bellies of the digastric muscle and the mandibular body). The mylohyoid muscle divides the gland into superficial and deep lobes. In the surgical field from the neck, retraction of the mylohyoid muscle

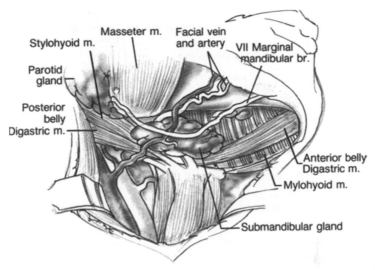

Fig. 15.3 Anatomy of the submandibular triangle. (From Johnson JT, Rosen CA: *Bailey's Head & Neck Surgery: Otolaryngology,* 5th ed, Philadelphia, 2014, Wolters Kluwer/Lippincott Williams & Wilkins.)

reveals the lingual nerve, Wharton's duct (submandibular duct), and hypoglossal nerve lying superficial to the hyoglossus muscle.

The facial artery travels obliquely and deep to the posterior belly of the digastric muscle along the posterior surface of the submandibular gland. The facial artery curves over the mandible body at the superior aspect of the gland. The facial vein travels anterior to the gland.

Parasympathetic innervation: superior salivatory nucleus –> nervus intermedius –> chorda tympani –> submandibular ganglion –> lingual nerve.

7. **Describe the anatomy, parasympathetic innervation, and ducts of the sublingual gland.**
   The sublingual gland (Fig. 15.4) is located adjacent to the lingual frenulum, lateral to the genioglossus and genio-hyoid muscles, and superficial to the mylohyoid muscle. The blood supply is from the branches of the facial and lingual arteries. Parasympathetic innervation is the same as for the submandibular gland. The sublingual gland drains into the oral cavity through the ducts of Rivinus or into Wharton's duct via the Bartholin duct.

8. **What is the most common bacteria in acute suppurative sialadenitis? How is it treated?**
   Staphylococcus aureus is the most common bacteria that causes sialadenitis. Treatment consists of antibiotics effective against β-lactamase-producing bacteria (i.e., amoxicillin-clavulanate) or culture-directed antibiotics plus hydration, warm compresses, gland massage, and sialagogues.

9. **Sialolithiasis affects which salivary gland primarily? List available treatment options.**
   The submandibular gland is most affected by sialolithiasis due to the more viscous/mucinous saliva that travels superiorly against gravity in Wharton's duct. Treatment options include the following:
   1. Conservative management with sialagogues, warm compresses, antibiotics, massage, and hydration
   2. Open sialolithotomy
   3. Sialendoscopy (<6 millimeter sialoliths)
   4. Lithotripsy
   5. Excision of salivary gland

10. **What is the most common viral infection of the parotid?**
    Mumps is still the most common cause of viral parotitis, although most infections have been eliminated by vaccination.

11. **What is the most common parotid abnormality associated with HIV and its treatment?**
    Benign lymphoepithelial cystic disease. HIV should be ruled out in any patient with cystic parotid disease. Treatment includes observation or serial drainage with needle aspiration of symptomatic disease and antiretroviral medication.

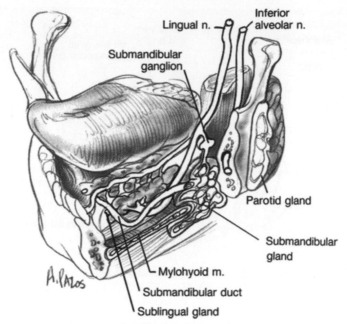

Fig. 15.4 Anatomy of the sublingual gland and surrounding structures. (From Johnson JT, Rosen CA: *Bailey's Head & Neck Surgery: Otolaryngology*, 5th ed, Philadelphia, 2014, Wolters Kluwer/Lippincott Williams & Wilkins.)

12. **Describe granulomatous diseases of the salivary glands, causative organisms, and treatment.**
    1. Tuberculosis: diagnosed by FNA with acid-fast bacilli (culture or PCR) and patients may be PPD positive with cavitary lesions on chest x-ray (CXR). Treated with isoniazid, rifampin, pyrazinamide, and ethambutol for 2 months, followed by isoniazid and rifampin (4 months).
    2. Atypical mycobacteria: diagnosed by culture or PCR; PPD is typically nonreactive and CXR negative. Definitively treated with surgical excision with antibiotic adjunct (macrolide +/- rifamycin or ethambutol).
    3. Actinomycosis: caused by gram-positive, anaerobic actinomyces (pathognomonic sulphur granules). Treatment includes penicillin G, doxycycline, or clindamycin.
    4. Cat-scratch disease: caused by *Bartonella henselae*. Affects parotid-associated lymph nodes. Treated with azithromycin.
    5. Toxoplasmosis: caused by *Toxoplasma gondii*. Treated with pyrimethamine, sulfadiazine, and folinic acid.
    6. Sarcoidosis: Noncaseating granulomas. Usually responds to steroids. Can present as Heerfordt disease/uveoparotid fever consisting of parotitis, uveitis, and CN VII paralysis.

13. **What are the laboratory and biopsy diagnostic tests for Sjögren's syndrome?**
    Sjögren's is an immune-mediated destruction of exocrine glands. Laboratory tests include Ro/SS-A and La/SS-B antibodies, rheumatoid factor (RF), and antinuclear antibodies (ANA). Lymphocytic infiltration on minor salivary gland biopsy (three to five glands) is diagnostic.

14. **Sjögren's syndrome increases the risk of developing which disease?**
    Lymphoma.

15. **Where do salivary gland tumors most commonly present? What is the rate of malignancy for each gland?**
    Most tumors are found in the parotid gland but they are the least likely to be malignant.
    Location: parotid > submandibular > sublingual/minor salivary glands.
    Rate of malignancy: minor salivary glands (80%) > submandibular (50%) > parotid (20%).

16. **What is a ranula? What is the difference between a simple and plunging ranula?**
    A ranula is a mucous retention cyst that arises from the sublingual gland. A simple ranula is confined to the sublingual space, while a plunging ranula has herniated through the mylohyoid muscle into the neck.

Table 15.1 World Health Organization Classification (4th ed. 2018) of Benign Salivary Gland Tumors and Combined Incidence Based on Two Epidemiologic Studies

HISTOLOGY	# PATIENTS (%) (TOTAL = 2807)	# PATIENTS (%) (TOTAL = 918)
Pleomorphic adenoma	1274 (45.4)	651 (70.9)
Warthin's tumor	183 (6.5)	203 (22.1)
Oncocytoma	20 (0.7)	10 (1.1)
Basal cell adenoma	N/A	22 (2.4)
Myoepithelioma	N/A	10 (1.1)
Canalicular adenoma	N/A	6 (0.7)
Cystadenoma	N/A	4 (0.4)

N/A indicates that histologic subtype was not assessed in the epidemiologic study. Other benign tumors include sebaceous adenoma, lymphadenoma, and ductal papillomas (not assessed in the included studies).
(From Spiro RH: Salivary neoplasms: overview of a 35-year experience with 2807 patients, *Head Neck Surg* 8:177–184, 1986; Bradley PJ, McGurk M: Incidence of salivary gland neoplasms in a defined UK population, *Br J Oral Maxillofac Surg* 51:399–403, 2013.)

17. **List physical exam findings that can distinguish a benign salivary gland mass from a malignant salivary gland mass.**
   Benign masses are usually slow-growing, well-defined, nontender, and freely mobile with normal nerve function (i.e., CN VII, XII, lingual nerve). Malignant masses are associated with pain, fixation, rapid growth, cervical lymphadenopathy, and nerve paresis/paralysis.

18. **List benign tumors of the salivary glands. Which is most common? Which can present bilaterally?**
   See Table 15.1.
   The most common benign tumor is pleomorphic adenoma in adults and hemangioma in pediatric patients. Warthin's tumors present bilaterally in up to 10% of cases.

19. **Warthin's tumor is an eponym for what? What are some epidemiologic features?**
   Warthin's tumor is an eponym for papillary cystadenoma lymphomatosum. It is more often found in men in the sixth or seventh decade of life and is related to cigarette smoke exposure despite being benign.

20. **List malignant tumors of the salivary glands. Which is most common in the parotid gland?**
   See Table 15.2.
   The most common malignancy of the parotid gland is mucoepidermoid carcinoma.

21. **Which benign salivary gland tumor can degenerate into a malignant tumor over a prolonged period of time?**
   A pleomorphic adenoma can undergo malignant transformation to a carcinoma ex pleomorphic adenoma. Rapid enlargement of a long-standing mass is very suggestive of malignant transformation.

22. **Which malignant salivary gland tumor has the highest propensity for perineural spread?**
   Adenoid cystic carcinoma (ACC) has the highest rate of perineural spread. ACC can have late recurrence, presenting 15 to 20 years after the initial presentation.

23. **Describe the initial workup of a salivary gland mass.**
   The combination of FNA and imaging (contrasted CT or MRI) can help differentiate benign from malignant processes and often provide a diagnosis. MRI provides higher soft tissue resolution, revealing tumor characteristics and perineural invasion. PET/CT cannot reliably distinguish benign from malignant tumors.

24. **A diagnosis of squamous cell carcinoma (SCC) of the parotid demands what additional workup?**
   It is essential to ensure that SCC of the parotid is not metastatic disease as primary SCC of the salivary glands is rare.

25. **Describe the TNM classification of salivary gland tumors.**
   TX: Primary tumor cannot be assessed.
   T0: No evidence of primary tumor.

Table 15.2 World Health Organization Classification (4th ed. 2018) of Malignant Salivary Gland Tumors and Combined Incidence Based on Four Epidemiologic Studies

HISTOLOGY	# PATIENTS (%) (TOTAL = 2807)	# PATIENTS (%) (TOTAL = 147)	# PATIENTS (%) (TOTAL = 1831)	# PATIENTS (%) (TOTAL = 2737)
Mucoepidermoid carcinoma	439 (15.7)	38 (25.9)	290 (15.8)	373 (13.6)
Adenoid cystic carcinoma	281 (10.0)	32 (21.8)	214 (11.7)	455 (16.6)
Adenocarcinoma NOS	225 (8.0)	25 (17.0)	228 (12.5)	451 (16.5)
Acinic cell carcinoma	84 (3.0)	18 (12.2)	147 (8.0)	406 (14.8)
Polymorphous low grade adenocarcinoma	N/A	17 (11.6)	N/A	N/A
Epithelial-myoepithelial carcinoma	53 (1.9)	N/A	N/A	165 (6.0)
Carcinoma ex pleomorphic adenoma	N/A	5 (3.4)	128 (7.0)	207 (7.6)
Salivary duct carcinoma	N/A	N/A	N/A	55 (2.0)
Clear cell adenocarcinoma	N/A	1 (0.7)	N/A	N/A
Other*	35 (1.3)	9 (6.1)	N/A	348 (12.7)

*Other includes basal cell adenocarcinoma, sebaceous carcinoma, sebaceous lymphadenocarcinoma, cystadenocarcinoma, low-grade cribriform cystadenocarcinoma, mucinous adenocarcinoma, oncocytic carcinoma, carcinosarcoma NOS, metastasizing pleomorphic adenoma, small cell carcinoma, large cell carcinoma, lymphoepithelial carcinoma, and sialoblastoma (not otherwise specified). N/A indicates that the histologic subtype was not assessed in the epidemiologic study.

(From Spiro RH: Salivary neoplasms: overview of a 35-year experience with 2807 patients, *Head Neck Surg* 8:177–184, 1986; Bradley PJ, McGurk M: Incidence of salivary gland neoplasms in a defined UK population, *Br J Oral Maxillofac Surg* 51:399–403, 2013; Fu JY, et al: Salivary gland cancer in Shanghai (2003–2012): an epidemiological study of incidence, site and pathology, *BMC Cancer* 19:350–355, 2019; de Ridder M, et al: An epidemiological evaluation of salivary gland cancer in the Netherlands (1989-2010), *Cancer Epidemiol* 39:14–20, 2015.)

Tis: Carcinoma in situ.
T1: Tumor ≤2 centimeters in greatest dimension without extraparenchymal extension.
T2: Tumor >2 centimeters but ≤4 centimeters in the greatest dimension without extraparenchymal extension.
T3: Tumor >4 centimeters and/or tumor having extraparenchymal extension.
T4a: Moderately advanced disease. The tumor invades the skin, mandible, ear canal, and/or facial nerve.
T4b: Very advanced disease. Tumor invades the skull base and pterygoid plates and/or encases the carotid artery. (Extraparenchymal extension is a clinical or macroscopic evidence of invasion into soft tissues).
NX: Regional lymph nodes cannot be assessed.
N0: No regional lymph node metastasis.
N1: Metastasis in a single ipsilateral lymph node, ≤3 centimeters in greatest dimension and extranodal extension negative (ENE[−]).
N2:
  N2a: Metastasis in a single ipsilateral lymph node >3 centimeters but ≤6 centimeters in the greatest dimension and ENE(−).
  N2b: Metastases in multiple ipsilateral lymph nodes, ≤6 centimeters in greatest dimension and ENE(−).
  N2c: Metastases in bilateral or contralateral lymph nodes, ≤6 centimeters in the greatest dimension and ENE(−).
N3:
  N3a: Metastasis in a lymph node >6 centimeters in the greatest dimension and ENE(−).
  N3b: Metastases in any node(s) with clinically overt ENE(+).
M0: no distant metastases.
M1: distant metastases.

26. **What incisions are used for a parotidectomy and submandibular gland excision?**
A modified Blair incision is used for parotidectomy and can be extended to the neck if neck dissection is indicated. The incision for submandibular gland excision is made two fingerbreadths (approximately 3 centimeters) below the angle of the mandible to protect the marginal mandibular branch of the facial nerve.

27. **During a parotidectomy, what are some ways the facial nerve can be identified?**
   1. 1–1.5 centimeters deep and inferior to the tragal pointer.
   2. 6–8 millimeters deep to the tympanomastoid suture line.
   3. Attachment of the posterior belly of the digastric muscle to the digastric ridge identifies the plane of the facial nerve.

4. Superficial/lateral to the styloid process.
5. Retrograde dissection of any facial nerve branch back to the pes anserinus and main trunk.
6. Mastoidectomy with anterograde nerve dissection.

28. **List the indications for postoperative radiotherapy of a salivary neoplasm.**
   - High-grade tumors
   - Gross or microscopic residual disease, positive margins
   - Lymph node metastasis
   - Extraparenchymal extension
   - Tumors involving the facial nerve
   - Recurrent disease

29. **What is Frey's syndrome? How is it diagnosed and treated?**
   Frey's syndrome is gustatory sweating and flushing of the skin overlying the parotidectomy surgical site caused by postoperative aberrant reinnervation of postganglionic parasympathetic neurons to sweat glands and cutaneous blood vessels. It can be diagnosed with the starch iodine test, and treatments include Botox injection and topical antiperspirants.

30. **What is the role of elective neck dissection in treating salivary gland malignancies?**
   Elective neck dissection is generally reserved for high-grade tumors or tumors of significant size (T3–T4) as the risk of microscopic metastasis to the neck is greater than 20%.

CONTROVERSIES

31. **What adjuvant treatment should be used for high-risk salivary gland malignancies?**
   Recent evidence demonstrates that adjuvant radiation improves locoregional control and overall survival. Thus far adjuvant chemotherapy has not shown any benefit, but a clinical trial (RTOG 1008) is underway to determine the efficacy of adjuvant radiation and weekly cisplatin for high-risk tumors.

32. **How should a functioning or paretic facial nerve be managed during parotid surgery?**
   The facial nerve should be preserved unless grossly infiltrated or embedded in the tumor and only the infiltrated portion of the nerve should be resected. Immediate nerve grafting should be performed if the facial nerve is sacrificed. The great auricular nerve is an excellent donor nerve for grafting.

33. **Is extracapsular dissection a reasonable alternative to superficial parotidectomy for benign tumors?**
   Extracapsular dissection involves careful dissection around a mobile, <4-centimeter benign tumor capsule without identifying the facial nerve. Retrospective studies have shown similar recurrence rates and decreased rates of facial nerve paresis/paralysis and Frey's syndrome compared to superficial parotidectomy. Appropriate patient selection and surgeon experience are critical factors.

BIBLIOGRAPHY

Bradley PJ, McGurk M: Incidence of salivary gland neoplasms in a defined UK population, *Br J Oral Maxillofac Surg* 51:399–403, 2013.
Carlson ER, Schlieve T: Salivary gland malignancies, *Oral Maxillofac Surg Clin North Am* 31:125–144, 2019.
Cummings CW, Flint PW: *Cummings Otolaryngology Head & Neck Surgery*, 5th ed, Philadelphia, 2010, Elsevier-Mosby.
de Ridder M, Balm AJM, Smeele LE, Wouters MWJM, van Dijik BAC: An epidemiological evaluation of salivary gland cancer in the Netherlands (1989–2010), *Cancer Epidemiol* 39:14–20, 2015.
Drake R, Vogl AW, Mitchell AWM: *Gray's Anatomy for Students*, Philadelphia, 2009, Elsevier.
Fu JY, Wu CX, Shen SK, Zheng Y, Zhang CP, Zhang ZY: Salivary gland carcinoma in Shanghai (2003–2012): an epidemiological study of incidence, site, and pathology, *BMC Cancer* 19:350–355, 2019.
Gooi Z, Agrawal N: *Difficult Decisions in Head and Neck Oncologic Surgery*, Switzerland, 2019, Springer.
Guntinas-Lichius O, Silver CE, Thielker J, Bernal-Sprekelsen M, Bradford CR, De Bree R, et al: Management of the facial nerve in parotid cancer: preservation or resection and reconstruction, *Eur Arch Otorhinolaryngol* 275:2615–2626, 2018.
Johnson JT, Rosen CA: *Bailey's Head and Neck Surgery Otolaryngology*, 5th ed, Philadelphia, 2014, Wolters Kluwer/Lippincott Williams & Wilkins.
Kochhar A, Larian B, Azizzadeh B: Facial nerve and parotid gland anatomy, *Otolaryngol Clin North Am* 49:273–284, 2016.
Lalwani AK: *Current Diagnosis and Treatment Otolaryngology Head and Neck Surgery*, 3rd ed, New York, 2012, McGraw-Hill.
Mehta V, Nathan CA: Extracapsular dissection versus superficial parotidectomy for benign parotid tumors, *Laryngoscope* 125:1039–1040, 2015.
Sokoya M, Leem TH: Diseases of the salivary glands. In: *ENT Secrets*, 4th ed, Philadelphia, 2016, Elsevier, pp. 94–99.
Spiro RH: Salivary neoplasms: overview of a 35-year experience with 2807 patients, *Head Neck Surg* 8:177–184, 1986.

CHAPTER 16

THYROID AND PARATHYROID DISEASE

Erin J. Buczek, MD, FACS

KEY POINTS

1. Thyroid cancer occurs in 5% to 10% of palpable nodules.
2. Most thyroid cancers are papillary thyroid cancer (70%–80%) and follicular thyroid cancer (15%–20%).
3. In medullary thyroid cancer, the age of surgery is determined by specific gene mutations. For the highest risk mutations, surgery is recommended before 6 months of age (MEN IIB). Surgery for moderate risk mutations is usually recommended before age 5 (MEN IIa).
4. The superior parathyroid glands develop from the fourth branchial pouch and the inferior parathyroid gland develops from the third pharyngeal pouch along with the thymus.

Pearls

1. Mutation panel testing: Tests for DNA mutations most commonly seen in thyroid cancer, including *BRAF* V000E, *RAS*, *RET/PTC*, and *PAX8/PPARG* rearrangements. When these mutations are detected, the test helps to "rule in" cancer with a positive predictive value of 83%.
2. Gene sequencing classifier testing: Tests for RNA expression of several different genes for benign and malignant nodules. Has a greater than 95% negative predictive value and essentially "rules out" cancer.
3. All anaplastic thyroid tumors are classified as stage IV, regardless of tumor size, location, or metastasis.
4. The classic symptoms of hypercalcemia are often described as "moans, groans, stones, and psychic overtones."

QUESTIONS: THYROID DISEASE

1. **What is the incidence of a thyroid nodule?**
   Clinically palpable nodules occur in 4% to 7% of the population, though the rate of incidental nodule founds on ultrasound is higher (20%–67% of patients), with more than half of thyroids containing more than one nodule. Nodules are more common in women (female-to-male ratio of 4:1). Thyroid cancer occurs in 5% to 10% of palpable nodules.

2. **What is the workup of a thyroid nodule?**
   - Comprehensive history and physical including a visualization of the vocal cords (laryngoscopy) to evaluate recurrent laryngeal nerve function
   - Thyroid function assay
   - Ultrasound evaluation of nodule
   - Possible fine-needle aspiration (FNA) if concern for malignancy

3. **What features of thyroid nodules indicate a higher risk of malignancy?**
   - Age less than 30 and over 60 years old
   - Male
   - Positive family history
   - Radiation exposure
   - Hashimoto's thyroiditis
   - Rapid growth
   - Pain
   - Dysphonia
   - Cervical lymphadenopathy
   - Firm, fixed nodules

4. **What ultrasound features are concerning for malignancy?**
   - Microcalcification
   - Irregular margins
   - Solid rather than cystic nodules
   - Internal vascularity
   - Multiple nodules
   - Hypoechoic or isoechoic
   - Enlarged cervical lymph nodes, particularly on the same side of the neck

5. **What is the diagnostic accuracy of FNA cytology?**
   Accuracy 95%; false-negative rate 2.3%; false-positive rate 1.1%.

6. **What is the Bethesda Classification for Thyroid Cytopathology and associated risk of malignancy?**
   - Bethesda I: nondiagnostic or unsatisfactory (n/a)
   - Bethesda II: benign (<5%)
   - Bethesda III: atypia of undetermined significance (AUS) or follicular lesion of unknown significance (FLUS) (5%–15%)
   - Bethesda IV: follicular neoplasm (15%–30%)
   - Bethesda V: suspicious for malignancy (60%–75%)
   - Bethesda VI: malignancy (97%–99%)

7. **What is the role of molecular testing for thyroid cancer?**
   Genetic molecular testing is used for Bethesda III and IV thyroid nodules to either "rule in" a cancer or "rule out" a benign nodule. These tests should help to further risk stratify patients to improve diagnostic accuracy preoperatively, save unnecessary surgery, and help determine the extent of surgery when indicated.

8. **What molecular tests are currently available for thyroid nodules?**
   1. Mutation panel testing: Tests for DNA mutations most commonly seen in thyroid cancer, including *BRAF* V000E, *RAS*, *RET/PTC*, and *PAX8/PPARG* rearrangements. When these mutations are detected, the test helps to "rule in" cancer with a positive predictive value of 83%.
   2. Gene sequencing classifier testing: tests for RNA expression of several different genes for benign and malignant nodules. Has a greater than 95% negative predictive value and essentially "rules out" cancer.

9. **What is the recommended follow-up for benign thyroid nodules?**
   Pending characteristics on ultrasound, most authors recommend repeat ultrasound at 6 months for concerning nodules. Significant changes often warrant repeat FNA. Suppression with exogenous thyroxine is NOT recommended.

10. **What is the differential diagnosis of thyroid cancers?**
    - Papillary carcinoma: 70%–80%
    - Follicular carcinoma: 15%–20%
    - Hurthle cell carcinoma: 3%–5%
    - Medullary carcinoma: 3%–10%
    - Anaplastic carcinoma: less than 2%
    - Insular or poorly differentiated carcinoma: rare
    - Other: lymphoma, squamous cell carcinoma, metastases from other sites (renal cell carcinoma, melanoma, breast cancer)

11. **What is the TNM staging for well-differentiated thyroid cancer?**
    See Table 16.1.

12. **What is the staging for well-differentiated thyroid cancers?**
    See Table 16.2.

13. **What are the clinical prognostic indicators for thyroid cancer?**
    - **AMES**: Age; Metastasis; Extent and Size of primary tumor
      - Low risk: Age less than 40 (M) or 50 (F); tumor less than 4 centimeters and within thyroid gland
      - High risk: Age over 41 (M) or 51 (F); size >5 centimeters; extrathyroidal extension
    - **MACIS**: Metastasis; Age; Completeness of resection; Invasion; Size of tumor
      - High risk: Age over 40; incomplete tumor resection; local invasion beyond thyroid (recurrent laryngeal nerve, trachea, esophagus, strap muscles) or angioinvasion; size >4 centimeters

Table 16.1 TNM Staging for Well-Differentiated Thyroid Carcinoma

T0: No evidence of primary tumor

T1:
T1a: Tumor <1 cm, without extrathyroidal extension
T1b: Tumor <1 cm but ≤2 cm in greatest dimension, without extrathyroidal extension

T2: Tumor >2 cm but ≤4 cm in greatest dimension, without extrathyroidal extension

T3: Tumor >4 cm in greatest dimension limited to the thyroid or any size tumor with minimal extrathyroidal extension (e.g., extension into sternothyroid muscle or perithyroidal soft tissues.)

T4:
T4a: Tumor of any size extending beyond the thyroid capsule to invade subcutaneous soft tissues, larynx, trachea, esophagus, or recurrent laryngeal nerve
T4b: Tumor of any size invading prevertebral fascia or encasing carotid artery or mediastinal vessels

N0: No metastatic nodes

N1:
N1a: Metastases to Level VI (pretracheal, paratracheal, and prelaryngeal/Delphian lymph nodes)
N1b: Metastases to unilateral, bilateral, or contralateral cervical (Levels I–V) or retropharyngeal or superior mediastinal lymph nodes (Level VII)

M0: No distant metastases

M1: Distant metastases

Source: AJCC seventh edition.

Table 16.2 Staging for Papillary and Follicular Thyroid Cancer

Papillary or follicular thyroid tumors <45 years old
Stage I: Any T, any N, M0
Stage II: Any T, Any N, M1

Papillary or follicular thyroid tumors >45 years old
Stage I: T1N0M0
Stage II: T2N0M0
Stage III: T1–2 N1a M0 or T3 N0–1a M0
Stage IVA: T1–3 N1b M0 or T4a any N M0
Stage IVB: T4b, any N, M0
Stage IVC: Any T, any N, M1

14. **What is the difference between a total thyroidectomy (TT), hemithyroidectomy or lobectomy, near-total thyroidectomy (NT), and subtotal thyroidectomy?**
    TT is the complete removal of all visible thyroid tissue. Hemithyroidectomy is complete removal of all thyroid tissue on one side of the thyroid (left or right) with or without isthmusectomy. In an NT, the surgeon elects to leave a very small amount of thyroid tissue around the parathyroid glands or recurrent laryngeal nerve to reduce morbidity. A subtotal thyroidectomy is poorly defined and results in large amounts of thyroid tissue left behind. A subtotal thyroidectomy is NOT an acceptable surgery for thyroid cancer.

15. **What is the treatment for early-stage papillary or follicular thyroid cancers?**
    The treatment for isolated T1 lesions is a typically lobectomy. Guidelines for T2 lesions suggest that either lobectomy or total thyroidectomy can be used to treat, pending concerning features on pathology, contralateral thyroid disease, and patient considerations. Any evidence of macroscopic nodal disease warrants total thyroidectomy to facilitate radioactive iodine (RAI) treatment.
    Advantages of total thyroidectomy include allowing for adjuvant RAI (^{131}I) ablation, improving the specificity of thyroglobulin assays for cancer surveillance, and the use of total body scanning with nuclear medicine scanning. Disadvantages include the need for lifelong thyroid replacement therapy and potentially increased surgical risk.

16. **What is the treatment for Stage III papillary or follicular thyroid cancer?**
    - TT plus removal of involved lymph nodes. Consider prophylactic central neck dissection for T3 cancers.
    - ^{131}I ablation is typically given following TT.

17. **What is the treatment for Stage IV papillary or follicular thyroid cancer?**
    - Surgery: TT and neck dissection as indicated. Treatment of distant metastases is usually not curative but may be treated with ^{131}I. External beam radiation is considered for localized lesions that are unresponsive to RAI.
    - Resection of limited metastases, especially symptomatic metastases, should be considered when the tumor has no uptake of ^{131}I. Removal of structures that will cause functional deficits (i.e., larynx, pharynx, trachea) should be thoroughly discussed with the patient.
    - Patients with unresectable disease who are also unresponsive to ^{131}I should be considered for chemotherapy such as tyrosine kinase inhibitors.

18. **What is the role of neck dissection in well-differentiated thyroid cancer?**
    Papillary and medullary thyroid cancers have a high propensity to spread to regional lymph nodes compared to follicular thyroid carcinoma, which tends to spread hematogenously. A careful assessment of the central compartment (level VI) and lateral neck (levels II–V) should be done prior to surgery. Elective neck dissection beyond the central compartment is controversial. Cancers that have spread to the lateral neck without evidence of central neck disease on imaging should also get an ipsilateral central neck dissection at the same time as total thyroidectomy. Level I (submandibular gland) is rarely involved by locoregional metastasis and can be preserved in thyroid cancer surgery.

19. **What is multiple endocrine neoplasia?**
    The term "multiple endocrine neoplasia" (MEN) encompasses several distinct syndromes featuring tumors of endocrine glands, each with its own characteristic pattern.
    - MEN type I: pancreas, pituitary, parathyroid adenomas
    - MEN type IIa: medullary carcinoma of thyroid, pheochromocytoma, parathyroid hyperplasia
    - MEN type IIb: MEN IIa and mucosal neuromas; no parathyroid involvement

20. **What is the staging for medullary thyroid cancer?**
    See Table 16.3.

21. **What important characteristics are unique to medullary thyroid cancer?**
    - More aggressive than well-differentiated thyroid cancers (i.e., papillary and follicular)
    - Derived from parafollicular or C cells and can secrete calcitonin and carcinoembryonic antigen (CEA) as well as prostaglandins, histaminases, and serotonin
    - High propensity for invasion into muscle and trachea as well as hematogenous spread to lungs and viscera (50% at presentation)
    - *RET* proto-oncogene mutation at codon 634 results in MEN IIa; codon 918 mutation results in MEN IIb
    - MEN IIb type is the most aggressive; familial medullary thyroid carcinoma has the best prognosis and MEN IIa has an intermediate prognosis
    - Sporadic unifocal lesions: 70%; familial/genetic: 30%

22. **What is the workup for medullary thyroid cancer?**
    Patients positive for *RET* mutation should be screened for MEN type II tumors: (1) pheochromocytoma: plasma fractionated metanephrines and abdominal scan to rule out pheochromocytoma and (2) parathyroid adenoma: serum calcium and parathyroid hormone (PTH). Family members should have genetic screening for *RET* protooncogene and MEN type II tumors. Imaging should evaluate both locoregional and distant metastasis with computed tomography (CT) or magnetic resonance imaging (MRI) pending calcitonin and CEA levels. High levels of calcitonin or CEA indicate distant metastasis and may prompt additional imaging.

Table 16.3 Staging for Medullary Thyroid Cancer

Stage I: T1 N0 M0
Stage II: T2–T3 N0 M0
Stage III: T1–3 N1a M0
Stage IVa: T4a, any N, M0 or T1–3 N1b M0
Stage IVB: T4b, any N, M0
Stage IVC: Any T, any N, M1

23. **What is the treatment for medullary thyroid cancer?**
TT and neck dissection (as needed) with resection of any additional structures involved is recommended. Children with MEN II are recommended to undergo prophylactic TT. Age of surgery is determined by specific gene mutations. For the highest risk mutations, surgery is recommended before 6 months of age (MEN IIB). Surgery for moderate risk mutations is usually recommended before age 5 (MEN IIa). Long-term follow-up with serial serum calcitonin and CEA levels is recommended.

24. **What is anaplastic thyroid cancer?**
    * Extremely aggressive malignancy; usually occurs in older patients
    * Eighty percent occur in preexisting thyroid mass, suggesting malignant de-differentiation within existing tumor
    * Presents as sudden growth in preexisting mass, associated with pain, hoarseness, dysphagia, and dyspnea

25. **What is the staging for anaplastic thyroid cancer?**
    * **Stage IV:** All anaplastic thyroid tumors are classified as stage IV, regardless of tumor size, location, or metastasis.
    * **IVA:** Anaplastic tumor that has spread to nearby structures, T4a
    * **IVB:** Tumor that has spread beyond nearby structures, T4b
    * **IVC:** There is evidence of metastasis (any N or M)

26. **What is the treatment for anaplastic thyroid cancer?**
Almost all cases are advanced at time of presentation and median survival is less than 6 months. Doxorubicin, radiation, and palliative surgery (debulking and airway management) can be considered for palliation and to improve quality of life. Incidentally found anaplastic cancer and locally limited disease have somewhat better prognosis.

27. **How is RAI given?**
RAI is given with thyroid hormone withdrawal or recombinant human thyroid stimulating hormone (rhTSH). Studies show that rhTSH maintains quality of life and reduces the radiation dose delivered to the body compared with thyroid hormone withdrawal alone.

28. **What is the treatment for recurrent thyroid cancer?**
    * Ten to 30% of patients develop recurrence and/or metastases.
    * Eighty percent develop recurrence with disease in the neck alone; 20% develop recurrence with distant metastases (primarily lung or bone).
    * Fifty percent of patients operated on for recurrent tumors can be rendered free of disease with a second operation.
    * Recurrences detected by ^{131}I scan or increasing thyroglobulin and not clinically apparent can be treated with ^{131}I ablation with excellent prognosis.
    * Patients with iodine-refractory advanced thyroid cancer may respond to multi-tyrosine kinase inhibitor therapy or external beam radiation.

QUESTIONS: PARATHYROID TUMOR

29. **What is the embryology of the parathyroid glands?**
The superior parathyroid glands develop from the fourth branchial pouch and the inferior parathyroid gland develops from the third pharyngeal pouch along with the thymus. Although most people have four parathyroid glands, 3% to 7% have five to seven glands, and 3% to 5% have fewer than four glands.

30. **What are the normal characteristics of parathyroid glands?**
The average parathyroid gland weighs 35 to 50 mg and is 1 to 5 millimeters in diameter. Its primary blood supply is from the inferior thyroid artery or, more rarely, from the posterior branch of the superior thyroid artery.

31. **What is primary hyperparathyroidism?**
Primary hyperparathyroidism is caused by the overproduction of PTH. Etiology is usually due to the following:
    * Solitary parathyroid adenoma (85%)
    * Multiple hyperplastic glands (10%–15%)
    * Multiple adenomas (3%–4%)
    * Parathyroid carcinoma (<1%)
        Primary hyperparathyroidism may be related to overexpression of *PRAD1* oncogene or low-dose radiation exposure, but the true etiology is unknown.

32. **What are secondary and tertiary hyperparathyroidism?**
Secondary hyperparathyroidism is seen in patients with chronic renal failure causing elevated phosphate and decreased 1-α-hydroxylase in the kidney, resulting in low vitamin D. It is associated with mild hypercalcemia but

high PTH. Surgery is recommended if refractory to medical management (phosphate binders, vitamin D treatment, or calcimimetics). The goal of surgery is to prevent long-term bone damage (osteopenia). Surgical treatment is either a subtotal (three and one-half glands) parathyroidectomy or four-gland parathyroidectomy with autotransplant of a small portion into the brachioradialis or sternocleidomastoid muscle.

Tertiary hyperparathyroidism is the result of long-term secondary hyperparathyroidism that results in autonomous parathyroid function, even when the underlying causes are corrected. Cinacalcet (calcimimetic agent) can be effective in treating patients with secondary hyperparathyroidism.

33. What are the classic symptoms of hypercalcemia?
"Moans, groans, stones, and psychic overtones": The most common symptoms include gastrointestinal disturbance (nausea, constipation, peptic ulcer, pancreatitis), muscle weakness, renal stones, hypertension, cardiac arrhythmia, polydipsia, and neuropsychiatric symptoms including depression, fatigue, and memory loss. Renal stones and severe bone disorders such as osteitis fibrosa cystica are rare since the advent of routine PTH testing. Long-term hypercalcemia can lead to osteopenia or osteoporosis.

34. What is the differential diagnosis for hypercalcemia?
See Table 16.4.

35. How is the diagnosis of primary hyperparathyroidism made?
- Increased serum total calcium and increased or very high PTH
- Serum phosphate is decreased or low-normal
- If PTH is elevated *but* serum calcium is normal or low normal, rule out vitamin D insufficiency or malabsorption
- If both calcium and phosphate levels are elevated, rule out hypervitaminosis D

36. What are available localization imaging studies for primary hyperparathyroidism?
- Noninvasive Localization
  - Technetium 99m sestamibi (Tc99m MIBI): Sestamibi localizes into the mitochondria of parathyroid cells. Late-phase images at 2 hours allow for sestamibi to clear from the thyroid gland but not the parathyroid. Single adenoma detection is high with sensitivity of 100% and specificity of 90%. Less useful for four-gland hyperplasia.
  - Tc99m MIBI plus single-photon emission CT (SPECT): Addition of SPECT gives a higher resolution three-dimensional image, and some report superior detection of adenomas within the carotid sheath or mediastinum.
  - Tc99m + thallium-201 subtraction: Thallium is taken up by the parathyroid and less by the thyroid gland. Subsequent subtraction image can detect enlarged parathyroid glands. Sensitivity rates are varied (30%–90%) but more widely available than MIBI.
  - Ultrasound (US): Superior to other techniques for identifying intrathyroid parathyroid adenomas, quicker, and involves no radiation. Ectopic adenomas of retroesophageal, tracheal, and mediastinal origin are more difficult to localize with US. False-positive rate is 15% to 20%.
  - MRI: Adenomas appear with high signal intensity on T2-weighted images. May be useful in identifying ectopic adenomas and in patients requiring reexploration after initial surgery.
  - CT angiography (CTA) neck with parathyroid protocol (i.e., 4D-CT) involves acquisition of images during two or more contrast enhancement phases. Parathyroid glands quickly wash out contrast (bright on arterial phases but not on venous phases).

Table 16.4 Causes of Hypercalcemia
Iatrogenic: Calcium supplementation
Idiopathic infantile hypercalcemia
Benign familial hypocalciuric hypercalcemia
Primary hyperparathyroidism (adenoma, hyperplasia, carcinoma, multiple endocrine neoplasias I and II)
Parathyroid hormone–secreting tumors (paraneoplastic, mediated by parathyroid hormone–related protein): small cell lung cancer, ovarian cancer, thymoma
Multiple myeloma, leukemia, lymphoma
Granulomatous disease: Sarcoidosis, tuberculosis, histoplasmosis, leprosy, granulomatosis with polyangiitis
Drugs: Thiazide diuretics, lithium, theophylline, hypervitaminosis A and D
Immobilization, total parenteral nutrition
Milk alkali syndrome
Adrenal insufficiency
Paget's bone disease, hyperphosphatemia

- Invasive Localization
  - Intraoperative gamma probe: Tc99m MIBI is injected 2 hours prior to surgery and radioactive parathyroid glands are localized using handheld gamma probes.
  - Parathyroid angiography/arteriography.
  - Venous sampling of PTH: Angiographic sampling of selective veins preferred, but even large vein sampling (internal jugular vein) can help lateralize the gland and can be useful in reexploration.
  - US-guided parathyroid FNA with PTH washout

37. **What are the most common ectopic locations of parathyroid glands?**
    Ectopic parathyroid glands can be found in the superior mediastinum, in the thymic capsule, retroesophageal, within the carotid sheath, and medial to the superior thyroid pole. The inferior parathyroid gland has more variability in its final location because it descends with the thymus gland. The superior parathyroid gland tends to be more closely associated with the lateral lobe of the thyroid.

38. **What is the most recent NIH recommendation for surgery in the asymptomatic primary hyperparathyroidism patient?**
    See Table 16.5.

39. **How is intraoperative PTH monitoring used in parathyroid surgery?**
    PTH has a half-life of 3 to 5 minutes. In parathyroid surgery, the goal is to see a decrease in PTH level by more than 50% at 10 minutes after removal of a parathyroid(s) and a drop into the normal range. Intraoperative PTH monitoring allows focused parathyroid surgery (i.e., one-gland surgery) and can prevent unnecessary bilateral four-gland exploration.

40. **How is autotransplantation of parathyroid tissue performed?**
    Parathyroid tissue can either be autotransplanted at the time of surgery or cryopreserved for up to 18 months and transplanted later. Transplantation occurs most commonly into the sternocleidomastoid (SCM) of the neck or into the brachioradialis of the arm. Transplanted parathyroid tissue usually functions within 3 months and has a success rate of 50%. One advantage of transplanting into the arm is the ability to remove parathyroid tissue under local anesthetic if it becomes hyperplastic.

41. **What are the surgical options for hyperparathyroidism?**
    - Primary hyperparathyroidism: Pending preoperative workup (including imaging), a targeted approach with utilization of intraoperative PTH levels is preferred to minimize complications. If intraoperative PTH does not drop as expected after resection, strongly consider four-gland exploration
    - MEN syndrome: Bilateral cervical exploration and four-gland identification
    - Secondary or tertiary hyperparathyroidism: Subtotal parathyroidectomy (3- or 3.5-gland resection) or 4-gland parathyroidectomy with autotransplantation

42. **What strategies are used for parathyroid reexploration?**
    In reexploration, the strategy is to dissect lateral to medial, from the SCM to retroesophageal tissue overlying the cervical spine. Inferiorly, the thymus is resected. Medially, the prevertebral space (retroesophageal, retropharyngeal) is explored. The thyroid lobe is mobilized and palpated for an intrathyroidal parathyroid. If only one gland can be found on a given side, the ipsilateral thyroid lobe is often resected as intrathyroidal parathyroid glands are common. The carotid sheath is opened from the hyoid to the mediastinum. If unilateral exploration is negative, contralateral exploration is then performed. Mediastinal exploration should be performed only after imaging (i.e., MIBI and MRI) has been done.

Table 16.5 NIH Guidelines for Surgery in Asymptomatic Primary Hyperparathyroidism

Age <50
Serum calcium >1.0 mg/dL above the upper limit of normal
T score <2.5 at any site and/or previous fragility fracture
Renal function: estimated glomerular filtration rate <60 mL/min
Patient desires surgery or cannot be reliably followed
24-hour urine calcium: only recommended at initial workup to evaluate for familial hypocalciuric hypercalcemia but no longer an indication for surgery

CONTROVERSIES

43. **Does the presence of lymph node metastasis in well-differentiated thyroid cancers worsen the prognosis?**
This is unclear. Some studies demonstrate increased risk of local recurrence and lower disease-specific survival with nodal metastasis, while other studies demonstrate survival difference only in patients older than 45 years old. While survival may not be impacted by lymph node metastasis, disease-free survival is lower in patients with lymph node involvement.

44. **What is the optimal surgery for micropapillary thyroid cancer (<1 centimeters)?**
According to the National Cancer Institute, thyroid lobectomy alone is sufficient treatment for small (<1 centimeters), low-risk, unifocal, intrathyroidal papillary carcinomas in the absence of prior head and neck irradiation or radiologically or clinically involved cervical nodal metastases. Lobectomy is associated with a lower incidence of complications, but approximately 5% to 10% of patients will have a recurrence in the contralateral thyroid. Completion thyroidectomy is often curative in these cases.

45. **What is the role of RAI in patients with low-risk thyroid cancer?**
In low-risk patients (complete tumor resection; no nodal involvement; patients with T1 or T2 stage I younger than 45 years), there was no difference in overall survival and disease-specific survival between those receiving RAI and those without. Long-term complications of RAI include second malignancies, sialadenitis, and lacrimal and salivary gland dysfunction. Reducing the amount of radiation exposure by lowering the dosage of RAI and giving it in combination with rhTSH have been explored for patients with low-risk thyroid cancer.

46. **Is molecular diagnostics for thyroid cancer cost-effective?**
This is unclear. Recent studies show that if unnecessary surgery and two-surgery approaches are eliminated by molecular testing, there is a cost savings even with the high cost of the tests. Additional value of molecular testing may be as a quality control for cytopathology and as a prognostic test for the aggressiveness of a thyroid cancer.

BIBLIOGRAPHY

Amin MB, Edge S, Greene F, Byrd DR, Brookland RK, Washington MK, Gershenwald JE, Compton CC, Hess KR, et al. (Eds.). AJCC Cancer Staging Manual (8th edition). Springer International Publishing: American Joint Commission on Cancer; 2017 [cited 2016 Dec 28].

Bilezikian JP, Khan AA, Potts JT Jr: Guidelines for the management of asymptomatic primary hyperparathyroidism: summary statement from the third international workshop, *J Clin Endocrinol Metab* 94(2):335–339, 2009.

Bilimoria KY, Bentrem DJ, Ko CY, et al: Extent of surgery affects survival for papillary thyroid cancer, *Ann Surg* 246(3):375–381, 2007, discussion 381–384.

Carling T, Udelsman R: Thyroid tumors. In: DeVita VT Jr, Lawrence TS, Rosenberg SA, eds: *Cancer: Principles and Practice of Oncology*, 9th ed, Philadelphia, 2011, Lippincott Williams & Wilkins, pp 1457–1472.

Fazeli SR, Zehr B, Amraei R, et al: Thyroseq v2 testing: impact on cytologic diagnosis, management, and cost of care in patients with thyroid nodule, *Thyroid* 30(10):1528–1534, 2020.

Kebebew E, Clark OH: Medullary thyroid cancer, *Curr Treat Options Oncol* 1(4):359–367, 2000.

Mazzaferri EL, Jhiang SM: Long-term impact of initial surgical and medical therapy on papillary and follicular thyroid cancer, *Am J Med* 97(5):418–428, 1994.

Mazzaferri EL: Management of a solitary thyroid nodule, *N Engl J Med* 328(8):553–559, 1993.

Mazzaferri EL: Thyroid cancer in thyroid nodules: finding a needle in the haystack, *Am J Med* 93(4):359–362, 1992.

Schlumberger M, Catargi B, Borget I, et al: Strategies of radioiodine ablation in patients with low-risk thyroid cancer, *N Engl J Med* 366(18):1663–1673, 2012.

Shaha AR: Controversies in the management of thyroid nodule, *Laryngoscope* 110(2 Pt 1):183–193, 2000.

Walsh RM, Watkinson JC, Franklyn J: The management of the solitary thyroid nodule: a review, *Clin Otolaryngol Allied Sci* 24(5):388–397, 1999.

CHAPTER 17

NECK DISSECTION

Farshad N. Chowdhury, MD and Carissa M. Thomas, MD, PhD, FACS

KEY POINTS

1. The presence of cervical lymphadenopathy is a significant negative prognostic indicator in head and neck squamous cell carcinoma.
2. Knowledge and identification of first echelon nodes for various primary head and neck tumor sites allows for selective neck dissection of nodes at greatest risk for metastatic disease.
3. A thorough knowledge of key anatomic relationships allows the surgeon to preserve important anatomic structures while proceeding efficiently with an oncologic neck dissection.
4. In certain contexts, controversies remain in the approach and extent of surgical management of neck disease where evidence that weighs the risks and morbidity of the procedure versus the procedure's impact on survival is not yet available.

Pearls

1. Plan the neck incision appropriately. Consider the lymph node basins to be dissected, be at least two finger breadths below the mandible to protect the marginal mandibular nerve and for improved cosmesis, and avoid incisions with trifurcations, especially a trifurcation over the carotid. Also consider the need for cervicofacial advancement flaps, supraclavicular artery island flaps, submental flaps, and other reconstructive options.
2. Raise superior and inferior neck skin flaps in the subplatysmal plane to preserve the vascular supply and viability of the skin flaps. The superior limit is the inferior border of the mandible and the inferior limit is the clavicle.
3. The digastric muscle is often referred to as the "resident's friend" because it is lateral to many of the most important structures of the neck, including the internal jugular vein (IJV), carotid artery, and the hypoglossal nerve. Dissecting systematically along the digastric muscle prevents injury to these structures.
4. Cranial nerve (CN) XI is located at the junction of the upper one-third and lower two-thirds of the sternocleidomastoid muscle and is typically accompanied by a vessel that is encountered first. The relationship of CNXI and the IJV is variable. CNXI is most commonly superficial to the vein but can also be posterior to or travel between the IJV. In Level V, CNXI is identified deep to Erb's point and travels obliquely to the trapezius muscle. It is important not to confuse CNXI with superficial branches of the cervical plexus.
5. It is important that the fibrofatty tissue of Level IIb be passed underneath CNXI to be removed *en bloc* with the rest of the neck dissection specimen.
6. The floor of the neck dissection is formed by the fascia overlying the splenius capitis and levator scapulae muscles superiorly, the deep cervical rootlets in the mid-portion, and the scalene muscles (anterior, middle, posterior) inferiorly.
7. The phrenic nerve can be preserved by not violating the vertebral layer (or deep layer) of the deep cervical fascia at the level of the scalene muscles.
8. The deep branches of the cervical plexus should be preserved as well as the transverse cervical artery and vein.
9. A dissection too far medial along the deep muscles of the neck may result in injury to the sympathetic chain, which runs posterior to the carotid artery and should be preserved.
10. The best way to prevent a chyle leak is to dissect laterally from the IJV as you dissect below the omohyoid muscle (i.e., Level IV). Lymphatic vessels must be handled and ligated carefully when identified. Dissecting and ligating the Level IV tissues in segments may aid in capturing crossing lymphatic vessels. Increasing the intrathoracic pressure via Valsalva maneuver during surgery can test for and identify the source of a chyle leak.

QUESTIONS

1. **According to the American Joint Committee on Cancer (AJCC), what constitutes the Level I nodal group?**
   Level I includes both submental (Ia) and submandibular (Ib) lymph node basins. Anatomically, Ia includes the triangle formed by the anterior bellies of the digastric muscle bilaterally and the hyoid bone, and the mylohyoid muscle forms the floor. Level Ib is bound by the posterior belly of the digastric muscle and the mandible and includes lymph nodes around the facial artery and vein (Fig. 17.1).

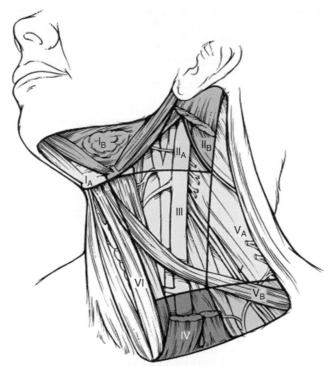

Fig. 17.1 The six levels of the neck for describing the location of lymph nodes. *IA*, Submental group; *IB*, submandibular group; *IIA*, upper jugular nodes; *IIB*, upper jugular nodes in the submuscular recess; *III*, mid-jugular nodes; *IV*, inferior jugular nodes; *VA*, spinal accessory nodes; *VB*, the supraclavicular and transverse cervical nodes. (Redrawn from art provided courtesy of Douglas Denys, MD. From Flint PW, Haughey BH, Lund VJ, et al, eds: *Cummings Otolaryngology – Head and Neck Surgery*, 5th ed, Philadelphia, 2010, Mosby Elsevier, p 1705.)

2. **What constitutes the Level II nodal group?**
    Level II includes the uppermost jugular nodes and is divided into Level IIa (nodes anteromedial to the spinal accessory nerve/cranial nerve XI) and Level IIb (nodes posterior lateral to CNXI). This includes all nodes adjacent to the great vessels from the skull base to the carotid bifurcation and from the sternohyoid muscle to the posterior border of the sternocleidomastoid muscle (SCM) (Fig. 17.1).

3. **What constitutes the Level III nodal group?**
    Level III includes the mid-jugular nodes extending from the carotid bifurcation to the omohyoid muscle and from the sternohyoid muscle to the posterior border of the SCM (Fig. 17.1).

4. **What constitutes the Level IV nodal group?**
    Level IV includes the inferior-most jugular nodes extending from the omohyoid muscle to the clavicle and from the sternohyoid muscle to the posterior border of the SCM (Fig. 17.1).

5. **What constitutes the Level V nodal group?**
    Level V includes the posterior triangle bounded by the posterior border of the SCM, the anterior edge of the trapezius muscle, and the clavicle. Level V is divided into two subgroups by a horizontal plane at the level of the cricoid: Level Va (spinal accessory nodes) and level Vb (supraclavicular and transverse cervical nodes) (Fig. 17.1).

6. **What serves as the boundary between Levels II to IV and Level V?**
    The plane delineated by the cervical plexus rootlets serves as the deep boundary of Levels II to IV and the corresponding superficial boundary of level V.

7. **What constitutes the Level VI nodal group?**
    Level VI includes the central compartment nodes extending from the hyoid bone to the suprasternal notch and laterally by the carotid arteries. These include pretracheal, paratracheal, and Delphian (precricoid) nodes. Perithyroidal nodes and nodes occurring along the recurrent laryngeal nerves are also in Level VI (Fig. 17.1).

8. Which primary sites are most likely to metastasize to these nodal groups?
   1. Level Ia: Anterior oral tongue, floor of mouth, lower alveolar ridge/gingiva, lower lip
   2. Level Ib: Oral cavity (including tongue, lateral floor of mouth, buccal mucosa), anterior nasal cavity, maxillary sinus, submandibular gland
   3. Level II: Most primary head and neck sites including oral cavity, nasal cavity, nasopharynx, oropharynx, hypopharynx, larynx, parotid gland
   4. Level III: Oral cavity, oropharynx, nasopharynx, hypopharynx, larynx
   5. Level IV: Hypopharynx, thyroid, larynx, cervical esophagus
   6. Level V: Cutaneous malignancies of posterior scalp and neck, nasopharynx, oropharynx
   7. Level VI: Thyroid, larynx (glottic and subglottic), cervical esophagus, apex of piriform sinus (Fig. 17.1)

9. What is the AJCC eighth edition clinical staging for nodal disease for head and neck tumors (excluding human papillomavirus (HPV)-positive oropharynx, nasopharynx, and thyroid)? How does it differ from pathologic staging?

Regional Lymph Nodes (N), Clinical N (cN)

NX Regional lymph nodes cannot be assessed

N0 No regional lymph node metastasis

N1 Metastasis in a single ipsilateral lymph node, 3 centimeters or smaller in greatest dimension, extranodal extension (ENE)(−)

N2 Metastasis in a single ipsilateral node, 3 to 6 centimeters in greatest dimension, ENE(−); *or* metastases in multiple ipsilateral lymph nodes, none larger than 6 centimeters in greatest dimension, and ENE(−); *or* in bilateral or contralateral lymph nodes, none larger than 6 centimeters in greatest dimension, and ENE(−)

    N2a Metastasis in a single ipsilateral lymph node, 3 to 6 centimeters in greatest dimension and ENE(−)

    N2b Metastases in multiple ipsilateral lymph nodes, none larger than 6 centimeters in greatest dimension, and ENE(−)

    N2c Metastases in bilateral or contralateral lymph nodes, none larger than 6 centimeters in greatest dimension, and ENE(−)

N3 Metastasis in a lymph node larger than 6 centimeters in greatest dimension and ENE(−); *or* metastasis in any node(s) and clinically overt ENE(+)

    N3a Metastasis in a lymph node larger than 6 centimeters in greatest dimension and ENE(−)

    N3b Metastasis in any node(s) and clinically overt ENE(+)

pN2 and **pN3** pathologic staging differs as outlined below. **pNX, pN0,** and **pN1** is the same as clinical staging.

pN2 Metastasis in a single ipsilateral node, 3 centimeters or smaller in greatest dimension, and ENE(+); *or* 3 to 6 centimeters in greatest dimension and ENE(−); *or* metastases in multiple ipsilateral lymph nodes, none larger than 6 centimeters in greatest dimension, and ENE(−); *or* in bilateral or contralateral lymph node(s), none larger than 6 centimeters in greatest dimension, and ENE(−)

    pN2a Metastasis in a single ipsilateral node, 3 centimeters or smaller in greatest dimension, and ENE(+); *or* a single ipsilateral node, 3 to 6 centimeters in greatest dimension, and ENE(−)

    pN2b Metastases in multiple ipsilateral lymph nodes, none larger than 6 centimeters in greatest dimension, and ENE(−)

    pN2c Metastases in bilateral or contralateral lymph nodes, none larger than 6 centimeters in greatest dimension, and ENE(−)

pN3 Metastasis in a lymph node larger than 6 centimeters in greatest dimension and ENE(−); *or* metastasis in a single ipsilateral node larger than 3 centimeters in greatest dimension and ENE(+); *or* multiple ipsilateral, contralateral, or bilateral nodes any with ENE(+); *or* a single contralateral node of any size and ENE(+)

    pN3a Metastasis in a lymph node larger than 6 centimeters in greatest dimension and ENE(−)

    pN3b Metastasis in a single ipsilateral node larger than 3 centimeters in greatest dimension and ENE(+); *or* multiple ipsilateral, contralateral, or bilateral nodes any with ENE(+); *or* a single contralateral, node of any size and ENE(+)

10. What is the AJCC eighth edition clinical nodal staging for nasopharyngeal tumors?

Regional Lymph Nodes (N)

NX Regional lymph nodes cannot be assessed

N0 No regional lymph node metastasis

N1 Unilateral metastasis in cervical lymph node(s) and/or unilateral or bilateral metastasis in retropharyngeal lymph node(s), 6 centimeters or smaller in greatest dimension, above the caudal border of cricoid cartilage

N2 Bilateral metastasis in cervical lymph node(s), 6 centimeters or smaller in greatest dimension, above the caudal border of cricoid cartilage

N3 Unilateral or bilateral metastasis in cervical lymph node(s), larger than 6 centimeters in greatest dimension, and/or extension below the caudal border of cricoid cartilage

11. **What is the AJCC eighth edition clinical nodal staging for HPV+ oropharyngeal tumors? How does it differ from pathologic staging?**
Regional Lymph Nodes (N), Clinical N (cN)
NX Regional lymph nodes cannot be assessed
N0 No regional lymph node metastasis
N1 One or more ipsilateral lymph nodes, none larger than 6 centimeters
N2 Contralateral or bilateral lymph nodes, none larger than 6 centimeters
N3 Lymph node(s) larger than 6 centimeters
Regional Lymph Nodes (N), Pathologic N (pN)
NX Regional lymph nodes cannot be assessed
pN0 No regional lymph node metastasis
pN1 Metastasis in four or fewer lymph nodes
pN2 Metastasis in more than four lymph nodes

12. **What is the AJCC eighth edition clinical nodal staging for thyroid tumors?**
See thyroid and parathyroid (Chapter 16).

13. **What are the overarching principles of surgical management of the neck in head and neck cancers?**
In general, the extent of the primary tumor will dictate surgical management of neck lymph nodes. Ipsilateral neck dissection is frequently done along with resection of the primary tumor. Bilateral neck dissection is indicated for tumor primary sites that often have bilateral lymphatic drainage such as the base of tongue, supraglottic larynx, etc. Patients with oral cavity tumors that approximate or cross midline should be considered for a bilateral neck dissection.

14. **What is a radical neck dissection (RND)?**
This neck dissection, first popularized by George Crile in the early 20th century and later by Hayes Martin in the 1950s, espoused the concept of radical *en bloc* resection of cervical lymph nodes for cancers of the head and neck. RND includes removal of lymph node Levels I through V, along with the SCM, internal jugular vein (IJV), and spinal accessory nerve (CN XI).

15. **What morbidity is associated with RND?**
Shoulder dysfunction is a significant morbidity of RND. Symptoms include shoulder tilt/drop, constant pain, winged scapula, and limited range of motion, including anterior flexion, abduction, and retraction. In bilateral neck dissections, removal of both IJVs can result in significant venous edema and chronic lymphedema of the face and can be fatal in 10% of patients when performed simultaneously. At least one IJV should be preserved in bilateral procedures. If both IJVs are involved by disease, a staged neck dissection separated by at least 2 weeks should be performed to allow for collateral circulation to develop.

16. **What are the indications for RND?**
Today, RND is indicated for patients whose cervical node metastases has extended beyond the capsule of the lymph node (ENE) to invade the SCM, CNXI, or IJV such that the removal of these structures is necessary to remove the disease in its entirety.

17. **What is a modified RND (MRND)?**
In an MRND, lymph node Levels I through V are removed, but one or more of the nonlymphatic structures (CNXI, SCM, or IJV) are spared.

18. **What is the rationale for an MRND?**
Unless there is fixation or infiltration of the SCM, IJV, and/or CNXI, these structures are preserved to significantly reduce morbidity. In addition, removal of an uninvolved SCM, IJV, and/or CNXI does not improve oncologic outcomes.

19. **What is a selective neck dissection (SND)?**
In a SND, an *en bloc* resection of one or more nodal groups is performed while preserving nonlymphatic structures. Only the nodal groups determined to be at highest risk for metastasis are removed. A *comprehensive* neck dissection resects all I to V nodal basins while preserving the SCM, IJV, and CNXI.

20. **What are the indications for an SND?**
In previously untreated patients with head and neck cancer, the level of nodal metastasis typically occurs in a predictable pattern. This allows for the identification of highest-risk, first-echelon lymph nodes for a variety of primary tumor sites. SND can be used for treatment in conjunction with resection of tumors with limited neck

disease, for surgical staging of the neck in the clinically N0 neck, or to direct further adjuvant therapy if multiple nodes or the presence of ENE is found.

21. **What is the extent of SND in these primary head and neck cancer sites?**
    - Oral cavity: Levels I, II, III (supraomohyoid neck dissection)
    - Oropharynx, hypopharynx, larynx: Levels II to IV (lateral neck dissection)
    - Posterior scalp: Levels II to V, retroauricular and suboccipital nodes (posterolateral neck dissection)
    - Preauricular, anterior scalp: Levels II to Va, parotid and facial nodes
    - Anterior and lateral face: Levels I to III, parotid and facial nodes
    - Thyroid, esophagus, advanced laryngeal or hypopharyngeal tumor: Level VI (anterior or central neck dissection)
      Additional levels may also be dissected with advanced tumors based on surgical discretion.

22. **What is an elective neck dissection (END)?**
    In general, a patient without clinical evidence of nodal metastasis should receive END when the probability of occult nodal metastasis exceeds 20%. This threshold was established in a decision tree analysis conducted by Weiss et al. In this context, single modality treatment with either surgery or radiation was equally effective.

23. **What is a sentinel lymph node?**
    The first lymph node in a primary nodal drainage basin for a malignancy and the most likely site for regional metastasis. The sentinel lymph node can be identified with a combination of lymphoscintigraphy imaging and lymphatic mapping with gamma detection.

24. **What is the role of lymphoscintigraphy and sentinel lymph node biopsy (SLNB) in neck dissection?**
    Lymphoscintigraphy is performed by injecting radiotracer into the primary site of interest to determine the primary echelon nodal basin. In head and neck mucosal malignancies, SLNB can be used to (1) stage neck disease in clinically N0 necks, (2) identify lymphatic flow into atypical nodal basins that would not be addressed in classic SNDs, and (3) determine lymphatic flow changes as a result of surgery and radiation that are at risk for metastasis from recurrent or residual disease.

25. **What is the role of SLNB in head and neck cutaneous melanoma?**
    The use of SLNB in head and neck melanoma is well established as a therapeutic instrument and staging tool. Multicenter clinical trials (MSLT-I, DECOG-SLT, MSLT-II) support the use of SLNB as a method to address first-echelon nodal disease, and complete neck dissection can be avoided in the setting of a negative SLNB.

26. **How should the neck be managed in early-stage, clinically node-negative (cT1-2N0) oral squamous cell carcinoma (SCC)?**
    A clinical trial by D'Cruz et al. in 2015 provided Level 1 evidence that an END had superior overall and disease-free survival in clinically node-negative early-stage oral SCC compared to monitoring and performing a therapeutic neck dissection if lymph node metastases occurred. The benefit was observed in tumors with 3 millimeters or greater depth of invasion (DOI). In the literature, oral tongue DOI greater than 2 to 4 millimeters and floor of mouth greater than 1.5 millimeters are commonly cited indications for neck dissection in clinically lymph node–negative patients.

27. **What are some complications after a neck dissection?**
    - **Chylous fistula:** The thoracic duct transports chyle composed of chylomicrons, long-chain fatty acids, and lymphocytes. A chylous fistula (or chyle leak) is caused by an injury to the thoracic duct as it enters the IJV laterally just superior to the junction of the IJV and subclavian vein. Most commonly associated with a left Level IV dissection and occurs in 1% to 3% of neck dissections. Daily output greater than 500 mL (high-output leak) will require surgical exploration and ligation of the duct. Thoracoscopic and interventional radiology approaches to ligating the thoracic duct are possible. Total parenteral nutrition may be considered in high-output leaks. Output of less than 500 mL (low-output leak) may be managed conservatively with activity restriction, pressure dressing, and diet modification with restriction to nonfat, low-fat, or medium-chain fatty acid–only diets. Pharmacologic intervention with octreotide, a somatostatin analogue thought to reduce chyle production and lymph flow, can be done. Electrolytes should be monitored, fluid losses repleted, and the patient assessed for possible chylothorax.
    - **Facial and cerebral edema:** Associated with bilateral ligation of IJV and in patients with previous radiation therapy. This can be avoided by staged neck dissections and by preserving one or more external jugular veins. Cerebral edema resulting from IJV ligation can cause syndrome of inappropriate secretions of antidiuretic hormone (SIADH). Intravenous fluids should be carefully administered in bilateral neck dissections where the IJV is ligated and serum and urine osmolarity carefully monitored perioperatively. In addition, increased intracranial pressure, altered mental status, blindness, and cranial nerve VI palsy have been reported.

- **Phrenic nerve injury:** Injury to the phrenic nerve can occur during the Level IV neck dissection and results in paralysis of the ipsilateral hemidiaphragm.
- **Carotid rupture/blowout:** This catastrophic complication is associated with salivary fistula, neck skin flap breakdown due to previous radiation, malnutrition, infection, and diabetes. Poorly placed and designed neck incisions can expose the carotid and increase risk of rupture. Placement of vascularized tissue over the carotid is indicated in cases of large salivary fistulas or carotid exposure. Patients at risk of carotid rupture should be on "carotid blowout precautions" including IV access with two large-bore IVs, intubation tray at bedside, two units of packed red blood cells typed and crossed, and an educated nursing staff.

28. **What are the types of neck dissection after chemoradiation or radiation therapy?**
Neck dissection after chemoradiation falls into one of three categories:
    - **Failure at the primary site:** Neck dissection is performed at the same time as salvage surgery for the primary site. Can be done regardless of nodal status at completion of treatment and frequently because vessel access is needed for microvascular reconstruction of the primary site.
    - **Salvage neck dissection:** Neck dissection is performed if there is persistent nodal disease after treatment. Assessment of nodal disease is performed 12 weeks posttreatment using positron emission tomography scan or computed tomography and magnetic resonance imaging.
    - **Planned/staged neck dissection:** Some surgeons will recommend a planned neck dissection for high-volume nodal disease (N3) regardless of response to therapy. However, a prospective randomized controlled trial was performed by Mehanna et al. that compared image-guided surveillance to planned neck dissection in patients with advanced nodal disease (N2–3) treated primarily with chemoradiation and found surveillance was not inferior to planned neck dissection, with similar survival and quality of life regardless of HPV status. In their study, approximately 80% of patients were spared a neck dissection, and surveillance had significant cost savings compared to a planned neck dissection.

29. **What are indications for postoperative radiation to the neck after a neck dissection?**
Multiple positive lymph nodes or ENE.

30. **What is the recommended number of lymph nodes to sample in a unilateral neck dissection?**
Retrospective reviews utilizing large national databases indicate that at least 18 lymph nodes are needed for an adequate assessment of occult metastatic disease. Removing at least 18 lymph nodes in an unilateral neck dissection is associated with improved survival.

31. **Regional lymph node metastases reduces 5-year overall survival by how much compared to early-stage disease?**
50%

CONTROVERSIES

32. **Role of END in the setting of salvage laryngectomy**
END for the management of the clinically N0 neck in the setting of salvage laryngectomy is often controversial. Historically, the reported rate of occult nodal metastasis has varied widely in single-institution studies (4%–27%), as have reported rates of postoperative complications (salivary fistula, wound infection, carotid blowout, etc.) and the benefit in overall survival derived from END. Recent meta-analyses have reported a pooled rate of occult nodal metastasis in laryngeal cancers between 11% and 14%, with higher rates of occult nodal metastases for supraglottic and T3/T4 glottic cancers. Pooled data on rates of perioperative complications and overall survival remain inconclusive. Prospective data are needed to better determine whether END confers a survival benefit that would outweigh the risks associated with END in the salvage setting.

33. **Role of SLNB in oral cavity SCC for neck management**
Several multicenter prospective trials on the use of SLNB in oral SCC have demonstrated high rates of SLN identification (>97.6%) and high negative predictive values (88%–97.8%). In these studies, regional recurrence ranged from 4.7% to 12%. An advantage to lymphatic mapping and SLNB is that contralateral drainage patterns can be identified that might not be addressed with a standard END. Currently, it appears that SLNB can be a safe alternative to END in early-stage cN0 oral SCC; however, there are no prospective randomized data comparing SLNB to END on survival. The NRG-HN006 trial is currently ongoing to address this question.

34. **Role of completion lymph node dissection (CLND) in patients with melanoma and a positive SLN**
The second Multicenter Selective Lymphadenectomy Trial (MSLT-II) randomized positive SLNB to completion lymphadenectomy or observation with ultrasound. Only 13.7% of each arm was composed of patients with head and neck melanoma. There was no difference in melanoma-specific survival (MSS) between dissection and observation. Disease-free survival was higher in the dissection group. CLND improved regional control but did not

improve MSS. The morbidity associated with CLND in the head and neck is less significant than CLND of the groin or axilla. Regional recurrence in the head and neck can cause CN palsies, bleeding, airway compromise, and other significant sequelae; therefore CLND is still a consideration in head and neck melanoma.

BIBLIOGRAPHY

Agrawal A, Civantos FJ, Brumund KT, et al: [99mTc]Tilmanocept accurately detects sentinel lymph nodes and predicts node pathology status in patients with oral squamous cell carcinoma of the head and neck: results of a Phase III multi-institutional trial, *Ann Surg Oncol* 22(11):3708–3715, 2015.

Bello DM, Faries MB: The Landmark Series: MSLT-1, MSLT-2 and DeCOG (management of lymph nodes), *Ann Surg Oncol* 27(1):15–21, 2020.

Byers RM, Wolf PF, Ballantyne AJ: Rationale for elective modified neck dissection, *Head Neck Surg* 10(3):160–167, 1988.

D'Cruz AK, Vaish R, Kapre N, et al: Elective versus therapeutic neck dissection in node-negative oral cancer, *N Engl J Med* 373(6):521–529, 2015.

Deschler DG, Day T, eds: *TNM Staging of Head and Neck Cancer and Neck Dissection Classification,* 3rd ed, Alexandria, VA, 2008, American Academy of Otolaryngology-Head and Neck Surgery Foundation.

Divi V, Chen MM, Nussenbaum B, et al: Lymph node count from neck dissection predicts mortality in head and neck cancer, *J Clin Oncol* 34(32):3892–3897, 2016.

Faries MB, Thompson JF, Cochran AJ, et al: Completion dissection or observation for sentinel-node metastasis in melanoma, *N Engl J Med* 376(23):2211–2222, 2017.

Flach GB, Bloemena E, Klop WM, et al: Sentinel lymph node biopsy in clinically N0 T1–T2 staged oral cancer: the Dutch multicenter trial, *Oral Oncol* 50(10):1020–1024, 2014.

Gavilán J, Castro A, Rodrigáñez L, et al: *Functional and Selective Neck Dissection*, 2nd, New York, 2020, Thieme.

Head and Neck Cancer (Version 2.2021), 2021 National Comprehensive Cancer Network.

Huang SH, Hwang D, Lockwood G, et al: Predictive value of tumor thickness for cervical lymph-node involvement in squamous cell carcinoma of the oral cavity, *Cancer* 115(7):1489–1497, 2009.

Martin H, Del Valle B, Ehrlich H, et al: Neck dissection, *Cancer* 4(3):441–499, 1951.

Mehanna H, Wong WL, McConkey CC, et al: PET-CT surveillance versus neck dissection in advanced head and neck cancer, *N Engl J Med* 374(15):1444–1454, 2016.

Morton DL, Thompson JF, Cochran AJ, et al: Final trial report of sentinel-node biopsy versus nodal observation in melanoma, *N Engl J Med* 370(7):599–609, 2014.

Morton DL, Thompson JF, Cochran AJ, et al: Sentinel-node biopsy or nodal observation in melanoma, *N Engl J Med* 355(13):1307–1317, 2006; erratum in: *N Engl J Med* 355(18):1944, 2006.

Pynnonen MA, Gillespie MB, Roman B, et al: Clinical practice guideline: evaluation of the neck mass in adults, *Otolaryngol Head Neck Surg* 157(2_suppl):S1–S30, 2017.

Robbins KT, Shaha AR, Medina JE, et al: Consensus statement of the classification and terminology of neck dissection, *Arch Otolaryngol Head Neck Surg* 134(5):536–538, 2008.

Schilling C, Stoeckli SJ, Haerle SK, et al: Sentinel European Node Trial (SENT): 3-year results of sentinel node biopsy in oral cancer, *Eur J Cancer* 51(18):2777–2784, 2015.

Shah JP, Candela FC, Poddar AK: The patterns of cervical lymph node metastases from squamous carcinoma of the oral cavity, *Cancer* 66(1):109–113, 1990.

Shah JP: Patterns of cervical lymph node metastasis from squamous carcinomas of the upper aerodigestive tract, *Am J Surg* 160(4):405–409, 1990.

Weiss MH, Harrison LB, Isaacs RS: Use of decision analysis in planning a management strategy for the stage N0 neck, *Arch Otolaryngol Head Neck Surg* 120(7):699–702, 1994.

CHAPTER 18

VASCULAR TUMORS OF THE HEAD AND NECK

Kenny D. Rodriguez, MD and Brook K. McConnell, MD

KEY POINTS

1. Most head and neck paragangliomas are nonfunctional, although suspected sympathetic symptoms (flushing, palpitations, sweating) should be evaluated thoroughly.
2. Treatment of head and neck paragangliomas involves observation, surgery, or radiotherapy depending on patient-specific factors, tumor growth rate, and suspicion for malignancy.
3. The natural history of a hemangioma is rapid growth followed by involution; therefore a conservative approach is recommended for most lesions unless there is significant ocular or airway involvement.

Pearls

1. Carotid body paragangliomas are the most common head and neck paragangliomas.
2. Carotid body paragangliomas present as a pulsatile neck mass with characteristic computed tomography, magnetic resonance imaging, and angiographic signs including characteristic flow voids and splaying of the external and internal carotid arteries (lyre sign).
3. Genetic testing is recommended for all patients with paragangliomas.
4. Familial paragangliomas are inherited in an autosomal dominant fashion modified by genomic imprinting. Affected offspring will develop paragangliomas only if the gene is paternally inherited. Maternally inherited genes are inactive, and offspring develop no tumors.
5. A teenage male with unilateral nasal obstruction, epistaxis, and a bluish mass filling the nasal cavity is the typical presentation of a juvenile nasopharyngeal angiofibroma.

QUESTIONS

1. **What are paragangliomas and from which tissues do they arise?**
   Paragangliomas (PGLs) are slow-growing neuroendocrine neoplasms derived from paraganglia cells. These cells are extra-adrenal neuroectoderm-derived cells located in the adventitia of blood vessels. Paraganglia in the head and neck are typically related to the parasympathetic system, classified as nonchromaffin, non-catecholamine-secreting cells. Paraganglia related to the sympathetic system are classified as chromaffin, catecholamine-secreting neoplasms and are more common outside of the head and neck.

2. **How are head and neck PGLs different than PGLs outside of the head and neck?**
   The most common site of involvement is the adrenal medulla (pheochromocytoma, 90%), followed by the abdomen (8.5%), the thorax (1.2%), and the head and neck (0.3%). Head and neck PGLs are typically nonsecreting neoplasms with less than 1% producing catecholamines.

3. **What is the current standard terminology for head and neck PGLs?**
   PGLs have previously been referred to as carotid body tumors, nonchromaffin tumors, chemodectomas, glomus tympanicum, and glomus jugulare. *Glomus* is the most frequently misused term in the literature as it is technically a term for a histologically different benign cutaneous tumor. Proper nomenclature classifies head and neck PGLs based on anatomic location (e.g., carotid body, vagal, jugulotympanic paragangliomas).

4. **What are carotid body PGLs and what are their typical characteristics?**
   The carotid body is the largest, most compact collection of paraganglia in the body. Carotid body PGL is the most common in the head and neck, accounting for 60% of cases. Due to the physiologic function of the carotid body as a chemoreceptor, PGLs were known as chemodectomas. Although the term chemodectoma has been used in connection with all PGLs, it only applies to carotid body PGLs because the carotid body and aortic body are the only paraganglia that act as chemoreceptors. Carotid body PGLs typically present in the fifth or sixth decade of life, although hereditary forms tend to present 1 or 2 decades earlier, often by age 30 to 40. Bilateral tumors are found in 10% to 25% of cases.

5. **What is a major recognized risk factor for the development of a PGL?**
   Chronic hypoxia has long been recognized as a significant risk factor for development of a PGL. Interestingly, there is a dose-dependent relationship between incidence and altitude. At higher altitudes, female predominance is markedly elevated at 8:1 compared to 3:1 at lower altitudes.

6. **What are the two major types of middle ear PGLs?**
   Middle ear PGLs are commonly referred to as glomus jugulare and glomus tympanicum tumors and account for 30% of head and neck PGLs. They typically present in the sixth decade of life. Jugular neoplasms arise from jugular bulb paraganglia along the medial promontory wall, whereas tympanic neoplasms arise from paraganglia associated with Jacobson's nerve. Jugular neoplasms tend to invade the petrous bone and their growth leads to bony destruction. Tumors of the jugular foramen can result in cranial IX to XI nerve dysfunction, and resection in this region involves a combined skull base procedure that can result in significant cranial nerve–related morbidity.

7. **What are vagal PGLs? What are laryngeal PGLs?**
   Vagal PGLs arise from the inferior vagal ganglion (nodose ganglion) in the vagal trunk approximately 2 centimeters distal to its exit from the brainstem, although they can also arise from the superior vagal ganglion. These tumors comprise 10% of head and neck PGLs. Tumors associated with peripheral vagus nerve branches are categorized based on their anatomical locations. Laryngeal PGLs are very rare neoplasms derived from the superior or inferior paraganglia of the larynx. Laryngeal PGLs are most often located in the supraglottis and are more common in women.

8. **How do head and neck PGLs present?**
   Head and neck PGLs are typically asymptomatic and are frequently discovered incidentally on imaging. All PGLs demonstrate a female predominance. Carotid body PGLs typically present with a pulsatile neck mass that is mobile in the horizontal direction but limited vertically – an exam finding known as Fontaine's sign. They occur near the anterior border of the sternocleidomastoid muscle and the angle of the mandible and are rubbery and well-circumscribed upon palpation. The growth rate is estimated at 5 millimeters per year. Vagal PGLs can present with Fontaine's sign but are generally not pulsatile, although they can transmit pulsations. These tumors commonly present with an ipsilateral Horner's syndrome or vocal cord paralysis. A comprehensive cranial nerve exam is critical for all patients with head and neck PGLs. Middle ear PGLs commonly present with pulsatile tinnitus, hearing loss, and aural fullness, and larger tumors can present with lower cranial nerve involvement (cranial nerves IX, X, and XI). Tympanic PGLs can be visualized on otoscopy as a vascular mass behind or protruding through the eardrum. Laryngeal PGLs present with symptoms of laryngeal obstruction, including shortness of breath, hoarseness, and stridor.

9. **What are the symptoms of a functional PGL tumor and which laboratory tests should be performed to evaluate for them?**
   Primary head and neck PGLs do not typically produce catecholamines. Functional tumors are rare and comprise approximately 1% to 3% of head and neck PGLs, but the presence of a second primary tumor must be ruled out. It is important to gather a thorough history to assess for a functional tumor. The presence of headaches, hypertension, flushing, heat intolerance, or palpitations should be further evaluated with 24-hour urine norepinephrine and fractionated metanephrines. Alpha- and beta-adrenergic blockade is indicated for patients with functional neoplasms to reduce the risk of sudden catecholamine release.

10. **What imaging modalities can be used to evaluate PGLs?**
    Computed tomography (CT) with contrast or magnetic resonance imaging (MRI) with gadolinium (and CT/MRI angiography if needed) will often contribute to the diagnosis and provide anatomic detail. Vascular flow voids are often demonstrated on imaging, which strongly predicts a PGL. Ultrasonography may be helpful on initial examination to determine the difference between a vascular tumor and lymph node. Conventional angiography was very common prior to CT or MRI angiography technology but is now reserved for preoperative embolization, if indicated. Imaging of carotid body PGLs classically demonstrates splaying of the internal and external carotid arteries with displacement of the internal carotid posteriorly and external carotid anteriorly, resulting in the classic "lyre sign" (Fig. 18.1). Vagal PGLs can be differentiated on imaging because they are superior to the bifurcation and displace the vessels anteriorly and medially. Vagal PGLs located at the jugular foramen can exhibit a dumbbell shape representing intracranial and extracranial extension. Additional imaging modalities, including radioisotope imaging, can be helpful when other cross-sectional scans fail to demonstrate a lesion or when malignant disease is likely.

11. **What is the predominant molecular pathogenesis for the development of head and neck PGLs? What are the recommendations for genetic testing? What is the inheritance pattern of familial PGLs?**
    Mutations in the succinate dehydrogenase (SDH) enzyme, a multiprotein complex found in the mitochondrial matrix, comprise the prevailing pathway for the development of head and neck PGLs. PGLs have a high association with germline mutations, with at least 14 identified susceptible genes. SDH mutations account for most hereditary

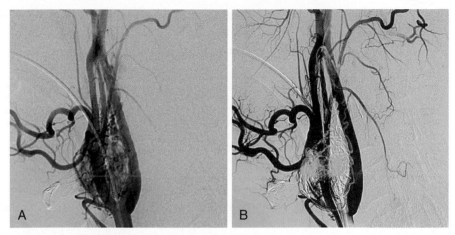

Fig. 18.1 Conventional angiography performed for the purpose of embolization that nicely demonstrates splaying of the internal and external carotid arteries known as the "lyre sign."

cases, followed by those associated with von Hippel Lindau disease, multiple endocrine neoplasia types 2A and 2B, and neurofibromatosis type 1. With the identification of these germline mutations, PGLs have been found to represent the most common hereditary neoplasms, with 30% to 40% of head and neck PGLs being familial. As a result, the Endocrine Society guidelines recommend genetic testing for all patients with a PGL. Familial PGLs are inherited in an autosomal dominant fashion modified by genomic imprinting. Affected offspring will develop PGLs only if the gene is paternally inherited. When maternally inherited, the gene is not expressed, and offspring will not exhibit the disease. Gene mutations of SDHB carry the highest risk of malignancy.

12. **What are the treatment options for PGLs? What are the possible postsurgical morbidities?**
    Options for PGL treatment include observation, surgery, and radiation. Treatment depends on patient-specific factors such as age, neoplasm growth rate, suspicion for malignancy, and multicentricity. Carotid body PGLs are typically treated with early surgical intervention if the patient is a good surgical candidate. However, PGLs often remain stable for many years or grow very slowly, and for older patients, those with multiple lower cranial nerve involvement, or those with bilateral carotid body PGLs, observation via serial imaging may be reasonable management to avoid surgical morbidity. Damage to lower cranial nerves can result in aspiration, dysphagia, facial nerve injuries, and vocal cord paralysis. Radiotherapy through several modalities can be effective in arresting growth of PGLs, with 10-year local progression-free rates between 92% and 100%. No permanent neuropathy has been reported with radiotherapy management, but the potential for secondary malignancies limits its use in younger patients.

13. **What is the classic histology of a PGL?**
    There are three types of cells: capillaries, chief cells (type I), and sustentacular cells (type II). Type I cells are the predominant cell type and form organized nests of cells in a pattern known as *zellballen.* Type II cells are identified in the periphery around type I cells.

14. **How are malignant PGLs diagnosed?**
    Malignant PGLs are histologically indistinct from benign tumors. Malignancy is determined purely based on the presence of regional and distant metastasis.

15. **How common is metastasis with head and neck PGLs?**
    Vagal PGLs have the highest metastatic potential (16%) compared to carotid body (4%-6%) and middle ear (5%) tumors.

16. **What can happen if bilateral carotid tumors are excised?**
    Baroreflex failure is an impairment of autonomic regulation resulting in extremely labile blood pressure caused by various abnormalities related to glossopharyngeal or vagal nerves, carotid bodies, brainstem connections, or damage to brainstem nuclei. Damage may occur in the presence of a neoplasm, traumatic injury, stroke, high-dose radiation therapy, or surgical intervention for bilateral PGLs. Special planning is warranted for bilateral PGLs to avoid bilateral surgical excision. Treatment of baroreflex failure is difficult and includes medications to manage hypertension, including clonidine, which acts to reduce sympathetic activity. Benzodiazepines are also useful because hypertension is often partially cortically driven. In general, vasodilators should be avoided because they can result in life-threatening hypotension in the setting of absent baroreflexes. Hypotension can also occur and is

managed with increasing dietary salt and pharmacologic agents such as fludrocortisone. Compensation can occur but the rate and timing is variable.

17. **Describe juvenile nasopharyngeal angiofibroma including the common presenting characteristics and predominant affected population.**

    Juvenile nasopharyngeal angiofibromas (JNAs) are rare benign vascular lesions, composed of complex endothelium-lined vessels embedded in fibrous stroma. They account for 0.05% to 0.5% of all head and neck neoplasms, although there is still debate as to whether JNAs represent true neoplasms or congenital vascular malformations. The most common presenting symptoms are unilateral nasal obstruction and epistaxis. Other related symptoms are due to mass effect, including sinusitis, hearing loss, otitis media, and ocular symptoms. These tumors classically arise in the pterygopalatine fossa and spread through the skull base, resulting in nasopharyngeal and nasal cavity involvement. Physical exam typically demonstrates a large, bluish mass in the nasopharynx and/or nasal passage. Additional growth can result in the infratemporal fossa, maxillary sinus, orbital, or intracranially.

    JNAs frequently express androgen receptors resulting in growth almost exclusively in adolescent males.

18. **How are JNAs diagnosed?**

    Both MRI and CT are common imaging modalities to diagnose a JNA and to determine the extent of the lesion. CT is important to determine bony involvement and growth pattern. Additionally, CT is helpful for surgical planning. MRI demonstrates flow voids, which further aids in the diagnosis. MRI is also critical to evaluate the degree of soft tissue involvement, including orbital and intracranial spread. MRI is typically preferred for posttreatment monitoring. The Holman–Miller sign is a classic CT finding demonstrating anterior bowing of the posterior wall of the maxillary antrum frequently seen with JNAs.

    Due to the characteristic findings on history, physical exam, and imaging, together with the high risk of life-threatening hemorrhage, diagnostic biopsy of these vascular tumors should be avoided.

19. **What is the typical treatment for a JNA?**

    Although they are histologically benign, they may be locally invasive and have the potential to extend intracranially. JNAs may be treated via open or endoscopic approaches, but endoscopic resection generally results in decreased intraoperative blood loss and lower recurrence rates. Angiography is often used to identify feeding vessels and perform preoperative embolization to reduce intraoperative blood loss. Low-dose radiation therapy can be used successfully but is reserved for unresectable cases due to potential secondary malignancies later in life. JNAs have been associated with a significant recurrence rate of 5% to 39%, although there are reports of spontaneous involution after adolescence.

20. **What is a hemangioma and what are the most common types?**

    Hemangiomas are benign vascular neoplasms that can occur in patients of all ages.
    - Infantile hemangiomas are absent at birth and present in infancy. They occur with a female predominance and are notable for the presence of GLUT1 by immunohistochemistry.
    - Congenital hemangiomas are present at the time of birth and present in a rapidly involuting and noninvoluting variety.
    - Lobular capillary hemangiomas are proliferations of capillaries arranged in lobules.
    - Cavernous hemangiomas are composed of multiple thin-walled blood-filled cysts.

21. **What treatment options are available for an infantile hemangioma and when are they indicated?**

    Infantile hemangiomas typically present with a period of rapid growth and subsequent involution. Without treatment, 50% will involute completely by age 5 and 70% by age 7. Common treatment options include propranolol (first-line treatment), systemic and intralesional steroids, sclerotherapy, and surgical excision. Treatment is indicated for hemangiomas that impair vision or impact breathing or for those unresponsive to medical therapy and those with hemorrhagic complications.

22. **A child with a rapidly enlarging hemangioma develops a coagulopathy. What is this entity and how is it managed?**

    Kasabach–Merritt syndrome is a disseminated intravascular coagulation-like syndrome with platelet trapping within vascular lesions. This condition is seen in vascular lesions including tufted angioma and kaposiform hemangioendothelioma. It is treated by transfusing clotting factors and platelets as necessary and addressing the responsible lesion.

23. **What pattern of infantile hemangioma involvement carries the risk of associated airway hemangiomas?**

    Hemangiomas in a beard distribution (V3) carry a high risk of airway hemangioma, which occurs in up to 50% of cases. Direct laryngoscopy and bronchoscopy are warranted, and severe airway compromise may necessitate tracheostomy.

24. **What is Sturge–Weber syndrome?**

    This is a congenital neurocutaneous syndrome characterized by port wine stains, facial capillary malformation most commonly in the V1 distribution, abnormal blood vessels known as leptomeningeal angiomas, and abnormal blood vessels in the eye. Affected individuals may experience neurologic symptoms such as seizures, headaches, stroke-like episodes, focal neurologic deficits, and cognitive deficits. Multidisciplinary management is important and requires involvement of neurologists and ophthalmologists. Port wine stains can be managed with laser therapy.

25. **What types of lasers are used to treat cutaneous vascular lesions?**

    Development of light-based treatments led to selective photothermolysis to target hemoglobin, transfer energy to vessel walls, and minimize collateral damage. Argon lasers were the first treatments used; however, melanin absorption limits use of this laser. A pulsed dye laser with a target wavelength of 595 nanometers is the gold standard for port wine stains and many other cutaneous vascular lesions such as facial telangiectasias hemangiomas, rosacea, and cherry angiomas. Side effects of treatment are rare but occur more commonly in darker-skinned patients and include abnormal pigmentation and scarring. Potassium-titanyl-phosphate (KTP) lasers can also target oxyhemoglobin and are effective for superficial lesions. KTP lasers are preferred treatments for rosacea and telangiectasias. Neodymium-doped yttrium aluminum garnet (Nd:YAG) and near-infrared lasers can target oxyhemoglobin at 700 to 1200 nm with deeper penetration and lower absorption by melanin. These lasers can be effective in targeting resistant or deeper lesions.

26. **Name the most common malignant vascular tumors of the head and neck.**

    - Angiosarcoma is a rare malignant vascular tumor that can occur in the skin, superficial soft tissue of the head and neck, and sinonasal cavity.
    - Epithelioid hemangioendotheliomas arise from endothelial cells and are extremely rare tumors uncommonly involving the head and neck. These tumors are variable in their behavior ranging from benign to aggressive forms.

27. **What is a Kaposi sarcoma, and which viral infections is it related to?**

    Kaposi sarcoma is a locally aggressive vascular neoplasm that is caused by γ-2 human herpesvirus 8. There are four variants of Kaposi sarcoma, including indolent/sporadic, endemic, iatrogenic, and epidemic. The epidemic form is associated with human immunodeficiency virus (HIV), with up to 20% of individuals developing oropharyngeal Kaposi sarcoma. The epidemic form tends to be more aggressive where the course of disease is improved with antiretroviral therapy.

BIBLIOGRAPHY

Blount A, Riley KO, Woodworth BA: Juvenile nasopharyngeal angiofibroma, *Otolaryngol Clin North Am* 44(4):989–1004, 2011.

Boghani Z, Husain Q, Kanumuri VV, et al: Juvenile nasopharyngeal angiofibroma: a systematic review and comparison of endoscopic, endoscopic-assisted, and open resection in 1047 cases, *Laryngoscope* 123(4):859–869, 2013.

Day TA, Bewley AF, Joe JK: Neoplasms of the neck. In: Flint P, Haughey B, Lund V, et al, eds: *Cummings Otolaryngology—Head and Neck Surgery,* 6th ed, Philadelphia, 2015, Elsevier, pp 1787–1804.

Dinulos JGH: Vascular tumors and malformations. In: Dinulos JGH, ed: *Habif's Clinical Dermatology,* Philadelphia, 2021, Elsevier, pp 905–926.

El-Naggar AK, Chan JKC, Grandis JR, et al, eds: *WHO Classification of Head and Neck Tumours,* Lyon, 2017, International Agency for Research on Cancer.

Garden BC, Garden J, Goldberg DJ: Light-based devices in the treatment of cutaneous vascular lesions: an updated review, *J Cosmet Dermatol* 16(3):296–302, 2017.

Lack EE, Kozakewich HPW: Tumors of the autonomic nervous system, including paraganglia. In: Fletcher CDM, ed: *Diagnostic Histopathology of Tumors,* 5th ed, Philadelphia, 2021, Elsevier, pp 2201–2224.

Lenders JWM, Duh QY, Eisenhofer G, et al: Pheochromocytoma and paraganglioma: an Endocrine Society clinical practice guideline, *J Clin Endocrinol Metab* 99(6):1915–1942, 2014.

Nicolai P, Castelnuovo P: Benign tumors of the sinonasal tract. In: Flint PW, Haughey BH, Lund V, et al,eds: *Cummings Otolaryngology—Head and Neck Surgery,* 6th ed, Philadelphia, 2015, Elsevier, pp 740–751.

Perkins JA: Vascular anomalies of the head and neck. In: Flint PW, Haughey BH, Lund V, et al, eds: *Cummings Otolaryngology—Head and Neck Surgery,* 6th ed, Philadelphia, 2015, Elsevier, pp 3065–3081.

Persky M, Tran T: Acquired vascular tumors of the head and neck, *Otolaryngol Clin North Am* 51(1):255–274, 2018.

Persley M, Manolidis S: Vascular tumors of the head and neck. In: Johnson JT, Rosen CA, eds: *Bailey's Head & Neck Surgery: Otolaryngology,* 5th ed, Philadelphia, 2014, Lippincott, Williams, and Wilkins, pp 1999–2043.

Roberson D, Robertson RM: Cardiovascular manifestations of autonomic disorders. In: Zipes DP, Libby P, Bonow RO, et al, eds: *Braunwald's Heart Disease,* 11th ed, Philadelphia, 2019, Elsevier, pp 1930–1944.

Shah JP, Patel SG, Singh B, et al: Neurogenic tumors and paragangliomas. In: Shah JP, Patel SG, Singh B, et al, eds: *Jatin Shah's Head and Neck Surgery and Oncology* 5th ed, Philadelphia, 2020, Elsevier, pp 609–646.

Williams MD: Paragangliomas of the head and neck: an overview from diagnosis to genetics, *Head Neck Pathol* 11(3):278–287, 2017.

CHAPTER 19

SINONASAL TUMORS

Thad W. Vickery, MD and Jeffrey D. Suh, MD

KEY POINTS

1. Sinonasal tumors are rare and account for 3% of upper aerodigestive tract cancers.
2. Squamous cell carcinoma is the most common sinonasal malignancy.
3. Occupational exposures are the main risk factors for sinonasal malignancies. Risk factors for adenocarcinoma are wood dust exposure and leather working.
4. Sinonasal malignancies typically present at a late stage because diagnosis is delayed due to nonspecific clinical presentation, which often mimics benign conditions.
5. Surgery followed by radiation therapy is the mainstay of treatment for sinonasal malignancies. For both benign and malignant tumors, obtaining clear margins is critical to reduce the risk of local recurrence. The best approach (endoscopic versus open) depends on a variety of factors including tumor location, type, size, and surgeon comfort.

Pearls

1. Ohngren's line is an imaginary line drawn from the medial canthus to the angle of the mandible. The significance of this marker is that maxillary sinus tumors that are located above this line on presentation are associated with a poor prognosis and tend to spread superiorly and posteriorly and are more prone to perineural invasion and skull base invasion.
2. Adenocarcinoma is associated with exposure to wood and leather dust. Squamous cell carcinoma is associated with exposure to chromium, nickel, mustard gas, and aflatoxin.
3. The classic radiographic findings for JNA are expansion of the PPF on axial view (Holman-Miller sign), widening of the sphenopalatine and Vidian foramina, and bony destruction of the pterygoid process.

QUESTIONS

GENERAL/EPIDEMIOLOGY

1. **What are the important epidemiologic aspects of sinonasal cancer?**
   Sinonasal cancer is rare, accounting for only 3% of upper aerodigestive tract malignancies. There are varied histologic subtypes of sinonasal cancer, which at least in part explains the diverse behavior and presentation of these tumors. Sinonasal malignancies tend to be diagnosed in the fifth and sixth decades of life. The disease is most common in Caucasians, and men are affected at twice the rate of women. A number of occupational exposures are associated with these cancers, including industrial fumes, nickel, leather, and wood dust (more details later in this chapter). There is also a higher rate of sinonasal cancers in cigarette smokers and heavy alcohol users. The 5-year survival for all nasal and paranasal malignancy is 40%, although this varies based on the histopathology of the tumor.

2. **What are the most common presenting symptoms of sinonasal tumors? What symptoms are particularly concerning for malignancy?**
   Unilateral nasal symptoms are the most common presenting symptoms of sinonasal tumors, including obstruction, discharge, congestion, and epistaxis. These symptoms are often overlooked because they can mimic chronic sinusitis or allergies. However, persistent or worsening unilateral nasal symptoms or development of orbital symptoms, such as vision loss, tearing (epiphora), diplopia, or exophthalmos warrant a detailed examination.

   Paresthesia or pain along V2 (maxillary nerve), cheek swelling, and numbness of the face or palate would be unusual for sinusitis and are symptoms that are concerning for malignancy. Cavernous sinus invasion by sphenoid tumors can lead to dysfunction of cranial nerves III, IV, V1, V2, and VI. Thus, the most important indicators of malignancy include cranial neuropathies and orbital complications.

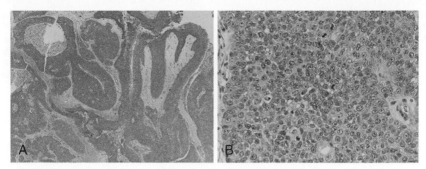

Fig. 19.1 A, Hematoxylin and eosin (H&E) stain 4× : epithelial proliferation demonstrating an endophytic growth pattern characteristic of Schneiderian papilloma, inverted type. **B**, H&E stain 40× : the epithelial proliferation exhibits a disorganized architecture and the epithelial cells demonstrate frank atypical features including marked pleomorphism, increased nuclear-to-cytoplasmic ratio, prominent nucleoli, increased mitotic activity, and atypical mitotic figures indicative of severe dysplasia.

BENIGN SINONASAL TUMORS

3. **What are the different types of nasal papillomas?**
   Nasal papillomas are characterized based on their histologic appearance.
   - **Exophytic (fungiform) papilloma:** the most common subtype, accounting for 50% of nasal papillomas. These papillomas typically arise from the nasal septum and resemble papillomas found at other locations on the body in terms of histopathology. In contrast to the other types of nasal papillomas, the exophytic papilloma does not have malignant potential.
   - **Inverted (endophytic) papilloma:** these arise from Schneiderian mucosa, which is ectodermally derived ciliated columnar epithelium with goblet cells, though it is different from similarly appearing respiratory epithelium, which is endodermally derived. These papillomas are most commonly located on the lateral nasal wall or maxillary sinus; however, any paranasal sinus can be involved (Fig. 19.1). These papillomas account for 47% of nasal papillomas and are associated with high rates of recurrence if not completely resected. Inverted papillomas are associated with an 8% to 10% chance of malignant transformation to squamous cell carcinoma. Inverted papillomas can be associated with HPV infection.
   - **Oncocytic (cylindrical) papilloma:** oncocytic papillomas usually arise from the lateral nasal wall and are the rarest of the three papilloma types, accounting for only 3% of nasal papillomas. These tumors are thought to have rare malignant potential, usually reported at between 4% and 17% (Fig. 19.1).

4. **What is the standard treatment for inverting papilloma?**
   Complete surgical resection with clear margins is the treatment of choice for all sinonasal papillomas. Identification and removal of the tumor site of attachment (origin) gives the highest chance of cure. Radiation with or without chemotherapy is reserved for tumors with malignant transformation.
   Traditional open surgery utilizes a lateral rhinotomy or midface degloving to provide access to the nasal cavity for tumor removal. Endoscopic or endoscopic-assisted approaches have largely replaced open approaches for most IPs and have reduced the tumor recurrence rate from 20% to 12%.

5. **What is a juvenile nasopharyngeal angiofibroma (JNA)?**
   JNA is a benign vascular tumor, seen exclusively in adolescent males. These tumors are slow growing, are locally invasive, and do not metastasize. However, these tumors can be quite large at presentation and can involve the intracranial cavity, orbit, pterygopalatine fossa, or infratemporal fossa. JNAs often present with unilateral, recurrent epistaxis. CT/MRI adding angiography can be helpful to visualize the vascularity of the tumor and confirm the diagnosis. Biopsy carries a high risk of hemorrhage and is not recommended, and preoperative embolization is often warranted to reduce intraoperative blood loss.

6. **What is Fisch's classification system for JNA?**
   Fisch I: limited to nasal cavity
   Fisch II: extends to pterygomaxillary fossa or sinuses with bony destruction
   Fisch III: invades orbit, infratemporal fossa, or parasellar area
   Fisch IV: extends to cavernous sinus, optic chiasm, or pituitary fossa

7. **What is the treatment of JNA?**
   Tumors are typically embolized prior to surgical removal to reduce intraoperative bleeding. Endoscopic techniques are typically used for Fisch I and II, whereas more advanced lesions may require a craniofacial or endoscopic-assisted resection. Radiation therapy may be used for unresectable tumors.

8. **What other benign tumors are found in the nasal cavity? What are the unique features of these tumors?**
   - **Osteomas** are the most common benign sinonasal tumors and are slow-growing tumors of mature bone. Multiple osteomas can be associated with Gardner's syndrome. These are most often incidentally discovered on CT scans of the sinus, although they can cause symptoms by obstruction of normal sinus drainage or through direct mass effect. The most common location of osteomas in the paranasal sinuses is in the frontal sinuses, with more than 80% presenting in this location.
   - **Hemangiomas** are rare and most often present on the septum or inferior turbinate.
   - **Pyogenic granulomas** are benign, friable polypoid lesions often found on the septum that can be caused by irritation, physical trauma, and hormonal factors. There is a female predilection and increased incidence during the first trimester of pregnancy.
   - **Hemangiopericytomas** are vascular tumors derived from pericyte cells (Zimmerman pericytes) that surround capillaries and postcapillary venules, accounting for approximately 1% of all vascular tumors. Hemangiopericytomas are usually well-differentiated tumors with a low potential for recurrence with complete resection. The treatment of choice is surgical resection.
   - **Salivary gland tumors** arising from minor salivary glands in the sinuses are rare. The most common is pleomorphic adenoma.
   - **Chordomas** are benign, locally aggressive tumors arising from notochord. They are usually found in the clivus and often present with cranial nerve palsy.

MALIGNANT SINONASAL TUMORS

9. **Describe the epidemiology of sinonasal malignancy.**
   Sinonasal malignancies are rare and represent 3% of head and neck malignancies, typically presenting in the fifth to sixth decades of life.

10. **What are the most common pathologic types of sinonasal malignancy?**
    Squamous cell carcinoma and adenocarcinoma are the most common histologic subtypes. Others include esthesioneuroblastoma, adenoid cystic, mucoepidermoid, mucosal melanoma, sinonasal undifferentiated carcinoma, sarcoma, and lymphoma.

11. **What are the distinctive features of the following malignant sinonasal tumors?**
    - **Squamous Cell Carcinoma:** the most common sinonasal malignancy, representing approximately 80% of these tumors.
    - **Adenocarcinoma:** presents most commonly in the ethmoid sinuses, with increased incidence in wood and leather workers.
    - **Sinonasal Undifferentiated Carcinoma (SNUC):** these tumors typically arise near the olfactory groove and portend a very poor prognosis because they are rapidly progressive, cause extensive local tissue destruction, and commonly metastasize.
    - **Esthesioneuroblastoma (or olfactory neuroblastoma):** these tumors arise from olfactory epithelium and show bimodal distribution in teenage and elderly populations. They frequently involve the skull base and orbit. There are two staging systems for these tumors: Kadish and Dulguerov-Calcaterra.
    - Kadish
      A: tumors confined to the nasal cavity
      B: tumor in nasal cavity with extension to the paranasal sinuses
      C: tumor extending to the orbit, skull base, or brain or with distant metastasis
    - Dulguerov-Calcaterra
      T1: tumor involving the nasal cavity or paranasal sinuses (excluding sphenoid or superior ethmoid air cells)
      T2: tumor involving the nasal cavity or paranasal sinuses including the sphenoid or with extension to the cribriform plate
      T3: extension to orbit or anterior cranial fossa
      T4: extension to the brain
    - **Mucoepidermoid:** salivary gland tumors that rarely present in the nasal cavity.
    - **Adenoid Cystic Carcinoma:** characterized by insidious growth, distant metastasis, and perineural invasion. Long-term surveillance is important due to a higher risk of late tumor recurrence.

12. **Are there occupational exposures that increase the risk of certain sinonasal tumors?**
    Adenocarcinoma is associated with exposure to wood and leather dust, as well as organic solvents. Squamous cell carcinoma is associated with exposure to chromium, nickel, mustard gas, and aflatoxin. Exposure to tobacco smoke, alcohol, and salted or smoked foods increases the risk of all types of sinonasal malignancy.

13. **What is the most common sinonasal tumor in the pediatric population?**
    Sinonasal tumors are rare in the pediatric population. Sarcomas represent approximately 75% of sinonasal malignancies in this demographic.

14. **What is the prognosis of sinonasal malignancy?**
    Five-year survival has been reported ranging from 20% to 50%, but this can vary based on location and histology. Tumors in the maxillary sinus located superior to Ohngren's line (a line drawn from the medial canthus to the angle of the mandible) are associated with poorer survival (see Question 25 for more details).

15. **What are the subsites of sinonasal malignancy?**
    - **Paranasal sinuses:** each sinus can be involved with a tumor. The maxillary sinus is the most common subsite (70%), followed by the ethmoid sinus (20%), sphenoid sinus (3%), and frontal sinus (less than 1%).
    - **Nasal cavity:** the second most common subsite overall but associated more with benign tumors.
      Sinonasal malignancy may also spread into the anterior cranial fossa via the frontal and ethmoid sinuses, the middle cranial fossa via the sphenoid sinus, pterygopalatine fossa, infratemporal fossa, and orbital cavity.

16. **What are the treatment modalities for sinonasal malignancy, and what are the limitations of adjuvant treatments?**
    Surgical resection is the mainstay of therapy for early-stage disease. Radiation therapy is given postoperatively based on tumor histology (high-grade tumors) and positive margins or if there is evidence of perineural invasion. Chemotherapy is also considered in advanced disease or when there are metastases. Radiation therapy is limited by close proximity to the orbit and brain. Unresectable tumors can be managed with chemoradiation.

17. **What are the contraindications for surgery?**
    Sisson outlined four factors that make sinonasal tumors inoperable due to significant morbidity or inability to obtain clear margins.
    1. Significant involvement of brain parenchyma (superior extension)
    2. Invasion of prevertebral fascia (posterior extension)
    3. Invasion into the cavernous sinus (lateral extension)
    4. Involvement of the bilateral orbits or optic chiasm

18. **What are the benefits of proton therapy in the treatment of sinonasal malignancy?**
    Sinonasal tumors may be difficult to treat with conventional radiotherapy protocols given the proximity of multiple sensitive organs in the vicinity, including the optic nerves, orbit, and brain. Proton therapy has a potential advantage over conventional electron - or photon-based therapy, as it has a finite penetration range and it is easier to contour a uniform dose to a target tumor volume. It has been applied in multiple situations in which tumors are in close proximity to vital organs. Several case series have indicated improved tumor control with decreased complication rates when comparing proton therapy to conventional radiotherapy in the treatment of esthesioblastoma and skull base chordomas. Despite these early successes, clinical trials directly comparing conventional treatment to proton therapy have not been performed to date.

19. **What is the nodal drainage pattern of sinonasal malignancy? How is the neck typically treated?**
    The nodal drainage pathway depends on the subsite. The anterior nasal cavity follows an anterior drainage pathway to the perifacial and Level IA/IB nodes. In contrast, the middle and posterior nasal cavity as well as the paranasal sinuses drain into the retropharyngeal and upper jugulodigastric nodes with a relatively low rate of occult neck metastasis (<10%). When tumors invade the orbit, they may also drain to periparotid lymph nodes. In accordance with this information, the N0 neck is typically not treated with an elective neck dissection. Clinical nodal disease, on the other hand, is a grim prognostic indicator and should be addressed with a neck dissection and postoperative radiation.

SURGICAL AND ANATOMIC CORRELATES

20. **What symptoms are associated with orbital invasion and what are the indications for orbital exenteration?**
    Orbital invasion is associated with rapidly progressive symptoms, including diplopia, proptosis, worsening acuity, lid edema, chemosis, and epiphora. Orbital exenteration is indicated for tumors located within the orbital apex or demonstrated erosion of the orbital bone with invasion through the periorbita (periosteum of the orbit) and into the extraocular muscles. Severe, intractable eye pain can be an indication. However, the prognosis for these patients is poor even after orbital exenteration, so palliative measures can also be considered.

21. **What are the surgical approaches used to treat sinonasal malignancies?**
    - Endoscopic approach: previously limited to benign tumors, now increasingly used in malignant disease and advanced disease. Advantages of the endoscopic approach include decreased morbidity, no external incisions, shorter hospitalizations, and improved visualization of structures and margins.
    - Transfacial open approaches
    - Lateral rhinotomy: the incision begins at the medial brow and extends along the lateral nasal sidewall, around the alar cartilage to the philtrum and through the lip. This is the classic approach to a medial maxillectomy

providing access to the maxillary sinus, medial orbital wall, nasal cavity, and ethmoid and sphenoid sinuses (Fig. 19.2). Lip split is performed to improve exposure of the hard palate. Can be combined with a sublabial or transpalatal approach for tumors involving the floor of the nose or inferior portion of the maxilla.

- Weber-Ferguson: lateral rhinotomy approach in combination with a lip-splitting incision that extends sublabially. A subciliary/transconjunctival incision is also made, which provides improved access to the maxilla for a total maxillectomy.
- Midface degloving: involves gingivobuccal incisions as well as bilateral intercartilaginous incisions. The advantage of this approach is avoiding an external scar and adequate visualization of the inferior and medial maxillary walls.
- Facial translocation: involves extensive facial flaps with sacrifice of the frontal branch of the facial nerve. The approach affords wide exposure of the skull base, infratemporal fossa, and pterygopalatine fossa.
- Infratemporal approach: access though a preauricular or postauricular incision that extends coronally. High risk of damage to the frontal branch of the facial nerve.
- Craniofacial resection: combined approach from above and below. Involves en bloc tumor removal of the anterior cranial base including the dura, cribriform plate, and ethmoid sinuses (Fig. 19.3).

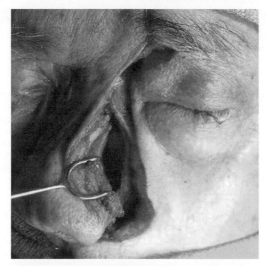

Fig. 19.2 Lateral rhinotomy incision used to gain access to the nasal cavity and paranasal sinuses.

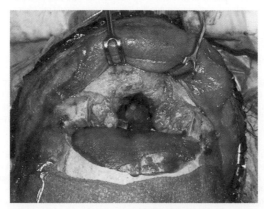

Fig. 19.3 Coronal incision and frontal craniotomy used as part of the craniofacial resection. The cribriform plate has been removed and the frontal lobe is exposed.

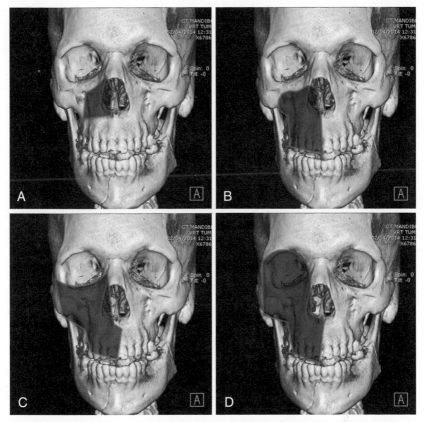

Fig. 19.4 Illustration of maxillectomy defects. Medial maxillectomy **(A)**, inferior maxillectomy **(B)**, total maxillectomy **(C)**, and radical maxillectomy **(D)**.

22. **What are the anatomic boundaries of the different types of maxillectomies? What are the indications for these surgeries?**
    - **Medial maxillectomy:** removal of the lateral nasal wall and medial maxilla, with or without sphenoethmoidectomy. May be performed endoscopically or open. This technique is commonly utilized for tumors in the maxillary sinus.
    - **Inferior maxillectomy:** involves removal of the inferior portion of the maxillary sinus. Indicated for tumors involving the maxillary alveolar process or limited hard palate lesions.
    - **Total maxillectomy:** includes en bloc removal of the entire maxilla. Indicated for tumors involving the maxillary antrum.
    - **Radical maxillectomy:** total maxillectomy with orbital exenteration (Fig. 19.4).

23. **What are the most common surgical complications?**
    Complications can usually be predicted based on the origin of the tumor. The general complications that can occur after any sinonasal tumor removal are bleeding, postoperative infection, and loss of olfaction. Intracranial complications can include meningitis, CSF leak, and tension pneumocephalus. Orbital complications include hematoma, emphysema, optic nerve injury, epiphora from injury to the nasolacrimal duct, and diplopia from injury to any of the extraocular muscles. Injury can also occur to cranial nerves III, IV, V1, V2, and VI (see Question 3).

ANATOMIC CORRELATES

24. **What is Ohngren's line? What is the importance of this anatomic marker?**
    Ohngren's line (Fig. 19.5) is an imaginary line drawn from the medial canthus to the angle of the mandible. The significance of this marker is that maxillary sinus tumors that are located above this line on presentation are associated with a poor prognosis, tend to spread superiorly and posteriorly, and are more prone to perineural invasion and skull base invasion.

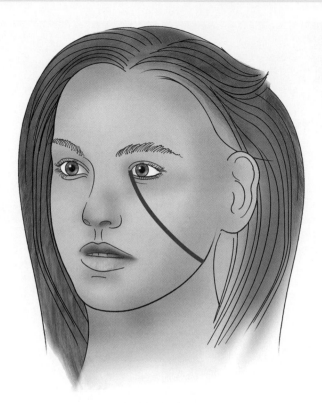

Fig. 19.5 Ohngren's Line. Tumors located superior to this line are associated with a worse prognosis given the proximity to the skull base.

25. **What is the pterygopalatine fossa? What important structures are located in this space?**
    The pterygopalatine fossa (PPF) is a pyramidal space located below the apex of the orbit.
    - Boundaries: superiorly, apex of the orbit; anteriorly, the posterior wall of the maxillary sinus; posteriorly, the pterygoid plates. It opens laterally into the infratemporal fossa.
    - Contents: fat, foramen rotundum (contains the maxillary nerve V2), Vidian nerve, pterygopalatine ganglion and nerve, lesser and greater palatine nerves, and the internal maxillary artery.

26. **What is the infratemporal fossa and what important structures are located in this space?**
    - Boundaries: anteriorly bounded by the maxilla, posteriorly bounded by the glenoid fossa and mandible, and medially bounded by the lateral pterygoid plates. Connects to the PPF via the pterygomaxillary fissure.
    - Contents: Pterygoid muscles and venous plexus, foramen ovale and V3, foramen spinosum, and the internal maxillary artery.

27. **Which subsite of paranasal cancer is associated with more frequent injuries to cranial nerves?**
    The sphenoid sinus, given its proximity to the cavernous sinus and optic nerve. Contents of the cavernous sinus include the internal carotid artery and CNs III, IV, V1, V2, and VI. The abducens nerve is located most medially in the cavernous sinus, and is usually affected first by sphenoid sinus tumors spreading to the cavernous sinus.

28. **What is cavernous sinus syndrome?**
    Cavernous sinus syndrome (CSS) is characterized by ophthalmoplegia caused by compression of CNs III/IV and VI. It is also characterized by numbness in the distribution of V1 and V2 and, potentially, ipsilateral Horner's syndrome. A complete lesion results in a fixed dilated pupil and hypesthesia of V1/V2. This can be caused by the mass effect from a skull base tumor or secondary to thrombosis from a retrograde spreading infection.

BIBLIOGRAPHY

Batsakis JG: Pathology consultation: nasal papillomas, *Ann Otol Rhinol Laryngol* 90(2):190–191, 1981.
Bhattacharyya N: Cancer of the nasal cavity: survival and factors influencing prognosis, *Arch Otolaryngol Head Neck Surg* 128(9): 1079–1083, 2002.

Binazzi A, Ferrante P, Marinaccio A: Occupational exposure and sinonasal cancer: a systematic review and meta-analysis, *BMC Cancer* 15:49, 2015.

Busquets JM, Hwang PH: Endoscopic resection of sinonasal inverted papilloma: a meta-analysis, *Otolaryngol Head Neck Surg* 134(3):476–482, 2006.

Leong SC: A systematic review of surgical outcomes for advanced juvenile nasopharyngeal angiofibroma with intracranial involvement, *Laryngoscope* 123(5):1125–1131, 2013.

Nishimura H, Ogino T, Kawashima M, et al: Proton-beam therapy for olfactory neuroblastoma, *Int J Radiat Oncol Biol Phys* 68(3):758–762, 2007.

Patel SH, Wang Z, Wong WW: Charged particle therapy versus photon therapy for paranasal sinus and nasal cavity malignant diseases: a systematic review and meta-analysis, *Lancet Oncol* 15:1027–1038, 2014.

Reder LS, Kokot N: Management of the neck in sinonasal malignancy. In Chiu AG, Ramakrishnan VR, Suh JD, editors: *Sinonasal Tumors*, 2020, Jaypee Brothers Medical Publishers, pp 142–144.

Rokade A, Sama A: Update on management of frontal sinus osteomas, *Curr Opin Otolaryngol Head Neck Surg* 20(1):40–44, 2012.

Suh JD, Ramakrishnan VR, Chi JJ, et al: Outcomes and complications of endoscopic approaches for malignancies of the paranasal sinuses and anterior skull base, *Ann Otol Rhinol Laryngol* 122(1):54–59, 2013.

Vorasubin N, Vira D, Suh JD, et al: Schneiderian papillomas: comparative review of exophytic, oncocytic, and inverted types, *Am J Rhinol Allergy* 27(4):287–292, 2013.

Weymuller EA, Davis GA: Malignancies of the paranasal sinus. In Flint P, Haughey B, Lund V, et al, editors: *Cummings Otolaryngology: Head and Neck Surgery*, 5th ed., Philadelphia, 2010, Mosby Elsevier, pp 1636–1642.

Zevallos JP, Jain KS, Roberts D, et al: Sinonasal malignancies in children: a 10-year, single-institutional review, *Laryngoscope* 121(9):2001–2003, 2011.

Zheng W, McLaughlin JK, Chow WH, et al: Risk factors for cancers of the nasal cavity and paranasal sinuses among white men in the United States, *Am J Epidemiol* 138(11):965–972, 1993.

CHAPTER 20

SKULL BASE SURGERY

William C. Yao, MD, Jeffrey D. Suh, MD and Vijay R. Ramakrishnan, MD

KEY POINTS

1. Proper selection of the surgical approach requires thorough evaluation to meet the surgical goals, while attempting to minimize injury to adjacent neurovascular structures.
2. A multidisciplinary team is helpful in the management of skull base tumors, including an otolaryngologist, neurosurgeon, head and neck or neuroradiologist, neuropathologist, radiation oncologist, and medical oncologist.
3. The nasoseptal flap is a popular method of reconstruction that can provide reliable closure for large, complex defects.
4. If there is a CSF leak following a repair, consider conservative management using a lumbar drain if the leak is small *and the repair is sound*. In addition, recognize the potential need for early intervention for continued leaks due to risk of postoperative meningitis. Exercise caution with lumbar drains in some cases due to risk of tension pneumocephalus and active CSF leaks with inadequate repairs.
5. Clinically significant pneumocephalus should address closure of the skull base defect. More aggressive evacuation is sometimes necessary to prevent major neurologic compromise.
6. Endoscopic skull base surgery has a learning curve for both the otolaryngologist and neurosurgeon. It is best to begin with simple cases or those in which the endoscope is used as an adjunct to an open approach.

Pearls
1. CN VI is the most medial nerve in the cavernous sinus and the most commonly injured or affected by sinus pathology.
2. CNs III, IV, V1, V2, VI, internal carotid artery, and venous channels are present in the cavernous sinus.
3. The Vidian nerve consists of parasympathetic and sympathetic fibers from the greater petrosal nerve and deep petrosal nerve. The canal lies medial to the foramen rotundum along the greater wing of the sphenoid sinus. The maxillary branch of the trigeminal (V2) nerve runs through the foramen rotundum.
4. CSF production is approximately 20 mL/hour.
5. The crista ethmoidalis is a reliable landmark for endoscopically locating the sphenopalatine artery.
6. A Weber-Ferguson incision consists of a lip-splitting extension of a lateral rhinotomy and a subciliary incision extended to the lateral canthus.

QUESTIONS

BASICS

1. **What are the compartments of the skull base?**
   The skull base is separated into three compartments, or fossae: anterior, middle, and posterior. The anterior compartment extends from the frontal sinus to the anterior clinoid process and planum sphenoidale (sphenoid roof). The middle cranial fossa extends from the greater wing of the sphenoid to the clivus, including the sella turcica. The posterior fossa consists of the occiput and begins from the basal aspect of the occipital bone (Fig. 20.1).

2. **What are the most common pathologies in which skull base surgery (SBS) is performed?**
   Benign sinonasal pathologies include inverted papilloma, juvenile nasal angiofibroma, fibrous dysplasia, and osteoma. Common intracranial skull base tumors include pituitary tumor, craniopharyngioma, and meningioma. Sinonasal malignancies include olfactory neuroblastoma (esthesioneuroblastoma), sinonasal undifferentiated carcinoma (SNUC), squamous cell carcinoma, adenocarcinoma, and melanoma.

3. **How can the skull base be accessed?**
   The skull base can be accessed using open, endoscopic, microscopic, or combined open-endoscopic approaches. The goal of any approach is to provide the best visualization and exposure to surrounding neurovascular structures and the tumors.

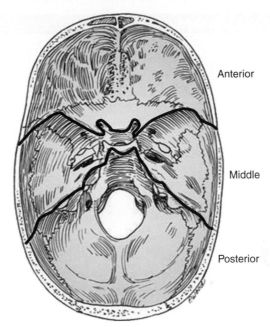

Anterior

Middle

Posterior

Fig. 20.1 Axial section of the skull base. Dark lines separate the three skull base compartments: anterior, middle and posterior. (Image edited from Flint PW: *Cummings Otolaryngology: Head and Neck Surgery*, Philadelphia, 2010, Mosby Elsevier.)

4. **What types of approaches are used to access the skull base?**
See Table 20.1.

5. **What incisions may be used to access the anterior skull base?**
Open approaches to the anterior fossa may use the coronal, lid crease, brow, gullwing, Lynch (medial orbital), lateral rhinotomy, Weber-Ferguson, or midface degloving incisions (Fig. 20.2).

6. **What tests and examinations are helpful prior to resecting a skull base malignancy?**
For surgical planning, basic laboratory studies including CBC, BMP, and coagulation studies should be performed, as well as imaging of the primary site (fine-cut CT and MRI). Other data may be obtained depending on tumor type (e.g., for pituitary tumor: ACTH, PRL, LH/FSH, GH, TRH) and location (arteriography). If indicated, a thorough evaluation for distant metastases should be performed.

7. **What imaging studies should be performed?**
Fine-cut CT scans (at least 1-mm section) should be performed for evaluation of bony anatomy of the skull base; the use of contrast may be helpful in defining the lesion and nearby vasculature. MRI with and without contrast is useful to delineate the lesion from surrounding structures, intracranial evaluation, help create a radiologic differential diagnosis, and evaluate for soft tissue invasion and perineural spread. CT, MR, or fused CT-MR images are helpful for intraoperative image guidance. PET scans can be used to rule out distant metastases.

8. **What is endoscopic skull base surgery (ESBS)?**
Endoscopic skull base surgery is an extension of endoscopic sinus surgery. A rigid endoscope is used to improve visualization and illumination and may obviate the need for facial incisions such as a lateral rhinotomy. Recent reports have demonstrated that endoscopic resections of skull base tumors may yield similar oncologic results to traditional open approaches in appropriately selected cases.

9. **When is the endoscopic skull base approach appropriate?**
Indications for endoscopic transnasal skull base surgery are increasing. The technique is utilized in pathology from the frontal sinus, entirety of the anterior skull base, much of the middle cranial fossa, and portions of the posterior fossa. ESBS performed through small incisions also allows minimally invasive lateral and neurosurgical approaches.

Table 20.1 Open Approaches to the Skull Base

Anterior Skull Base
Subfrontal approach
Transfrontal sinus – osteoplastic flap
Frontotemporal – orbitozygomatic
Transmaxillary sinus
Transfacial
LeFort osteotomy
Facial translocation
Lateral infratemporal fossa approach Fisch type approaches Type A: Anterior transposition of CN VII Type B: Sigmoid to petrous tip Type C: Extended approach to include cavernous sinus
Middle Skull Base
In addition to the anterior skull base approaches:
Transoral
Transseptal
Palatal split
Mandibular split
Middle cranial fossa subtemporal
Posterior Skull Base
Transoral approach
Palatal split
Translabyrinthine approach
Retrosigmoid
Suboccipital

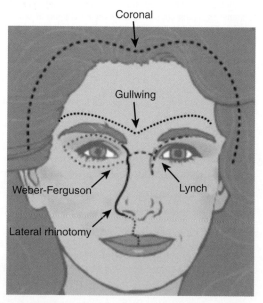

Fig. 20.2 Image depicting various external incisions that allow access to the skull base.

10. **What are the advantages of the endoscopic skull base approach?**
Compared to open surgery, the endoscopic approach allows for a more direct visualization with less manipulation of the surrounding soft tissues. This can allow for a more precise resection of the lesion due to better visualization for more posterior lesions and minimal manipulation of nearby neurovascular structures. Compared to the traditional microscopic view, endoscopes give a dynamic operative view with the added ability to see around corners using angled endoscopes. ESBS can avoid external incision, decrease hospital stays, and cause less postoperative pain.

11. **What are the limitations of endoscopic skull base surgery?**
Not all areas of the skull base can be visualized and safely instrumented via a transnasal endoscopic route. Malignancies involving the orbit, lateral frontal sinus, and facial skin are considered contraindications to endoscopic skull base surgery. As a general rule, the endoscopic approach should not compromise the ability to achieve appropriate oncologic resection, and crossing major neurovascular structures is not advised.

12. **In what situations should adjuvant radiotherapy and/or chemotherapy be considered?**
The primary modality of treatment for the majority of skull base malignancies is surgical resection. There are some exceptions to the rule (e.g., lymphoma and plasmacytoma). Adjuvant radiotherapy is considered when there is a high propensity for tumor recurrence, which includes presence of perineural invasion, high-grade tumor, and close or positive margins. Chemotherapy can be considered for induction therapy and metastatic disease or may be used as adjuvant therapy for chemosensitive histology. Radiation therapy may have a role in the management of certain benign skull base pathologies, such as meningioma, schwannoma, vascular tumors, and chordoma.

13. **What is stereotactic radiosurgery?**
Stereotactic radiosurgery utilizes ionizing radiation to treat well-defined targets with high accuracy and precision. This can be applied to areas with adjacent critical neurovascular structures such as in the skull base. It is most often used for pituitary adenoma, schwannoma, meningioma, AV malformations, and isolated intracranial metastases.

14. **Where is CSF produced and absorbed?**
CSF is produced by the choroid plexus in the lateral ventricles and is reabsorbed into the dural venous sinuses through the arachnoid villi. Total CSF volume is approximately 150 mL. An adult produces approximately 20 mL/hour and 550 mL/day. Normal adult intracranial pressure ranges from 10 to 20 centimeters H_2O.

15. **What are the three layers of the meninges?**
The dura mater, arachnoid, and pia mater. The dura mater is separated into the superficial layer and the meningeal layers.

16. **Describe the segments of the carotid artery.**
The internal carotid artery can be separated into seven anatomic segments: C1, cervical; C2, petrous; C3, lacerum; C4, cavernous; C5, clinoid; C6, ophthalmic; and C7, communicating. A mnemonic for remembering branches in the skull is **P**lease **L**et **C**hildren **C**onsume **O**ur **C**andy (Fig. 20.3).

APPROACH

17. **How are approaches classified in endoscopic transnasal skull base surgery?**
Approaches to the ventral skull base are classified according to their location in the sagittal or coronal plane (Table 20.2 and Figs. 20.4 and 20.5).

18. **What is the crista ethmoidalis?**
The crista ethmoidalis is a bony landmark located just anterior to the sphenopalatine foramen. It is identified for sphenopalatine artery ligations and endoscopic approaches to the pterygopalatine fossa.

19. **How can the lateral aspect of the sphenoid sinus be accessed?**
The lateral recess of a pneumatized sphenoid sinus can be accessed by the use of angled instruments following a wide sphenoidotomy or via the transpterygoid approach through the posterior wall of the maxillary sinus and pterygopalatine fossa.

20. **What is the Vidian canal?**
The Vidian canal runs through the inferolateral aspect of the sphenoid sinus, transmitting the Vidian nerve and an arterial branch from the internal carotid artery. It can be used as a surgical landmark for locating the internal carotid artery (Fig. 20.6).

21. **What structures are present in the cavernous sinus?**
Within the cavernous sinus lie cranial nerves III, IV, and VI as well as the ophthalmic/maxillary branch of the trigeminal nerve (CN V1 + V2) and the carotid artery. CN VI is the most medial and therefore the most commonly injured (Fig. 20.7).

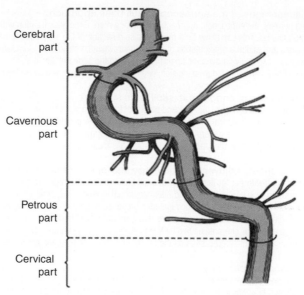

Cerebral part

Cavernous part

Petrous part

Cervical part

Fig. 20.3 Image of the internal carotid artery traversing through the skull base. (Image from Myers EN: *Operative Otolaryngology: Head and Neck Surgery*, 2nd ed, Philadelphia, 2008, Elsevier.)

Table 20.2 Endonasal Approaches to the Ventral Skull Base
Sagittal Plane
Transfrontal
Transcribriform
Transplanum/tuberculum
Transsellar
Transclival
Transodontoid
Coronal
Anterior coronal plane
• Supraorbital
• Transorbital
Middle coronal plane
• Medial petrous apex
• Petroclival approach
• Quadrangular space
• Cavernous sinus
• Transpterygoid/Infratemporal approach
Posterior coronal plane
• Infrapetrous
• Transcondylar
• Transhypoglossal
• Parapharyngeal space
• Medial (jugular foramen)
• Lateral

RECONSTRUCTION

22. **How is a skull base defect reconstructed?**

A skull base defect can be repaired in layers using autologous or synthetic materials. The dural layer can be reconstructed using temporalis fascia or fascia lata or allogeneic materials. The bony defect may be reconstructed with cartilage or bone from the septum, turbinate, or split calvarial grafts, if desired. The mucosal surface may be repaired using free mucosal grafts, fascia, autologous fat, or pedicled rotational flaps (i.e., nasoseptal flap). If the

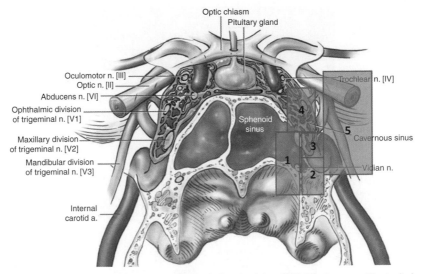

Fig. 20.4 Schematic description of endonasal surgical approaches in the coronal plane. [1] Medial petrous apex, [2] petroclival, [3] quadrangular space, [4] superior cavernous sinus, and [5] transpterygoid/infratemporal. (Image edited from Palmer JN: *Atlas of Endoscopic Sinus and Skull Base Surgery*, Philadelphia, 2013, Saunders Elsevier.)

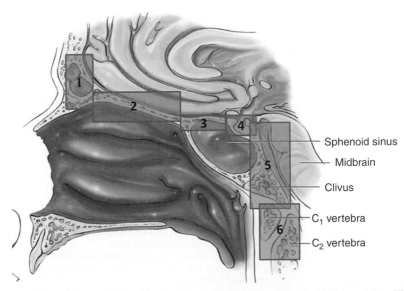

Fig. 20.5 Schematic description of endonasal surgical approaches in the sagittal plane. [1] Transfrontal, [2] transcribiform, [3] transplanum, [4] transsphenoid, [5] transclival, and [6] transodontoid. (Image edited from Palmer JN: *Atlas of Endoscopic Sinus and Skull Base Surgery*, Philadelphia, 2013, Saunders Elsevier.)

need arises, external approaches utilizing the pericranium may also be considered. Packing material, tissue glues, or direct suture techniques may be used to fix graft materials in place.

23. **Describe the nasoseptal flap.**
The nasoseptal flap is the workhorse pedicled mucosal flap based on the posterior septal branch of the sphenopalatine artery. The size can be customized, and its wide arc of rotation makes it versatile to reconstruct skull base defects.

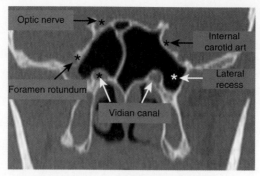

Fig. 20.6 Coronal section of the sphenoid bone. The white arrow represents the Vidian canal. The black stars are labeled accordingly. The white * depicts the lateral recess of the sphenoid bone.

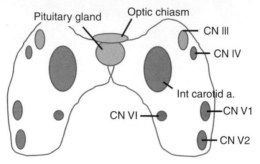

Fig. 20.7 Coronal diagram of the cavernous sinus.

24. **What is a free mucosal transfer?**
    A free mucosal transfer utilizes a mucosal graft harvested from another area in the nasal cavity, similar to a skin graft. Common sites of graft harvest include the inferior or middle turbinate, septum, or nasal floor.

25. **Which free flaps are preferred for reconstruction of larger defects?**
    Common flap options include anterolateral thigh, radial forearm, latissimus dorsi, and rectus myocutaneous flaps. If an osseocutaneous flap is required, options include a free fibula flap and scapular flap.

COMPLICATIONS

26. **What are the complications of skull base surgery?**
    Common complications of open skull base surgery include anosmia and associated taste dysfunction, poor aesthetic results, and neurologic complications such as cranial nerve injury or those secondary to brain retraction. Major skull base surgery complications include CSF rhinorrhea, meningitis, intracranial hemorrhage, orbital complications such as diplopia or vision loss, vascular injury, stroke, and death.
    Complications from endoscopic approaches are similar to those from the open approach; however, there is improved cosmesis and less brain retraction. The most common complications are hyposmia and associated taste disturbance, epistaxis, and prolonged local wound healing.

27. **What are the rates of complications of open and endoscopic skull base surgery?**
    The rate of surgical complications between 5% and 20% and the rate of medical complications is between 8% and 40%. Several studies have demonstrated that both medical and surgical complications are more frequent and severe using open approaches compared with endoscopic approaches.

28. **What are signs of failure in reconstruction?**
    Symptoms include clear rhinorrhea and constant postnasal drip. Other signs may include meningitis, severe headaches, seizures, and worsening pneumocephalus.

29. **If a CSF leak is identified, what nonoperative management options exist?**
    If the defect is small and there is confidence in the original reconstruction, conservative management with bed rest, stool softeners, and lumbar drainage can be considered. Antibiotics are sometimes administered for

meningitis prophylaxis. Medications may be prescribed to decrease CSF production (acetazolamide, furosemide, digoxin, topiramate) or decrease ICP (corticosteroids).

30. **What causes postoperative pneumocephalus?**
Nearly all patients undergoing skull base surgery will have some degree of postoperative pneumocephalus on initial imaging. Significant pneumocephalus is reported in 5% to 10% of patients when a ball valve action occurs along the reconstruction, from either increased negative pressure from the intracranial side (excessive CSF drainage from lumbar drain) or increased extracranial pressure (coughing, nose-blowing, CPAP use).

31. **What are the consequences of a pneumocephalus?**
Patients with pneumocephalus may present with headaches, dizziness, nausea and vomiting, seizures, depressed neurologic status, or neurologic symptoms from mass effects on nearby structures.

32. **What is the treatment of symptomatic or tension pneumocephalus?**
Nasal packing should be removed and the lumbar drain should be clamped. If severe, emergent drainage with needle aspiration should be performed if the area is safely accessible. The skull base reconstruction may require revision or, in refractory cases, airway diversion (tracheotomy) can be considered.

CONTROVERSIES

33. **Oncologic outcomes for endoscopic versus open surgery for malignancies.**
Endoscopic management of skull base tumors appears to have similar outcomes to open approaches in properly selected cases. True en bloc resection does not appear necessary to achieve good oncologic outcomes. The surgeon must evaluate whether complete tumor resection with negative margins can be accomplished through an endoscopic approach.

34. **What is the role of lumbar drains?**
Lumbar drains can decrease intracranial pressure and thereby reduce the pressure applied to the skull base reconstruction; however, they may be associated with significant morbidity and potential for complications. The use of lumbar drain primarily following a repair varies by surgeon and should not be universally utilized in a routine fashion. When used, the duration of drainage is also according to surgeon discretion.

35. **Best type of reconstruction.**
Most reconstructive methods appear to have similar efficacy, and there is therefore no universal "best type of reconstruction." In general, small defects (<1 centimeter) can be closed in a single layer, and multilayer repair is preferred for larger defects. Some surgeons prefer to use a rigid layer of bone or cartilage to reconstruct the skull base, although this is not required. Vascularized mucosal tissue (e.g., nasoseptal flap) has been demonstrated to improve repair results for larger defects; however, single-layer nonvascularized tissue can also be successful in this setting.

36. **Use of perioperative antibiotics.**
Postoperative antibiotics are an important consideration for skull base surgery because of the temporary connection between the intracranial space and external environment. The rate of postoperative wound infection following ESBS is approximately 2% and appears to be higher in open skull base surgery. Broad coverage with IV cephalosporins with or without vancomycin (or oral amoxicillin/clavulanate) is most often recommended. Studies that support the use of perioperative antibiotics are lacking and their use is more likely to benefit patients with a CSF leak or resection of malignant tumor. That said, most surgeons prefer to use systemic or topical antibiotics in some form after surgery.

BIBLIOGRAPHY

Bleier BS: Comprehensive techniques in CSF leak repair and skull base reconstruction, *Adv Otorhinolaryngol* 74:1–11, 2013.
Bolger WE, Borgie RC, Melder P: The role of the crista ethmoidalis in endoscopic sphenopalatine artery ligation, *Am J Rhinol* 13(2):81–86, 1999.
Kennedy DW, Hwang PH: *Rhinology: Disease of the Nose, Sinuses and Skull Base*, 2012, Thieme.
Lund VJ, Stammberger H, Nicolai P, et al: European position paper on endoscopic management of tumours of the nose, paranasal sinuses and skull base, *Rhinol Suppl* 1(22):1–143, 2010.
Myers EN: *Operative Otolaryngology: Head and Neck Surgery*, 2nd ed, 2008, Elsevier.
Teknos TN, Smith JC, Day TA, et al: Microvascular free tissue transfer in reconstructing skull base defects: lessons learned, *Laryngoscope* 112(10):1871–1876, 2002.
Timperley DG, Banks C, Robinson D, et al: Lateral frontal sinus access in endoscopic skull base surgery, *Int Forum Allergy Rhinol* 1(4):290–295, 2011.
Schirmer CM, Heilman CB, Bhardwaj A, et al: Pneumocephalus: case illustrations and review, *Neurocrit Care* 13(1):152–158, 2010.
Simmen DB, Raghavan U, Briner HR, et al: The anatomy of the sphenopalatine artery for the endoscopic sinus surgeon, *Am J Rhinol* 20(5):502–505, 2006.
Suh JD, Ramakrishnan VR, Chi JJ, et al: Outcomes and complications of endoscopic approaches for malignancies of the paranasal sinuses and anterior skull base, *Ann Otorhinolaryngol* 122(1):54–59, 2013.
Wang EW, Zanation AM, Gardner PA, et al: ICAR: endoscopic skull-base surgery, *Int Forum Allergy Rhinol* 9(Suppl 3):S145–S365, 2019.
Wormald PJ: *Endoscopic Sinus Surgery: Anatomy, Three-Dimensional Reconstruction, and Surgical Technique*, 3rd ed, 2013, Thieme.

CHAPTER 21

HEMATOLOGIC MALIGNANCY

Sarah A. Gitomer, MD

KEY POINTS

1. Painless lymph node enlargement is the most common head and neck manifestation of lymphoma.
2. Hematologic malignancies can involve extranodal tissues of the sinuses, salivary glands, and thyroid.
3. "B" symptoms include fever, weight loss, and night sweats. They are associated with poor prognosis.
4. Excisional lymph node biopsy is the preferred method of obtaining tissue diagnosis in lymphoma, although flow cytometry from core needle aspirate specimens may be diagnostic in some cases.
5. Severe oral mucositis is a dreaded complication of intensive chemotherapy regimens and hematopoietic stem cell transplantation.
6. Ototoxicity due to chemotherapeutic agents may be irreversible. This adverse reaction requires screening and early recognition, along with possible concurrent treatment with sodium thiosulfate for prevention.
7. Patients with neutropenia (including those undergoing treatment) are at risk for invasive fungal sinusitis, a potentially fatal disease.

Pearls
1. Excisional lymph node biopsy is the gold standard for the diagnosis of lymphoma and subtyping, but core needle biopsy may obtain enough tissue for diagnosis and can be used to direct further workup.
2. Sore throat can be the earliest symptom of severe neutropenia.
3. The use of ice chips in the mouth during chemotherapy can prevent mucositis by causing vasoconstriction, and rinsing the mouth with buffered saline can treat mucositis.

QUESTIONS

CLASSIFICATION, HISTORY, AND EXAM

1. **What are the broad classes of hematologic malignancies?**
   Hematologic malignancies include leukemia, lymphomas, and multiple myeloma. Leukemias are either acute or chronic and are classified based on the myeloid or lymphoid lineage. Lymphomas are further categorized as B-cell (Hodgkin's and non-Hodgkin's) or T-cell neoplasms.

2. **What are the head and neck manifestations of hematologic malignancies?**
   This can be broadly divided into nodal and extranodal manifestations.
   - **Nodal:** Cervical lymphadenopathy is a common presentation of lymphomas and is also observed in chronic lymphocytic leukemia (CLL). Certain lymphomas present with Waldeyer's ring involvement (clinically apparent as adenotonsillar hypertrophy).
   - **Extranodal:** Involvement of lymphoid tissues in the salivary glands, thyroid, and paranasal sinuses may present as masses in these regions. Endemic Burkitt's lymphoma has a distinct propensity to present as a mass of facial bones. Extramedullary plasmacytomas can originate in the sinonasal tissues. Mediastinal lymphadenopathy could cause compression of the trachea or superior vena cava with findings of dyspnea, airway compression while lying supine, or facial edema. Other presentations are summarized in Table 21.1.

3. **In a patient with cervical lymphadenopathy, what features should alert the clinician to the possibility of lymphoma?**
   Generalized symptoms along with lymphadenopathy raise the suspicion of malignancy. (1) Unexplained fevers (temperature > 38°C during previous month), (2) unintentional weight loss (>10% of body weight during the previous 6 months), and (3) drenching night sweats during the previous month are the classically designated "B" symptoms and portend a poor prognosis. Although nonspecific, approximately 25% of patients with Hodgkin's lymphoma and up to 40% of patients with non-Hodgkin's lymphoma present with "B" symptoms. Fatigue is an additional symptom. Hodgkin's lymphoma is uniquely associated with pruritus and pain after alcohol consumption.

Table 21.1 ENT Manifestations of Hematologic Malignancies

I. Nodal	Lymphadenopathy Involvement of Waldeyer's ring
II. Extranodal	Nasal obstruction Paranasal sinus involvement Facial bone erosion Thyroid infiltration Salivary gland involvement Airway obstruction (direct or from tracheal compression)
III. Vascular	Superior vena cava (SVC) syndrome
IV. Neurologic	Cranial nerve palsy (if CNS involvement) Mental nerve involvement Recurrent laryngeal nerve palsy
VI. Cytopenias	Anemia: mucosal pallor Thrombocytopenia: epistaxis, mucosal petechiae, purpura Neutropenia: sore throat

4. **What are the physical exam characteristics of lymphadenopathy in lymphomas?**
   Lymphoma-involved nodes are nontender and could be matted and fixed to underlying structures; one of the physical examination findings is multiple, bulky lymph nodes in several locations. It is important to examine the supraclavicular, axillary, and inguinal areas for lymphadenopathy.

5. **What is lethal midline granuloma?**
   This term is used to describe an aggressive form of extranodal natural killer/T-cell lymphoma mediated by Epstein-Barr virus infection. It is common in East Asia and Latin America. Patients present with destructive masses involving the nasal cavity, sinuses, or palate, sometimes with extension into the upper airway and Waldeyer's ring. The tumors are fast growing and may cause airway obstruction. Biopsy of these lesions usually reveals extensive necrosis with lymphomatous infiltration and vascular invasion. Localized disease is responsive to concurrent chemoradiotherapy, but advanced-stage disease is rapidly fatal despite treatment.

DIAGNOSIS

6. **Should adult patients with cervical lymphadenopathy be given a trial of empiric antibiotics?**
   Empiric antibiotics are generally not useful due to the multitude of possible etiologies and could result in a delay in diagnosis. There are insufficient data to support this practice in adults. Biopsies of suspicious lymph nodes should be performed without delay.

7. **What are the indications for cervical lymph node biopsy in suspected lymphomas?**
   In adults, the most common concern with cervical lymphadenopathy is malignancy, very commonly from squamous cell carcinoma but also potentially from hematologic malignancy. The American Academy of Otolaryngology–Head and Neck Surgery (AAO-HNS) clinical practice guidelines define patients at increased risk of malignancy as those who:
   - Lack infectious etiology
   - Have a neck mass for more than 2 weeks
   - Have one or more of the following physical examination findings: fixation to adjacent tissues, firm consistency, size >1.5 centimeters, ulceration of the overlying skin
       The guidelines recommend thorough head and neck examination, including laryngeal examination, for any adult presenting with concerning neck masses and recommend FNA as the first-line diagnostic biopsy for patients at increased risk of malignancy.

8. **What are the criteria for biopsy in children?**
   Painless cervical lymphadenopathy in children is most commonly secondary to reactive hyperplasia. Children presenting with 6 to 8 weeks or more of persistent lymphadenopathy (greater than 2 centimeters) should undergo thorough evaluation for evaluation of lymphoma. Risk factors for malignancy include age >10 years, multiple subsites of lymphadenopathy, supraclavicular lymph nodes, and large size.

9. **What is the importance of performing an excisional lymph node biopsy in suspected lymphomas?**
   Excisional biopsy remains the gold standard for diagnosing lymphoma because it ensures an adequate quantity of tissue to perform various histologic, immunologic, and molecular biological tests. With excisional biopsy, the

capsule of the lymph nodes is included to allow examination of the entire lymph node architecture, including normal and abnormal zones and capsular integrity. This is crucial for the precise classification of the lymphoma subtype, which can have implications for treatment.

10. **What is the role of core needle biopsy and fine needle aspiration of suspicious lymph nodes?**
Fine needle or core needle biopsy may be used as a first step in diagnosis if excisional biopsy is increased risk (for instance, lymph nodes adjacent to the facial nerve) or if other malignancies are expected. A core needle is preferred because of its increased ability to evaluate the lymph node capsule. However, if lymphoma cells are present, an excisional biopsy may still be necessary for subtyping to direct treatment.

11. **Which blood tests are indicated in patients with suspected hematologic malignancies?**
A complete blood count with differential counts, peripheral blood smear evaluation, erythrocyte sedimentation rate, coagulation profile (PT/INR and PTT), comprehensive metabolic panel, and serum lactate dehydrogenase (LDH) levels are useful basic tests in patients with suspected hematologic malignancies. Evaluation of HIV status, viral hepatitis panel, and uric acid levels might also be warranted. Based on history, additional labs including *Bartonella*, EBV, CMV titers, or PPD may also be included.

COMPLICATIONS OF TREATMENT

12. **Name some of the early head and neck indicators of complications from treatment of hematologic malignancies.**
Sore throat is one of the earliest manifestations of agranulocytosis. Mucosal pallor results from severe anemia due to myelosuppression. Epistaxis and palatal petechiae may indicate thrombocytopenia due to chemotherapy. When managing epistaxis in a patient with lymphoma and associated thrombocytopenia, the least invasive absorbable packing is recommended as the first line to avoid causing trauma and recurrent nasal bleeding with packing removal.

13. **Which toxicities pertaining to the head and neck result from the treatment of hematologic malignancies?**
Ototoxicity, radiation-induced xerostomia, hypothyroidism, fibrosis of neck muscles, carotid injury, and secondary malignancies (especially skin cancers) are some complications of chemotherapy and radiation. Chronic graft-versus-host disease after hematopoietic stem cell transplantation can cause severe xerostomia and ear canal obstruction.

14. **Can treatment of hematologic malignancies cause ototoxicity?**
Yes. Cisplatin, vinblastine, nitrogen mustard, arsenic trioxide, and bleomycin have been implicated in the development of hearing loss. It is usually dose dependent and symptoms vary from mild tinnitus to high-frequency sensorineural hearing loss and vestibular injury. Routine screening for high-frequency hearing loss can help detect early changes. New clinical practice guidelines recommend the use of systemic sodium thiosulfate to help prevent cisplatin-induced ototoxicity in nonmetastatic cancers.

15. **What is mucositis and how is it graded?**
Mucositis is a term used to describe inflammation and loss of mucosal integrity of the gastrointestinal tract. Mucositis is a common complication in patients undergoing hematologic stem cell transplantation, especially with conditioning regimens that use high-dose melphalan and radiation. The mouth and oropharynx are frequently involved, and clinical manifestations range from mild pain that does not limit oral intake to severe ulcerations that could result in profound weight loss and even death (Table 21.2).

16. **Describe the management of mucositis.**
Preventive measures: (1) oral hygiene, (2) cryotherapy during infusion (ice chips swished around the mouth for 30 minutes) can cause vasoconstriction and reduced drug concentration in the oropharyngeal mucosa, (3) calcium phosphate rinse (Caphosol® artificial saliva), (4) intravenous glutamine, and (5) keratinocyte growth factor.

Table 21.2 Grades of Oral Mucositis	
Grade 1	Asymptomatic or mild symptoms; no intervention required
Grade 2	Moderate pain, not interfering with oral intake. Dietary modifications required
Grade 3	Severe pain, interfering with oral intake
Grade 4	Life-threatening, requires urgent intervention
Grade 5	Death

Treatment of established mucositis: (1) salt and baking soda rinse every 4 hours, prepared by adding one teaspoon of baking soda and one-half teaspoon of salt to a quart of water; (2) viscous lidocaine; (3) "magic mouthwash" rinse that includes equal parts of viscous lidocaine, diphenhydramine, sodium bicarbonate, and magnesium aluminum hydroxide; and (4) systemic analgesics.

17. **Describe risk factors for and clinical presentation of invasive fungal sinusitis.**
A new diagnosis of lymphoma or leukemia and induction chemotherapy are risk factors for invasive fungal sinusitis. This disease process is rapidly progressive and may quickly involve the orbit and skull base and at times may be fatal specifically, an absolute neutrophil count <1000 is associated with an increased risk of invasive fungal sinusitis. Symptoms include facial pressure/pain, swelling, and/or congestion. Early and thorough evaluation (including nasal endoscopy and biopsies when indicated) and prompt diagnosis are essential for effective treatment. Physical examination findings include mucosal pallor and loss of sensation, progressing to necrotic eschar of the sinonasal mucosa (particularly the middle turbinate) and/or the hard palate.

BIBLIOGRAPHY

Ackerman BH, Kasbekar N: Disturbances of taste and smell induced by drugs, *Pharmacotherapy* 17(3):482–496, 1997.

Amador-Ortiz C, Chen L, Hassan A, et al: Combined core needle biopsy and fine-needle aspiration with ancillary studies correlate highly with traditional techniques in the diagnosis of nodal-based lymphoma, *Am J Clin Pathol* 135(4):516–524, 2011.

Anderson T, Chabner BA, Young RC, et al: Malignant lymphoma: the histology and staging of 473 patients at the National Cancer Institute, *Cancer* 50(12):2699–2707, 1982.

Common terminology criteria for adverse events (CTCAE) Version 4.0. Available at: http://evs.nci.nih.gov/ftp1/CTCAE/CTCAE_4.03_2010-06-14_QuickReference_5x7.pdf. Accessed February 2013.

Freyer DR, Brock PR, Chang KW, et al: Prevention of cisplatin-induced ototoxicity in children and adolescents with cancer: a clinical practice guideline, *Lancet Child Adolesc Health*, 4(2):141–150, 2019.

Kwong YL: The diagnosis and management of extranodal NK/T-cell lymphoma, nasal-type and aggressive NK-cell leukemia, *J Clin Exp Hematop* 51(1):21, 2011.

Lister TA, Crowther D, Sutcliffe SB, et al: Report of a committee convened to discuss the evaluation and staging of patients with Hodgkin's disease: Cotswolds meeting, *J Clin Oncol* 7(11):1630–1636, 1989.

Nolder AR: Paediatric cervical lymphadenopathy: when to biopsy? *Curr Opin Otolaryngol Head Neck Surg* 21(6):567–570, 2013.

Orient JM: Sapira's art and science of bedside diagnosis. In: *Examination of Lymph Nodes*, 3rd ed, Philadelphia, 2005, Lippincott Williams, Wilkins, pp. 165.

Pynnonen MA, Gillespie MB, Roman B, et al: Clinical practice guideline: evaluation of the neck mass in adults, *Otolaryngol Head Neck Surg* 157(Suppl 2):S1–S30, 2017.

Suzuki R: NK/T-cell lymphomas: pathobiology, prognosis and treatment paradigm, *Curr Oncol Rep* 14(5):395–402, 2012.

Swerdlow SH, Campo E, Harris NL, et al, eds: *World Health Organization Classification of Tumours of Haematopoietic and Lymphoid Tissues*, Lyon, France, 2008, IARC Press.

Worthington HV, Clarkson JE, Bryan G, et al: Interventions for preventing oral mucositis for patients with cancer receiving treatment, *Cochrane Database Syst Rev* 13(4):CD000978, 2011.

CHAPTER 22

RADIATION AND SYSTEMIC THERAPY FOR HEAD AND NECK CANCER

Douglas E. Holt, MD, Sana D. Karam, MD, PhD and Timothy V. Waxweiler, MD

KEY POINTS

1. Radiation therapy (RT) uses ionizing radiation to locally treat cancers, while systemic therapy uses cytotoxic chemotherapy or molecular targeted biologics to systemically treat cancers.
2. Compared to surgical treatment of head and neck (HN) cancers, radiation potentially offers a curable alternative or adjunct, sometimes with the added benefit of organ preservation.
3. Prompt dental evaluation with necessary tooth extractions and optimal lifetime dental hygiene are critical for patients with HN cancer who may receive radiation to the mandible to minimize the risk of long-term osteoradionecrosis.
4. In the combined setting, chemotherapy potentiates the effects of RT, exerts cytotoxic effects on cancer cells, and may modulate the antitumor immune response to improve both local and systemic disease control.
5. Bolus cisplatin is generally the standard of care for systemic therapy for HN cancer with concurrent radiation, although the final choice of systemic therapy is at the discretion of the medical oncologist.

Pearls
1. Postoperative chemoradiation is indicated for positive margins or nodal extracapsular extension.
2. Definitive HN cancer radiation doses generally range from 66 to 70 Gy.
3. Definitive radiation is an effective treatment alternative for nonmelanomatous skin lesions.
4. Risk for long-term complications is a function of the total dose of radiation delivered, the dose per fraction, the time frame over which it was given, the anatomic sites included within the radiation fields, and potential added effects from concurrent therapies.
5. Induction chemotherapy has been shown to improve disease control and overall survival in nasopharyngeal cancers and improve larynx preservation in some patients, but the value in improving overall survival in HN cancers remains unclear.

QUESTIONS

1. **What is radiation therapy (RT), and what are the common techniques used in treating cancers of the head and neck (HN)?**

   Radiotherapy, also called radiation therapy (RT), is the localized treatment of cancer and other diseases with ionizing radiation. Ionizing radiation induces mitotic cell death via damage to DNA through a variety of atomic interactions, including free radical generation and direct DNA strand breaks. The primary goal of all RT is to maximize cancer cell death while minimizing damage to healthy normal tissues. Radiation is most often delivered by an external source (i.e., external beam RT [EBRT]) using photons, protons, electrons, and other heavy particles but may also be administered by temporarily or permanently placing radioactive sources into a patient's body (i.e., brachytherapy). The most frequently used modern EBRT techniques for treatment of head and neck (HN) cancers are a complex method of volumetric-modulated arc therapy (VMAT) and occasionally three-dimensional conformal RT (3DCRT). Varying dose rates/energies, multiple beam angles/arcs, and dynamic multileaf collimator shapes combine to optimize delivery of the radiation. Image-guided RT (IGRT) uses imaging capabilities on the treatment machine (e.g., cone beam computed tomography [CT] and x-ray) to verify patient setup. Stereotactic body RT (SBRT) is an additional technique often used in the palliative or re-irradiation setting that delivers high doses of radiation in five or fewer treatments (Fig. 22.1).

2. **Who should evaluate a patient prior to initiating RT with or without systemic therapy?**

   Patients undergoing RT for HN cancers require timely coordination and support from a multitude of care providers. The following specialists are often involved:
   - **Radiation oncologist:** A formal history and physical evaluation and review of all available imaging are necessary to determine the appropriate radiation targets, dosing, and schedule.
   - **Medical oncologist:** A formal medical oncology evaluation is recommended for any patient who may be a candidate for systemic therapies.

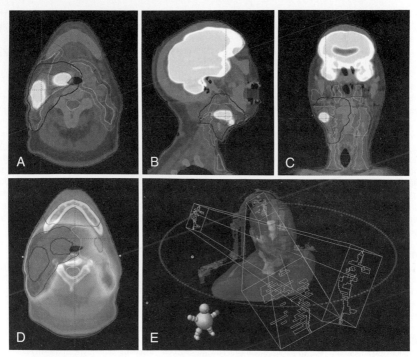

Fig. 22.1 Overview of planning volumes drawn on CT images with PET fusion **(A–C)**, visualization of expected dose delivery with inner circles being the highest dose **(D)**, and 3D visualization of beam arcs and shapes with respect to patient **(E)**. *CT*, Computed tomography; *PET*, positron emission tomography.

- **Dentist or oral surgeon:** Any patient who may receive radiation in the region of the mandible, maxilla, or teeth should receive a formal evaluation and any necessary dental work (e.g., extraction of unhealthy teeth, fillings, fluoride trays) prior to initiating RT, if possible. RT should not start until 2 weeks or more after a dental procedure to ensure proper healing. A delay in the dental evaluation is one of the most common yet significant causes of delay in initiating RT. For this reason, patients with clearly unhealthy teeth who undergo initial surgical resection may have concurrent dental extractions performed in anticipation of adjuvant RT.
- **Nutritionist:** Regular assessments of nutritional status for patients with HN cancer before, during, and after RT and systemic therapy are critical. Nutritionists can also provide teaching and support for patients with and without feeding tubes.
- **Speech and swallow therapy:** A baseline evaluation is recommended for patients with current or anticipated speech or swallowing problems.
- **Pathology, radiology, and otolaryngology:** Involvement is recommended to help with RT planning.
- **Additional consultants:** May include interventional radiology, audiology, ophthalmology, neurosurgery, plastic surgery, physical medicine and rehabilitation, social work, addiction services, smoking cessation, psychology, and palliative care.

3. **What are the initial steps undertaken for a patient with HN cancer prior to receiving radiation?**
   - **CT simulation:** Planning, or simulation, CT scans are performed in the radiation oncology department, at which time immobilization devices customized to the patient are made, including a thermoplastic molded mask, a mouthpiece, and a head rest. Magnetic resonance imaging (MRI), positron emission tomography (PET)/CT, and additional scans may be performed to assist with both staging and treatment planning. Whenever possible, patients should receive these additional scans in the radiation treatment position using their mask, mouthpiece, and head rest to assist with immobilization. Having similar positions between all imaging modalities optimizes the accuracy of image fusions used for target delineation planning software (Fig. 22.1).
   - **Drawing volumes:** The radiation oncologist will then use planning software to outline gross tumor, areas of potential microscopic disease, and normal tissues. This process is known as "drawing volumes," or contouring, and often takes several hours and may involve more than 20 distinct volumes or structures.

- **Planning:** A dosimetrist, physicist, and the radiation oncologist then work together to create the optimal plan for delivering the radiation to the target while restricting the dose to normal tissues. These plans are often reviewed by multiple people and run through quality assurance checks on the treatment machine.
- **Treatment:** RT for patients with HN cancer may consist of a schedule such as daily single treatments for 6 to 7 weeks, with weekly check-up appointments with the radiation oncologist to evaluate and treat toxicities.

4. **How do RT and surgery compare to each other?**
Both RT and surgery are local therapies. Definitive RT strives for organ preservation to maintain critical functions such as swallowing, normal speech, and breathing while attempting to maximize the quality of life in patients who might otherwise undergo morbid surgical resection. RT is typically delivered daily (Monday through Friday) over 6 to 7 weeks on an outpatient basis without need of anesthesia, making it a more ideal treatment modality for poor surgical candidates. The protracted time commitment can be problematic for noncompliant or elderly patients and those living great distances from a radiation oncology facility. Surgery could be advantageous in providing a one-time procedure and optimal pathologic assessment of primary tumors and nodal disease. While acute side effects of surgery occur primarily in the immediate postoperative time frame, acute RT toxicities typically build up gradually throughout the course of treatment. Extent of disease and involvement of critical structures limit surgeons in their ability to achieve complete resection of disease and radiation oncologists in their ability to treat these disease sites to full definitive doses. Both specialties must balance aggressive treatment with acute and long-term local toxicities.

5. **What are the general doses used in RT for HN cancers?**
A gray (Gy) represents one joule per kilogram and is the standard unit of absorbed dose used in clinical radiation oncology. A variety of doses and fractionation schedules are used in treating HN cancers. In the typical daily radiation setting, daily doses of 180 to 225 cGy (1.8 to 2.25 Gy) are used. General, non-site-specific total doses vary based on the setting (definitive RT to gross disease $\approx$ 66 to 70 Gy; high-risk elective neck coverage $\approx$ 60 Gy; low-risk elective neck $\approx$ 54 Gy; and postoperative RT $\approx$ 54 to 66 Gy).

6. **Who cannot be treated with RT?**
Patients who should not receive RT are those with collagen vascular diseases, other hypersensitivity conditions (e.g., ataxia-telangiectasia), pregnant women particularly in the first two trimesters, and those who would exceed maximum safe cumulative doses of RT to critical structures. Some patients can be retreated, usually with a lower dose, after time has elapsed since the previous treatment. Additionally, disorders of DNA repair and conditions (e.g., Li-Fraumeni syndrome and xeroderma pigmentosum) put patients at high risk for radiation-induced secondary cancers.

7. **What is systemic therapy, and how does it work both with and without radiation?**
Chemotherapy, biologics, and immunotherapies are the three main groups of systemic therapies. Cytotoxic chemotherapy drugs interfere with DNA replication, microtubule formation, and other cellular processes to impair mitosis and/or induce apoptosis. While these agents tend to primarily damage cells with high mitotic rates (e.g., cancer, mucosal tissues, and bone marrow), they are fairly indiscriminate. Biologics, in turn, typically employ antibodies to specifically target proteins ubiquitous among a clonal cancer cell population, such as surface antigens and/or components critical to a cancer signaling pathway. Immunotherapies help activate the immune system to attack cancer cells through various mechanisms. Systemic therapies and RT may provide a synergistic effect, allowing for improved tumor control. Systemic therapy can put cancer cells into a radiosensitive state by manipulation of the proliferative pathways. At present, immunotherapies are approved as first-line therapy for recurrent or metastatic HN cancers, and trials are underway combining them with RT.

8. **What are the most common systemic agents used in treatment of nonmetastatic HN cancers and their associated toxicities?**
Cisplatin is the most used systemic therapy in concurrent setting. For concurrent chemoradiation, cisplatin bolus is preferred over weekly cisplatin. Systemic agents most often used for treatment of nonmetastatic HN cancers, along with their main adverse effects, are reported in Table 22.1.

9. **How is systemic therapy used in the treatment of HN cancers?**
Systemic therapy may be administered in the following settings with different goals:
- **Neoadjuvant or induction:** Given prior to definitive treatment to decrease tumor size, permitting less extensive local treatment, and in some cases allows for organ preservation.
- **Adjuvant:** Given after definitive treatment with hopes of decreasing recurrence either locally or distally (not currently the standard of care in HN cancers).
- **Concomitant or concurrent with radiation:** Used to augment the efficacy of radiation via radiosensitization. In this setting, systemic therapy is not thought to significantly improve control of undetectable metastatic disease.
- **Metastatic:** Primarily used to prolong disease control and palliate symptoms.

Table 22.1 Common Systemic Agents Used in Head and Neck Cancer Treatments and Their Associated Toxicities

AGENT	NOTABLE TOXICITIES
Cisplatin	Hearing loss, renal failure, peripheral neuropathy, electrolyte abnormalities, gastrointestinal toxicity
Carboplatin	Electrolyte abnormalities, myelosuppression
5-Fluorouracil	Mucositis, hand-foot syndrome, photosensitivity, maculopapular rash
Paclitaxel	Peripheral neuropathy, arthralgia, myalgia
Docetaxel	Peripheral neuropathy, edema, asthenia
Cetuximab	Acneiform rash, dermatitis, hypomagnesemia, neutropenia
Pembrolizumab	Arthralgia, myalgia, dermatitis, edema, electrolyte abnormalities, gastrointestinal toxicity, pancytopenia, hepatitis, elevated serum creatinine
Nivolumab	Arthralgia, peripheral neuropathy, myalgia, dermatitis, edema, asthenia, electrolyte abnormalities, gastrointestinal toxicity, pancytopenia, hepatitis, fever, elevated serum creatinine

NOTE: Additional side effects seen in many of these agents include myelosuppression, diarrhea, nausea/vomiting, alopecia, and hypersensitivity reactions.

10. Who should receive induction therapy?

Induction chemotherapy has been shown to improve disease control or overall survival (OS) in nasopharyngeal cancers. For the remaining HN cancers, the value of induction chemotherapy remains unclear. Evidence exists for a reduction of distant metastases and improved organ preservation in hypopharynx cancers and a trend to ward improved OS for locally advanced HN cancers. Currently, induction chemotherapy should be considered only in clinical trials or in select conditions where there may otherwise be a delay in initiation of definitive treatment. Multidisciplinary tumor board review and treatment at experienced tertiary care centers are highly recommended when considering induction therapy.

11. What is the role of cetuximab in treating HN cancers?

Cetuximab is a monoclonal antibody that targets the extracellular domain of endothelial growth factor receptor (EGFR). EGFR is frequently mutated and/or overexpressed in HN cancers. While cisplatin remains the gold standard systemic therapy in concurrent chemoradiation setting with superior outcomes in patients with human papillomavirus (HPV), cetuximab is an FDA-approved alternative with a different side effect profile, making it a suitable alternative in select situations (e.g., a patient with contraindications to cisplatin therapy). Cetuximab and chemotherapy combinations are also under active investigation.

12. Which tumors can be definitively treated with RT as the sole treatment modality, and when should concurrent systemic therapy be added?

Surgery is often preferred in settings where complete resection with sufficient margins can be expected without causing significant morbidity; however, many early-stage HN cancers that are T1 to 2 and N0 to 1 are candidates for definitive RT alone. These include primary tumors of the tongue, tonsil, larynx, and hypopharynx. Exceptions include cancers of the nasopharynx, in which EBRT is the standard treatment regardless of T or N stage. Tumors of the salivary glands and floor of the mouth are generally managed primarily with surgery, even if diagnosed at an early stage. Concurrent systemic therapy should be added to RT for more advanced (e.g., T3–T4, N2–N3) HN tumors. Multiple randomized trials and meta-analyses have shown an absolute survival benefit in this setting.

13. What are the standard indications for adjuvant RT and/or systemic therapy after surgical resection of an HN squamous cell carcinoma?

Positive margins, T3 to 4 tumors, multiple or bulky positive lymph nodes, nodal extracapsular extension (ECE), perineural invasion (PNI) greater than 0.1 millimeter, lymphovascular invasion (LVI), or nodal disease in levels IV or V. Additionally, oral cavity cancers with depth of invasion greater than 5 millimeters or close margins should receive adjuvant RT. In most cases, patients with recurrent disease treated with salvage surgery should be offered adjuvant RT when feasible.

14. What are the standard indications for concurrent chemotherapy with RT after surgical resection of an HN squamous cell carcinoma?

The addition of concurrent chemotherapy to adjuvant RT is typically recommended for patients with positive margins or ECE. Two major randomized trials (i.e., RTOG 95-01 and EORTC 22931) have examined adjuvant RT with or without concomitant cisplatin, with results showing local control, disease-free survival, and possibly OS benefits when using combined modality treatment.

15. **What are the indications for adjuvant RT after surgical resection for salivary gland tumors?**
For salivary gland tumors, adjuvant RT should be offered to patients with close or positive margins, pT3 to 4 tumors, intermediate- or high-grade tumors, adenoid cystic carcinoma histology, bone invasion, PNI, LVI, and pathologic node-positive disease. The addition of concurrent chemotherapy may be considered on a case-by-case basis and is the subject of multiple ongoing trials. For salivary gland tumors, postoperative RT also improves OS in addition to local regional control in patients with high-grade histology or locally advanced tumors.

16. **What is the recommended time between surgery and initiation of adjuvant RT for most HN cancers?**
Generally, 4 to 6 weeks is recommended because there is a direct correlation between the time to initiation of postoperative RT and tumor control outcomes, but patients must be well-healed before starting radiation. Several studies have validated the importance of a "package time" being approximately 13 weeks from date of surgery to completion of adjuvant RT. Delays or breaks in treatment are associated with poor outcomes for two primary reasons: (1) HN cancers exhibit accelerated repopulation and (2) an inherent bias exists that patients with advanced disease tolerate treatment poorly and require these delays and breaks.

17. **When delivering RT for an HN cancer of unknown primary, which areas should be treated?**
Possible primary mucosal sites that commonly metastasize, including the nasopharynx and oropharynx, and bilateral neck (unilateral coverage is controversial). The larynx, hypopharynx, and oral cavity may be treated if the patient is suspected to be at high risk in those areas.

18. **Does HPV or p16 status affect the recommended doses for RT?**
No. While HPV(+) and p16(+) oropharynx patients have better outcomes, and retrospective data show favorable outcomes with dose deescalation, no level 1 evidence exists for deescalation. Treatment deintensification with reduced dose for p16(+) is an active area of research.

19. **Which patients with HN skin cancer should be considered for definitive RT?**
Patients with large lesions who would require significant morbid surgeries, those with lesions of the central face or other locations for which surgery would result in significant cosmetic defects (e.g., nasal ala), and nonsurgical candidates.

20. **What are the indications for adjuvant therapy after surgical resection for HN skin cancers?**
Extensive or large nerve PNI, positive surgical margins, T3 and T4 tumors (including deep invasion >6 millimeters or into subcutaneous fat, muscle, or bone), recurrent disease after prior margin-negative resection, desmoplastic or infiltrative tumors in the setting of chronic immunosuppression, or an ear primary with high-risk features (i.e., depth of invasion >2 millimeters for skin cancer, Clark's level ≥IV, poor differentiation).

21. **What features of a primary skin cancer warrant elective nodal irradiation?**
Multiple positive lymph nodes (>3), ECE, large tumors (>4 centimeters), deep invasion greater than 6 millimeters, or cancer of the ear (particularly preauricular).

22. **What are the common acute adverse effects of RT to the HN region, and how are they managed?**
The acute side effects of RT usually appear in weeks 2 to 3, gradually progress through the week after the last radiation treatment, and resolve within 4 to 6 weeks after completion. Toxicities are often worse with concurrent systemic therapy. Optimal supportive management is necessary to avoid treatment breaks, which have been proven to decrease treatment efficacy. Supportive treatments for the most common symptoms include the following:
- Fatigue: An active exercise regimen and general healthy lifestyle practices, psychostimulants, and antidepressants
- Skin reactions: Nonperfumed moisturizers and humectants
- Mucositis, dysphagia, odynophagia: Dietary modifications, gabapentin, nonsteroidal anti-inflammatory drugs, steroids, lidocaine, opioids, and optimal hydration/nutrition support, which sometimes includes feeding tube placement
- Xerostomia: Mouthrinses (including combinations of water, baking soda, salt, hydrogen peroxide), Biotène, and optimal oral hygiene
    Hoarseness, otitis media, dry eyes, conjunctivitis/keratitis, sinonasal congestion, and epistaxis may also occur, depending on the site receiving radiation.

23. **Why is hydration/nutrition important for patients receiving RT and/or systemic therapies for HN tumors?**
Most of these patients are nutritionally depleted due to the morbidity of the tumor itself. Mucositis, nausea, vomiting, and anorexia from multimodal treatments add to the nutritional depletion. Poor nutrition or hydration may lead

to hospitalization and treatment breaks. In addition, patients who lose significant amounts of weight may not align correctly in their positioning masks for RT, which can require replanning with treatment breaks. Treatment breaks, while sometimes necessary, decrease cure rates and should be avoided when at all possible. Enteral gastrostomy feedings are often used when patients receive bilateral neck RT to support nutrition and hydration either prior to or during RT when necessary.

24. **What are the potential long-term complications of RT?**

Serious RT complications are unusual (with an incidence of less than 10%) but are difficult to manage when they occur. The likelihood of a given patient developing long-term complications depends on the total dose of radiation delivered, the dose per fraction, the time frame over which it was given, and the anatomic sites included within the radiation portal. In general, the risk increases with increasing doses delivered over shorter time periods to greater volumes of tissue. Complications include xerostomia, dysgeusia, skin changes, hypothyroidism, osteoradionecrosis, bone exposure, laryngeal edema with voice changes, esophageal stenosis, vision/hearing deficits, lymphedema, fibrosis including trismus, and induction of secondary cancers. Xerostomia is one of the most common and bothersome long-term side effects of HN irradiation. When possible, attempts should be made to minimize doses to parotid, submandibular glands, and minor salivary glands of the oral cavity and upper enterogastric track without sacrificing tumor coverage. Dry mouth also causes an increased risk of developing dental caries with subsequent increased risk for osteoradionecrosis.

25. **What is the benefit of Volumetric Modulated Arc Therapy (VMAT) in treating HN cancers?**

VMAT has become the standard RT technique for HN cancers in the past 10 years, and multiple trials have shown an ability to achieve similar rates of local control while lowering the incidence of acute and long-term toxicities by decreasing the radiation dose to critical organs (e.g., salivary glands for xerostomia, constrictor muscles for dysphagia).

26. **When should a neck dissection be performed after definitive RT or CRT?**

Neck dissection is reserved for high-risk concern of clinical or radiographic progressive or persistent disease with adequate surveillance. The response to radiation is generally assessed by PET/CT at 12 or more weeks posttreatment, although patients may take additional months to fully respond to RT. HPV(+) disease in particular has a longer treatment involution process and may require extended surveillance.

27. **When should re-irradiation be considered?**

Recurrent disease, when the patient is not eligible for salvage surgery or with post-salvage surgery high-risk features, may be considered for re-irradiation. In the re-irradiation setting, the risks for both acute and long-term toxicities are increased. SBRT is one technique under investigation for use in the re-irradiation setting as a means of delivering highly conformal high-dose radiation to areas of relapse while sparing normal tissues.

BIBLIOGRAPHY

Bonner JA, Harari PM, Giralt J, et al: Radiotherapy plus cetuximab for locoregionally advanced head and neck cancer: 5-year survival data from a phase 3 randomized trial, and relation between cetuximab-induced rash and survival, *Lancet Oncol* 11(1):21–28, 2010.

Cooper JS, Zhang Q, Pajak TF, et al: Long-term follow-up of the RTOG 9501/intergroup phase III trial: postoperative concurrent radiation therapy and chemotherapy in high-risk squamous cell carcinoma of the head and neck, *Int J Radiat Oncol Biol Phys* 84(5):1198–1205, 2012.

Koyfman SA, Ismaila N, Crook D, et al: Management of the neck in squamous cell carcinoma of the oral cavity and oropharynx: ASCO Clinical Practice Guideline, *J Clin Oncol* 37(20):1753–1774, 2019.

Likhacheva A, Awan M, Barker CA, et al: Definitive and postoperative radiation therapy for basal and squamous cell cancers of the skin: executive summary of an American Society of Radiation Oncology Clinical Practice Guideline, *Pract Radiat Oncol* 10(1):8–20, 2020.

Mahmood U, Koshy M, Goloubeva O, et al: Adjuvant radiation therapy for high-grade and/or locally advanced major salivary gland tumors, *Arch Otolaryngol Head Neck Surg* 137(10):1025–1030, 2011.

Mehanna PH, Robinson M, Hartley A, et al: Radiotherapy plus cisplatin or cetuximab in low-risk human papillomavirus–positive oropharyngeal cancer (De-ESCALaTE HPV): an open-label randomized controlled phase 3 trial, *Lancet* 393(10166):51–60, 2018.

Noronha V, Joshi A, Patil VM, et al: Once-a-week versus once-every-3-weeks cisplatin chemoradiation for locally advanced head and neck cancer: a phase III randomized noninferiority trial, *J Clin Oncol* 26(11):1064–1072, 2018.

NCCN Clinical Practice Guidelines in Oncology: Head and Neck Cancers Version 3, 2019. Available at https://www.nccn.org/professionals/physician_gls/pdf/head-and-neck.pdf.

Pignon JP, le Maître A, Maillard E, et al: Meta-analysis of chemotherapy in head and neck cancer (MACH-NC): an update on 93 randomized trials and 17,346 patients, *Radiother Oncol* 92(1):4–14, 2009.

Terhaard CH, Lubsen H, Rasch CR, et al: The role of radiotherapy in the treatment of malignant salivary gland tumors, *Int J Radiat Oncol Biol Phys* 61(1):103–111, 2005.

Zhang Y, Chen L, Hu GQ, et al: Gemcitabine and cisplatin induction chemotherapy in nasopharyngeal carcinoma, *N Engl J Med* 381(12):1124–1135, 2019.

CHAPTER 23

SINONASAL ANATOMY AND EMBRYOLOGY WITH RADIOLOGY CORRELATES

Jeremiah A. Alt, MD, PhD, Daniel M. Beswick, MD and Richard R. Orlandi, MD

KEY POINTS

1. While there can be great variation in sinus anatomy, the drainage patterns of the sinuses are fairly consistent.
2. Embryologic patterns of pneumatization of the paranasal sinus lamellae aid in understanding of related anatomy.
3. The blood supply to the nose and sinuses originates from both internal and external carotid branches. Knowledge of the arterial blood supply to the nose and sinuses facilitates understanding how to avoid and treat bleeding during and following sinus surgery.
4. Diseases of the paranasal sinuses can extend hematogenously or via direct extension into adjacent structures.

Pearls

1. The paranasal sinuses form as evaginations from the nasal cavity. The ethmoid and maxillary sinuses are present at birth, and all of the sinuses continue to develop postnatally, with the sphenoid and frontal sinuses developing last.
2. The osteomeatal unit (OMU) is a functional anatomic unit. Obstruction in this area can lead to anterior ethmoid and maxillary sinusitis and possibly frontal sinusitis.
3. CT with triplanar reconstruction is the preferred method for evaluating the sinuses radiographically.
4. Sinus disease can spread via vascular channels into the intracranial cavity and orbit.

QUESTIONS

1. Describe the septum and the turbinates.

   The nasal septum is the midline partition that separates the left and right sides of the nasal cavity. It is composed of the quadrangular cartilage, perpendicular plate of the ethmoid bone, vomer, and maxillary crest. There are three paired turbinates, or *concha*, on each side. The middle and superior turbinates are part of the ethmoid bone, whereas the inferior turbinate is its own bone. Occasionally, a fourth paired turbinate, the supreme turbinate, is present.

2. Define the paranasal sinuses.

   The paranasal sinuses are pneumatized areas of the facial and skull base bones. They communicate with the nasal cavity through small ostia, allowing air exchange and drainage of secreted mucus.

3. Which epithelium lines the paranasal sinuses?

   The sinuses are lined by pseudostratified ciliated columnar or respiratory epithelium. Cilia beat in a coordinated fashion to transport mucus from the point of its secretion in the sinus toward its natural ostium. From there, cilia within the nasal cavity move the secretions toward the nasopharynx. A portion of the nasal cavity near the superior turbinates and superior portion of the septum is lined with olfactory neuroepithelia.

4. What is the function of the paranasal sinuses?

   A number of theories exist about the possible function of the sinuses, including decreasing the mass of the skull, enhancing vocal resonance, absorption of mechanical force during trauma in order to protect the orbits and brain, and production of a reservoir for nitric oxide, a postulated aerocrine substance that may regulate pulmonary function. There is evidence for and against all of these theories.

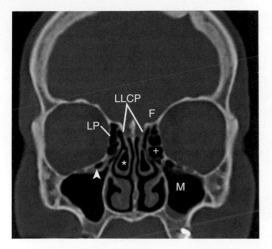

Fig. 23.1 Coronal computed tomography (CT) scan image in a bone window algorithm showing pneumatization in the head of the middle turbinate (*), also called a concha bullosa. Infraorbital ethmoid air cells (Haller cells) are seen as pneumatized air cells off the inferior orbital floor (arrow). This can narrow the drainage of the maxillary sinus (M). The lateral wall of the ethmoid cavity is the lamina papyracea (LP), lateral to which is the orbit. The olfactory cleft and lateral lamella of the cribriform plate (LLCP) are depicted. Note the relationship of the LLCP with the insertion of the basal lamella of the middle turbinate, as well as the fovea ethmoidalis (F) laterally. The LLCP is commonly asymmetric. This asymmetric anatomic variation should be recognized on presurgical planning to prevent iatrogenic cerebrospinal fluid leaks. The ethmoid bulla is seen adjacent to the LP (+).

5. **Where is the maxillary sinus located?**
   The maxillary sinus is located within the body of the maxilla. Medially it is bounded by the lateral nasal wall, superiorly by the floor of the orbit (containing the infraorbital nerve and artery), posteriorly by the pterygopalatine and infratemporal fossae, and inferiorly by the alveolar process and hard palate. Maxillary tooth roots commonly reach to the floor of the maxillary sinus (Fig. 23.1).

6. **Where are the ethmoid sinuses located?**
   The ethmoid sinuses form a lattice-like series of cells medial to the orbits and inferior to the anterior cranial base. They are functionally divided into the anterior and posterior ethmoid cells by a portion of the middle turbinate termed the basal lamella. The anterior ethmoid cells are bounded medially by the middle turbinate and drain into the middle meatus. The posterior ethmoid cells are bounded medially by the superior turbinate and drain into the superior meatus. The ethmoid cells are bounded laterally by the lamina papyracea of the orbit. Posterior to the posterior ethmoid cells are the sphenoid face and sphenoid bone containing the sphenoid sinus. The nasal cavity is inferior to the ethmoid air cells and the frontal bone and skull base are superior. As the ethmoid cells form embryologically, they expand into the frontal bone superiorly and make shallow depressions in it, called fovea ethmoidalis. The frontal bone abuts the cribriform plate of the ethmoid medially, and a small portion of the cribriform plate sits superior to the ethmoid cells. This area tends to be very thin and easily injured during sinus surgery, which can lead to a cerebrospinal fluid leak.

7. **Where is the sphenoid sinus located?**
   The sphenoid sinus pneumatizes the sphenoid bone and is posterior to the ethmoid sinus. The sella turcica and pituitary gland lie superior to the sphenoid sinus. The optic nerve lies within the lateral wall of the sphenoid sinus. The venous cavernous sinus, near the sphenoid sinus, contains the internal carotid artery and cranial nerves III, IV, V_1, V_2, and VI. Posterior to the sphenoid sinus is the posterior cranial fossa (Fig. 23.2). The sphenoid sinus can pneumatize laterally into the pterygoid region of the sphenoid and thus lies inferior to the temporal lobes of the brain.

8. **Where is the frontal sinus located?**
   The frontal sinuses are air spaces within the frontal bones. The frontal bone thus has an anterior wall and a posterior wall, which are referred to as tables. The anterior table lies deep to the forehead skin. The frontal lobes of the brain lie posterior to the frontal sinus.

9. **At which point during gestation do the sinuses begin to develop?**
   The sinuses begin to form in the third fetal month. Only the ethmoid and maxillary sinuses are present at birth (remember: "ME at birth"). They form as evaginations from the developing nasal cavity that invade into the surrounding bones.

10. **Do the sinuses continue to develop postnatally?**
    Yes. The maxillary sinus continues to grow in size as the face grows overall. The maxillary sinus enlarges again after eruption of the permanent dentition. The ethmoid sinuses continue to develop postnatally until approximately 12 years of age. The frontal sinus pneumatizes slowly postnatally, rarely reaching any significant size during the first decade of life. Thereafter, the frontal sinus rapidly pneumatizes into the frontal bone, reaching its final size

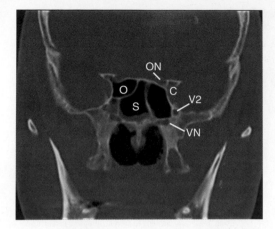

Fig. 23.2 Coronal computed tomography (CT) scan in a bone window algorithm showing a right sphenoethmoidal air cell (Onodi cell) located superior and lateral to the sphenoid sinus (S). The optic nerve (ON) and carotid artery (C) are seen as bony protrusions in the sphenoethmoidal air cell (O) rather than the sphenoid sinus. The Vidian nerve (VN) and the maxillary division of the trigeminal nerve (V2) can be seen inferiorly and laterally.

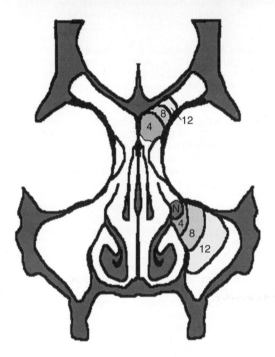

Fig. 23.3 Coronal representation of the development of the frontal and maxillary sinus. The frontal sinus begins to develop at the age of 4 years and does not fully mature until after the age of 12 years. The newborn (N) has a small maxillary sinus that continues to expand in a lateral inferior direction, reaching adult pneumatization after 12 years of age.

near the end of the second decade of life. Likewise, the sphenoid sinus develops little until approximately 7 years of age, after which it rapidly pneumatizes and reaches its final size during adolescence (Fig. 23.3).

11. **How are the sinuses evaluated radiographically?**
    High-resolution thin-cut multiplanar computed tomography (CT) is commonly used to evaluate the complex bony anatomy of the paranasal sinuses. Direct acquisition in the axial plane with reconstruction in the coronal and sagittal planes is now commonplace. Such triplanar imaging allows for the study of complex anatomic relationships throughout the paranasal sinuses and cranial base. Of the three views, the coronal images can be considered the most useful because they closely resemble the surgeon's endoscopic surgical view, although all three views are complementary. Inflammation of the sinuses is seen on CT as thickening of the mucoperiosteum of the paranasal sinuses. Plain radiographs of the sinuses are rarely used nowadays due to the lack of anatomic detail compared with CT imaging. MRI can augment CTs by providing soft tissue analysis, such as when secretions cannot be differentiated from a neoplasm. Due to the lack of bony detail, MRI is not commonly used for standard initial sinus evaluations.

12. **What is the osteomeatal unit and which structures make up this area?**
    The osteomeatal unit (OMU) is a functional anatomic area within the middle meatus comprised of the ethmoid bulla, uncinate process, ethmoid infundibulum, and hiatus semilunaris. The OMU is the common drainage pathway of the anterior ethmoid and maxillary sinuses. Depending on the superior attachment of the uncinate process, it may also drain the frontal sinus. Inflammation within the OMU may lead to obstruction of and inflammation within these draining sinuses.

13. **What is the ethmoid bulla?**
    The ethmoid bulla is the most consistent and typically largest anterior ethmoid cell. Its lateral wall is the lamina papyracea. It usually has a rounded shape anteriorly, running parallel to the uncinate process (see Fig. 23.1).

14. **What is the uncinate process?**
    The term *uncinate process* means "hook-shaped" bone. It is a crescent- or hook-shaped fold of bone that sweeps from superior to posterior, just anterior to the ethmoid bulla within the anterior ethmoid sinuses. The uncinate process and anterior face of the bulla tend to run parallel to each other, forming a small window termed the hiatus semilunaris. The uncinate process is attached to the lateral wall of the nose and has a free edge posteriorly. It therefore forms a trough-shaped space that runs from superior to posterior within the anterior ethmoid sinuses. This space is called the *ethmoid infundibulum*.

15. **What is the difference between the hiatus semilunaris and the ethmoid infundibulum?**
    The hiatus semilunaris is a two-dimensional gap (remember: *hiatus* means "gap") between the ethmoid bulla and the uncinate process. The ethmoid infundibulum is a three-dimensional trough between the uncinate process and lateral nasal wall/lamina papyracea. Surgically, the ethmoid infundibulum can be accessed through the hiatus semilunaris. In other words, the trough is reached through the semilunar gap.

16. **What is the agger nasi?**
    The term agger nasi means "nasal mound" and refers to the area in the lateral wall of the nasal cavity that projects medially, just superior to the middle turbinate's anterior superior attachment. It is commonly pneumatized, forming an agger nasi cell (Fig. 23.4).

17. **How do the sinuses drain into the nasal cavity?**
    Each sinus communicates with the nasal cavity through an ostium. The sizes of the ostia vary but generally measure from 1 to 3 mm. Each ethmoid cell has a variably placed ostium but the anterior and posterior ethmoid cells as groups have consistent drainage patterns. The anterior ethmoid cells as a group drain into the middle meatus and the posterior ethmoid cells drain collectively into the superior meatus.

    The maxillary, sphenoid, and frontal sinuses have relatively consistent drainage patterns. The maxillary sinus ostium drains into the ethmoid infundibulum. From there it drains into the middle meatus of the nasal cavity. The sphenoid sinus ostium drains into the sphenoethmoidal recess, between the superior turbinate and the nasal septum. The frontal sinus may also drain into the ethmoid infundibulum of the anterior ethmoid sinus. If, however, the uncinate process attaches to the lamina papyracea, the frontal sinus will bypass the ethmoid infundibulum and drain directly into the middle meatus. Once the secretions have reached the nasal cavity, they are carried into the nasopharynx by cilia.

18. **What variations are seen in the anatomy of the ethmoid sinuses?**
    Infraorbital ethmoid air cells, termed Haller cells, may be present laterally within the ethmoid sinus, adjacent to the inferior orbital floor and at the medial extent of the roof of the maxillary sinus. It is important to identify these cells because they have the potential to narrow the ethmoid infundibulum and maxillary sinus drainage. Coronal CT is the best for identifying these air cells (see Fig. 23.1). The term *concha bullosa* is used to describe pneumatization of the middle turbinate. A concha bullosa of the middle turbinate can narrow the OMU by compressing the uncinate process laterally (see Fig. 23.1). A concha bullosa of the superior turbinate may also exist.

19. **What variations are seen in the anatomy of the sphenoid sinus?**
    Sphenoethmoidal cells, termed Onodi cells, are posterior ethmoid cells that pneumatize into the sphenoid bone. An Onodi can extend superiorly, posteriorly, and laterally and therefore have an intimate relationship with the optic nerve and carotid artery in its lateral wall. The sphenoethmoidal cell is visualized on coronal CT views with the appearance of a horizontal split of the sphenoid sinus. Coronal, sagittal, and axial views should be reviewed to clarify whether the origin of the cell is from the posterior ethmoids rather than the sphenoid, which is medial and inferior (see Fig. 23.2).

20. **Which structures make up the frontal recess?**
    The frontal outflow tract is an hourglass-shaped space formed and impinged upon by a number of variable structures surrounding it. The frontal recess outflow is not a discrete or singular duct. Generally, these boundary structures are:
    • Agger nasi cell, anterior
    • Middle turbinate, medial

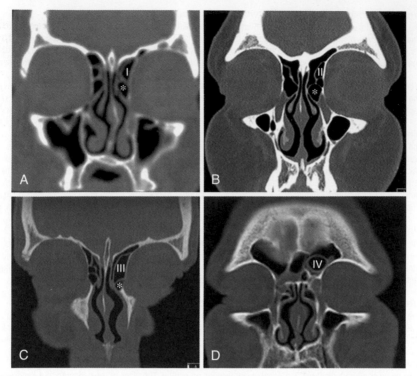

Fig. 23.4 Computed tomography (CT) images in bone window algorithms demonstrating types of frontal cells (Kuhn classification I–IV): **A**, Type I cell directly above the agger nasi cell (*). **B**, Type II cell. **C**, Type III Kuhn cell. The coronal CT imaging shows bilateral Type III Kuhn frontal air cells. **D**, Type IV Kuhn frontal cell is isolated within the left frontal sinus.

- Anterior fossa cranial base, posterior-superior
- Lamina papyracea, lateral
- Ethmoid bulla, posterior-inferior

21. **What are frontal cells?**

The pattern of pneumatization within the ethmoid sinuses is highly variable. Sometimes ethmoid or other air cells can be present superiorly within the frontal sinus drainage. Frontal cells have been grouped according to two classification systems. The original system (Kuhn classification) includes four principal patterns (see Fig. 23.4):
- Type 1: A single ethmoid cell resting immediately superior to the agger nasi cell
- Type 2: More than one ethmoid sitting atop the agger nasi cell
- Type 3: A significantly pneumatized ethmoid cell that extends beyond the frontal recess into the frontal sinus
- Type 4: An air cell that is isolated within the frontal sinus

Recently, an international consensus effort was undertaken to establish a naming convention for frontal cells based on their anatomical location and to facilitate communication and education. In addition to the agger nasi, this classification of frontal cells includes supra agger cell, supra agger frontal cell, supra bulla cell, supra bulla frontal cell, supraorbital ethmoid cell, and frontal septal cell. All of these cells can narrow the frontal sinus drainage.

22. **Explain the concepts of endoscopic sinus surgery (ESS).**

Functional endoscopic sinus surgery stresses restoring the normal drainage ("function") of the sinuses through their natural ostia. Part or all of the ethmoid partitions may be removed to promote drainage of the ethmoid cells. The ostia of the affected frontal, sphenoid, or maxillary sinuses may then be widened to promote their drainage into the nasal cavity. The remaining mucosa is maximally preserved to restore normal mucociliary clearance patterns. Prior to ESS, mucosa was thought to be irreversibly diseased and was therefore removed. This removal destroyed the normal mucociliary clearance, leading to dysfunctional sinuses that depended on gravity to drain. A large body of prospective evidence shows that ESS results in quality of life improvements for appropriately selected patients with chronic rhinosinusitis.

23. **Describe the blood supply to the nose and paranasal sinuses.**
    The nose and ethmoid sinuses are principally supplied by three arteries whose branches form anastomoses with one another:
    - The anterior and posterior ethmoid arteries are branches of the ophthalmic artery, which branches from the internal carotid artery. They arise in the orbit and pass into the roof of the ethmoid sinuses through foramina in the lamina papyracea. They supply much of the ethmoid sinuses and the superior nasal septum.
    - The sphenopalatine artery is a terminal branch of the internal maxillary artery, which arises from the external carotid artery. It has two principal branches, one of which passes just inferior to the sphenoid sinus ostium and supplies the posterior nasal septum. A second branch enters into the middle turbinate. Smaller branches supply the nasal floor and inferior turbinate.
    - The frontal, maxillary, and sphenoid sinuses are supplied by small arteries that perforate their bony walls.

24. **Describe the venous drainage of the nose and paranasal sinuses.**
    The venous drainage of the nose and sinuses passes into venous sinuses in the pterygopalatine fossa, which then communicate with the venous cavernous sinus lateral to the sphenoid sinus. Some of the venous drainage can pass through the lamina papyracea. The frontal sinus drains intracranially through small veins that perforate the posterior table of the frontal bone. Infection in the sinuses can pass into the orbit or cranial cavity through these venous drainage pathways.

25. **Name and describe the lamellas that originate from the bony ridges (ethmoturbinals) in the lateral nasal wall during embryologic development.**
    - First lamella is made up of both an ascending and descending portion and becomes the agger nasi cell and the uncinate process, respectively.
    - Second lamella becomes the bulla ethmoidalis.
    - Third lamella becomes the basal lamella of the middle turbinate. It provides a clear distinction between the anterior and posterior ethmoid air cells.
    - Fourth lamella becomes the superior turbinate.
    - Fifth lamella is more varied but arises from the fusion of the fifth and sixth ethmoturbinals to become the supreme turbinate (if one is present).

26. **Which areas of a CT scan should be specifically evaluated prior to ESS?**
    Inflammation within the sinuses is assessed by examining the scan for any mucosal thickening. The frontal, anterior ethmoid, posterior ethmoid, maxillary, and sphenoid sinuses and OMU are assessed bilaterally. Anatomic variants that may contribute to obstruction or that may impact surgery are noted.
    The following areas can be involved in potential complications and should be investigated during the planning stages of surgery:
    - Lamina papyracea integrity
    - Cribriform plate anatomy – specifically, the depth of the olfactory fossa and the symmetry between the two sides
    - Ethmoid skull base integrity
    - Anterior ethmoid artery location – does it run along the skull base or does it run in a more inferiorly positioned bony mesentery?
    - Sphenoethmoidal (Onodi) cell presence
    - Are the sphenoid sinuses asymmetric in size or shape?
    - Optic nerve anatomy – covered by bone or dehiscent?
    - Internal carotid anatomy – covered by bone or dehiscent?
    An acronym to recall areas to evaluate on preoperative CT scan is CLOSE: Cribriform place, Lamina papyracea, Onodi cell, Sphenoid sinus pneumatization, and anterior Ethmoid artery.

CONTROVERSIES

27. **How much does anatomy contribute to rhinosinusitis?**
    Chronic rhinosinusitis is an inflammatory process that involves inflammation within the paranasal sinuses and nasal cavity. Its etiology remains elusive and is likely multifactorial. Anatomic variations may play a role in some cases but, overall, the impact appears to be small. Correction of sinus anatomic issues without attention to accompanying mucosal inflammation only occasionally resolves chronic rhinosinusitis.
    Recurrent acute rhinosinusitis (RARS) is a less common form of sinus inflammation centered on repeated episodes of acute bacterial rhinosinusitis (ABRS). Recent studies have implicated narrowing of the ethmoid infundibulum as a possible risk factor for this condition, and appropriately selected patients usually have good outcomes following endoscopic sinus surgery. It is imperative that patients who are considered for a diagnosis of RARS meet full diagnostic criteria before being given this diagnosis, as symptoms due to many other conditions, such as allergic rhinitis, migraines, headaches, and other disorders, can mimic the symptoms of ABRS.

Bibliography

Deutshmann MW, Yeung J, Bosch M, et al: Radiologic reporting for paranasal sinus computed tomography: a multi-institutional review of content and consistency, *Laryngoscope* 123:1100–1105, 2013.

Orlandi RR, Kingdom TT, Hwang PH, et al: International consensus statement on allergy and rhinology: rhinosinusitis, *Int Forum Allergy Rhinol* 6(Suppl 1):S22–209, 2016.

Rosenfeld RM, Piccirillo JF, Chandrasekar SS, et al: Clinical practice guidelines (update): adult sinusitis, *Otolaryngol Head Neck Surg* 152(2S):S1–S39, 2015.

Stammberger H: *Functional Endoscopic Sinus Surgery*, 1991, BC Decker.

Stammberger HR, Kennedy DW: Paranasal sinuses: anatomic terminology and nomenclature, *Ann Otol Rhinol Laryngol Suppl* 167:7–16, 1995.

Wise S, DelGaudio J, Orlandi RR: Sinonasal anatomy and development. In Kennedy DW, Hwang PH, editors: *Rhinology: Diseases of the Nose, Sinuses, and Skull Base*, 2012, Thieme.

Wormald PJ, Hoseman W, Callejas C, et al: The International Frontal Sinus Anatomy Classification (IFAC) and Classification of the Extent of Endoscopic Frontal Sinus Surgery (EFSS), *Int Forum Allergy Rhinol* 6(7):677–696, 2016.

CHAPTER 24

EPISTAXIS

Laylaa Ramos Arriaza, MD, MS and Vijay R. Ramakrishnan, MD

KEY POINTS

1. Anterior epistaxis is the most common and often originates from Little's area in Kiesselbach's plexus, whereas posterior bleeds commonly originate from the sphenopalatine artery distribution.
2. The most important initial evaluation is a rough gauge of epistaxis severity and, if needed, status of ABCs (airway, breathing, and circulation) and vital signs. This plays the key initial role in evaluation and planning.
3. There are a number of modifiable factors that should be kept in mind in the treatment of chronic epistaxis, such as current medications, home/work environment, and indoor humidity at place of residence.
4. In cases of repeated epistaxis without an identified cause, conditions such as coagulopathy, vascular abnormality, drug use, hereditary disorders, and inflammatory and autoimmune conditions should be considered.
5. When considering intervention for posterior epistaxis, SPA ligation is a more efficacious and cost-effective means of controlling epistaxis compared to posterior packing and hospitalization or embolization. The latter may be preferred in the poor surgical candidate.

Pearls

1. Wegener granulomatosis, now referred to as granulomatosis with polyangiitis (GPA), affects the upper airway, kidneys, and lungs and can present to the otolaryngologist as epistaxis, nasal obstruction, olfactory dysfunction, hearing loss, or subglottic stenosis.
2. Conditions to be considered in a patient with epistaxis and thrombocytopenia: massive hemorrhage, disseminated intravascular coagulation (and associated underlying medical issues such as sepsis), thrombotic microangiopathy, heparin- or other drug-induced thrombocytopenia, idiopathic thrombocytopenic purpura, and bone marrow suppression.
3. A patient who requires posterior nasal packing should be admitted to the hospital and placed on telemetry and continuous pulse oximetry.
4. In general, endoscopic sphenopalatine artery ligation for posterior epistaxis is both more effective and more cost beneficial than arterial embolization.
5. A teenage male presenting with unilateral nasal obstruction and epistaxis should raise suspicion for juvenile nasopharyngeal angiofibroma (JNA). JNA is a highly vascularized benign tumor that originates near the medial pterygopalatine fossa (PPF). Diagnosis is made by classic history and radiology (widening of the PPF and anterior bowing of the posterior maxillary sinus wall or Holman-Miller sign); biopsy should be avoided due to risk of hemorrhage.

QUESTIONS

1. Discuss the epidemiology of epistaxis.

   Epistaxis occurs in 60% of the population in the United States; approximately 6% of people who experience epistaxis will seek medical attention. The vast majority of episodes are benign and self-limited. Epistaxis accounts for 0.5% of all emergency department visits and one-third of all otolaryngology-related emergency department encounters. Epistaxis occurs in all age groups with a bimodal distribution in the young and elderly; it is categorized into childhood versus adult epistaxis, or primary versus secondary epistaxis, which is important for diagnostic and therapeutic decision-making.

2. Which blood vessels supply the nasal mucosa?

   The anterior and posterior ethmoid arteries supply the superior nasal cavity and septum; they arise from the ophthalmic branch of the internal carotid artery. The sphenopalatine artery is the terminal branch of the internal maxillary artery (from the external carotid circulation) and supplies the posterior lateral nasal wall and nasal cavity. The facial artery, also from the external carotid distribution, provides additional supply to the anterior nasal cavity (Fig. 24.1).

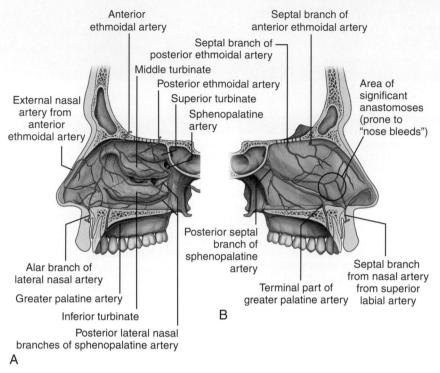

Fig. 24.1 Arterial supply of the nasal cavities. **A**, Lateral wall of the right nasal cavity. **B**, Septum (medial wall of right nasal cavity). (From Drake RL, Vogl AW, Mitchel AWM: *Gray's Anatomy for Students*, 2nd ed, St. Louis, 2009, Elsevier.)

3. **What is Kiesselbach's plexus? What is Woodruff's plexus? Where are they located?**
   Kiesselbach's plexus is a confluence of vessels arising from both the internal and external carotid artery systems. It supplies an area on the anterior-inferior nasal septum known as Little's area, the most common site for epistaxis.
   Woodruff's plexus is a confluence of thin-walled veins located posteriorly in the inferior meatus. This area was previously thought to be arterial and also thought to be a main contributor to posterior bleeds, but this does not appear to be the case.

4. **What is meant by "anterior" and "posterior" epistaxis?**
   The majority of bleeds (90% to 95%) originate anteriorly; many of the anterior bleeds occur in Little's area within Kiesselbach's plexus. Occurring much more often than posterior bleeds because of their location (nose picking/local trauma, dryness), anterior bleeds are easily accessible and managed with conservative measures such as moisturization, pressure, decongestion, or topical cautery. Posterior bleeds are generally from the distribution of the sphenopalatine artery and are the cause of 5% to 10% of epistaxis. The exact focus of origin is more challenging to identify, and these bleeds are therefore more likely to require nasal packing as part of intervention.

5. **What should be included in the history evaluation of a patient with new-onset epistaxis?**
   In an emergent setting, emphasis should be placed on managing airway, breathing, and circulation with volume replacement as needed and a focused history to expedite locating the source by nasal endoscopy and controlling hemorrhage. In the nonemergent setting, a careful and thorough history and physical exam can be obtained. The history should include timing, frequency, sidedness, and severity of epistaxis (which can be quantified by volume of observed blood or number of tissues), exploring predisposing conditions such as trauma, recent surgery, coagulopathy, cancer, medications and illicit drug use, contributory chronic medical issues, and current symptoms indicative of blood loss such as lightheadedness or dyspnea. Family history of bleeding disorder or epistaxis is also worthy of inquiry.

6. **What are the initial measures utilized to control mild epistaxis?**
   (1) Instruct the patient to gently blow the nose. This removes blood/clots. (2) Intranasal administration of nasal decongestant spray such as oxymetazoline (a selective alpha-1 agonist/partial alpha-2 agonist). (3) Instruct the

patient to pinch the nasal alae against the septum to apply hemostatic pressure and hold for 10 to 15 minutes, or longer if needed. (4) Place a cold compress over the bridge of the nose, if available.

7. **Why is it helpful to have the patient lean forward in addition to the measures suggested in the previous question?**
Having the head tilted posteriorly may result in posterior drainage of blood, increasing the potential for aspiration and/or gastric irritation with resultant bloody emesis. Additionally, having the blood fall back into the throat and be swallowed makes it difficult to quantify the amount of bleeding.

8. **What are the key components of the initial physical examination for patient with epistaxis?**
Initial physical evaluation should include ensuring patency of the airway, appropriate breathing, and circulation; obtaining vital signs; and checking mental status. Check for signs of anemia or shock (anxiety, cool/clammy skin, oliguria or anuria, weakness, pallor, diaphoresis, altered mentation) or signs of coagulopathy such as petechiae or purpura.

9. **How is the nose examined in the epistaxis evaluation?**
Anesthetic and a vasoconstrictive agent can be provided through topical sprays or soaked cotton strips, with preparations such as 2% lidocaine or 4% cocaine. Oxymetazoline or phenylephrine spray can be given for vasoconstrictive effect. The patient may expectorate blood/clots as tolerated to better visualize the nasal cavity and maintain the sniffing position. A nasal speculum should be used initially, and suction can be used to help remove blood and clots. Inspect relevant anatomic locations such as Kiesselbach's plexus, septum, and turbinates. In addition to bleeding, the clinician can discover ulcerations, excoriations, and erosion of the mucosa. This will be sufficient for most anterior bleeds but may not be for many posterior bleeds. Endoscopy should be utilized if the source of bleeding is not clear on anterior rhinoscopy, posterior epistaxis is suspected on history, conservative measures have not been successful, or a tumor or lesion is suspected on history.

10. **Should you obtain bloodwork in the above evaluation?**
It is not currently recommended to obtain routine CBC or coagulation studies in the initial assessment, unless the history is suggestive of significant blood loss, repeated large episodes, suspicion of coagulopathy, or current use of anticoagulant medication.

11. **What is primary versus secondary epistaxis? After determining if the bleed is primary or secondary in nature, how should you proceed?**
Primary (idiopathic) epistaxis is a spontaneous bleed without any identified precipitant, while those with an identified cause are termed secondary. Primary epistaxis with an identified source, especially when anterior, should be treated with direct therapy measures such as topical emollients, application of topical hemostatic agents, and/or focal cauterization if necessary. Posterior primary bleeds can be treated with nasal packing, chemical and/or electrocautery, arterial ligation, or embolization.
    In secondary epistaxis, the underlying disorder needs to be addressed in addition to resuscitative efforts and local modalities. Common causes of secondary epistaxis include liver disease, hematologic disorders (e.g., leukemia), and use of anticoagulant medications such as warfarin or antiplatelet agents (see Controversies section for further discussion). Other causes of secondary epistaxis include trauma, recent surgery, hereditary disorders, and neoplasms.

12. **Describe the treatment of recurrent epistaxis in the pediatric population.**
In children with recurrent epistaxis, a recommended treatment option is antiseptic cream (chlorhexidine/neomycin). Unilateral cauterization with silver nitrate also appears to be safe and effective. It is rare for children to require surgical intervention.

13. **Describe the placement of an anterior nasal pack.**
Anterior packing can be performed with either gauze or nasal tampons that expand with the addition of saline. A nasal tampon is placed by first applying topical anesthetic/analgesic intranasally and coating the pack with antibiotic ointment (this serves as both lubrication and possible prevention of toxic shock syndrome), sliding the tampon into place, and expanding it with saline application. Balloon/Merocel combinations have also been utilized and are another effective method for temporary epistaxis control. Petroleum-impregnated gauze can also be used with antibiotic ointment, placed intranasally with bayonet forceps and layered top to bottom/back to front until tamponade is achieved. Other custom-fashioned hemostatic packs can be used in similar fashion, such as an absorbable gelatin sponge wrapped in oxidized cellulose dressing.

14. **How is silver nitrate chemical cautery applied?**
Bleeding must be of minimal severity for silver nitrate to be successful, and ideally unilateral to avoid bilateral cauterization, which can carry a risk of septal perforation. The mucosa needs to be relatively dry for the silver nitrate to take effect, so a topical decongestant is administered and pressure is applied first to slow bleeding. The

silver nitrate stick should be focally placed at the origin of the bleed, holding the tip of the applicator stick against the mucosa until the mucosa becomes gray, working from the periphery to the center of the bleeding site. Topical saline or decongestant is applied to halt the chemical reaction once the desired effect is achieved.

15. **Describe the placement of posterior packs and their associated complications.**
A posterior pack can be performed with insertion of a cotton pack or Foley catheter. A small red rubber tube is carefully inserted in the nose and passed through the oropharynx and the end is retrieved through the mouth using a ring forceps. On the oral end of the tube, a cotton pack is attached with silk ties. The tube is gently pulled antero-inferiorly from the nasal side until the pack passes through the oropharynx to a resting place in the naso-pharynx and posterior choana. The anterior nasal cavity may be packed subsequently, and the tube is fastened externally while care is taken not to exert excessive pressure on the nasal ala. The patient should be admitted for telemetry, pulse oximetry, and antibiotic therapy.

   Potential complications include pain, discomfort, respiratory difficulty (including aspiration of the packing material), infection (as well as toxic shock syndrome, sinusitis from blocking outflow tracts), alar/septal necrosis, and pharyngeal fibrosis/stenosis. Supplemental oxygen may be required; telemetry monitoring is required given the risk of arrhythmia and syncope.

16. **What are the surgical interventions for persistent epistaxis?**
Endoscopic diathermy, laser photocoagulation, septal surgery, arterial ligation, and embolization can be used for persistent bleeding. Endoscopic sphenopalatine artery ligation or internal maxillary artery ligation is now frequently used in the management of posterior epistaxis. Endoscopic sphenopalatine artery ligation is successful and cost-effective when compared to nasal packing or embolization.

17. **How do SPA ligation and embolization compare in the management of epistaxis?**
Embolization results in almost twice the hospital cost compared to that of surgical ligation and may be less effective than SPA ligation in some scenarios. Although it carries a low risk of major complication, embolization may be an appropriate alternative in patients who cannot tolerate general anesthesia or are otherwise not good surgical candidates.

18. **List a broad differential for new-onset nasal bleeding.**
   - Environmental: cold air/dry air can be compounded by central heating systems for rooms that are not humidified (dryness results in mucosal irritation)
   - Trauma: most commonly digital trauma (nose picking) but can also be from other local trauma/facial trauma, foreign body, surgery
   - Inflammatory (exacerbated by upper respiratory infections, sinusitis, environmental or other allergies, drugs/chemicals) or autoimmune
   - Medications: antiplatelet agents or anticoagulants, nasal sprays
   - Vascular: arterial aneurysm or pseudoaneurysm
   - Congenital/developmental: septal abnormality such as deviation or perforation
   - Genetic: Osler-Weber-Rendu syndrome/hereditary hemorrhagic telangiectasia (HHT)
   - Systemic disorders: arteriosclerosis, hypertension, blood dyscrasias (von Willebrand, paraneoplastic effects, liver disease, hemophilia, thrombocytopenia)
   - Neoplastic: benign or malignant processes

19. **What are some medications that may contribute to epistaxis?**
Aspirin, clopidogrel, warfarin, or other forms of anticoagulation; intranasal steroids; nasal cannula oxygen; and chemotherapy. Herbal medicines that confer antiplatelet effects or affect the liver's CYP3 A4 enzymes, including fish oil, evening primrose, garlic, cranberry juice, vitamin E, echinacea, ginseng, St. John's wort, gingko biloba, ginger, kava, and saw palmetto.

20. **What is Osler-Weber-Rendu syndrome/hereditary hemorrhagic telangiectasia (HHT)?**
HHT is an autosomal dominant disorder characterized by vascular malformations that does not manifest at birth but rather as one ages. Diagnostic criteria include spontaneous/recurrent epistaxis, mucocutaneous and fingertip telangiectasias, visceral involvement (e.g., hepatic, pulmonary, cerebral, or gastrointestinal arteriovenous malformations), and an affected first-degree relative (known as Curacao criteria). Diagnosis is confirmed if three or more criteria are met. Generally, epistaxis is the first manifestation of the disease. Epistaxis management includes utilization of topical emollients, topical cautery, or packing in acute events and laser photocoagulation or coblation of lesions, septodermoplasty, or nasal closure in extreme cases. Newer experimental therapies, including antiangiogenic medications and sclerotherapy, are being investigated.

21. **A patient presents with epistaxis from a nasal mucosal ulcer. What is the differential diagnosis? Describe the workup.**
Nasal cavity ulcerations should be treated conservatively and worked up if they do not spontaneously resolve or when suspicion for underlying disorder is present (pain, numbness, smoking history, irregularities on exam).

Epistaxis may be the first sign of malignancy, autoimmune disease, or rare infectious disorders like syphilis, leprosy, and tuberculosis.

Nasal biopsies should always be performed when malignancy or autoimmune disorder is suspected. Recent studies suggest that biopsies to rule out autoimmune disease are not mandatory in the absence of any nasal or systematic signs of vasculitis and with negative c-ANCA and ACE test results.

CONTROVERSIES

22. **What is the recommended medical management for a patient with epistaxis currently on anticoagulation therapy for cardiac disease?**
    1. Obtain a complete blood count including platelets for all patients and PT/INR if taking warfarin.
    2. If the patient has a metal heart valve, INR dictates warfarin administration (if supratherapeutic, hold until INR is therapeutic; if INR is therapeutic, continue current regimen).
    3. If life-threatening bleeding occurs in a patient with a metal heart valve, care planning should be discussed with the cardiologist prior to discontinuing aspirin if a coronary stent is in place, as platelet transfusions may be utilized.
    4. For all other patients (without a metal heart valve), aspirin or clopidogrel should be continued, but if a life-threatening bleed occurs, the utility of platelet transfusion should also be discussed with the cardiologist.

23. **What is the role of antibiotic prophylaxis with nasal packing?**
    Toxic shock syndrome is an extremely rare complication occurring in 0.002% to 0.032% of nasal and sinus surgery cases; appropriate studies on antibiotic prophylaxis are lacking. Although controversial, antibiotic administration with nasal packing is commonly performed. If used, the antibiotic chosen should have staphylococcal coverage (e.g., amoxicillin-clavulanate).

24. **What is the link between hypertension and epistaxis?**
    Several case series demonstrate a relationship between hypertension and epistaxis, although population-based studies have not confirmed this relationship. Even if not a causative factor, elevated blood pressure may be associated with patient anxiety surrounding epistaxis and intervention and may slow the resolution. The best approach is to offer reassurance and treat the hypertension whenever possible.

BIBLIOGRAPHY

Dedhia RC, Desai SS, Smith KJ, et al: Cost-effectiveness of endoscopic sphenopalatine artery ligation versus nasal packing as first-line treatment for posterior epistaxis, *Int Forum Allergy Rhinol* 7:563–566, 2013.

Kuhn D, Hospowsky C, Both M, et al: Manifestation of granulomatosis with polyangiitis in head and neck, *Clin Exp Rheumatol* 2:78–84, 2018.

Kuhnel T, Wirsching K, Wohlgemuth W, et al: Hereditary hemorrhagic telangiectasia, *Otolaryngol Clin North Am* 51:237–254, 2018.

Lange JL, Peeden EH, Stringer SP: Are prophylactic systemic antibiotics necessary with nasal packing? A systematic review, *Am J Rhinol Allergy* 31:240–247, 2017.

Lopez F, Triantafyllou A, Snyderman CH, et al: Nasal juvenile angiofibroma: current perspectives with emphasis on management, *Head Neck* 39:1033–1045, 2017.

Min HJ, Kang H, Choi GJ, et al: Association between hypertension and epistaxis: systematic review and meta-analysis, *Otolaryngol Head Neck Surg* 157:921–927, 2017.

Sylvester MJ, Chung SY, Guinand LA, et al: Arterial ligation versus embolization in epistaxis management: counterintuitive national trends, *Laryngoscope* 127:1017–1020, 2017.

Tunkel DE, Anne S, Payne SC, et al: Clinical practice guideline: nosebleed (epistaxis), *Otolaryngol Head Neck Surg* 162:S1–S38, 2020. Available at uptodate.com.

CHAPTER 25

RHINITIS, IMMUNOTHERAPY, AND BIOLOGICS

Anjeli Prabhu Kalra, MD and Lorelei Bourla, MD, MS

KEY POINTS

1. Allergic rhinitis can present with seasonal or perennial symptoms.
2. Beta 2- transferrin present on nasal discharge indicates cerebrospinal fluid (CSF) leak.
3. Rhinitis medicamentosa is associated with the use of over-the-counter intranasal decongestants that contain α-adrenergic compounds for more than 3 to 5 days.
4. Allergen immunotherapy is the only disease-modifying treatment available for allergic rhinitis.

Pearls
1. There is a strong overlap of asthma and allergic nasal disease in patients.
2. Smoking and work exposures can trigger nonallergic rhinitis.
3. Surgery is reserved for refractory cases of rhinitis that have failed medical management.
4. Skin testing is rarely associated with anaphylaxis and is a relative contraindication in pregnant patients.

QUESTIONS

1. **What is rhinitis?**
   Rhinitis is inflammation of the nasal passages resulting in one of the following: nasal congestion, rhinorrhea, sneezing or nasal pruritus. It affects both children and adults and is categorized as allergic or non-allergic. Rhinitis may be inflammatory, non-inflammatory or structural in nature.

2. **What are the causes of inflammatory rhinitis?**
   Inflammatory rhinitis may be allergic, drug-induced, infectious or irritant. Allergic rhinitis affects 10-30% of adults and 40% of children in the United States. Causes of allergic rhinitis are commonly pollens (trees, grasses and weeds), animal dander, dust mites, cockroaches and molds. Skin prick testing in these patients is typically positive, although an entity called local allergic rhinitis may also be present in which allergen specific IgE is only present in the nasal mucosa. This condition may occur in up to 25% of patients with rhinitis and can be confirmed through a nasal allergen provocation challenge. Nonsteroidal anti-inflammatory drugs (NSAIDs) and aspirin can induce an acute inflammatory reaction involving the nasal mucosa in patients with aspirin exacerbated respiratory disease (AERD) along with symptoms of acute asthma. Infectious rhinitis is most commonly due to viral upper respiratory tract infections. However, in patients who are immunocompromised, fungal infections should be considered. Patients who are susceptible to infectious rhinitis include those with anatomic abnormalities, ciliary dysfunction, chronic rhinosinusitis with nasal polyps, cystic fibrosis, primary immunodeficiency and children. Irritant rhinitis can occur due to exposure to an airborne irritant such as solvents, chemicals, fumes, construction materials and workplace irritants (occupational rhinitis).

3. **What are the causes of non-inflammatory rhinitis?**
   There are a variety of causes of non-inflammatory rhinitis, including vasomotor rhinitis, gustatory rhinitis, medication-induced rhinitis, NARES, atrophic rhinitis and rhinitis of pregnancy. Vasomotor rhinitis is triggered by cold air, temperature changes, exercise, strong odors and/or airborne irritants. Gustatory rhinitis involves clear rhinorrhea following ingestion of spicy or hot foods. Rhinitis medicamentosa is characterized by severe rebound nasal congestion caused by chronic or frequent use of intranasal decongestants. Other medications such as NSAIDs, alpha antagonists, oral contraceptives and antihypertensive agents can also cause non-inflammatory rhinitis. Non-allergic rhinitis with eosinophilia (NARES) is a condition characterized by high eosinophil numbers on nasal smear. Atrophic rhinitis may occur in some patients due to multiple sinus or nasal surgeries, systemic disease or infection. Finally, rhinitis of pregnancy is a common cause of non-inflammatory rhinitis due to hormonal changes.

4. **What are causes of structural rhinitis?**
In patients who report their primary complaint as nasal obstruction, causes such as septal deviation, turbinate or adenoid hypertrophy, nasal polyposis, sinonasal tumors, and foreign bodies should be considered. Foreign bodies are most common in younger patients. The likelihood of nasal polyps increases if the patient complains of a lack of sense of smell and sensitivity to aspirin or other NSAIDs. For patients who report primarily rhinorrhea, CSF leak should be considered, and history should be obtained regarding sinus surgery and head trauma. CSF leaks tend to be unilateral and can be diagnosed by measurement of beta2-transferrin in the nasal discharge, as this should be present in CSF only.

5. **What are the treatment options for rhinitis?**
Topical corticosteroids remain the mainstay of rhinitis therapy. Patients with chronic rhinitis, both allergic and non-allergic, may benefit from topical antihistamine nasal sprays, such as azelastine and olopatadine. First-generation antihistamines are discouraged for treatment of rhinitis. In addition, leukotriene receptor antagonist therapies (LTRAs) are also not recommended as initial treatment of chronic rhinitis. Use of intranasal decongestants should be limited due to concern for rhinitis medicamentosa. Intranasal cromolyn can be offered as a therapy for patients with allergic rhinitis and should be taken prior to allergen exposure. For vasomotor and gustatory rhinitis, Ipratropium nasal sprays can be useful.

6. **What are the surgical options for rhinitis?**
I would not change this section but would like to get Dr. Ramakrishnan's opinion on updates here.

7. **What is allergen immunotherapy?**
Subcutaneous allergen immunotherapy (aka "allergy shots") is the act of giving small and incrementally increasing doses of an allergen to which a patient is sensitized with the aim of desensitization. Allergen immunotherapy is used in patients with clinical symptoms consistent with allergic rhinitis, allergic conjunctivitis, allergic asthma, and venom (hymenoptera) allergy.

8. **Who first described allergen immunotherapy?**
Leonard Noon and John Freeman in 1911.

9. **How does allergen immunotherapy work?**
There are data to support multiple mechanisms including the development of regulatory B and T cells that act to suppress allergen-specific lymphocytes, downregulation of mast cells and basophils, resulting in suppression of allergic responses, an increase in allergen-specific IgG4 level (deemed the "blocking antibody"), and an increase followed by a subsequent decrease in allergen-specific IgE.

10. **What are the indications for allergen immunotherapy?**
Allergen immunotherapy can be considered in patients with specific IgE antibodies, usually proven through skin prick testing to clinically relevant allergens, such as pollens and animal dander. Suboptimal control of nasal, ocular, or respiratory symptoms with standard medications, severity of symptoms, and patient preferences should all be considered before starting allergen immunotherapy.

11. **How is allergen immunotherapy administered?**
Clinically, allergen immunotherapy is most often administered through a subcutaneous or sublingual route. Subcutaneous allergen immunotherapy may be administered using different protocols that vary in how quickly a patient can reach a maintenance dose.

12. **How is subcutaneous allergen immunotherapy designed?**
Allergen immunotherapy is dependent on findings obtained from skin prick testing and is therefore patient-dependent and individualized. Mixes are typically made in 5 or 10 mL vials and care must be taken when placing certain allergens together. Molds and cockroach allergens tend to be proteolytic and will degrade other extracts, such as pollens.

13. **Which allergens can be administered by standardized sublingual therapy?**
There are currently four sublingual immunotherapy (SLIT) tablets that are FDA approved in the United States. Grastek is a timothy grass tablet, Oralair is a five-grass mixture tablet, Ragwitek is a ragweed tablet, and Odactra is a house dust mite tablet. Sublingual immunotherapy via liquid formulation ("allergy drops") is not currently approved by the FDA.

14. **How long should a patient be treated with allergen immunotherapy?**
Patients should be treated with allergen immunotherapy for at least 3 to 5 years. The decision to discontinue allergen immunotherapy should be a joint decision between the patient and the physician.

15. **What are the other benefits of allergen immunotherapy?**
   In addition to improvement in both allergic rhinitis and allergic conjunctivitis symptoms, allergen immunotherapy may help to prevent asthma and further sensitize children to other allergens.

16. **Who is not a candidate for subcutaneous immunotherapy?**
   Patients receiving beta blockers are at an increased risk of a severe systemic reaction when concurrently receiving subcutaneous immunotherapy. Patients with severe, suboptimally controlled asthma are also poor candidates because of the risk of anaphylaxis with pulmonary involvement. Allergen immunotherapy should not be initiated in pregnant patients. However, if allergen immunotherapy has already been initiated, the dose received can be continued throughout pregnancy. Dose escalation is avoided during pregnancy because of the risk of anaphylaxis.

17. **What are biologic therapies?**
   Biologic therapies can be used to describe any product that can be obtained from a living organism. In allergy, these therapies are often monoclonal antibodies designed to bind specific molecules in the body, but they may also be vaccines, tissues, blood or blood components, proteins, or even cells.

18. **Which biologic therapies can be used in the treatment of nasal polyps and chronic sinusitis?**
   Dupilumab (Dupixent) is a monoclonal antibody against the IL-4 receptor, which is FDA-approved for use in chronic sinusitis with nasal polyps (CRSwNP), as well as for use in atopic dermatitis and asthma. Mepolizumab (Nucala) and Benralizumab (Fasenra) are both monoclonal antibodies directed against IL-5 and have shown benefit in patients with CRSwNP. Mepolizumab is FDA approved for the treatment of CRSwNP. Omalizumab (Xolair) is a monoclonal antibody against IgE and is also approved to treat CRSwNP.

19. **How does dupilumab work?**
   Dupilumab is a monoclonal IgG antibody that binds the IL-4 receptor alpha subunit, which is shared between the I-L4 and IL-13 receptor complexes, thereby blocking signaling through both IL-4 and IL-13. This mechanism blocks the release of inflammatory cytokines, chemokines, and IgE.

20. **How do Mepolizumab and Benralizumab work?**
   Mepolizumab is a monoclonal antibody against IL-5. By binding to IL-5, Mepolizumab prevents this interleukin from binding to its receptor. Benralizumab binds to the alpha-chain of the IL-5 receptor, thereby preventing IL-5 from binding. Both medications lead to decreased eosinophils, since IL-5 is critical for eosinophil development and survival.

21. **How does omalizumab work?**
   Omalizumab is a monoclonal antibody against IgE and an allergic antibody. By binding free IgE, omalizumab prevents it from binding to the high-affinity IgE receptor on mast cells and basophils and prevents signaling to release allergic mediators. Omalizumab results in lower free IgE levels and lower numbers of high-affinity IgE receptors.

BIBLIOGRAPHY

Blaser K, Akdis CA: Interleukin-10, T regulatory cells and specific allergy treatment, *Clin Exp Allergy* 34:328–331, 2004.
Chhabra N, Houser SM: Surgical options for the allergic rhinitis patient, *Curr Opin Otolaryngol Head Neck Surg* 20:199–204, 2012.
Corren J, Baroody FM, Pawankar R: Allergic and nonallergic rhinitis. In: *Middleton's Allergy: Principles and Practice*, 664–685.
Cox L, Nelson H, Lockey R: Allergen immunotherapy: a practice parameter third update, *J Allergy Clin Immunol* 127:S1–S55, 2011.
Creticos PS, Van Metre TE, Mardiney MR, Rosenberg GL, Norman PS, Adkinson NJ Jr: Dose response of IgE and IgG antibodies during ragweed immunotherapy, *J Allergy Clin Immunol* 73:94–104, 1984.
Daigle BJ, Rekkerth DJ: Practical recommendations for mixing allergy immunotherapy extracts, *Allergy Rhinol* 6:e1–e7, 2015.
Durham SR, Varney VA, Gaga M, et al: Grass pollen immunotherapy decreases the number of mast cells in the skin, *Clin Exp Allergy* 29:1490, 1999.
Eifan AO, Durham SR: Pathogenesis of rhinitis, *Clin Exp Allergy* 46:1365–2222, 2016.
Hoyt AEW, Borish L, Gurrola J, Payne S: Allergic fungal rhinosinusitis, *J Allergy Clin Immunol Pract* 4:599–604, 2016.
Nelson HS: Injection immunotherapy for inhalant allergens. In: *Middleton's Allergy: Principles and Practice*, 2014, pp. 1416–1437.
Penagos M, Eifan AO, Durham SR, Scadding GW: Duration of allergen immunotherapy for long-term efficacy in allergic rhinoconjunctivitis, *Curr Treat Options Allergy* 5:275–290, 2018.
Rhinitis 2020: A practice parameter update
Tsetsos N, Goudakos JK, Daskalakis D, Donstantinidis I, Markou K: Monoclonal antibodies for the treatment of chronic rhinosinusitis with nasal polyposis: a systematic review, *Rhinology* 56:11–21, 2018.
van de Veen W, Stanic B, Yaman G, et al: IgG4 production is confined to human IL-10 producing regulatory B cells that suppress antigen-specific immune responses, *J Allergy Clin Immunol* 131:1204–1212, 2013.
Wilson DR, Irani AM, Walker SM, et al: Grass pollen immunotherapy inhibits seasonal increases in basophils and eosinophils in the nasal epithelium, *Clin Exp Allergy* 31:1705, 2001.

CHAPTER 26

ACUTE RHINOSINUSITIS AND INFECTIOUS COMPLICATIONS

Daniel M. Beswick, MD and Jeffrey Chain, MD

KEY POINTS

1. Antibiotics are frequently administered to treat acute rhinosinusitis. Guidelines for appropriate antibiotic use should be followed.
2. Infectious complications of rhinosinusitis extending beyond the paranasal sinuses are rare. These include orbital, intracranial, and, less commonly osseous complications.
3. Acute invasive fungal sinusitis must be suspected in immunocompromised patients with acute, rapidly progressive disease and must be managed expeditiously.

Pearls
1. Acute rhinosinusitis is more commonly viral than bacterial, especially within the first 10 days of symptoms.
2. The Chandler classification for orbital extension of rhinosinusitis is used to categorize infections: I, preseptal cellulitis; II, orbital cellulitis; III, subperiosteal abscess; IV, orbital abscess; and V, cavernous sinus thrombosis.
3. Acute intracranial complications of the frontal lobe may result from the spread of infection through the venous channels directly communicating with the frontal sinus.

QUESTIONS

1. **How is acute rhinosinusitis (ARS) defined?**
   ARS is a symptomatic inflammation of the nasal cavity and paranasal sinuses for up to 4 weeks. The most common causes of this condition are viral and bacterial infections, with viral etiologies predominating in the first 10 days. Symptoms include nasal congestion, postnasal drainage, facial pain/pressure, decreased olfaction, sore throat, hoarseness, cough, and/or fever. Recurrent acute rhinosinusitis (RARS) is defined as four or more episodes of acute bacterial rhinosinusitis (ABRS) annually; all episodes must meet the criteria for ABRS.

2. **What is the pathophysiology of ARS?**
   Inflammation of the nasal and paranasal sinus mucosa with subsequent edema is an initiating factor in this disease. Most often this inflammation is caused by viral infections and/or allergic rhinitis. This edema can cause obstruction of normal sinus drainage, impaired mucociliary clearance, and altered local immune system function. These changes create an ideal environment for pathogen colonization and growth.

3. **How common is rhinosinusitis (RS)?**
   RS is a major burden on the health care system, with 12% to 15% of adults diagnosed with acute or chronic rhinosinusitis annually in the United States. ARS is the fifth leading indication for antibiotic prescriptions and is responsible for over 5 million ambulatory visits each year in the United States.

4. **How common are infectious complications of ARS?**
   Infectious complications of ARS are rare in immunocompetent individuals, with a rate of less than 0.01% per episode of ARS in children and even less in adults. Orbital complications are more common in children, and in immunocompromised patients (diabetes mellitus, human immunodeficiency virus, immunosuppression due to chemotherapy) the complication rate is likely higher.

5. **How can the clinician differentiate acute viral rhinosinusitis (AVRS) from ABRS?**
   Identifying the presence of ABRS is important for providing appropriate therapy. The main determination is based on the time course of the symptoms. Symptoms of RS that are present for <10 days are more commonly due to viral etiologies. Symptoms that are present for longer or symptoms that initially improved and then worsened are more likely to be bacterial. Symptoms associated with ABRS include purulent nasal discharge and unilateral, localized facial pain.

6. **What bacteria are the most common pathogens in ABRS?**
   Understanding the bacteriology of ARS is paramount for choosing the most effective antibiotic regimen to treat the disease. *Streptococcus pneumoniae, Haemophilus influenzae,* and *Moraxella catarrhalis* (more common in children) are generally accepted as the most common pathogens in this disease. *Streptococcus pyogenes, Staphylococcus aureus,* gram-negative bacilli, and anaerobes are less common.

7. **What is the relevance of antibiotic resistant organisms in ABRS?**
   H. influenzae (30%) and *M. catarrhalis* (90%) have a high prevalence of beta-lactamase-producing organisms. The prevalence of *S. pneumoniae* seems to be decreasing due to pneumococcal vaccination. However, its resistance to penicillin and macrolides is approximately 30%. Knowledge of regional antibiotic resistance is important for guiding therapy.

8. **What are the goals of treatment of ABRS?**
   In treating ABRS, the clinician's primary goals are to decrease the duration and severity of symptoms, prevent infectious complications, prevent progression to chronic rhinosinusitis (CRS), and restore the patient's quality of life. Secondary goals include minimizing the side effects of medications and unnecessary antibiotics that could promote resistant organisms.

9. **When should antibiotics be prescribed for ABRS?**
   Studies in both adult and pediatric patients confirm that patients with ABRS treated with antibiotics experience more rapid resolution of symptoms when compared with placebo; however, initially withholding antibiotics and providing close follow-up is an option in cases of suspected uncomplicated ABRS. Some studies cite a 60% to 70% chance of spontaneous improvement in patients with ABRS by 7 to 12 days, which supports the "watchful waiting" approach.

10. **Which antibiotic should be prescribed for ABRS?**
    In both children and adults amoxicillin or amoxicillin-clavulanate is recommended as an initial empiric antimicrobial therapy. The preference for amoxicillin-clavulanate is due to the increasing prevalence of beta-lactamase-producing *H. influenzae* and *M. catarrhalis* since the use of pneumococcal vaccines. Second-line antibiotics for those who failed amoxicillin/amoxicillin/clavulanate include trimethoprim-sulfamethoxazole (TMP-SMX), doxycycline, and respiratory fluoroquinolones (levofloxacin or moxifloxacin). TMP-SMX has 30% to 40% resistance to both *S. pneumoniae* and *H. influenzae.* Doxycycline can be used only in adults due to risk of dental discoloration in children younger than 8 years of age. Fluoroquinolones also carry risks, especially in children.

11. **How long should antibiotics be prescribed and when should empiric antibiotics be changed if ineffective?**
    The optimal duration of antibiotic treatment remains controversial. Guidelines recommend empiric antibiotics for 5 to 10 days in adults (termed "short-term" antibiotics) and 10 to 14 days in children with uncomplicated ABRS. Other studies performed in ABRS require patients to complete a 2-week course of antibiotics. If symptoms worsen after 48 to 72 hours or fail to improve after 3 to 7 days, patients should be evaluated for resistant pathogens or a noninfectious etiology.

12. **What other treatments, in addition to antibiotics, should be considered in ARS?**
    Nasal saline irrigation and intranasal corticosteroids are usually recommended as adjuvant treatments for ARS. Topical or oral decongestants, antihistamines, and mucolytics are also commonly considered. Some type of analgesia, usually initially in the form of acetaminophen and ibuprofen, should also be considered.

13. **Which tests can be performed to help diagnose ABRS?**
    The diagnosis of ABRS is based on history and is centered on the patient's symptoms. Computed tomography (CT) is not routinely performed for uncomplicated ABRS. Studies indicate that during uncomplicated viral upper respiratory infections, the majority of patients will have significant abnormalities seen on imaging. Endoscopically guided cultures can help confirm the diagnosis of ABRS; however, this is not routinely required.

14. **When is testing appropriate in patients with ABRS?**
    CT or MRI should be performed if suppurative complications are suspected and can be considered in cases of RARS. CT is generally the preferred initial modality and is superior for defining the bony anatomy of the paranasal sinuses. Contrast should be used if the intraorbital or intracranial extent of the disease is suspected. MRI with gadolinium is recommended if the clinician suspects central nervous system complications. Endoscopic culture of the middle meatus can be helpful in these situations to guide antibiotic therapy. An allergy/immunology evaluation can be considered in patients with RARS if supported by history to identify concurrent predisposing factors causing mucosal inflammation.

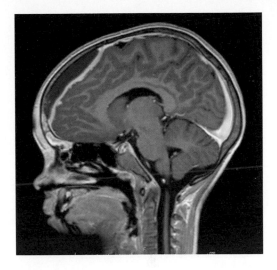

Fig. 26.1 Large epidural abscess in MRI in 7-year-old with frontal sinusitis.

15. **What are the suppurative complications of ABRS?**

Sequelae of ABRS can be divided into intraorbital, intracranial, and osseous complications. The most common complication is orbital involvement. Intracranial complications are the next most common (Fig. 26.1), although they are still quite rare. Osseous complications such as osteomyelitis of the frontal bone (Pott's puffy tumor) are rare.

16. **How are orbital complications of ABRS classified?**

The Chandler classification is used to classify the orbital complications of ABRS. Stage 1, *preseptal cellulitis,* is caused by infection anterior to the orbital septum and is thought to be due to impaired venous outflow from sinusitis and edema. Stage II, *orbital cellulitis,* occurs with infectious spread posterior to the orbital septum and causes impaired extraocular movements, proptosis, and chemosis. Stage III, *subperiosteal abscess,* is defined by the accumulation of purulence in the extracellular space between the lamina papyracea and the medial periorbita (Fig. 26.2). Visual acuity can be impaired. Stage IV, *orbital abscess,* involves abscess formation in the intraconal space and is usually accompanied by severe visual impairment and complete ophthalmoplegia. Stage V, *cavernous sinus thrombosis,* which can also be considered an intracranial complication, is characterized by bilateral ocular symptoms among other central nervous system signs and symptoms. Cavernous sinus thrombosis is confirmed radiologically by the absence of venous flow on the MR venogram. Progression between Chandler classes does not necessarily occur in a stepwise manner.

17. **Is surgery required for subperiosteal orbital abscesses in children?**

Generally, it is reasonable to trial medical management for small medially located subperiosteal abscesses without a decrease in visual acuity or systemic involvement. These patients require ophthalmologic evaluation and close monitoring. Surgery is indicated if there is failure to improve within 24 to 48 hours, decreasing visual acuity, and/ or progressive systemic involvement. Generally, drainage of the abscess and endoscopic sinus surgery for source control is the surgery of choice.

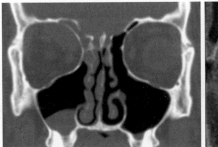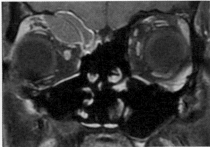

Fig. 26.2 Right subperiosteal abscess of the orbit. Note the sinus disease in the right frontal sinus.

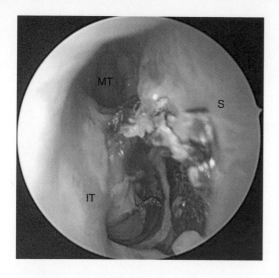

Fig. 26.3 Rigid nasal endoscopy of the right nasal cavity in a patient with invasive fungal sinusitis. MT, middle turbinate; IT, inferior turbinate; S, septum.

18. What are the intracranial complications of ABRS?

These include meningitis, cerebritis, epidural or subdural abscess, brain abscess, superior sagittal and cavernous thrombosis, and, more rarely, oculomotor or abducens palsy. Patients may present with nonspecific signs, such as fever or headache, and commonly have neck stiffness, nausea/vomiting, or altered mental status.

19. How are intracranial complications of ABRS managed?

Management of these complicated problems generally requires collaboration between a neurosurgeon and an infectious disease specialist. Broad-spectrum antibiotics with adequate penetration through the blood-brain barrier are required. Lumbar puncture may be useful if not contraindicated; usually, the sinuses that harbor the infection require endoscopic surgical drainage. In addition, surgery may be required to drain intracranial abscesses. For patients with thrombosis, anticoagulation remains controversial and should be considered on a case-by-case basis. Frequently, these patients require intensive care unit monitoring.

20. What is the role of fungus in acute rhinosinusitis?

Allergic fungal rhinosinusitis occurs when atopic patients inhale fungus, causing type I IgE-mediated hypersensitivity and mucosal inflammation. Diagnosis is made based on the Bent and Kuhn criteria in patients with nasal polyposis, type I hypersensitivity, characteristic CT findings, eosinophilic mucus without fungal invasion, and positive fungal stain. *Fungus ball* or *mycetoma* is a noninvasive fungal infection usually occurring in nonatopic immunocompetent patients. These are usually chronic processes.

Invasive fungal sinusitis (IFS) occurs in immunocompromised patients and involves fungal invasion of blood vessels and bony/soft tissue erosion. This process most commonly presents in an acute manner but can also take a chronic or granulomatous form. Treatment for IFS must be implement quickly and involves antifungal therapy (often with input from infectious disease specialists), surgical debridement, and reversal of the underlying etiology of immunosuppression (Fig. 26.3).

BIBLIOGRAPHY

Chow AW, Benninger MS, Brook I, et al: IDSA clinical practice guideline for acute bacterial rhinosinusitis in children and adults, *Clin Infect Dis* 54(8):e72–e112, 2012.

Coenraad S, Buwalda J: Surgical or medical management of subperiosteal orbital abscess in children: a critical appraisal of the literature, *Rhinology* 47(1):18–23, 2009.

Fokkens WJ, Lund VJ, Mullol J, et al: European position paper on rhinosinusitis and nasal polyps 2012, *Rhinology* 50(S23):1–298, 2012.

Meltzer EO, Hamilos DL, Hadley JA, et al: Rhinosinusitis: developing guidance for clinical trials, *Otolaryngol Head Neck Surg* 135(5): S31–S80, 2006.

Orlandi RR, Kingdom TT, Hwang PH, et al: International consensus statement on allergy and rhinology: rhinosinusitis, *Int Forum Allergy Rhinol* 6(Suppl 1):S22–209, 2016.

Rosenfeld RM, Piccirillo JF, Chandrasekar SS, et al: Clinical practice guidelines (update): adult sinusitis, *Otolaryngol Head Neck Surg* 152(2 Suppl):S1–S39, 2015.

Rosenfeld RM, Singer M, Jones S: Systematic review of antimicrobial therapy in patients with acute rhinosinusitis, *Otolaryngol Head Neck Surg* 137(3):S32–S45, 2007.

Sinus and Allergy Health Partnership: Antimicrobial treatment guidelines for acute bacterial rhinosinusitis, *Otolaryngol Head Neck Surg* 130(1):S1–S45, 2004.

Wald ER, Applegate KE, Bordley C, et al: Clinical practice guideline for the diagnosis and management of acute bacterial sinusitis in children aged 1 to 18 years, *Pediatrics* 132(1):e262–e280, 2013.

CHAPTER 27

CHRONIC RHINOSINUSITIS

Conner J. Massey, MD and Todd T. Kingdom, MD

KEY POINTS

1. Chronic rhinosinusitis (CRS) in both adults and children is defined based on specific guidelines including both subjective and objective criteria.
2. CRS is a multifactorial inflammatory process characterized by a dysfunctional host–environment interaction.
3. Medical management of CRS involves nasal saline irrigation, topical anti-inflammatory agents, oral antibiotics, and systemic corticosteroids.
4. Patients with CRS who fail to respond to appropriate medical therapy may be candidates for endoscopic sinus surgery, which has been shown to significantly improve symptom-related quality of life.

Pearls
1. There is an important association between the presence of asthma, CRS, airway inflammation, and nasal polyposis, especially in the case of aspirin-exacerbated respiratory disease (AERD).
2. The importance of bacteria (and all microbes) in the etiology of CRS and the role of antibiotics in its management remain to be defined.
3. Surgery in patients who have failed medical therapy has an important role in the management of CRS.

QUESTIONS

1. **Define chronic rhinosinusitis (CRS).**
   CRS is chronic inflammation of the mucosal lining of the paranasal sinuses that persists for at least 12 weeks. Clinically, rhinosinusitis is defined by clinical symptoms (subjective) plus characteristic endoscopic and/or CT changes (objective). CRS is generally further categorized as with nasal polyps (CRSwNP) or without nasal polyps (CRSsNP).

2. **What are the symptoms associated with CRS in adults and children?**
   The most common symptoms include nasal congestion or blockage, nasal discharge (either anterior or posterior), facial pain and pressure, and hyposmia. Other symptoms that may be associated are cough, headache, throat discomfort, laryngeal irritation, hoarseness, halitosis, ear pressure, dental pain, and malaise. In general, the same symptoms are seen with acute and chronic rhinosinusitis, but the symptom pattern and chronicity are different.

3. **What are the endoscopic and CT findings that are typical with CRS?**
   Endoscopic signs may include nasal polyps (Fig. 27.1), mucopurulent discharge (primarily from the middle meatus) (Fig. 27.2), and/or mucosal edema (also primarily in the middle meatus). CT findings include mucosal thickening of the paranasal sinuses and ostiomeatal complex, and fluid or debris in the paranasal sinuses (opacification) (Fig. 27.3).

4. **How is CRS diagnosed in adults?**
   The diagnosis requires both subjective and objective findings (Table 27.1).

5. **How is CRS diagnosed in children?**
   The diagnostic criteria in children are very similar to those in adults, however, cough is accepted as a symptom of CRS in the pediatric population. In addition, CT scans are ordered less frequently due to concern for unnecessary radiation exposure (Table 27.2).

6. **How common is CRS?**
   Based on a National Health Interview Survey, about 13% of the U.S. population reports that they suffer from "sinusitis." However, an analysis of the 2007 Medical Expenditure Panel Survey of 225 million Americans demonstrated the prevalence of physician-diagnosed CRS to be 4.9%. Many patients have symptoms they attribute to

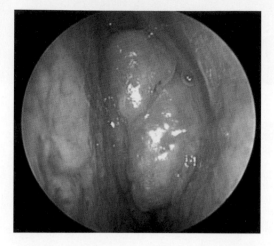

Fig. 27.1 Nasal endoscopy, left nasal cavity. Nasal polyps arising from middle meatus.

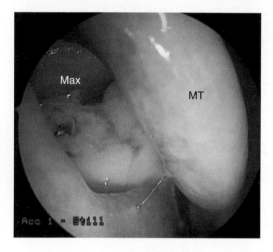

Fig. 27.2 Nasal endoscopy, right nasal cavity showing purulent secretions pooling in right maxillary sinus. *MT* = middle turbinate, *Max* = maxillary sinus.

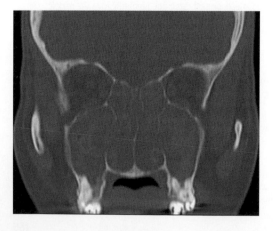

Fig. 27.3 Coronal noncontrast CT scan showing opacification of all paranasal sinuses.

Table 27.1 Diagnosis of CRS in Adults

Subjective

Sinonasal inflammation persisting for ≥12 weeks with at least two or more of the following symptoms:

Nasal blockage/congestion/obstruction
Nasal discharge (anterior/posterior)
Facial pain/pressure
Reduction/loss of sense of smell

Objective: Confirmation of diagnosis

Evidence of inflammation on paranasal sinus examination or CT
Evidence of purulence emanating from the paranasal sinuses or ostiomeatal complex
CRS is divided into CRSwNP or CRSsNP based on the presence or absence of polyps

Source: Table is derived from the International Consensus Statement on Allergy and Rhinology: Rhinosinusitis (ICAR:RS), International Forum of Allergy and Rhinology, 2016.

Table 27.2 Diagnosis of CRS in Children

Subjective	
≥12 weeks of two or more symptoms:	
Either	• Nasal blockage/obstruction/congestion *OR* • Anterior nasal discharge/posterior nasal drip
+/−	Facial pain/pressure
+/−	Cough
Objective	
Either endoscopic signs and/or CT changes	
Endoscopic signs	• Nasal polyps • Mucopurulent discharge • Mucosal edema
CT changes	• Obstruction of the ostiomeatal complex • Mucosal thickening or opacification of the paranasal sinuses

Source: Table derived from the European Position Paper on Rhinosinusitis, Rhinology, 2012.

CRS, which in actuality may be due to other causes – most commonly allergic rhinitis and chronic headaches or other facial pain syndromes.

7. **Describe the pathophysiology of CRS.**

The cause of CRS continues to be a topic of much research and debate; however, in general it is a multifactorial process characterized by a dysfunctional local host–environment interaction that leads to persistent mucosal inflammation. In general, the pathophysiology between CRSsNP and CRSwNP is thought to differ; the former is thought to be governed by a Th1-driven response, whereas the latter is characterized as mainly Th2-driven, although more heterogeneous. Possible contributing factors include abnormal host production of pro- and anti-inflammatory cytokines (as is seen with nasal polyps), eosinophilic tissue infiltration, defects in the sinonasal epithelial mechanical barrier or immune response, aberrant ciliary function, allergies, and asthma. Genetic factors may also be important and include primary immunodeficiencies and cystic fibrosis. The role of microbes in the development of CRS remains unclear, but it is accepted that bacteria contribute to initiation or propagation of the inflammatory response in some way. The makeup of the bacterial community (microbiome), biofilm production, presence of intracellular or intramucosal bacteria, and staphylococcal superantigens have all been implicated in CRS.

Perhaps the two most important potential triggers underlying sinusitis are upper respiratory viral infection and upper airway inflammation from other causes. These factors may include allergy (atopy), environmental hypersensitivities, mucociliary dysfunction (primary and acquired), anatomic relationships (e.g., frontal sinus outflow obstruction), immunodeficiencies, and fungal hypersensitivities. In general, the result of this inflammatory process is mucosal edema, the end stage of which is polyposis. Similar to acute sinusitis, this may lead to obstruction of the drainage routes of the sinuses, causing stasis of secretions and an overall physiologic change within the sinus cavity.

8. **Which sinus is most often involved in CRS?**

The anterior ethmoid sinuses are the most commonly affected in CRS, followed by maxillary, posterior ethmoid, sphenoid, and frontal sinuses. CRS from odontogenic causes typically manifests first in the maxillary sinuses, while primarily allergy-driven CRS occurs in the central compartment (middle and superior turbinates, superior nasal septum).

9. **Which inflammatory pathways are characteristic of CRS?**

There are multiple inflammatory markers that are characteristic of CRS. In general, CRSwNP and CRSsNP have distinct inflammatory pathways; however, both show an increase in pro-inflammatory leukotrienes and a decrease in anti-inflammatory prostaglandins. CRSwNP is characterized by an increase in serum and tissue eosinophils and the Th2-mediated pathway (including IL-4, IL-5, and IL-13), while CRSsNP is characterized by a predominance of Th1-mediated pathway, fibrosis, and high levels of TGF-β. Those patients with asthma have increased tissue eosinophilia and predominance of Th2-mediated inflammation similar to those with CRSwNP. It appears, however, that eosinophilic inflammation is important in most forms of CRS.

10. **Which bacterial organisms are associated with CRS?**

The same organisms found in acute disease are also prevalent in CRS, but coagulase-negative *Staphylococcus* species, *S. aureus*, *Pseudomonas aeruginosa*, gram-negative rods, and anaerobes are more frequently associated with CRS. Generally speaking, gram-negative rods and *Staphylococcus* species are important pathogens in CRS. It is important to note that while culture-based diagnostic methods remain the clinical standard today, they may detect only a small proportion of resident sinonasal bacteria.

11. **What is the relationship between allergy and CRS?**

Atopy and allergic rhinitis lead to the elaboration of multiple early- and late-phase inflammatory mediators, many of which are also active in CRS. Theoretically, active allergies can contribute to nasal inflammation and therefore could be a disease modifier in CRS; however, this has been extensively studied and only approximately half of the studies have observed an association between the two. Therefore, the role of allergy in CRS remains controversial. In general, when patients with allergy symptoms are well managed, this may theoretically reduce triggering effects on CRS.

12. **How does fungus play a role in CRS?**

The role of fungus in CRS continues to be an area of active research. *Allergic fungal rhinosinusitis* (AFRS) and *fungus ball* (mycetoma) represent two subsets of CRS in which fungus plays a clear role. Both are found in immunocompetent patients, in contrast to acute invasive fungal sinusitis.

Diagnostic criteria of AFRS include nasal polyposis, CT with evidence of hyperdense sinus infiltrates, eosinophilic mucin, and noninvasive fungal identification by culture or histopathology. These patients tend to have significant polyp burden, and over a prolonged period of time the thick, eosinophilic mucin can exert expansile mass effect into nearby structures, including the orbit and cranium. Treatment is with a combination of medical and surgical therapy. Neither systemic nor topical antifungal therapy has definitively been shown to improve treatment outcomes in this population.

A fungus ball (mycetoma) is a collection of inspissated fungal debris and mucus in an isolated paranasal sinus. Symptoms are similar to CRS or patients can occasionally be asymptomatic. The maxillary and sphenoid sinuses are the most common location. Characteristic CT appearance is a heterogeneous hyperdensity with microcalcifications. Intraoperatively, fungal balls appearing as a mass of thick, crumbly debris and fungal hyphae are often appreciable. Treatment is endoscopic removal. Antifungal medications are not typically required.

13. **What is the association of asthma with CRS?**

As the upper and lower airways (nose and bronchi) are connected anatomically and both are lined by pseudostratified respiratory epithelia, they are often affected by similar disease processes. This is seen specifically in CRS and asthma. Asthma is present in up to 50% of patients with CRSsNP; this figure rises to 80% in the setting of CRSwNP. In general, management of CRS improves asthma symptoms and vice versa. This linkage has led to the "unified airway" theory that conceptually considers the entire respiratory airway as a single functional unit.

14. **What is aspirin-exacerbated respiratory disease (AERD)?**

Previously known as Samter's triad, aspirin-exacerbated respiratory disease (AERD) is a subset of CRS characterized by nasal polyps, aspirin sensitivity, asthma, and eosinophilic inflammation. These findings are present in approximately 10% to 25% of patients with CRSwNP and 25% to 40% of patients with CRSwNP and comorbid asthma. Patients with AERD are thought to have a dysfunction in the arachidonic acid metabolism pathway, with a resultant increase in pro-inflammatory leukotrienes and a decrease in anti-inflammatory prostaglandins in both serum and respiratory mucosa. Bronchospasm, mucosal edema, and an influx of eosinophils result upon exposure to aspirin or nonsteroidal anti-inflammatory medications. These patients also tend to have more severe polyposis than others with CRSwNP. In addition to standard treatment for CRSwNP, aspirin desensitization may be necessary and is more effective when initiated in the weeks following sinus surgery.

15. **What is cystic fibrosis and how is it associated with CRS?**
    Cystic fibrosis (CF) is an autosomal recessive genetic disorder resulting from mutation of the cystic fibrosis transmembrane regulator gene (CFTR). A defective chloride channel results in thick secretions and impaired mucociliary function. Manifestations include chronic pulmonary disease, pancreatic insufficiency, and CRS (with or without NPs). CF patients often have severe sinus disease requiring multiple surgeries and aggressive medical therapy. Exacerbations of lung and sinus disease are often concurrent. Treatment of sinus exacerbation (including surgery) can improve lung symptoms. CRS can be the presenting symptom in some patients who are heterozygous for a CFTR mutation.

16. **How does the management of CRS differ from the management of acute bacterial rhinosinusitis (ABRS)?**
    The medical management of CRS differs from ABRS in that (1) the role of chronic inflammation is greater, (2) the bacterial pathogens may differ, and (3) the duration of therapy is typically longer. In addition, surgical management is a consideration in cases of CRS refractory to medical treatment.

17. **Discuss the role of anti-inflammatory agents in the treatment of CRS.**
    The majority of medical management of chronic rhinosinusitis is directed at controlling the inflammatory component of the disease and is often more important than antimicrobial treatment. Key treatment options include nasal saline rinses, prolonged intranasal steroids, systemic steroids, leukotriene modifiers, asthma management, and immunotherapy for allergic disease. Recently, there has been tremendous interest in biologic agents for patients with recalcitrant CRSwNP and asthma. These drugs, the first of which (dupilumab) was FDA-approved for CRSwNP in 2019, target specific immune cells or certain components of proinflammatory pathways. The length and type of anti-inflammatory therapy will depend on clinical symptoms and objective findings, stage of disease, and suspected underlying triggers.

18. **Describe the role of antimicrobial treatment in CRS.**
    There is a paucity of high-level evidence either supporting or refuting the role of oral antibiotics in CRS. Short-term (<3 weeks) antibiotics are a mainstay of treatment in acute exacerbations of CRS, but durations of more than 3 weeks are generally needed for clinical efficacy in managing baseline CRS disease. Limited data have shown effectiveness with macrolide antibiotics in patients with CRS (with or without NPs), although long-term benefit has not been assessed. Long-term nonmacrolide antibiotics (e.g., doxycycline) have been studied even less and are not routinely recommended. Frequent and prolonged use of antibiotics in the management of CRS may result in significant harm to the patient, including *Clostridium difficile* colitis, allergic reactions/anaphylaxis, and selection for drug-resistant organisms. Topical and intravenous antibiotics should not be routinely used. There is no role for antifungal therapy in CRS.

19. **What is the role of surgical intervention in CRS?**
    Medical management of CRS remains the primary treatment modality and is effective in the majority of patients. However, endoscopic sinus surgery (ESS) is a key therapeutic component and an important consideration in the comprehensive management of CRS. ESS is indicated for disease that is unresponsive to appropriate medical management of at least 3 to 4 weeks' duration. The goal of surgery is to facilitate the natural drainage of the sinuses, eradicate pathogenic bacteria, and remove nasal polyps or other mucosal disease. Generally speaking, surgery is not a cure for CRS but an adjunctive treatment option for select patients. Systematic reviews and meta-analyses have demonstrated significant improvements in symptom-related quality of life and endoscopic scores for patients who undergo surgery compared with those who opt for continued medical therapy.

BIBLIOGRAPHY

Bachert C, Han JK, Desrosiers M, et al: Efficacy and safety of dupilumab in patients with severe chronic rhinosinusitis with nasal polyps (LIBERTY NP SINUS-24 and LIBERTY NP SINUS-52): results from two multicentre, randomised, double-blind, placebo-controlled, parallel-group phase 3 trials, *Lancet* 394(10209):1638–1650, 2019.

Fokkens WJ, Lund VJ, Mullol J, et al: European position paper on rhinosinusitis and nasal polyps 2012, *Rhinol Suppl* 23:1–298, 2012.

Giklick RE, Metson R: The health impact of chronic sinusitis in patients seeking otolaryngologic care, *Otolaryngol Head Neck Surg* 113(1):104–109, 1995.

Kim JK, Kountakis SE: The prevalence of Samter's triad in patients undergoing functional endoscopic sinus surgery, *Ear Nose Throat J* 86(7):396–399, 2007.

Nicolai P, Lombardi D, Tomenzoli D, et al: Fungus ball of the paranasal sinuses: experience in 160 patients treated with endoscopic surgery, *Laryngoscope* 119(11):2275–2279, 2009.

Orlandi RR, Kingdom TT, Hwang PH, et al: International consensus statement on allergy and rhinology: rhinosinusitis, *Int Forum Allergy Rhinol* 1:S22–S209, 2016.

Rosenfeld RM, Piccirillo JF, Chandrasekhar SS, et al: Clinical practice guideline (update): adult sinusitis, *Otolaryngol Head Neck Surg* 152(2 Suppl):S1–S39, 2015.

Sacks PL, Harvey RJ, Rimmer J, et al: Antifungal therapy in the treatment of chronic rhinosinusitis: a meta-analysis, *Am J Rhinol Allergy* 26(2):141–147, 2012.

Smith TL, Kern RC, Palmer JN, et al: Medical therapy vs surgery for chronic rhinosinusitis: a prospective, multi-institutional study, *Int Forum Allergy Rhinol* 1(4):235–241, 2011.

Smith TL, Kern RC, Palmer JN, et al: Medical therapy vs surgery for chronic rhinosinusitis: a prospective, multi-institutional study with 1-year follow up, *Int Forum Allergy Rhinol* 3:4–9, 2013.

Soler ZM, Wittenberg E, Schlosser RJ, et al: Health state utility values in patients undergoing endoscopic sinus surgery, *Laryngoscope* 121:2672–2678, 2011.

Soler ZM, Oyer SL, Kern RC, et al: Antimicrobials and chronic rhinosinusitis with or without polyposis in adults: an evidence-based review with recommendations, *Int Forum Allergy Rhinol* 3(1):31–47, 2013.

Tan BK, Chandra RK, Pollak J, et al: Incidence and associated premorbid diagnoses of patients with chronic rhinosinusitis, *J Allergy Clin Immunol* 131(5):1350–1360, 2013.

Wilson KF, McMains C, Orlandi RR: The association between allergy and chronic rhinosinusitis with and without nasal polyps: an evidence-based review with recommendations, *Int Forum Allergy Rhinol* 4:93–103, 2014.

CHAPTER 28

SEPTOPLASTY AND TURBINATE SURGERY

Daniel M Beswick, MD and Vijay R. Ramakrishnan, MD

KEY POINTS

1. The various approaches to septoplasty include endonasal (Killian, hemitransfixion, transfixion incisions), open, endoscopic, and endoscopic-assisted. Many techniques exist for performing inferior turbinate reduction. Surgery on nondiseased middle turbinates is not commonly performed.
2. During septoplasty, care should be taken to leave at least a 1.5-centimeter strut of dorsal and caudal septal cartilage during resection to avoid loss of nasal tip support and saddle nose deformity.
3. During septoplasty, repairing rents or tears in the mucosal flaps and replacing the previously excised cartilage into the mucoperichondrial pocket can help to decrease the risk of septal perforation postoperatively.
4. An untreated septal hematoma may lead to septal perforation and saddle nose deformity and requires prompt management.
5. Medications used during nasal surgery are potentially dangerous if used improperly. Safe use of these medications requires familiarity with their pharmacology and dosing and knowledge of how to manage complications.

Pearls

1. The three major nasal tip support mechanisms include the size and shape of the lower lateral cartilage, attachment of the medial crura to the septum, and attachment of the upper and lower lateral cartilages. The minor tip support mechanisms include the interdomal ligament, dorsal septum, membranous septum, sesamoid complex, skin and subcutaneous tissue of the nasal tip, and maxillary spine.
2. The primary blood supply to the inferior turbinate is from a branch of the posterior lateral nasal artery, which originates from the sphenopalatine artery, a branch of the external carotid circuit.
3. How is the nose anomalous in a patient with unilateral cleft lip/palate? The ipsilateral lower lateral cartilage is displaced inferiorly, posteriorly, and laterally. The nasal tip, caudal septum, and columella are displaced toward the non-cleft side. The bony septum is deviated toward the cleft side.
4. The nasal cycle refers to the cyclic nature of blood flow and expansion of erectile tissue within the inferior turbinate and anterior septum. Related to an underlying autonomic process, blood flow increases on one side of the nasal cavity relative to the other side. This occurs imperceptibly for most individuals, although some patients will experience alternating nasal congestion related to this phenomenon.
5. During nasal surgery, medication is injected intranasally. Almost immediately, the patient becomes severely hypertensive and tachycardic. It is discovered that oxymetazoline was accidentally injected instead of a local anesthetic. What is the next step? Intravascular injection of oxymetazoline causes stimulation of alpha-1 receptors, resulting in vasoconstriction, hypertension, and tachycardia. Initial treatment should include administration of an alpha blocker, such as phentolamine, followed by other resuscitative therapies.
6. Toxic shock syndrome is a rare complication of *Staphylococcus aureus* infection characterized by high fever, rash, hypotension, vomiting, diarrhea, and multiorgan failure. Treatment consists of removal of the nasal packing, IV antibiotics, and supportive/resuscitative care.

QUESTIONS

1. **What is the clinical presentation of a patient with a deviated nasal septum and when should surgical correction be considered?**
   Nasal septal deviations can be congenital, developmental, or secondary to nasal trauma. Approximately 50% of the general population are thought to have some deviation in their nasal septum, and up to one third of individuals will seek medical care for nasal obstruction. Patients will often present with nasal congestion and can also present with nasal drainage, decreased sense of smell, and impaired sleep. If the deviation is severe, it can impinge on the turbinates, lateral nasal wall, and middle meatus and can predispose patients to recurrent and/or chronic

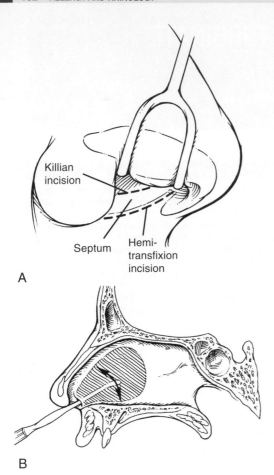

A

B

Fig. 28.1 A, B. Various approaches to the nasal septum when performing a septoplasty. (From Cummings C, Flint P, Harker L: *Cummings Otolaryngology Head & Neck Surgery*, 4th ed, St. Louis, 2005, Mosby, pp. 1001–1027.)

rhinosinusitis. Medical therapy in the form of intranasal steroids is the first-line treatment. If this fails, surgical correction should be considered in appropriate patients with chronic symptoms that are significantly affecting their quality of life.

2. **What are the various approaches to the nasal septum when performing a septoplasty?**
   Typically, a septoplasty is performed through an endonasal approach. A unilateral incision is made just beyond the mucocutaneous junction, known as a Killian incision, or more anterior at the mucocutaneous junction, known as a hemitransfixion incision. The latter type of incision allows better access to the caudal septum compared with a Killian incision and allows for elevation of bilateral mucoperichondrial flaps if needed. A full transfixion incision is one that is made at the mucocutaneous junction on one side and is extended through to the contralateral mucocutaneous junction. Again, this type of incision allows for access to the caudal septum, columella, and medial crura. The hemi- and full transfixion incisions can cause disruption of the septo-columellar ligamentous tissue and can theoretically lead to loss of nasal tip support. Finally, complete access to the entire septum can be achieved via a degloving, or external rhinoplasty, approach if more advanced maneuvers are required for addressing abnormalities of the dorsal and/or caudal septum (Fig. 28.1).

3. **What is an endoscopic septoplasty?**
   Most otolaryngologists perform a septoplasty using a headlight and direct vision for visualization of the surgical field. Many otolaryngologists are now using the endoscope for enhanced visualization. Outcomes are similar between approaches and choice of approach is best left to surgeon discretion in individual cases. Advantages of the endoscopic approach include magnification of the surgical field, improved access and visualization of the

posterior nasal cavity, and the potential for more limited dissection in specific cases. Disadvantages include a potential inability to adequately address severe deviations of the anterior and caudal septum. Since the endoscope is often used through incisions that are traditionally used for headlight visualization, a more accurate term for this procedure may be endoscopic-assisted septoplasty.

4. **What are the steps for performing a typical septoplasty?**
   1. Decongest nasal cavities with topical oxymetazoline spray. Inject lidocaine mixed with epinephrine into the septum bilaterally in a subperichondrial plane.
   2. Make an incision near the caudal septum. Elevate flap in the subperichondrial plane using broad, sweeping movements with the elevator. The elevation is carried posteriorly as required.
   3. Disarticulate septal cartilage from the bony septum and resect portions of bony septum as required.
   4. Resect deviated portions of septal cartilage as required, taking care to leave dorsal and caudal struts with a width of at least 1.5 centimeters for proper support of the nasal tip and dorsum.
   5. Repair any tears in the mucosal flaps primarily with dissolvable suture, if possible.
   6. If opposing tears exist, consider replacing excised cartilage into the mucoperichondrial pocket to decrease the risk of septal perforation, taking care not to cause further obstruction of the nasal cavity by doing so. Also consider documenting the precise amount of cartilage excised or remaining in the operative note, in case revision surgery is ever needed.
   7. The mucosal incision is then closed with absorbable suture. At this point, the septum can be quilted with absorbable suture and/or splints can be placed.

5. **What are the possible risks involved with septoplasty?**
   Risks include infection, bleeding, nasal dryness/crusting, persistent nasal congestion after surgery, septal hematoma/abscess, septal perforation, scarring, alteration of sense of smell/taste, numbness, CSF leak (rare), cosmetic deformity, complications of anesthesia, and need for further surgery.

6. **What is the anatomy of the inferior turbinate?**
   The inferior concha is its own bone and attaches to the medial maxilla. The medial submucosal tissue is composed mostly of venous channels and erectile tissue, whereas the lateral submucosal tissue is mostly glandular. Hasner's valve, which marks the opening of the nasolacrimal duct inferiorly, opens into the inferior meatus lateral to the inferior turbinate.

7. **What are the topical medications typically used during septoplasty/turbinate surgery?**
   Topical oxymetazoline and topical epinephrine are medications that are commonly used during nasal and septal surgery. These medications work as alpha-1 receptor agonists, causing vasoconstriction and decongestion of the nasal mucosa, resulting in decreased systemic absorption of local anesthetics, improved visualization and working space, and hemostasis. Topical cocaine is less commonly used nowadays but is a very effective decongestant and anesthetic. These medications can be applied preoperatively and/or intraoperatively as needed. Care should be taken to only use these medications topically. Intravascular administration can cause immediate and life-threatening hypertension, tachycardia, and arrhythmias and could lead to myocardial infarction or stroke.

8. **Which anesthetics are used during septoplasty/turbinate surgery? Can surgery be performed under local anesthesia?**
   Currently, most nasal surgery is performed under general anesthesia, although some surgeons prefer local anesthesia. During surgery, a local anesthetic mixed with dilute epinephrine is injected into the submucosal septum/turbinates. This results in hydrodissection of the injected plane, assisting with ease of surgical dissection and improved hemostasis as a result of vasoconstriction caused by the dilute epinephrine and helps with analgesia in the immediate postoperative period.

9. **Which techniques help with hemostasis during and after septoplasty/turbinate surgery?**
   Hemostasis is important during nasal surgery to ensure proper visualization, which allows for a more thorough and complete procedure. Topical decongestants and vasoconstrictors are applied immediately prior to surgery and/or during surgery as noted above. Local anesthetics mixed with dilute epinephrine are injected into the septum and turbinates, resulting in further vasoconstriction. The patient is positioned with the head elevated 20 to 30 degrees, decreasing venous congestion. Careful surgical technique with minimization of mucosal trauma is a must. Finally, dissolvable or nondissolvable nasal packing can be placed in the nasal cavities at the end of the procedure, but these have not been shown to significantly reduce rates of postoperative bleeding.

10. **What is the clinical presentation of a patient with inferior turbinate hypertrophy and when should surgery be considered?**
    Patients with inferior turbinate hypertrophy usually present with chronic complaints of nasal congestion and can also have symptoms of nasal drainage, facial pressure, ear fullness, and sleep impairment. A history of allergic rhinitis is common. The congestion is often described as bilateral, alternating from side to side, worse during

sleep in a supine position, and improved in the upright position, with exposure to steam (e.g., in the shower), with exercise, and with use of decongestants. Physical examination should be used to rule out septal abnormalities. Turbinate surgery should be considered when symptoms related to turbinate hypertrophy are adversely affecting quality of life despite medical treatments.

11. **How is inferior turbinate reduction surgery performed?**
Once the appropriate candidate is identified, surgery can be performed under local or general anesthesia. The surgery is often performed in conjunction with a septoplasty and is usually directed toward the inferior turbinates. The goal of surgery is to reduce the size of the turbinate, thereby improving the cross-sectional area inside the nasal cavity, without sacrificing function. There are a wide variety of techniques for turbinate reduction, and this is best accomplished by a submucous resection of soft tissue and/or bone, thereby preserving the overlying functional mucosa. Some of the various techniques that have been described include submucosal resection, (full/partial) turbinate resection, laser cautery, electrocautery (monopolar or bipolar), cryotherapy, coblation, radiofrequency ablation, and lateral outfracture.

12. **What is empty nose syndrome?**
Also called ozena or chronic atrophic rhinitis, empty nose syndrome is an uncommon condition in which the patient experiences chronic symptoms of nasal congestion despite a widely patent nasal airway. Additional symptoms can include dryness, crusting, bleeding, drainage, and pain. There is a significant association with depression. Typically, patients have a history of prior nasal surgery with turbinate resection. It is thought that the severe distortion of intranasal anatomy results in altered sensation of normal airflow, thereby resulting in a subjective sensation of congestion. Treatment options are limited and include nasal saline, topical ointments, and antibiotics when indicated. Surgical augmentation of the inferolateral nasal wall has been utilized in refractory cases. The best strategy is avoidance of this complication with careful preoperative planning and proper surgical technique.

13. **When is middle turbinate surgery indicated?**
The middle turbinate derives from the ethmoid bone and facilitates humidification, airflow, and sinus drainage. Unlike the inferior turbinates, middle turbinates do not commonly develop mucosal or submucosal hypertrophy and do not fluctuate as much in size with changes in blood flow. In some cases, the middle turbinate can have a concha bullosa, which is an air-filled cell of thin bone, causing it to be much larger than normal. This can contribute to symptoms of nasal obstruction and deviation of the septum and may obstruct the ostiomeatal complex, resulting in chronic rhinosinusitis. In cases of severe nasal polyps, the middle turbinate can develop polypoid degeneration. In these cases, excision of a concha bullosa or partial resection of the middle turbinate can be considered.

14. **What is the nasal valve?**
The nasal valve refers to the narrowest area in the anterior nasal cavity through which air flows. Abnormalities of the nasal valve result in symptoms of nasal obstruction. The valve has both internal and external components. The internal nasal valve refers to the area of the nasal cavity bounded by the septum, head of the inferior turbinate, and upper lateral cartilage. The external nasal valve refers to the area bounded by the columella, lateral crus of the lower lateral cartilage, and nasal ala.

15. **How is the nasal valve evaluated?**
When evaluating a patient with symptoms of nasal congestion, the external nose and nasal valve should be examined along with the intranasal anatomy. The nasal dorsum, nasal sidewalls, nasal tip, nasal alae, and columella are examined from an anterior view, profile view, and base view at rest and during inspiration. The Cottle maneuver is performed by displacing the cheek laterally. The modified Cottle maneuver is performed by supporting the lateral nasal wall intranasally with a cotton tipped applicator or ear curette during inspiration. In patients with abnormalities of the nasal valve, these maneuvers will result in improvement in nasal breathing. Abnormalities of the nasal valve are important to detect preoperatively, as they can cause persistent symptoms of nasal obstruction after septoplasty/turbinate surgery and require different management strategies.

16. **What is nasal valve collapse?**
Nasal valve collapse refers to nasal obstruction caused by an abnormality of the nasal valve. This can be congenital or acquired from prior surgery, trauma, or, more rarely, facial paralysis. Symptoms of congestion are usually constant, improve with the use of adhesive nasal strips placed over the dorsum or lateral displacement of the cheeks, and worsen with exercise. Nasal valve collapse can be either static or dynamic depending on the patient's anatomy.

17. **How is nasal valve collapse treated?**
Nonsurgical treatment options include use of adhesive nasal strips or disposable intranasal stent devices. There are a wide variety of surgical treatment options that can be employed for specific anatomic issues. These include placement of spreader grafts, flaring sutures, butterfly grafts, batten grafts, lateral crural strut grafts, alar rim

grafts, and bone-anchored suture techniques, among others. Surgery can be performed via a closed or open approach. Cartilage grafts are harvested from the septum, ear, or rib.

18. **What is the clinical presentation and treatment for a septal hematoma/abscess?**
A septal hematoma may occur as a result of recent nasal surgery or nasal trauma. Symptoms include acute onset of severe nasal congestion, pain, swelling, and possibly fever. Examination shows fluctuance of the septum that may occlude the nasal cavity. Treatment is immediate incision and drainage of the fluid collection under local or general anesthesia and usually antibiotics. Delay in treatment could result in necrosis of septal cartilage, septal perforation, and subsequent saddle nose deformity.

19. **What is the clinical presentation and treatment of a septal perforation?**
Septal perforations can cause symptoms including a whistling sound with respiration, dryness, crusting, bleeding, pain, congestion, and drainage or may be asymptomatic. The differential includes prior surgery, trauma, drug use (nasal sprays, recreational), vasculitis, atypical infection, granulomatous disease, or malignancy. On examination, the size and location of the perforation should be noted. Nonsurgical treatment options include nasal saline and topical ointment. Surgical treatment options include placement of a silastic septal button or surgical repair. Perforations of 5 millimeters or less can often be repaired primarily with placement of an interposition graft via an endonasal approach. For perforations of 5 millimeters to 2 centimeters, an open approach should be considered, and local mucosal flaps will be needed. Perforations of greater than 2 centimeters are more difficult to successfully repair. Surgical repair is contraindicated in patients actively abusing cocaine or with active infectious, inflammatory, or malignant disease.

20. **What is the clinical presentation and treatment of saddle nose deformity?**
Patients with saddle nose deformity present with a depression or concavity involving the nasal dorsum. This is typically caused by prior nasal trauma or overly aggressive nasal surgery during dorsal hump reduction or from overresection of the dorsal septal strut during septoplasty. Some patients with nasal manifestations of vasculitis will also develop this deformity. After treatment of any underlying disease process, surgical correction is performed using an open approach for exposure of the nasal dorsum. The deficient area is then augmented with either conchal (ear) or rib cartilage.

21. **What is toxic shock syndrome?**
Toxic shock syndrome is a rare complication of *S. aureus* infection. The TSST-1 toxin produced by the bacteria causes high fever, rash, hypotension, vomiting, diarrhea, and multiorgan failure. This has rarely been associated with nonabsorbable nasal packing. Patients with nasal packing or splints are typically covered with antistaphylococcal antibiotics, such as a first-generation cephalosporin. Treatment includes removal of the nasal packing, IV antibiotics, and supportive/resuscitative care for shock.

22. **What are some limitations to the endonasal approach for septoplasty?**
The endonasal approach to septoplasty refers to making a Killian or hemitransfixion incision to access the septal cartilage and bone. This approach allows limited access to and manipulation of the dorsal septum, septal angle, caudal septum, and nasal spine. Deviation from the midline in these areas is a common cause for failure of primary septoplasty. If deviation is noted in one or more of these areas, an open approach to the septum should be considered for adequate exposure. Deviation of the dorsal septum and septal angle can be corrected by conservative shaving and (extended) spreader grafts. A deviation of the posterior septal angle can be corrected by conservative shaving and/or repositioning of the cartilage on the nasal spine. A deviation in the caudal septum can be corrected with a septal batten graft, repositioning, tongue-in-groove technique, caudal septal extension graft, or other modifications.

23. **Is nasal surgery safe to perform in children?**
The nasal septum is important in development of the pediatric nose into the adult nose. Therefore, with few exceptions, septoplasty is usually not performed until at least 16 years of age when the development of the nasal structures is typically complete. Turbinate surgery can be safely performed in young children if needed but should be done conservatively to minimize the risk of long-term complications.

CONTROVERSIES

24. **What is Sluder's neuralgia?**
This is an antiquated term now referred to as sphenopalatine ganglion neuralgia or contact point headache. Symptoms include midfacial pain that is typically unilateral and localized. Decongestants sometimes provide symptom relief, while other medications typically do not. Examination and CT scan may show a deviated septum impinging into a turbinate and/or lateral nasal wall with no significant sinus disease. The pain may be exacerbated by manipulation of the septal deviation and relieved with application of topical anesthetic. Some consider this to be a structural problem and recommend septoplasty for treatment, while others consider this to be a neurologic condition requiring medical treatment. Optimal management remains controversial.

25. **Should the middle turbinate be preserved at all costs during nasal/sinus surgery?**
Consensus opinion on resection of the middle turbinate has evolved. In specific cases, some argue that it is beneficial to resect the middle turbinate, such as a large middle turbinate concha bullosa and severe polypoid degeneration. Advantages to resection include improved access to the sinuses postoperatively for surveillance, instrumentation, and penetration of topical irrigations. Recent studies have shown no major differences in outcomes between patients with and without middle turbinate resections. Most clinicians would argue against routine resection of the nondiseased middle turbinate during sinus and nasal surgery.

26. **Is the placement of nasal splints necessary after nasal surgery?**
Traditionally, splints have been placed as dressing/packing in the nasal cavities after nasal surgery, especially septoplasty. This serves to eliminate dead space between the mucosal flaps, minimize risk of septal hematoma, enhance healing of the mucosa, and prevent synechiae formation between the septum and lateral structures. When aggressive maneuvers have been performed to correct a severe deviation, splints can also serve to stabilize the remaining septal cartilage. The splints are usually removed about 1 week after surgery. The placement of splints can result in discomfort after surgery and potentially be a source of infection. Studies have shown that patients who did not have splints placed after septal surgery had similar success and complication rates compared with those who had splints placed, suggesting that splints may not be necessary at all.

BIBLIOGRAPHY

Ballert J, Park S: Functional rhinoplasty: treatment of the dysfunctional nasal sidewall, *Facial Plast Surg* 22:49–54, 2006.
Cummings C, Flint P, Harker L: *Cummings Otolaryngology Head & Neck Surgery*, 4th ed, 2005, Elsevier Mosby, pp. 1001–1027.
Kennedy D, Hwang P: *Rhinology Diseases of the Nose, Sinuses, and Skull Base*, 2012, Thieme Medical Publishers.
Kridel R: Considerations in the etiology, treatment, and repair of septal perforations, *Facial Plast Surg Clin North Am* 12:435–450, 2004.
Lee KJ: *Essential Otolaryngology Head & Neck Surgery*, 8th ed, McGraw-Hill, 2003.
Orlandi RR, Kingdom TT, Hwang PH, et al: International consensus statement on allergy and rhinology: rhinosinusitis, *Int Forum Allergy Rhinol* 6(Suppl 1):S22–S209, 2016.
Passali F, Passali G, Damiani V, et al: Treatment of inferior turbinate hypertrophy: a randomized clinical trial, *Ann Otol Rhinol Laryngol* 112:683–688, 2003.
Soler Z, Hwang P, Mace J, et al: Outcomes after middle turbinate resection: revisiting a controversial topic, *Laryngoscope* 120(4):832–837, 2010.

CHAPTER 29

FUNCTIONAL ENDOSCOPIC SINUS SURGERY

Henry P. Barham, MD and Anne E. Getz, MD

KEY POINTS

1. The goals of sinus surgery include atraumatic surgical technique, mucosal preservation, and restoration of normal sinus physiology.
2. The most common major complications of sinus surgery include hemorrhage, intracranial injury/cerebrospinal fluid (CSF) leak, and intraorbital injury.
3. Measures used to help improve visualization and decrease blood loss during sinus surgery include total intravenous anesthesia (TIVA), head of bed elevation >15 degrees, topical alpha-1 blockers (epinephrine or oxymetazoline), and local infiltration of epinephrine.

Pearls
1. Know the Keros classification of olfactory fossa depth (Class I: 1 to 3 millimeters, Class II: 4 to 7 millimeters, Class III: 8 millimeters and greater).
2. The most common complication of sinus surgery is hemorrhage.

QUESTIONS

1. **What is FESS?**

   Functional endoscopic sinus surgery. The goal of "functional" endoscopic sinus surgery is to correct underlying anatomic abnormalities or obstructions while preserving mucosa in order to restore mucociliary flow and normal sinus function. The term functional is directly related to techniques used to preserve the natural drainage pathway. The field of rhinology has undergone great advances in recent years with advances in endoscopic technology, instrumentation, image guidance, and understanding of the anatomy and pathophysiology of rhinosinusitis.

2. **What is the role of surgical intervention in rhinosinusitis?**

   Medical management is the primary, and often only, treatment modality in the majority of patients. When medical therapy fails to control symptoms adequately, surgery may be indicated. In cases of chronic or recurrent rhinosinusitis, surgical intervention should be directed at improving the natural drainage pathways of the sinuses and facilitating delivery of topical therapies such as saline rinses and topical steroid sprays. In cases of acute rhinosinusitis, surgical intervention is directed at decompression of the acutely infected sinus associated with possible complications, such as abscess formation.

3. **What measures should be taken prior to surgical intervention for the treatment of rhinosinusitis?**

   A detailed history and physical examination should be performed on any patient to help determine which patients would sufficiently benefit from surgical intervention. Nasal endoscopy should be performed preoperatively to evaluate the specific nasal anatomy along with assessment of the nasal mucosa. Fine-cut computed tomography (CT) is an important objective measure performed to identify a patient's specific anatomy used in preparation for sinus surgery. Imaging should ideally be studied in triplane (axial, coronal, and sagittal) orientation. As with any surgery, all preoperative medications (including over-the-counter medications) should be discussed with each patient to identify any medications that can increase the risk of bleeding.

4. **What are the main goals of functional endoscopic sinus surgery?**
   1. Thorough anatomic dissection of the paranasal sinuses to restore the normal drainage pathways. This dissection should be complete and apply mucosal-sparing techniques.
   2. Avoidance of complications. The paranasal sinuses reside in close proximity to critical structures including the orbit, skull base, carotid artery, and optic nerve.

5. **What are the most common causes of nasal airway obstruction and how are they addressed surgically?**
   Deviated nasal septum and inferior turbinate hypertrophy are two of the most common causes of nasal airway obstruction that can be surgically corrected. Septoplasty is a procedure performed to straighten the deviated septum. Reduction and outfracture of the obstructing inferior turbinates are commonly performed to improve the nasal airway.

6. **How should one proceed through dissection of the paranasal sinuses?**
   Based on its anterior location, the maxillary sinus is often addressed first. Osteomeatal complex obstruction is addressed by performing a maxillary antrostomy. The natural ostium of the maxillary sinus is exposed by removing the uncinate process. The natural ostium is enlarged (this ostium is enlarged to include accessory ostia when present). The anterior ethmoid cells are then addressed by opening the ethmoid bulla and proceeding anterior to posterior. The basal lamella of the middle turbinate is identified, which is the anatomic division between the anterior and posterior ethmoid sinuses. Dissection is then carried posteriorly until the anterior face (rostrum) of the sphenoid sinus is encountered, marking the posterior limit of the posterior ethmoid sinus in the absence of an Onodi cell (posterior ethmoid cell pneumatizing superiorly to the sphenoid sinus). Medially, the superior turbinate can be used to identify the sphenoid ostium in the sphenoethmoidal recess. If necessary, the inferior third of the superior turbinate may be removed to expose the sphenoid ostium. The sphenoid ostium is enlarged with care to avoid injury to the skull base superiorly and septal artery (medial terminal branch of the sphenopalatine artery) inferiorly. The remaining ethmoid partitions are dissected in a posterior to anterior direction from the anterior face of the sphenoid sinus along the ethmoid skull base superiorly with the limits of dissection including the lamina papyracea laterally, middle turbinate medially, and frontal recess anteriorly.

7. **How should one surgically address the frontal sinus?**
   Endoscopic frontal sinusotomy has become the standard approach to treating rhinosinusitis involving the frontal recess and sinus. While commonly considered the most difficult sinus to address surgically because of the anterior and superior location, surrounding anatomy, and associated risks, endoscopic surgery of the frontal sinus has become increasingly safe and successful. The successive approaches used to improve drainage of the frontal sinus include anterior ethmoidectomy, complete dissection of all anterior ethmoid and frontal cells within the frontal recess (also known as the Draf I procedure), widely opening the frontal ostium (Draf IIa), resection of the floor of the frontal sinus from the nasal septum medially to the lamina papyracea laterally (also known as the Draf IIb procedure), and connection of the two frontal sinuses from orbit to orbit with removal of each frontal sinus floor, inferior portion of the frontal intersinus septum, and superior part of the nasal septum (also known as the Draf III procedure, modified Lothrop, or transseptal frontal sinusotomy). External or open approaches may be used in select cases including a trephine, Lynch incision, or bicoronal approach with osteoplastic flap, which can be used for tumor removal, cranialization, or obliteration procedures. Open approaches are now rarely used for inflammatory disease.

8. **What is maxillary sinus "recirculation?"**
   Failure to incorporate the true maxillary ostium with the surgical antrostomy can result in two separate openings. This is a setup for recirculation of mucus from the natural ostium to the surgical ostium resulting in dysfunction and stasis of secretions.

9. **What are the four lamellae that serve as anatomic landmarks to complete a sinus surgery?**
   - First lamella: uncinate process
   - Second lamella: ethmoid bulla
   - Third lamella: basal lamella of the middle turbinate (horizontal component of the middle turbinate; this represents the anatomic division between anterior and posterior ethmoid air cells)
   - Fourth lamella: superior turbinate

10. **What are common minor complications of sinus surgery? How can they be avoided?**
    Bleeding, hyposmia, numbness, nasal obstruction, and adhesions. It is normal to have small amounts of bleeding after sinus surgery, which rarely (less than 1%) require intervention. Preoperative evaluation and discussion of all medications (prescription, over-the-counter, and supplements) known to cause increased bleeding and strict adherence to the principles of hemostasis can help minimize the bleeding risk. Hyposmia can occur, and although this is generally considered a minor complication, it can be quite distressing to the patient. Avoiding overdissection of the superior aspects of the middle and superior turbinates and mucosal stripping within the olfactory cleft can help prevent this. Infection, allergy, and the presence of nasal polyps can lead to impaired sense of smell postoperatively. Numbness of the nose, upper lip, or central upper teeth can occur postoperatively but is usually self-limited. Nasal obstruction and pain are common self-limited minor complications. Postoperative crusting and adhesions may occur in both the nasal cavity and paranasal sinuses, which should be debrided during early postoperative visits to prevent mature scar formation. This complication can be mitigated by performance of frequent postoperative saline irrigations by the patient and endoscopic evaluation and debridement by the surgeon.

11. **What are the major complications of sinus surgery?**

Orbital injury, intracranial injury, anosmia (see discussion of hyposmia above), and hemorrhage. The lamina papyracea separating the ethmoid sinuses from the orbit is one of the thinnest bones in the human body. Transgression of this bone or bleeding into the bony orbit can cause complications ranging from periorbital ecchymosis and emphysema to orbital hematoma and blindness. Anisocoria, ophthalmoplegia, and proptosis are ominous signs demanding prompt action. In cases of increased orbital pressure, steroids, mannitol, and/or orbital decompression via lateral canthotomy and cantholysis or endoscopic decompression should be performed immediately to relieve the pressure and preserve vision. Damage to the extraocular muscles, most commonly the medial rectus, can occur, leading to permanent diplopia. Overly aggressive anterior dissection of the maxillary antrostomy can result in injury to the nasolacrimal system, with resultant epiphora or recurrent dacryocystitis

The bone separating the paranasal sinus from the intracranial cavity is also very thin. Injury most commonly occurs at the cribriform plate and roof of the ethmoid sinus where the bone is thinnest. Intracranial complications include CSF leak, meningitis, vascular injury, tension pneumocephalus, and direct brain injury. Intracranial entry should be identified immediately and repaired. Injury to the ethmoidal, sphenopalatine, or internal carotid arteries (ICAs) can result in major hemorrhage. Direct endoscopic repair of an ICA injury is technically difficult given the high-flow bleeding and difficult visualization. Management typically involves aggressive packing to tamponade the hemorrhage and transfer to interventional radiology for possible embolization. Injury to the anterior ethmoidal arteries along the skull base can result in intracranial hemorrhage as well as intraorbital hematoma and resultant vision loss.

12. **What are the indications for image-guided sinus surgery?**

Image-guided surgery is a computerized navigation system that tracks surgical instruments in space using a patient's preoperative CT (or magnetic resonance imaging) scan. Indications include nasal polyps, revision sinus surgery, frontal or sphenoid surgery, orbital surgery, surgery for skull base disorder, or CSF leak.

13. **What type of general anesthetic technique can improve visualization in FESS?**

TIVA has been shown to improve the surgical field visualization by correlating decreased heart rate and improved surgical field visualization. A lower heart rate has the added benefit of lower mean arterial pressures, avoidance of excess fluid shifts, and lower central venous pressures. Avoidance of inhalational anesthetics prevents the peripheral vasodilation that accompanies these agents.

14. **How does patient positioning affect visualization?**

Elevation of the patient's head, or reverse Trendelenburg positioning, has been shown to improve visualization of the surgical field visualization by improving venous return.

15. **How do topical vasoconstrictors influence sinus surgery?**

Nasal pledgets soaked in oxymetazoline, neosynephrine, or epinephrine (1:1000) can be placed into the nasal cavity to cause vasoconstriction and help improve generalized mucosal oozing. They carry a low complication rate (0.001%) but should be used with caution in pediatric patients and patients with cardiovascular risks or hypertension.

16. **Which local injections can be used in sinus surgery?**

Local vasoconstrictive/anesthetic injections are important for decreasing blood loss and optimizing visualization. Anterior injection into the lateral nasal wall at the insertion of the root of the middle turbinate is effective in anterior hemostasis during surgery of the maxillary, anterior ethmoid, and frontal sinuses. Posterior injection on the region of the sphenopalatine foramen or transoral injection via the greater palatine foramen is effective for posterior hemostasis during surgery of the posterior ethmoid and sphenoid sinuses. Typically, 1% lidocaine with 1:100K or 1:200K epinephrine is used.

17. **What is the most important factor in preventing major complications during endoscopic sinus surgery?**

Thorough knowledge of the anatomy is paramount for the prevention of major surgical complications. Meticulous and detailed review of the patient's CT imaging preoperatively is an absolute requirement prior to surgery.

18. **What is the incidence of major complications in endoscopic sinus surgery?**

The overall major complication rate is reported to be less than 1%.

19. **What are the important anatomic factors to consider in preoperative CT scan review?**

First, one should always verify the correct patient and left/right orientation of the scan. Verify the integrity of the lamina papyracea. Pay attention to the height of the maxillary sinus relative to the height of the ethmoid sinuses. Tall maxillary sinuses result in relatively short ethmoid height and may disorient the surgeon because the skull base may be lower than anticipated. Assess the configuration of the skull base in terms of height, slope, symmetry, and depth of the cribriform plate. Assess the position of the anterior ethmoidal artery and if it is within the

KEROS CLASSIFICATION

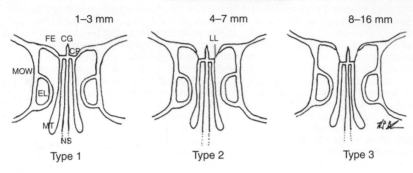

1–3 mm   4–7 mm   8–16 mm

Type 1   Type 2   Type 3

MOW: Medial orbital wall   FE: Fovea ethmoidalis
MT: Middle turbinate   CP: Cribiform plate
LL: Lateral lamella   CG: Crista galli
NS: Nasal septum   EL: Ethmoid labyrinth

Fig. 29.1 Keros classification of depth of olfactory fossa.

bony skull base or dehiscent. Verify the integrity of the bony skull base and note whether there are any areas of thinning. Within the sphenoid sinus, inspect the bone over the optic and carotid canals and look for an Onodi cell.

20. **Which radiologic staging system is used to assess the ethmoid skull base?**
The Keros classification is a method of classifying the depth of the olfactory fossa (Fig. 29.1). The depth of the olfactory fossa is determined by the height of the cribriform plate and is staged into three categories: type 1 has a depth of 1 to 3 millimeters (26% of the population), type 2 has a depth of 4 to 7 millimeters (73% of the population), and type 3 has a depth of 8 to 16 millimeters (1% of the population).

21. **What is a Caldwell-Luc procedure?**
This procedure was designed to treat the "irreversibly diseased" maxillary sinus by removing mucosa and creating a gravity-dependent drainage. The maxillary sinus is opened through a sublabial approach, the sinus mucosa is removed, and a large inferior meatal antrostomy is created. This technique is rarely used in the era of endoscopic functional sinus surgery and has been replaced by the modified endoscopic medial maxillectomy.

BIBLIOGRAPHY

Barham HP, Hall CA, Hernandez SC, et al: Impact of Draf III, Draf IIb, and Draf IIa frontal sinus surgery on nasal irrigation distribution, *Int Forum Allergy Rhinol.* 10(1):49–52, 2020.
Brunner JP, Levy JM, Ada ML, et al: Total intravenous anesthesia improves intraoperative visualization during surgery for high-grade chronic rhinosinusitis: a double-blind randomized controlled trial, *Int Forum Allergy Rhinol* 8(10):1114–1122, 2018.
Fraire ME, Sanchez-Vallecillo MV, Zernotti ME, et al: Effect of premedication with systemic steroids on surgical field bleeding and visibility during nasosinusal endoscopic surgery, *Acta Otorrinolaringol Esp* 64(2):133–139, 2013.
Hathorn IF, Al-Rahim RH, Jamil M, et al: Comparing the reverse Trendelenburg and horizontal position for endoscopic sinus surgery: a randomized controlled trial, *Otolaryngol Head Neck Surg* 148(2):308–313, 2013.
Higgins TS, Hwang PH, Kingdom TT, et al: Systematic review of topical vasoconstrictors in endoscopic sinus surgery, *Laryngoscope* 121:422–432, 2011.
Khosla AJ, Pernas FG, Maeso PA: Meta-analysis and literature review of techniques to achieve hemostasis in endoscopic sinus surgery, *Int Forum Allergy Rhinol* 3(6):482–487, 2013.
Krings JG, Kallogjeri D, Wineland A, et al: Complications of primary and revision functional endoscopic sinus surgery for chronic rhinosinusitis, *Laryngoscope* 124(4):838–845, 2014.
Ramakrishnan VR, Kingdom TT, Nayak JV, et al: Nationwide incidence of major complications in endoscopic sinus surgery, *Int Forum Allergy Rhinol* 2(1):34–39, 2012.
Senior BA, Kennedy DW, Tanabodee J, et al: Long-term results of functional endoscopic sinus surgery, *Laryngoscope* 108:151–157, 1998.
Stankiewicz JA: Complications of endoscopic sinus surgery, *Otolaryngol Clin North Am* 22:749–758, 1989.
Timperley D, Sacks R, Parkinson RJ, et al: Perioperative and intraoperative maneuvers to optimize surgical outcomes in skull base surgery, *Otolaryngol Clin North Am* 43:699–730, 2010.

CHAPTER 30

CEREBROSPINAL FLUID LEAKS AND ENCEPHALOCELES

Henry P. Barham, MD, Luke A. Corsten, MD and Anne E. Getz, MD

KEY POINTS

1. Trauma is the most common cause of CSF leaks.
2. Endoscopic repair of CSF leaks is effective and offers decreased morbidity compared to open approaches.
3. Meticulous technique is key to success in repair of skull base defects.
4. Materials used and procedures employed are less important than the quality of the repair.

Pearls

1. The lateral lamella of the cribriform plate is the most common site of iatrogenic CSF leak during functional endoscopic sinus surgery (FESS).
2. Conservative management is often the first step in managing CSF leaks resulting from acute nonsurgical trauma.
3. Spontaneous CSF leaks are frequently associated with idiopathic intracranial hypertension.

QUESTIONS

1. What are the most common causes of CSF leaks?
   - Trauma
   - Nonsurgical: most common etiology (70% to 80%). Between 1% and 3% of acute head injuries result in a CSF leak. Seventy percent of leaks close spontaneously with observation and conservative management, which may include bed rest, head of bed elevation, and lumbar drainage.
   - Surgical (planned and unplanned):
     FESS (<1% incidence of CSF leak): the most common site of skull base injury is the lateral lamella of the cribriform plate. The posterior ethmoid skull base is at greater risk when the maxillary sinus is highly pneumatized in the superior-inferior dimension, which creates a relatively decreased posterior ethmoid height (Fig. 30.1).
     Neurologic Surgery: transsphenoidal approach for sellar and suprasellar lesions (0.5% to 15% incidence of CSF leak)
   - Neoplasm: mechanisms include direct tumor invasion and/or mass effect leading to intracranial hypertension.
   - Congenital: failure of closure of developmental spaces with resultant herniation of intracranial contents. The foramen cecum is the most common location (50%).
   - Spontaneous: often the result of idiopathic intracranial hypertension (IIH) resulting from decreased CSF reabsorption.

2. What is empty sella syndrome and how is it treated?
   Empty sella syndrome is a radiographic appearance of CSF-filled sella and flattening of the pituitary gland (Fig. 30.2). The pituitary gland is an endocrine gland that resides in the sella turcica and functions to control other endocrine glands (adrenal glands, thyroid, ovaries, testicles) by secretion of controlling hormones. Empty sella syndrome can be seen in IIH, which typically affects women with obesity. Patients typically present with headaches, pulsatile tinnitus, and diplopia. A hallmark physical exam finding is bilateral optic disc edema (papilledema) secondary to increased intracranial pressure (ICP). Treatment is focused on decreasing ICP with pharmacologic therapy consisting of diuretics that lower ICP and headache management, which may include amitriptyline and propranolol. In severe cases with vision problems, surgical intervention may be required, including optic nerve decompression or CSF shunting. Empty sella syndrome can be seen in conjunction with spontaneous CSF leaks.

3. What is an encephalocele?
   An encephalocele is herniation of neural tissue through a defect in the skull base (Figs. 30.3 and 30.4) and is defined by the type of tissue that herniates through the defect. A meningocele contains herniated meninges, a

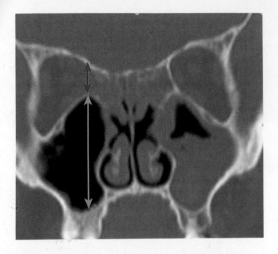

Fig. 30.1 A relatively short height of the ethmoid sinus (top arrow) as a result of a highly pneumatized tall maxillary sinus (bottom arrow).

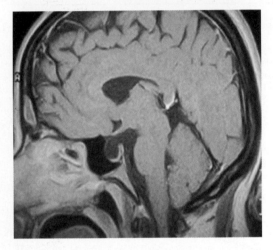

Fig. 30.2 Sagittal MRI of an "empty" sella turcica filled with CSF.

meningoencephalocele contains herniated brain matter and meninges, and a meningoencephalocystocele is composed of herniated brain matter and meninges that communicate with a cerebral ventricle.

4. **Where do encephaloceles occur?**
   Encephaloceles can occur in both the skull and spinal column. Twenty percent occur within the cranium and 15% of these are associated with the nasal cavity. Nasal encephaloceles are divided into two types: sincipital and basal. Sincipital (anterior and superior) encephaloceles comprise approximately 60% of nasal encephaloceles and typically present as a soft compressible mass over the glabella. Basal encephaloceles occur through the skull base more posteriorly and comprise approximately 40% of nasal encephaloceles. They may remain hidden for many years because they are located more posteriorly than the sincipital type.

5. **How is an encephalocele diagnosed?**
   Patients often present with rhinorrhea or recurrent meningitis and may have a broad nasal dorsum or hypertelorism. Encephaloceles may characteristically transilluminate, expand with the Valsalva maneuver, and demonstrate a positive Furstenberg sign (enlargement with compression of internal jugular veins). Radiologic imaging, including computed tomography (CT) and magnetic resonance imaging (MRI), may be used to evaluate the size and location of encephaloceles (see Figs. 30.3 and 30.4).

6. **Describe the physiology of CSF production.**
   CSF is produced by the choroid plexus of the lateral, third, and fourth ventricles at a rate of 0.35 mL/min (20 mL/hour or 350 to 500 mL/day) in the normal physiologic states. The total volume of circulating CSF is 90

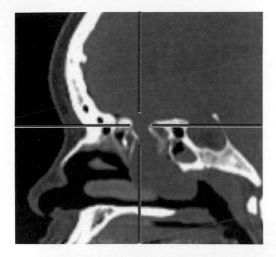

Fig. 30.3 Large encephalocele of the ethmoid skull base. Crosshairs localize the bony skull base defect.

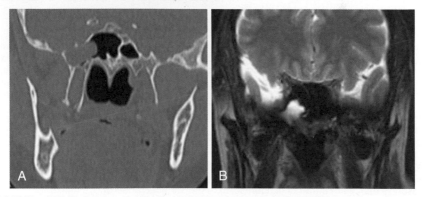

Fig. 30.4 CT **(A)** and MRI **(B)** of meningocele protruding into the lateral recess of the right sphenoid sinus.

to 150 mL. The entire volume of CSF turns over three to five times per day. Typical intracranial pressure is 5 to 15 centimeters H_2O and is considered elevated when it is greater than 15 centimeters H_2O.

7. **What is the most common complaint in patients presenting with concern for a CSF leak?**
Clear rhinorrhea that is unilateral, watery, and tastes salty or metallic is the most common feature. It may run out of the nose in more anterior leaks or down the back of the throat in more posterior leaks. Drainage can be exacerbated by the Dandy maneuver, which entails tilting the head forward into a chin-tuck position and straining.

8. **Which laboratory tests can be performed to diagnose a CSF leak?**
The classic test is qualitative β2-transferrin evaluation of the nasal drainage. β2-transferrin is detected in few fluids in the body including CSF, perilymph, and aqueous humor. Only 0.2 mL is needed for an adequate specimen. β2-Transferrin has a sensitivity of 97% and a specificity of 93%. False-positive results can occur with abnormal transferrin metabolism from chronic liver disease, glycogen metabolic disease, and carcinomas; results can therefore be verified with negative serum β2-transferrin. β-Trace protein is a newer laboratory test with higher sensitivity and specificity that offers faster results than β2-transferrin but is not universally available.

9. **Describe the radiologic evaluation of a patient with CSF rhinorrhea.**
The radiologic evaluation of a CSF leak often begins with a fine-cut maxillofacial CT scan to demonstrate bony abnormalities such as defects and fractures. CT is the mainstay for radiologic workup of CSF rhinorrhea with a sensitivity of 92% and a specificity of 92% to 96%. If the initial imaging does not show an obvious abnormality but suspicion is still high, a CT cisternogram may be useful. This study entails injection of radiopaque material through a lumbar drain into the intrathecal space to help delineate the CSF leak. Presence of contrast within the sinonasal cavity indicates a CSF leak. CT cisternography has a sensitivity of 92% with an active leak to 40% with an

intermittent leak. MR cisternography can be helpful in cases of neoplasm, meningoencephalocele, and encephalocele and in patients with an iodine allergy.

10. **Describe the workup of suspected CSF rhinorrhea.**
If β2-transferrin or β-trace protein is positive, obtain a fine-cut maxillofacial CT scan to assess for source. If β2-transferrin or β-trace protein is negative and clinical suspicion is low, workup is complete. If clinical suspicion remains high, evaluate with maxillofacial CT. If a single, small (less than 1 centimeter) bony defect is present on the CT in a patient with normal intracranial pressure, conservative therapy may be attempted, but surgical repair is also an option. If the bony defect is greater than 1 centimeter, or if the patient has elevated intracranial pressure and a high-pressure leak, surgical management is recommended. If more than one bony defect is seen on CT imaging, cisternography can be helpful in determining which site(s) are leaking. If no bony defect is detected on maxillofacial CT, repeat testing for β2-transferrin or β-trace protein may be performed. If positive, CT or MRI cisternogram is recommended. If negative and clinical suspicion is high, surgical exploration is indicated, possibly with utilization of intrathecal fluorescein. If a bony defect is present on CT with associated soft tissue mass, MRI or MRI cisternogram is recommended to further evaluate the characteristics of the soft tissue mass, which may represent a meningocele or other neoplasm.

11. **What does conservative therapy for CSF leak entail?**
In patients who have a traumatic leak and normal CSF pressure, conservative treatment consists of bed rest with head of bed elevation and lumbar drainage of CSF for 5 to 10 days. With conservative management, there is a reported risk of ascending meningitis ranging from 7% to 30%. The incidence of spontaneous resolution with conservative management is reported to be 70%.

12. **Should antibiotics be used in patients with known CSF rhinorrhea?**
The general consensus among practicing otolaryngologists is that antibiotics should not be used for conservative management unless there is a very large defect with comminuted bone of the skull base, as a simple CSF leak carries a 7% infection rate (meningitis, intracranial abscess, cellulitis/abscess, and osteomyelitis) and prophylactic antibiotics have not been shown to decrease the risk of infection. After endoscopic repair, antibiotics are generally recommended for 24 to 48 hours including cefazolin (1 g q8), vancomycin (1 g q12), or clindamycin (600 mg q8).

13. **How has surgical management of CSF leaks improved with the use of endoscopic surgery?**
Advancements in the endoscopic surgical repair of CSF leaks and encephaloceles have resulted from improvements in instrumentation, visualization, access, and technique. Improved diagnostic imaging and surgical navigation have also been beneficial. Advancements in endoscopic reconstructive techniques of the skull base, including utilization of local vascularized flaps, have improved success rates with endoscopic approaches.

14. **Describe the use of intrathecal fluorescein in the surgical repair of CSF leaks.**
Its advantages include the ability to stain defects that may be more difficult to identify clinically, through the visible CSF dye to a bright yellowish-green color. The surgeon can also use it to confirm a water-tight repair. It carries a 0% false positive rate. Its disadvantages include a moderate false-negative result. It requires a lumbar puncture, and the use of fluorescein intrathecally is not FDA approved. Rare complications including seizures (0.3%) and death have been reported; however, these have more commonly been associated with administration through a suboccipital puncture. If used to help localize a CSF leak it should be used with caution and should be dosed as 0.05 to 0.1 mL per 10 kg body weight up to maximum 0.1 mL 10% fluorescein. This is mixed in 10 mL preservative-free normal saline or CSF. The surgeon should inject slowly (over 5 to 10 minutes) without paralytics in the anesthetic regimen to assess for seizure activity. Fluorescein should be avoided in patients with abnormal renal function.

15. **What are the goals of skull base reconstruction?**
The primary goal in endoscopic repair of CSF leaks and skull base reconstruction is to definitively identify all leaks in order to completely reconstruct all defects. After identifying the leak (or leaks), the goals of reconstruction are creation of a safe barrier with separation of intracranial and sinonasal spaces and elimination of any dead space. As with any surgical intervention, meticulous surgical technique is paramount for success.

16. **What can be used to reconstruct the skull base?**
A reconstructive ladder should be used to help determine the type of repair performed. For simple, small (less than 1 centimeter) defects, a fat plug harvested from the earlobe or abdomen can be used to plug the defect. The next option includes a simple sinonasal overlay graft harvested from the nasal floor mucosa, turbinate mucosa, or nasal septum. If a more complex, larger reconstruction is in order, a composite (underlay and overlay) graft can be used consisting of an intracranial underlay of bone or cartilage from nasal septum, auricular cartilage, or turbinate bone and an overlay graft of mucosa (free or pedicled) as above. Local pedicled flaps should include the nasoseptal flap, which is supplied by the posterior nasal septal artery, a terminal branch of the sphenopalatine artery. Additional grafts that can be useful in larger defects include temporal fascia or tensor fascia lata grafts. These grafts are

often bolstered in the sinonasal cavity with abdominal fat, a nasoseptal flap, or both. In complex situations of extensive defects or poor local tissue, such as in chemo-radiated patients, a craniotomy with pericranial flap or free flap reconstruction of the skull base may be necessary.

17. What are the reported outcomes of endoscopic repair of CSF leaks?
A multitude of studies have shown high success rates of primary repair at approximately 92% and secondary repair at approximately 99%. These success rates compare favorably to traditional craniotomy approaches, with reported success rates between 70% and 80% that carry a higher morbidity profile.

BIBLIOGRAPHY

Bernal-Sprekelsen M, Alobid I, Mullol J, et al: Closure of cerebrospinal fluid leaks prevents ascending bacterial meningitis, *Rhinology* 43(4):277–281, 2005.

Bleier BS: Comprehensive techniques in CSF leak repair and skull base reconstruction, *Adv Otorhinolaryngol.* 74:1–11, 2013.

Brown SM, Anand VK, Tabaee A, et al: Role of perioperative antibiotics in endoscopic skull base surgery, *Laryngoscope* 117(9):1528–1532, 2007.

Hegazy HM, et al: Transnasal endoscopic repair of cerebrospinal fluid rhinorrhea: a meta-analysis, *Laryngoscope* 110(7):1166–1172, 2000.

Lanza DC, O'Brien DA, Kennedy DW: Endoscopic repair of cerebrospinal fistulae and encephaloceles, *Laryngoscope* 106(9 Pt 1):1119–1125, 1996.

Lund VJ, Stammberger H, Nicolai P, et al: European position paper on endoscopic management of tumours of the nose, paranasal sinuses and skull base, *Rhinol Suppl* 1(22):1–143, 2010.

May M, Levine HL, Mester SJ, et al: Complications of ESS: analysis of 2018 patients, *Laryngoscope* 104:1080–1083, 1994.

Mincy J: Posttraumatic cerebrospinal fluid fistula of the frontal fossa, *J Trauma* 6(5):618–622, 1966.

Schlosser RJ, Bolger WE: Nasal cerebrospinal fluid leaks, *J Otolaryngol Suppl* 1:S28–S37, 2002.

Suh JD, Ramakrishnan VR, Chi JJ, et al: Outcomes and complications of endoscopic approaches for malignancies of the paranasal sinuses and anterior skull base, *Ann Otorhinolaryngol.* 122(1):54–59, 2013.

Suwanwela C, Suwanwela N: A morphological classification of sincipital encephalomeningoceles, *J Neurosurg* 36:201–211, 1972.

Wolf G, Greistorfer K, Stammberger H, et al: Endoscopic detection of cerebral spinal fistulas with a fluorescence technique, Report of experiences with over 925 cases. Laryngorhinootologie 76(10):588–594, 1997.

Zweig JL, et al: Endoscopic repair of cerebrospinal fluid leaks to the sinonasal tract: predictors of success, *Otolaryngol Head Neck Surg* 123(3):195–201, 2000.

CHAPTER 31

ORBITAL SURGERY

Henry P. Barham, MD and Todd T. Kingdom, MD

KEY POINTS

1. Endoscopic sinus surgical techniques have advanced to include the treatment of select orbital pathology due to the close proximity of the orbit to the paranasal sinuses, advances in surgical instrumentation, and a working relationship with ophthalmologists.
2. Endoscopic approaches to the orbit require a deep knowledge and an accurate intraoperative identification of orbital anatomy.
3. Excess tearing (epiphora) can result from hypersecretion or failure of drainage (nasolacrimal system obstruction). Endoscopic dacryocystorhinostomy (DCR) is the preferred treatment for nasolacrimal duct obstruction.
4. Thyroid eye disease (TED) is the most common extrathyroidal manifestation of Graves' disease and is the leading cause of proptosis in adults. Endoscopic orbital decompression is often an important treatment approach to these patients.
5. Traumatic optic neuropathy is categorized as direct or indirect, and surgical intervention appears to be of limited benefit.

Pearls

1. Thyroid eye disease results from autoimmune inflammation of muscle and fat, where the thyroid-stimulating hormone (TSH) receptor is the autoantigen.
2. Dacryocystorhinostomy is an effective surgical management for nasolacrimal duct obstruction.
3. The medial rectus, superior rectus, inferior rectus, and inferior oblique muscles are innervated by cranial nerve III. The superior oblique muscle is innervated by cranial nerve IV. The lateral rectus muscle is innervated by cranial nerve VI.
4. The anterior and posterior ethmoid arteries are distal branches of the internal carotid circulation.

QUESTIONS

1. **Describe the important bony anatomy of the orbit.**
   The orbit is a pyramidal shaped space that is made up of seven bones: ethmoid, frontal, lacrimal, maxillary, palatine, sphenoid, and zygomatic (Fig. 31.1). The medial walls of each orbit lie parallel to each other and the lateral walls lie 45 degrees to the ipsilateral medial wall and 90 degrees to the contralateral lateral wall. The orbital walls are lined by periosteum called periorbita.

2. **Which bones make up each wall of the orbit?**
   The roof of the orbit is made up of the frontal bone and lesser wing of the sphenoid. The floor of the orbit is composed of the maxillary, palatine, and zygomatic bones. The medial wall of the orbit is composed of the ethmoid, lacrimal, maxillary, and sphenoid bones. The lateral wall of the orbit is composed of the greater wing of the sphenoid and the zygomatic bone.

3. **What are the dimensions of the orbit in adults?**
   The pyramidal shaped orbit has a typical volume of 30 mL. The entrance height is 35 millimeters and the entrance width is 40 millimeters. The width of the orbit is greatest 1-centimeter posterior to the entrance of the orbit, which corresponds to the equator of the globe. The medial wall length is 45 mm.

4. **What are the orbital foramina and which structures are contained within them?**
   The optic foramen passes through the lesser wing of the sphenoid extending from the middle cranial fossa to the orbital apex and contains the optic nerve, ophthalmic artery, and sympathetic fibers from the carotid plexus. The supraorbital foramen is located at the medial third of the superior margin of the orbital rim and contains the supraorbital nerve, artery, and vein. The anterior ethmoidal foramen is located at the frontoethmoidal suture 24 millimeters posterior to the orbital rim and contains the anterior ethmoidal vessels and nerve. The posterior ethmoidal foramen is located 12 millimeters posterior to the anterior ethmoidal foramen at the junction of the medial wall and orbital roof and contains the posterior ethmoidal vessels and nerve. The 24/12/6 rule is a nice reference to

Right orbit: frontal and slightly lateral view

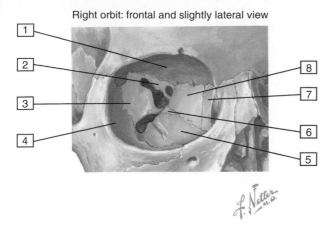

1. Frontal bone
2. Lesser wing of the sphenoid
3. Greater wing of the sphenoid
4. Zygomatic bone
5. Maxillary bone
6. Palatine bone
7. Lacrimal bone
8. Ethmoid bone

Bones creating the orbital margin include:
• Frontal
• Zygomatic
• Maxilla

Walls of the orbit

Superior	Frontal (orbital plate)
	Lesser wing of sphenoid
Inferior	Maxilla
	Zygomatic
	Palatine (orbital process)
Medial	Ethmoid (lamina papyracea)
	Lacrimal
	Sphenoid
	Maxilla
Lateral	Zygomatic
	Greater wing of sphenoid

Fig. 31.1 Bony anatomy of the orbit. (From Gentile MA, Tellington AJ, Burke WJ, et al: Management of midface maxillofacial trauma. *Atlas Oral Maxillofacial Surgery Clin North Am* 21(1):69–95, 2013.)

help remember foramina locations in the orbit, which stands for anterior ethmoid artery (24 millimeters), posterior ethmoid artery (12 millimeters), and optic nerve (6 millimeters) in sequential measurements from the posterior lacrimal crest. The zygomaticotemporal and zygomaticofacial foramina are located within the lateral wall of the orbit and transmit branches of the zygomatic nerve and artery.

5. **What are the orbital fissures and which structures are contained within them?**
   The superior orbital fissure is 22 millimeters in length and lies inferior and lateral to the optic foramen. It is formed by the greater and lesser wing of the sphenoid and is divided into superior and inferior parts by the lateral rectus. The superior part contains the frontal and lacrimal branches of cranial nerve V1 and cranial nerve IV. The inferior part contains the superior and inferior divisions of cranial nerve III, the nasociliary branch of V1, cranial nerve VI, the superior ophthalmic vein, and the sympathetic nerve plexus. The inferior orbital fissure lies between the lateral

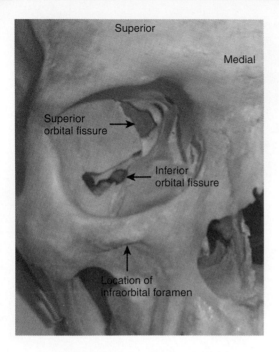

Superior

Medial

Superior orbital fissure →

← Inferior orbital fissure

↑ Location of infraorbital foramen

Fig. 31.2 Anterior view of the orbit on a dry skull. Foramina, or openings in the bone, can be seen. The superior orbital fissure is found at the orbital apex. The inferior orbital fissure is found on the orbital floor. The optic foramen is found on the superior-medial wall. (From Anderson BC, McLoon LK: Cranial nerves and autonomic innervation in the orbit. In Dartt DA, ed: *Encyclopedia of the Eye*, Oxford, 2010, Academic Press, pp. 537–548.)

wall and orbital floor (runs deep to the orbital floor) and contains branches of cranial nerve V2 and the inferior ophthalmic vein (Fig. 31.2).

6. **What are the extraocular muscles and where are they located?**
   There are six extraocular muscles within each orbit (Fig. 31.3) that control movement of the globe: inferior rectus, lateral rectus, medial rectus, superior rectus, superior oblique, and inferior oblique. With the inferior oblique as the exception, all extraocular muscles originate at the orbital apex. The four rectus muscles originate from the annulus of Zinn (a tendinous ring that encircles the inferior portion of the superior orbital fissure and optic foramen) and insert onto the anterior portion of the globe. The superior oblique travels from the orbital apex to the trochlea and makes a sharp turn (54 degrees) to insert on the globe. The inferior oblique travels from a shallow depression in the orbital plate of the maxillary bone, inferior to the lacrimal fossa, posteriorly laterally and superiorly to insert on the globe.

7. **Describe the innervation of the extraocular muscles.**
   The inferior rectus, medial rectus, superior rectus, and inferior oblique muscles are innervated by cranial nerve III. The superior oblique muscle is innervated by cranial nerve IV. The lateral rectus muscle is innervated by cranial nerve VI. The blood supply to the extraocular muscles is provided by the inferior and superior muscular branches of the ophthalmic artery, lacrimal artery, and infraorbital artery.

8. **Describe the vasculature to the orbit.**
   The arterial supply to the orbit is from the internal carotid artery via the ophthalmic branch with contributions from the external carotid artery system (superficial facial artery). The branches of the ophthalmic artery include the central retinal, lateral and medial posterior ciliary, lacrimal, muscular, supraorbital, anterior and posterior ethmoidal, supratrochlear, nasofrontal, and dorsonasal arteries. The lacrimal artery forms an anastomosis with the external carotid system via the transverse facial and superficial temporal arteries. Medially, the dorsonasal arteries anastomose with the external carotid system via the angular arteries. The maxillary artery contributes via its infraorbital branch. The venous drainage of the orbit is from the superior and inferior ophthalmic veins. The inferior ophthalmic vein originates from a plexus of vessels in the inferior orbit, joins the pterygoid plexus, and terminates at the superior ophthalmic vein to enter the cavernous sinus. The superior ophthalmic vein originates at the superior medial orbit and crosses midorbit below the superior rectus muscle. The lacrimal vein joins the superior ophthalmic vein prior to exiting the orbit to enter the cavernous sinus.

9. **Describe the anatomy of the lacrimal system.**
   The lacrimal gland, which is responsible for reflex tearing, is found within the lacrimal fossa in the orbital portion of the frontal bone. The gland is divided into the palpebral lobe and the orbital lobe by the lateral horn of the

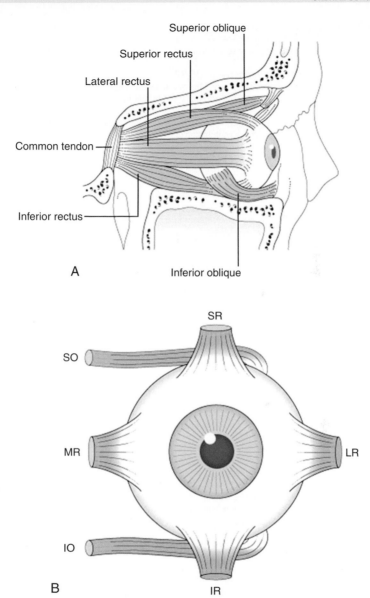

Fig. 31.3 Schematic diagrams depicting the extraocular muscles from lateral **(A)** and cut anterior **(B)** views. SO, superior oblique; IO, inferior oblique; MR, medial rectus; LR, lateral rectus; SR, superior rectus; IR, inferior rectus. In the lateral view **(A)**, the muscles are depicted attached to the common tendon. (From Carreiro JE: Ophthalmology. In Carreiro JE, ed: *An Osteopathic Approach to Children*, 2nd ed, Edinburgh, 2009, Churchill Livingstone, pp. 197–214.)

levator aponeurosis. Eight to twelve lacrimal gland ductules empty into the superior lateral conjunctival fornix. The accessory lacrimal glands (glands of Wolfring and Krause), which are responsible for basal tearing, are located in the eyelid. The lacrimal papillae are located medially on the posterior edge of the upper and lower eyelids and lead to the lacrimal canaliculi. The lacrimal canaliculi (superior and inferior) lead to the lacrimal sac within the lacrimal fossa, most often (>90%) forming a single common canaliculus prior to entering the sac. The valve of Rosenmuller is located at the medial end of the common canaliculus and prevents tear reflux. The nasolacrimal duct forms (exits) at the inferior portion of the lacrimal sac and lies within the bony nasolacrimal canal. The naso-lacrimal duct drains into the inferior meatus of the nose beneath the inferior turbinate through the valve of Hasner.

10. **What is a dacryocystorhinostomy (DCR)?**

DCR is a surgical procedure involving fistulization of the lacrimal sac into the nasal cavity. The procedure can be performed through an external incision or via a transnasal endoscopic approach.

11. **What are the advantages of endoscopic DCR?**

With the advances in endoscopic visualization and the development of improved instrumentation, endoscopic DCR has shown success rates (80% to 100%) that are similar to those of traditional external techniques. The advantages of endoscopic approaches include the absence of external skin incision and resultant scar, the preservation of the orbicularis oculi pump mechanism, decreased disruption of the medial canthal anatomy, decreased intraoperative bleeding, and the ability to address contributing nasal cavity or paranasal sinus abnormalities.

12. **What are the indications for endoscopic DCR?**

Excess tearing (epiphora) can result from hypersecretion (lacrimation) or failure of drainage. Bothersome epiphora due to nasolacrimal duct obstruction is the primary indication for DCR. Other causes include recurrent dacryocystitis, dacryolithiasis, tumors of the lacrimal system, nasal pathology, or anatomic abnormalities that obstruct the drainage pathway. Nasolacrimal duct obstruction often presents with epiphora or infection and can be confirmed via several diagnostic tests including the dye disappearance test, lacrimal system irrigation or probing, scintigraphy, and contrast dacryocystography.

13. **How does one perform an endoscopic DCR?**

The surgical approach is similar to performing endoscopic sinus surgery. Important landmarks include the maxillary line (corresponds to the suture line between the frontal process of the maxilla and the lacrimal bone), which serves as a landmark for the lacrimal sac, the uncinate process, and the superior attachment of the middle turbinate. A sickle knife is used to create a mucosal flap on the lateral nasal wall over the lacrimal sac, which may be debulked or trimmed. The lacrimal bone and frontal process of the maxilla are removed to expose the medial portion of the lacrimal sac. The sac is marsupialized into the nasal cavity, and silicone lacrimal intubation stents may be placed.

14. **What is the leading cause of proptosis in adults?**

Thyroid eye disease (TED or Graves' ophthalmopathy) is the most common extrathyroidal manifestation of Graves' disease and is the leading cause of proptosis in adults. It is considered an autoimmune process, with the thyroid-stimulating hormone (TSH) receptor as the likely autoantigen in both the thyroid gland and orbit. Fibroblasts and adipocytes act as effector cells, inducing a complex cytokine-mediated immunologic response marked by tissue inflammation and hypertrophy.

15. **What is the typical presentation of thyroid eye disease?**

Patients often complain of blurry vision, foreign body sensation, photophobia, tearing, diplopia, dull pain, and discomfort. Clinical features include eyelid retraction (90% of patients), periorbital soft tissue swelling, lid lag, lagophthalmos, conjunctival injection, exposure keratopathy, restrictive myopathy, exophthalmos, and optic neuropathy. Imaging usually reveals fusiform enlargement of the extraocular muscles. MRI is more sensitive than CT for showing optic nerve compression at the orbital apex. Approximately 5% of patients experience severe orbital inflammation and congestion resulting in compressive optic neuropathy, requiring urgent treatment.

16. **Describe the nonsurgical management of thyroid eye disease.**

In the majority of patients (80%), thyroid eye disease is self-limited, requiring only the supportive care of ocular lubrication, cool compresses, and sunglasses to manage light sensitivity and glare. Medical treatment should center on correction of thyroid dysfunction because this may improve orbitopathy. The goal of medical therapy is to minimize the severity and shorten the duration of inflammation and associated fibrosis. Corticosteroids (oral or IV) are often prescribed for clinically active thyroid eye disease. Additional immunomodulators including azathioprine, cyclosporin, and IV immunoglobulin have been used in several small studies with mixed results. Tepezza (teprotumumab-trbw) is an FDA-approved medicine for the treatment of TED. Tepezza is a fully human monoclonal antibody (mAb) and a targeted inhibitor of the insulin-like growth factor-1 receptor (IGF-1R). In selected patients, orbital radiation may be used to treat associated orbital inflammation and compressive optic neuropathy.

17. **What are the indications for surgical management of thyroid eye disease?**

Surgical intervention is indicated in cases of compressive optic neuropathy (CON), exposure keratopathy, and disfiguring proptosis. Diplopia is also a common clinical presentation for these patients. Multiple surgical approaches may be used to decompress the orbit, including transcranial, transconjunctival/transcaruncular, transantral, and endonasal (endoscopic). The degree of exophthalmos recession achieved by decompression is related to the number of orbital walls decompressed. In cases of compressive optic neuropathy, decompression of the posterior aspect of the medial, inferior, and/or lateral walls of the orbit is essential. Surgical intervention is typically staged with orbital decompression first, followed by strabismus surgery, followed by eyelid surgery.

18. **How is an orbital decompression performed?**
Decompression of the medial wall is best performed through a transnasal endoscopic approach, though a medial transorbital approach may be used. The inferior orbital decompression is best approached via a transconjunctival technique with an extended lid incision to provide access to the lateral wall for additional decompression. Removal of orbital fat inferiorly and/or laterally is often performed to varying degrees depending on the extent of reduction desired.

19. **Describe the anatomy of the optic nerve.**
The optic nerve is divided into four segments: intraocular, intraorbital, intracanalicular, and intracranial. The orbital segment of the optic nerve is 25 to 30 millimeters in length. The optic canal is formed by the two struts of the lesser wing of the sphenoid and contains both the optic nerve and ophthalmic artery. The optic nerve is a direct continuation of the brain and contains all three meningeal layers. The dural covering of the optic nerve is composed of two layers: an outer layer arising at the orbital apex where the dura splits to form the optic nerve sheath and the periorbita and an inner layer of arachnoid, which is attached to the inner portion of the dural sheath.

20. **When is endoscopic optic nerve decompression performed?**
Traumatic optic neuropathy (TON) is the most common indication for optic nerve decompression. Improvements in endoscopic instrumentation and growing surgical experience have made the endoscopic approach to the optic nerve possible. The endoscopic approach affords advantages over traditional external approaches including decreased morbidity, preservation of olfaction, faster recovery time, and more direct access to the relevant anatomy. Treatment for TON remains controversial due to limited evidence that surgical decompression is superior to medical management or observation.

21. **How is TON categorized?**
TON is categorized as direct or indirect. Direct TON commonly occurs as a result of penetrating injury and involves the intraorbital portion of the nerve. Indirect TON occurs from blunt head trauma with or without a resulting fracture of the orbital canal. Visual loss in cases of indirect TON can result from neural edema, hematoma, bone fragment nerve compression, shearing nerve injury, vascular compromise, or interruption of axonal transport. Optic nerve decompression is generally not indicated in direct TON but may be indicated in cases of indirect TON with hematoma, edema, or compression of the nerve within the bony canal.

22. **How is TON managed?**
There is no evidence-based consensus on the management of TON and management should be determined on a case-by-case basis. Systemic corticosteroids and surgical decompression are currently considered the mainstays of treatment, although neither has been shown to definitively improve outcomes. In patients with incomplete vision loss that fails to improve with systemic corticosteroids, surgical decompression is a reasonable treatment plan because studies have shown a potential benefit.

BIBLIOGRAPHY

Durairaj VD: Clinical perspectives of thyroid eye disease, *Am J Med* 119(12):1027–1028, 2006.

Kennedy DW, Goodstein ML, Miller NR, et al: Endoscopic transnasal orbital decompression, *Arch Otolaryngol Head Neck Surg* 116(3):275–282, 1990.

Kikkawa DO, Pornpanich K, Cruz RC Jr, et al: Graded orbital decompression based on severity of proptosis, *Ophthalmology* 109(7):1219–1224, 2002.

Kingdom TT, Barham HP, Durairaj VD: Long-term outcomes after endoscopic dacryocystorhinostomy without mucosal flap preservation, *Laryngoscope* 130(1):12–17, 2020.

Kingdom TT, Davies BW, Durairaj VD: Orbital decompression for the management of thyroid eye disease: an analysis of outcomes and complications, *Laryngoscope* 125(9):2034–2040, 2015.

Kingdom TT, Durairaj VD: Endoscopic applications in orbital surgery. In Kennedy DW, Hwang PH, eds: *Rhinology: Diseases of the Nose, Sinuses, and Skull Base*, 2012, Thieme, pp. 425–443.

Levin LA, Beck RW, Joseph MP, et al: The treatment of traumatic optic neuropathy: the International Optic Nerve Trauma Study, *Ophthalmology* 106(7):1268–1277, 1999.

Metson R, Dallow RL, Shore JW: Endoscopic orbital decompression, *Laryngoscope* 104(8 Pt 1):950–957, 1994.

Ramakrishnan VR, Hink EM, Durairaj VD, et al: Outcomes after endoscopic dacryocystorhinostomy without mucosal flap preservation, *Am J Rhinol* 21(6):753–757, 2007.

Tsirbas A, Davis G, Wormald PJ: Mechanical endonasal dacryocystorhinostomy versus external dacryocystorhinostomy, *Ophthalmic Plast Reconstr Surg* 20(1):50–56, 2004.

Wormald PJ, Kew J, Van Hasselt A: Intranasal anatomy of the nasolacrimal sac in endoscopic dacryocystorhinostomy, *Otolaryngol Head Neck Surg* 123(3):307–310, 2000.

CHAPTER 32

OTOLOGY ANATOMY AND EMBRYOLOGY WITH RADIOLOGY CORRELATES

Renee Banakis Hartl, MD, AuD

KEY POINTS

1. The ear is anatomically divided into the outer, middle, and inner ear. The outer ear begins at the auricle and ends at the tympanic membrane; the middle ear consists of the tympanic cavity, with the ossicular chain bridging the tympanic membrane to the cochlea; and the inner ear contains the organs of hearing and balance and the vestibulocochlear nerve (CN VIII).
2. The outer and middle ear structures are embryologically derived from the first and second branchial arches and the first branchial groove and pouch, while the bilateral otic placodes give rise to inner ear structures.
3. The end organ of hearing is the cochlea, which contains afferently innervated inner hair cells that are responsible for the transduction of auditory information.
4. The three semicircular canals are oriented in distinct planes to detect changes in angular acceleration, while the utricle and saccule detect linear acceleration and are oriented in the horizontal and vertical planes, respectively.
5. Auditory information passes through the central nervous system via the following pathway: auditory nerve, cochlear nucleus, superior olivary complex, lateral lemniscus, inferior colliculi, and medial geniculate body to the auditory cortex.

Pearls
1. Abnormalities of the external ear, including preauricular pits or tags, and malformations of the pinnae or ear canal can be associated with inner ear abnormalities and congenital syndromes and may indicate the need for additional otologic and genetic workup.
2. The ossicles transform acoustic energy to overcome the impedance mismatch between the aerated external ear canal and fluid-filled cochlea.
3. The cochlea is tonotopic, meaning that specific areas of the cochlea are stimulated by specific tone frequencies. The physical properties of the cochlear basilar membrane (thick, stiff, narrow base and thin, flexible, wide apex) are responsible for its tonotopic properties.
4. The severity of cochlear deformities depends significantly on the gestational age at growth arrest or disruption.

QUESTIONS

1. **Which structures comprise the outer ear?**
   The external ear is composed of the auricle and the external ear canal, terminating at the tympanic membrane (Fig. 32.1). The lateral one-third of the canal is cartilaginous and has hair follicles, along with ceruminous and sebaceous glands. The medial two-thirds of the canal is osseous and free of hair and adnexal structures. The length of the external canal, approximately 2.5 centimeters in adults, gives it a resonance frequency of 3 to 4 kHz.

2. **What are the hillocks of His? What structure do they ultimately form?**
   The hillocks are six small buds of mesenchyme surrounding the dorsal end of the first branchial cleft. Hillocks 1, 2, and 3 arise from the mandibular (or first) branchial arch, while 4, 5, and 6 develop from the hyoid (or second) arch. These mesenchymal structures ultimately rearrange to form the auricle. Although the exact embryology is controversial, it is classically taught that the first hillock forms the tragus, the second and third form the helix, the fourth and fifth develop into the antihelix, and the antitragus is formed from the sixth (Fig. 32.2).

3. **What is the function of the auricle? How does its unique structure contribute to auditory function?**
   The cone-shaped auricle collects and directs sound down the ear canal toward the tympanic membrane. The shape of the auricle also creates small, unique, high-pitched frequency resonances that contribute to the ability to localize sound in the vertical space.

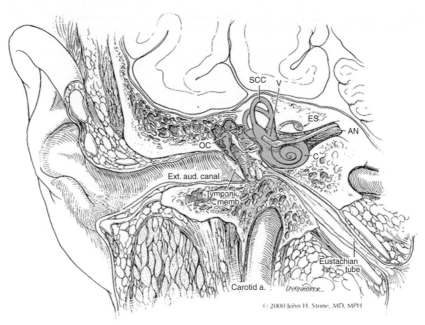

Fig. 32.1 Anatomy of the ear. (From Flint PW, et al: *Cummings Otolaryngology: Head & Neck Surgery*, 5th ed, Philadelphia, 2010, Mosby Elsevier, p. 1825.)

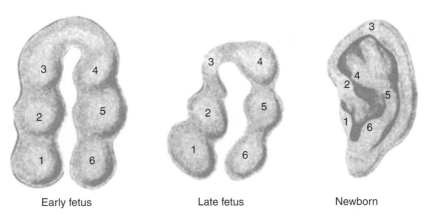

Early fetus   Late fetus   Newborn

Fig. 32.2 Auricular hillocks. By the fifth week of gestation, the area surrounding the first branchial groove becomes irregular, forming the six auricular hillocks of His. The following hillocks develop into the corresponding structures: 1 – tragus, 2 and 3 – helix, 4 and 5 – antihelix, 6 – antitragus. (From Flint PW, et al: *Cummings Otolaryngology: Head & Neck Surgery*, 5th ed, Philadelphia, 2010, Mosby Elsevier, p. 2742.)

4. **From which branchial structure does the external auditory canal develop?**
   The external auditory canal develops from the first (or mandibular) branchial groove.

5. **What are preauricular pits and tags? What is their clinical significance?**
   Preauricular pits and tags are benign preauricular soft tissue malformations. Pits are depressions in the skin located anterior to the ear canal. Epithelial mounds or pedunculated skin are known as preauricular tags. Structural abnormalities, including preauricular pits and tags, malformed pinnae, and stenotic or atretic ear canals, may indicate hearing loss and can be associated with congenital syndromes. Presence of these findings suggests the need for a thorough clinical examination for other congenital anomalies, audiometric evaluation, and possibly genetic testing.

6. **Which congenital syndromes are associated with external ear abnormalities?**
   - **Treacher-Collins syndrome (mandibulofacial dysostosis):** rare autosomal dominant condition with complete penetrance and variable expression consisting of downward-slanting palpebral fissures, auricular malformations with or without tags and preauricular blind fistulas, stenosis or atresia of the external ear canals, ossicular abnormalities, malar hypoplasia, flat nasal bridge, mandibular hypoplasia, cleft palate, and dental abnormalities.
   - **Goldenhar syndrome (oculo-auriculo-vertebral syndrome):** rare disorder of variable inheritance patterns characterized by anomalous development of the first and second branchial arches, which often results in unilateral craniofacial malformations, including hemifacial microsomia, eye anomalies, strabismus, anotia, preauricular skin tags, and stenotic or atretic ear canals. It is also associated with severe scoliosis.
   - **Branchio-oto-renal syndrome:** rare autosomal dominant disorder characterized by hypoplastic or absent kidneys, preauricular pits or tags, middle ear malformation or absence, and branchial cleft cysts or fistulae.
   - **CHARGE syndrome:** rare syndrome with a cluster of associated malformations, including coloboma of the eye, heart defects, atresia of the choanae, retardation of growth or development, genital defects (hypogonadism), and ear anomalies (asymmetric pinnae with low-set, lop ears).
   - **DiGeorge sequence:** 22q11 chromosomal deletion resulting in absence or hypoplasia of the thymus and/or parathyroid glands with cardiovascular and craniofacial anomalies, including low-set ears, micrognathia, hypertelorism, short philtrum, cleft palate, and choanal atresia.
   - **Crouzon syndrome:** rare autosomal dominant syndrome characterized by premature skull bone fusion (craniosynostosis). Other physical features include exophthalmos, hypotelorism, strabismus, beak-shaped nose, hypoplastic maxilla, low-set ears, and ear canal stenosis or atresia.

7. **Describe the middle ear. What structures can be found within the middle ear?**
   The middle ear is a 1 to 2 cm^3 air-filled cavity that houses the ossicles, the stapedius and tensor tympani muscles, and the chorda tympani nerve (containing taste fibers from the anterior two-thirds of the tongue and parasympathetic fibers to the submandibular and sublingual glands). The middle ear is bounded laterally by the tympanic membrane and medially by the lateral wall of the inner ear (otic capsule). It is continuous with the mastoid air cells via the antrum and nasopharynx via the eustachian tube (see Fig. 32.1).

8. **What are the ossicles? What is their embryologic origin? What is their function?**
   The ossicular chain is composed of the malleus, incus, and stapes. The malleus attaches laterally to the tympanic membrane, the stapes couples medially to the inner ear via the oval window, and the incus bridges these two bones. The first branchial arch gives rise to the head and neck of the malleus and the body of the incus. The second branchial arch gives rise to the long process of the malleus, the long process of the incus, and the stapes suprastructure. The stapes footplate derives from both the second branchial arch and the otic capsule. The ossicles transform acoustic energy to overcome the impedance mismatch between the aerated external ear canal and the fluid-filled cochlea.

9. **What is unique about the embryologic derivatives of the tympanic membrane?**
   The tympanic membrane consists of three layers, each of which is derived from a different germ layer. The outer epithelial layer derives from ectoderm, the middle fibrous layer derives from mesoderm, and the inner epithelial layer derives from endoderm. Neural crest–derived mesenchyme around the lateral margin of the membrane forms the tympanic annulus, which begins to ossify in the third month of gestation.

10. **Which muscles reside within the middle ear? Which cranial nerves innervate these muscles?**
    The stapedius and tensor tympani muscles are found in the middle ear. The stapedius is innervated by the facial nerve (CN VII), and a branch of the mandibular division of the trigeminal nerve (CN V3) innervates the tensor tympani.

11. **What is the function of the stapedius and tensor tympani muscles?**
    Contraction of both muscles can be induced with high-intensity acoustic stimuli, with a more pronounced effect at lower frequencies. When contracted, these muscles stiffen the ossicular chain, resulting in increased middle ear impedance and decreased sound transmission to the inner ear. The exact function of this musculature remains somewhat controversial, although it has been proposed that these reflexes serve either as a mechanism for protection of the cochlea from intense sounds or to reduce the intensity of low-frequency background noise to preserve higher-frequency speech information.

12. **Which structure provides aeration of the middle ear?**
    The eustachian tube, by its connection to the nasopharynx, aerates and drains the middle ear. Its dysfunction can cause a plugged feeling or popping of the ear and is implicated in the pathophysiology of otitis media. The immature anatomy of the eustachian tube in children predisposes them to ear infections.

13. **Describe the temporal bone. Which important structures does it contain?**
    The temporal bone is a pyramidal structure (apex pointing medially) that forms part of the base and lateral sides of the skull. Its major divisions are the squamous, petrous, tympanic, and mastoid bone segments. It houses the hearing and vestibular organs. Parts of the carotid, jugular, and facial nerves pass through it. It also includes the middle ear cavity and mastoid air cells.

14. **Describe the tortuous path of the facial nerve through the temporal bone.**
    The *meatal* segment of the facial nerve begins at the porus acusticus (medial internal auditory canal opening) and ends at the fundus (lateral opening). After exiting the internal auditory canal, the facial nerve courses through the temporal bone via a z-shaped course in three divisions: the *labyrinthine*, *tympanic*, and *mastoid* segments (Fig. 32.3). The labyrinthine segment begins as the nerve exits the internal auditory canal and travels superior to the cochlea. Just lateral and superior to the cochlea, it angles sharply forward to reach the geniculate ganglion and then makes an acute posterior and slightly inferior turn. This "hairpin" bend is the first genu of the facial nerve. The tympanic segment extends from this point posteriorly and laterally along the medial wall of the tympanic cavity, above the oval window and below the bulge of the lateral semicircular canal, until reaching the pyramidal eminence. At this point, the nerve drops sharply inferiorly to form the second genu. The mastoid segment passes downward in the posterior wall of the tympanic cavity and anterior wall of the mastoid to exit the base of the skull at the stylomastoid foramen.

15. **Why does complete radiologic evaluation of the facial nerve involve both CT and MRI studies?**
    When evaluating the facial nerve for a possible lesion, both a dedicated CT scan and MRI are useful. A CT scan can demonstrate the integrity of the osseous facial nerve (Fallopian) canal, while MRI can reveal enhancement of the facial nerve itself.

16. **Which structures comprise the inner ear?**
    The osseous and membranous labyrinthine systems comprise the inner ear. The osseous labyrinth consists of a layer of dense bone, known as the otic capsule, and the enclosed perilymphatic space, which contains perilymph

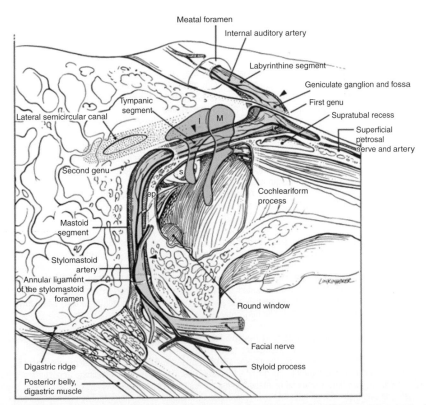

Fig. 32.3 Anatomy of intratemporal facial nerve. (From Flint PW, et al: *Cummings Otolaryngology: Head & Neck Surgery*, 5th ed, Philadelphia, 2010, Mosby Elsevier, p. 1826.)

fluid. The membranous labyrinth system is embedded in the osseous labyrinth and consists of a series of continuous cavities filled with endolymph fluid. This system consists of the auditory end organ (cochlea), which is responsible for the detection of sound, and the vestibular end organs (utricle, saccule, and semicircular canals), which sense linear and rotational acceleration.

17. **What is endolymph? What is perilymph? How do they differ?**
   Perilymph is the fluid contained within the osseous labyrinth that surrounds the membranous labyrinth. Endo-lymph is the fluid within the membranous labyrinth. Perilymph has an electrolyte composition similar to that of extracellular fluid (high in sodium, low in potassium), while the endolymph is high in potassium and low in sodium, similar to intracellular fluid. The difference in fluid characteristics sets up a large electrochemical gradient (approximately 80 to 100 mV) across the membranous labyrinth, which allows for the transduction of acoustic energy into a neural impulse. This gradient (or *endocochlear potential*) is maintained by the stria vascularis, which resides on the outer wall of the membranous labyrinth in the cochlea.

18. **What is the basilar membrane? What unique physical properties does it have?**
   The basilar membrane is the supporting structure on which the organ of Corti rests. The area below the basilar membrane contains perilymph, while the organ of Corti above is bathed in the endolymph. This membrane runs the length of the cochlea, and its physical properties are responsible for the tonotopic frequency arrangement of the cochlea. The base of the basilar membrane is stiff, thick, and narrow, while the apex is wide, thin, and flexible.

19. **What is the "traveling wave"?**
   G. von Bekesy is credited with describing the pattern of movement of the basilar membrane, or traveling wave, in response to sound. Each point on the basilar membrane moves at the same frequency as the acoustic stimulus; however, the amplitude and phase of the response vary considerably based on these physical properties. High frequencies cause the greatest physical displacement of the basilar membrane near the base of the cochlea, and the apex is the location of the largest amplitude response to low frequencies.

20. **What is the organ of Corti?**
   The organ of Corti contains auditory receptor cells, called hair cells, and a host of other structural and supporting cells. The hair cells sit on the basilar membrane and are overlaid by the tectorial membrane. There are two types of hair cells in the cochlea: inner hair cells and outer hair cells.

21. **How does the innervation of inner and outer hair cells of the cochlea differ?**
   Inner hair cells are predominantly afferently innervated. Afferent nerve fibers carry information from the hair cells to the brain. In contrast, outer hair cells are predominantly efferently innervated. Efferent fibers carry information from the brain to the hair cells. A single inner hair cell is innervated by numerous (up to 30) nerve fibers, whereas many outer hair cells are typically innervated by a single nerve fiber.

22. **How are the cochlear hair cells stimulated?**
   Hair cells are named for the presence of stereocilia, which are evaginations of the apical surface of the hair cell membrane that look like hair on the cell surface. The tectorial and basilar membranes are connected centrally. Sound moves these two structures differentially, causing a shear force that bends the stereocilia. Movement of the stereocilia opens and closes ion channels, producing a receptor potential in the inner hair cell. The receptor potential, in turn, releases neurotransmitters onto afferent nerve fibers, signaling the presence of a specific sound frequency to the brain. The specific hair cells stimulated by a given sound depend on the tonotopic map of the basilar membrane.

23. **What are the utricle and saccule? What are the semicircular canals?**
   The utricle and saccule are vestibular organs that are responsible for detecting acceleration in a linear plane. The utricle detects horizontal accelerations, and the saccule detects vertical accelerations, including gravitational force. The semicircular canals detect rotational or angular acceleration. There are three canals (lateral, horizontal, superior, anterior, and posterior) that are oriented in different planes. The vertical canals (superior and posterior) are oriented approximately 45 degrees relative to the sagittal plane and the horizontal canal is tilted upward approximately 30 degrees anteriorly from the horizontal plane.

24. **From which embryonic structure does the labyrinthine membrane of the inner ear develop? From which germ layer is this structure derived?**
   The structures of the inner ear and corresponding sensory innervation develop from bilateral otic placodes, which are ectodermal thickenings lateral to the rim of the neural tube. These placodes invaginate to become otic pits and subsequently become enveloped by mesenchyme as vesicular structures known as otocysts. These bilateral otocysts will eventually differentiate into the membranous structures of the labyrinth. The otic capsule ossifies around the labyrinthine membrane between weeks 16 and 24 of gestation to form the bony labyrinth. Fetal

Table 32.1 Osseous Malformations of the Inner Ear

NAME	LOCATION	GESTATIONAL AGE OF DEVELOPMENT ARREST	APPEARANCE
Cochlear aplasia	Osseous and membranous labyrinth of cochlea	5th week	Only a vestibule and SCCs present
Cochlear hypoplasia	Osseous and membranous labyrinth of cochlea	6th week	Hypoplastic cochlea consisting of a single turn or less
Incomplete partition (Mondini)	Osseous and membranous labyrinth of cochlea	7th week	Cochlea with 1.5 turns, partially or completely lacks interscalar septum
Common cavity	Entire osseous and membranous labyrinth	4th week	Cochlea and vestibule are confluent, forming an ovoid cystic space without internal architecture
Complete labyrinthine aplasia (Michel)	Entire osseous and membranous labyrinth	Prior to 4th week	Complete absence of inner ear structures

hearing is possible at approximately 2 to 3 m before birth because hair cell and auditory neural development are essentially complete by 26 to 28 weeks of gestation.

25. **What types of defects can result from abnormal cochlear development? Which imaging modality is preferred to diagnose these defects?**
Inner ear malformations are described as being limited to the membranous labyrinth or involving both the osseous and membranous labyrinth. Dysplasia of the membranous labyrinth may be complete, limited to the cochlea and saccule, or involve only the basal turn of the cochlea. Membranous dysplasia is assumed to account for more than 90% of congenital deafness but can only be identified histopathologically. Only approximately 5% to 15% of congenitally deaf individuals have involvement of the otic capsule and thus show abnormalities on imaging. These disorders include cochlear aplasia, cochlear hypoplasia, incomplete cochlear partition, and common cavity. The most severe agenesis is complete aplasia of the entire osseous labyrinth (both cochlear and vestibular). Table 32.1 describes the osseous malformations in detail. High-resolution CT is the preferred imaging modality for diagnosing combined malformations of the osseous and membranous labyrinth.

26. **Which rare disorder of the semicircular canals is associated with an anomaly of the temporal bone? Which imaging modality is preferred for diagnosis?**
Superior canal dehiscence syndrome (SCDS) is characterized by conductive hearing loss, sound- or pressure-induced vertigo, and autophony resulting from the absence of bone over the superior semicircular canal. The exact cause remains elusive, but dehiscent bone in SCDS has been proposed to be related to incomplete ossification of the otic capsule, leading to either absent or thinned bone susceptible to trauma-related injury. High-resolution CT is the imaging study of choice for diagnosing SCDS (Fig. 32.4).

27. **Which labyrinthine structure is thought to be a vestigial organ of hearing? Which electrophysiologic test is able to utilize this acoustic sensitivity?**
The saccule functions as an acoustic receptor in lower species that lack a cochlea. In humans it has been shown to respond to auditory stimuli. One proposed theory to explain this sensitivity in humans is that the saccule has retained acoustic sensitivity as a vestigial organ of hearing. The vestibular-evoked myogenic potential (VEMP) is an electrophysiologic test used clinically to evaluate balance function that capitalizes on this retained ability.

28. **Describe the orientation of the cochlear vestibular and facial nerves within the internal auditory canal.**
The internal auditory canal is approximately 1 centimeter in length and located along the medial aspect of the petrous portion of the temporal bone connecting the inner ear and the posterior cranial fossa. The transverse (or falciform) crest divides the canal into superior and inferior sections, while the vertical crest, known as Bill's bar, divides the canal anteriorly and posteriorly. The fundus (or lateral opening) is thus divided into four quadrants, each containing a major nerve branch: (1) anterior superior quadrant — facial nerve, (2) anterior inferior quadrant — cochlear nerve, (3) posterior superior quadrant — superior vestibular nerve, and (4) posterior inferior quadrant — inferior vestibular nerve (Fig. 32.5).

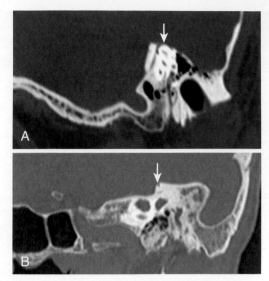

Fig. 32.4 Superior canal dehiscence. CT scan of the temporal bone in the parallel plane **(A)** and perpendicular plane **(B)**. Arrows demonstrate location of right superior canal dehiscence. (From Elmali M, et al: Semicircular canal dehiscence: frequency and distribution on temporal bone CT and its relationship with the clinical outcomes. *Eur J Radiol* 82(10):e607, 2013.)

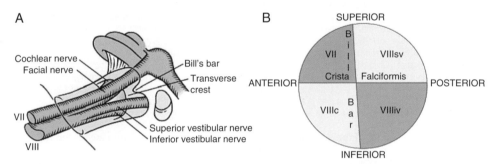

Fig. 32.5 Internal auditory canal anatomy. Contents of the canal shown in longitudinal view **(A)** and cross section **(B)**. (From Poulsgaard L: *Schmidek and Sweet's Operative Neurosurgical Techniques*, 6th ed, Philadelphia, 2012, Elsevier, pp. 555–564; Nadgir R, et al: *Neuroradiology: The Requisites*, 4th ed, Philadelphia, 2017, Elsevier, pp. 378–409.)

29. **Describe the neural pathway of auditory information from the periphery to the brain.**
    After hair cells are stimulated, afferent neurons of CN VIII relay information to the cochlear nuclei. From there, stimuli travel to the superior olivary complexes, lateral lemnisci, inferior colliculi, and medial geniculate bodies to the auditory cortex and association areas in the brain (Fig. 32.6). Auditory information from each ear remains ipsilateral until the level of the superior olivary nucleus, at which point there is significant signal crossover. The afferent pathway of the stapedial reflex synapses at the superior olivary complex, resulting in a reflex response that can be measured bilaterally.

30. **Where is auditory information processed in the brain?**
    Auditory information is processed in the temporal cortex of the brain. The primary auditory cortex is located in the area known as Heschl's gyrus on the superior surface of the temporal lobe close to the Sylvian fissure. This area is primarily responsible for the integration and processing of auditory information and is arranged in a tonotopic fashion, with high frequencies represented medially and low frequencies represented laterally. The auditory association cortex is located lateral to the primary auditory cortex and is part of Wernicke's area, which is responsible for language reception.

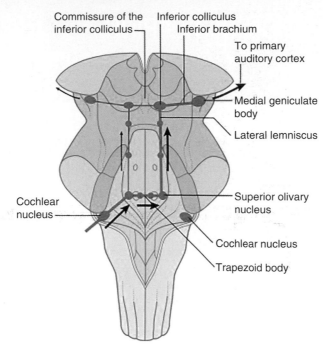

Fig. 32.6 Dorsal view of the brainstem showing the basic plan of central auditory pathways. (From Mtui E, et al: *Fitzgerald's Clinical Neuroanatomy and Neuroscience*, 7th ed, Oxford, 2016, Elsevier, pp. 207–211.)

BIBLIOGRAPHY

Bekesy GV: *Experiments in Hearing*, New York, 1960, McGraw-Hill.
Elmali M, Polat AV, Kucuk H, et al: Semicircular canal dehiscence: frequency and distribution on temporal bone CT and its relationship with the clinical outcomes, *Eur J Radiol* 82(10):e606–e609, 2013.
Flint PW, Haughey BH, Lund VJ, et al: *Cummings Otolaryngology: Head and Neck Surgery*, 5th ed, Philadelphia, 2010, Mosby Elsevier.
Gorlin RJ, Toriello HV, Cohen MM: *Hereditary Hearing Loss and Its Syndromes*, New York, 1995, Oxford University Press.
Lalwani AK: *Current Diagnosis and Treatment in Otolaryngology—Head and Neck Surgery*, 3rd ed, New York, 2012, McGraw Hill.
Lee KJ: *Essential Otolaryngology: Head and Neck Surgery*, 8th ed, New York, 2002, McGraw-Hill.
Mallo M: Embryological and genetic aspects of middle ear development, *Int J Dev Biol* 42:11–22, 1998.
Mtui E, Gruener G, Dockery P: *Fitzgerald's Clinical Neuroanatomy and Neuroscience*, 7th ed, Oxford, 2016, Elsevier.
Nadgir R, Yousem DM: *Neuroradiology: The Requisites*, 4th ed, Philadelphia, 2017, Elsevier.
Pasha R: *Otolaryngology Head and Neck Surgery, Clinical Reference Guide*, San Diego, 2000, Singular.
Poulsgaard L: *Schmidek and Sweet's Operative Neurosurgical Techniques*, 6th ed, Philadelphia, 2012, Elsevier.
Spoendlin H: Anatomy of cochlear innervation, *Am J Otolaryngol* 6(6):453–467, 1985.

CHAPTER 33

EVALUATION OF HEARING

Sanya Richardson, AuD, CCC-A, PASC, Sandra Abbott Gabbard, PhD, Stacy Claycomb, AuD and Kristin Uhler, PhD

KEY POINTS

1. There are two main types of hearing loss: conductive and sensorineural. Mixed hearing loss has both conductive and sensorineural components.
2. The patient's ability to understand speech is measured by word and sentence recognition tests.
3. The auditory brainstem response (ABR) evaluates electrical conductivity of the hearing signal through the brainstem.

Pearls

1. Decibel (dB) measurements of sound intensity are on a logarithmic scale.
2. Pure-tone average (PTA) is the average air conduction hearing threshold at three frequencies considered important for speech understanding (500, 1000, and 2000 Hz).
3. Masking is the simultaneous presentation of sound to the *non-test* ear (to "mask" it) while actually testing the other ear with the target stimulus.
4. A Stenger test can be performed to rule out nonorganic (functional hearing loss) or malingering when there is at least a 20 dB difference in air conduction thresholds between ears.
5. A tone 10 dB above the threshold (louder) in the better ear is presented while simultaneously presenting a tone 10 dB below the threshold (quieter) in the poorer-responding ear. The patient should respond if the hearing loss is genuine because the better ear will detect the sound presented to that side. This is reported as a negative Stenger test. Patients who are malingering or have nonorganic hearing loss will not respond, as the sound presented to the poorer ears is quieter than the volume at which they have decided to respond." This is reported as a positive Stenger test.
6. Patients with sudden sensorineural hearing loss should be evaluated urgently, and if there is not a medical contraindication, steroids should be administered transtympanically or systemically.

QUESTIONS

1. **What questions do you ask a patient presenting with hearing loss?**
   As with any evaluation, it is important to first obtain a history of the problem. Details such as onset, course since onset, ear(s) involved, exacerbating and relieving factors, and related symptoms are important. Also noted are the presence of tinnitus, dizziness and/or vertigo, aural fullness/pressure, and ear pain. A detailed family, medical, and social history, including noise exposure, should be obtained to identify risk factors. Also, patients should be asked about temporary or permanent functional changes involving other cranial nerves, in addition to a thorough cranial nerve examination. Recent trauma, either blunt or penetrating, may also produce hearing loss.

2. **Describe the two general types of hearing loss. How are they different?**
   1. Conductive hearing loss (CHL) results from disruption in the passage of sound from the external ear to the oval window. Anatomically, this pathway includes the ear canal, tympanic membrane, and ossicles. Such a loss may be due to cerumen impaction, tympanic membrane perforation, a foreign body, otitis media, or ossicular abnormality. CHL is often correctable with medical or surgical treatment.
   2. Sensorineural hearing loss (SNHL) results from otologic abnormalities beyond the oval window. Such abnormalities may affect the hair cells of the cochlea or the neural fibers of the eighth cranial nerve. Presbycusis, or hearing loss related to aging, is an example of SNHL. An eighth cranial nerve tumors may also lead to such a loss. SNHL are generally permanent and typically unmanageable medically. One exception is sudden SNHL which may respond to timely steroid treatment. Hearing aids usually benefit patients with SNHL. Patients could also have mixed hearing loss, a hearing loss with both a conductive and sensorineural component (e.g., chronic otitis media coexistent with cochlear damage) (Fig. 33.1).

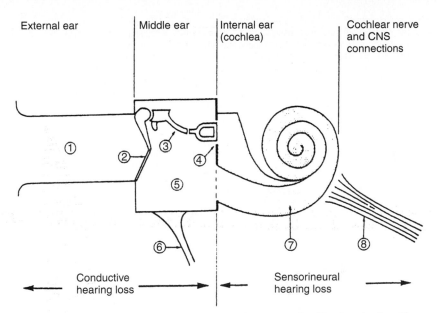

Fig. 33.1 Conductive and sensorineural hearing loss. Examples: (1) wax, inflammatory swelling; (2) perforated eardrum; (3) necrosed or immobile ossicles; (4) stapes fixation by otosclerosis; (5) otitis media; (6) eustachian tube block; (7) sensory presbycusis, mumps, noise injury; and (8) neural presbycusis, acoustic tumors. (Reproduced with permission from Coleman BH: *Diseases of the Nose, Throat, and Ear and Head and Neck*, Edinburgh, 1992, Churchill Livingstone, p. 106.) (From Goldstone H: *Netter's Surgical Anatomy and Approaches*, Philadelphia, 2014, Saunders, pp. 389–398.)

3. **What is the Weber tuning fork test? How is it performed and interpreted?**
   The Weber test is not a test of hearing, but it can provide information about the type of hearing loss. In the Weber test a tuning fork is struck and its base is placed midline on the patient's forehead. Commonly, a 512 Hz and/or 1024 Hz (hertz or Hz: a unit of measure for cycles per second) tuning fork is used. The patient is first asked where the tone is perceived and next whether the tone is louder in one ear or the other. With CHL, the tone is louder and localizes to the poorer hearing or affected ear. With SNHL, the patient perceives the tone as louder in the better hearing or unaffected ear. Patients with equal hearing or bilaterally symmetric hearing loss will localize the sound to the skull midline.

4. **What is the Rinne tuning fork test? How is it performed?**
   The Rinne test is also used to differentiate between CHL and SNHL. The test is performed by alternately placing the prongs of a vibrating tuning fork at the patient's ear canal and the base of the tuning fork on the patient's mastoid bone. The patient is asked whether the tone sounds louder at the ear canal or on the mastoid. In a patient with normal hearing and normal middle ear status, the tuning fork sounds louder at the ear canal or equally loud in both positions. Similar findings are expected in a patient with SNHL. Patients with CHL, however, hear the tuning fork sound louder at the mastoid position (because their bone conduction is better than their air conduction. This is referred to as a negative Rinne test.). A negative result is obtained when the CHL is at least 25 dB hearing level (dB HL).

5. **Why are tuning fork tests performed?**
   Tuning fork tests are primarily performed to assist in evaluating the possible type of hearing loss (CHL versus SNHL). They contribute little to evaluating the presence or degree of hearing loss, which should be assessed through a complete audiometric evaluation. However, they can be useful in a situation where the patient would not tolerate complete audiometric testing (e.g., a trauma patient in the ICU) or if audiometry is not available.

6. **How wide is the frequency range for normal hearing?**
   The young human ear can detect sound in the frequency range of 20 to 20,000 Hz. High-frequency hearing tends to deteriorate with age. Audiometric test procedures typically evaluate from 250 to 8000 Hz, due to the range of speech frequencies in spoken language.

7. What is a decibel?

A decibel (dB) is an arbitrary unit of measurement, for the intensity of sound, that is logarithmic in nature. There are several decibel scales used to measure sound intensity and hearing sensitivity, so it is necessary to identify the reference scale, when presenting a value in decibels. For example, hearing is measured on a biologic scale in decibels hearing level (dB HL), whereas environmental sounds are measured on a physical scale in decibels sound pressure level (dB SPL). The normal ear is not equally sensitive to all frequencies, as it is able to hear mid-frequencies better than low and high frequencies. Normal hearing is approximately 45 dB SPL at 125 Hz, 7 dB SPL at 1000 Hz, and 16 dB SPL at 6000 Hz. A reference level of 0 dB HL represents normal hearing across the assessed frequency spectrum.

8. What is an audiogram?

An audiogram is produced using a relative measure of the patient's hearing, as compared with an established "normal" value (Fig. 33.2). It is a graphic representation of auditory threshold responses that are obtained from testing a patient's hearing with pure-tone stimuli (Table 33.1). An auditory threshold is defined as the minimum intensity at which a patient perceives a sound stimulus 50% of the time. The parameters of the audiogram are frequency, as measured in cycles per second or hertz (Hz), and intensity, as measured in dB HL. The typical audiogram is determined by establishing hearing thresholds for single-frequency sounds at 250, 500, 1000, 2000, 4000, and 8000 Hz; the primary speech frequencies are 500, 1000, 2000, and 4000 Hz. The interoctave frequencies 3000 and 6000 Hz are also commonly measured.

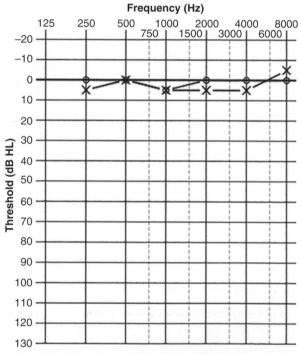

Fig. 33.2 A normal audiogram. (Reproduced with permission from Lee KJ: *Essential Otolaryngology – Head and Neck Surgery*, 5th ed, Norwalk, CT, 1995, Appleton and Lange, p. 37.)

Table 33.1 Commonly Used Audiometric Symbols

RIGHT EAR	INTERPRETATION	LEFT EAR
O	Unmasked air conduction	X
△	Masked air conduction	□
<	Unmasked bone conduction	>
[	Masked bone conduction	]
↙	No response	↘

Table 33.2 Degrees of Hearing Loss

DEGREE OF HEARING LOSS	HEARING LEVEL RANGE (dB HL)
Normal	−10 to 15
Slight	16 to 25
Mild	26 to 40
Moderate	41 to 55
Moderately severe	56 to 70
Severe	71 to 90
Profound	91+

9. **What is normal hearing?**

Normal adult hearing is between 0 and 20 dB HL. The measurement of hearing is based on threshold responses, with a threshold defined as the dB HL level at which a patient perceives a sound stimulus 50% of the time. Patients with hearing loss have audiograms with poorer thresholds, >20 dB HL (Table 33.2).

10. **What is the pure-tone average?**

The PTA is an estimate of a person's ability to hear within three important speech frequencies. The value is calculated by averaging the air conduction hearing thresholds at 500, 1000, and 2000 Hz. For individuals with a precipitously sloping hearing loss, Fletcher's average is commonly used, which is the average of the two best thresholds that are typically used to obtain the PTA. The PTA is used to assess reliability rather than functional hearing ability.

11. **When an audiologist says that a hearing loss requires masking to verify, what does this mean?**

Loud sounds presented to the test ear can travel, via bone conduction, through the skull, and be perceived in the opposite, non-test ear. This phenomenon, called crossover, can obscure measurement results in the test ear. Therefore, the non-test ear must be excluded from the test. Masking is the simultaneous presentation of sound to the *non-test* ear while testing the other ear with the target stimulus; this serves to prevent the non-test ear from interfering with sound perception in the test ear.

12. **How does the audiologist distinguish between air and bone conduction deficits?**

In measurements of air conduction hearing thresholds, headphones or insert earphones deliver sound to the patient. If a hearing loss is noted, bone conduction hearing thresholds are subsequently measured. Bone conduction is tested by placing a vibrating device (a bone oscillator), behind the ear, on the mastoid. The bone oscillator stimulates the cochlea, bypassing the outer and middle ear. Patients with SNHL have equal or near equal hearing thresholds by air and bone conduction, as the hearing loss originates from the cochlea or beyond. Patients with CHL have normal cochlear function, therefore, they have better hearing thresholds by bone conduction than they do by air conduction. This difference in air conduction and bone conduction thresholds is called the air-bone gap (ABG).

13. **What do you look for on an audiogram to determine whether hearing loss is sensorineural or conductive?**

When there is a hearing loss, look for an air-bone gap. An air-bone gap is present if there is a difference in hearing between the thresholds obtained using insert earphones/headphones (air conduction) and those obtained using bone oscillator (bone conduction). A significant air-bone gap (>10 dB) between a normal bone conduction threshold and an abnormal air conduction threshold indicates CHL (Fig. 33.3). Because the patient hears better through bone conduction than air conduction, a gap exists between the two measurements. With SNHL (Fig. 33.4), the air and bone conduction thresholds are approximately equal (≤10 dB) but, overall, both measurements show hearing loss (>20 dB HL). In cases of mixed hearing loss you will see abnormal bone conduction thresholds with significantly poorer air conduction thresholds (Fig. 33.5).

14. **What is the speech reception threshold test?**

The speech reception threshold (SRT) test is performed to confirm the pure-tone threshold findings. The patient is familiarized with a specific set of two-syllable words that are pronounced with equal emphasis on each syllable. These words are called spondees (e.g., airplane, popcorn, rainbow). The SRT is defined as the lowest intensity at which the patient correctly identifies the word in 50% of the presentations. The SRT should be within ±7 dB of the three-frequency PTA or Fletcher's average. If an SRT cannot be obtained, such as with babies, a speech awareness threshold (SAT) is evaluated instead.

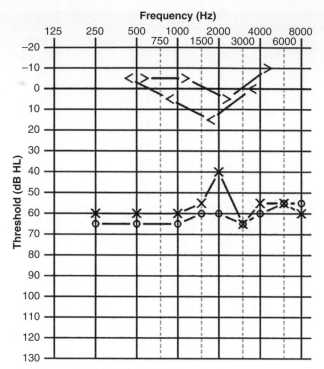

Fig. 33.3 Air-bone gap typical of a conductive hearing loss. (Reproduced with permission from Lee KJ: *Essential Otolaryngology – Head and Neck Surgery*, 5th ed, Norwalk, CT, 1995, Appleton and Lange, p. 37.)

15. **Describe word recognition and sentence recognition tests.**
    The purpose of speech recognition tests is to assess the patient's ability to repeat words or sentences when the stimulus loudness level is sufficient for the listener to perform maximally. A standardized list of single-syllable words or sentences is presented 40 dB above the SRT or at the patient's most comfortable listening level. The patient repeats each word or sentence, and the score is determined according to the percentage of words that are correctly identified. Good to excellent speech understanding results in scores between 80% and 100%; however, scores are dependent on the number of items in each list and the test method. Speech recognition is assessed in quiet or in the presence of varying degrees of background noise and is used to estimate functional performance with and without hearing aids, cochlear implants, and bone conduction hearing devices.

16. **What do you do when the patient's tuning fork test results do not agree with the audiogram?**
    Consider a number of factors. Has the audiometric equipment recently been producing questionable results? Do both insert earphones/headphones work? Is the examiner properly using the tuning forks? Is the examiner comfortable with the anatomy? Does the patient understand the instructions? Does the patient have a secondary gain? If available, prior audiograms should be obtained for comparison. Most importantly, the inconsistency needs to be resolved.

17. **What is the immittance test battery?**
    The immittance test battery is not a hearing test but rather an electroacoustic procedure that is used to evaluate the status of the auditory system. The test typically include tympanometry (a measurement of energy transmission through the middle ear) and ipsilateral and contralateral acoustic reflex thresholds (measurements of stapedius muscle contraction that provide information regarding the integrity of the acoustic reflex arc from the outer ear to the lower brainstem).

18. **How is the examiner's subjective evaluation of the tympanic membrane quantified objectively?**
    Tympanometry can be thought of as electronic pneumatic otoscopy. It is an objective test that measures the mobility, or compliance, of the middle ear system including the tympanic membrane. Tympanometry also provides

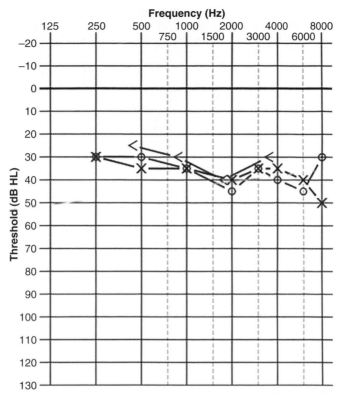

Fig. 33.4 Audiogram showing sensorineural hearing loss. (Reproduced with permission from Lee KJ: *Essential Otolaryngology – Head and Neck Surgery*, 5th ed, Norwalk, CT, 1995, Appleton and Lange, p. 38.)

information about the volume of the outer ear canal, from the tip of the tympanometric probe to the tympanic membrane, as well as the integrity of the tympanic membrane (e.g., presence of a Pressure Equalization [PE] tube or tympanic membrane perforation, patency status of a PE tube). To perform the test, a hermetic seal is obtained between the instrument probe and the opening to the external ear canal. The probe emits a tone, most commonly 226 Hz, although 1000 Hz is used for infants younger than 6 months of age (younger than 1 year for children with Down syndrome). Compliance is quantified by mechanically modifying air pressure in the ear canal and measuring the subsequent change in sound pressure level. Tympanometric results, including equivalent ear canal volume (ECV), tympanometric peak pressure (TPP), compliance, and tympanometric width, are displayed on a graph called a tympanogram. Normative values for the parameters of the tympanogram can vary depending on the clinical instrument, the probe stimulus, and whether the patient is a child or an adult. The compliance of the middle ear system is at its maximum when air pressure on both sides of the eardrum is equal. Normal compliance is typically considered to range from 0.2 to 1.5 mmho. TPP is relatively equal to the patient's middle ear pressure. Normal peak pressure is between +25 and −150 daPa and represents normal eustachian tube function. Negative peak pressure greater than −150 daPa is indicative of poor eustachian tube function.

19. **The chart of a patient says that she had a Type B tympanogram on her last visit. What does this mean?**
   Tympanograms are classified into five configurations (Table 33.3).

20. **How can I tell whether a "flat" tympanometric configuration is a Type B tympanogram or indicates a patent PE tube/tympanic membrane perforation?**
   Look at the ECV on the tympanogram. The ECV is typically reported in centimeters cubed (cm^3) and is the measured volume of air from the tympanometric probe to the eardrum, when the tympanic membrane is intact. However, in situations where the tympanic membrane is perforated or there is a patent PE tube in the eardrum, the ECV is large, as the volume of air through the middle ear space is also included. Normal ECVs for children range from approximately 0.5 to 1.0 cm^3, and normal ECVs for adults can be as large as approximately 3.0 cm^3.

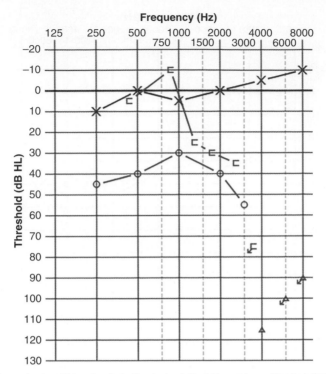

Fig. 33.5 An audiogram showing mild to profound mixed hearing loss in the right ear and normal hearing in the left ear.

Table 33.3	Tympanometric Configurations
Type A	Normal middle ear function (Normal ear canal volume [ECV], normal tympanometric peak pressure [TPP], normal compliance/movement)
Type A$_s$	Middle ear system is stiffer than normal (e.g., otosclerosis) (Decreased compliance/movement, normal ECV, normal TPP)
Type A$_d$	Middle ear system is more flaccid than normal (e.g., ossicular discontinuity) (Increased compliance/movement, normal ECV, normal TPP)
Type B	Middle ear system is maximally stiff (e.g., middle ear effusion, otitis media) Also known as a "flat" tympanogram, indicating that the middle ear system is not compliant/moving (No compliance/no movement, no TPP, normal ECV)
Type C	Eustachian tube dysfunction (Negative TPP [> -150 daPa], normal ECV, normal compliance/movement)

21. **What is the function of the stapedius muscle reflex?**
    The stapedius muscle, attached to the posterior crus of the stapes, contracts reflexively at the onset of a loud stimulus. The muscle contracts bilaterally, even when only one ear is stimulated. When the stapedius muscle contracts, it causes immediate stiffening of the ossicles and decreased compliance of the middle ear system and tympanic membrane. This movement can be measured as the acoustic reflex threshold (ART) or the lowest decibel level at which the contraction of the stapedius muscle is elicited. It is an important part of the immittance test battery.

22. **Describe the acoustic reflex neural pathways, also known as the acoustic reflex arc.**
    The acoustic reflex has both an ipsilateral and contralateral pathway. The majority of neurons run through the ipsilateral pathway. The ipsilateral pathway begins at the outer ear and proceeds through the middle ear space, eighth nerve, cochlear nucleus, trapezoid body, superior olivary complex, and facial motor nucleus to the ipsilateral stapedius muscle. The contralateral pathway crosses the brain stem at the superior olivary complex and continues to the opposite superior olivary complex, cochlear nucleus, trapezoid body, motor nucleus of the facial nerve, and stapedius muscle.

23. **How is the acoustic reflex measured?**
    The acoustic reflex is measured with the same immittance equipment used to complete tympanometry. A loud stimulus is presented through the probe, causing the stapedius muscle to contract and decreasing the compliance of the middle ear system. The ipsilateral reflex is both elicited and measured in the test ear. The contralateral reflex is elicited in the test ear but measured in the non-test ear. To be clear, right contralateral acoustic reflex thresholds are obtained by presenting the sound stimulus to the right ear and measuring the change in middle ear compliance in the left ear. Left contralateral acoustic reflex thresholds are obtained by presenting the sound stimulus to the left ear and measuring the change in middle ear compliance in the right ear. Measurement of the acoustic reflex threshold is a valuable tool used to determine the integrity of the neural pathways that are a part of the acoustic reflex arc. Acoustic reflex threshold testing provides information that can indicate a problem along the pathway such as an eighth nerve tumor, the presence of certain types and/or degrees of hearing loss, or a loudness tolerance issue.

24. **What is an auditory brainstem response?**
    An auditory brainstem response (ABR) is an objective physiologic measurement of auditory neural function. This auditory evoked potential (AEP) is used to assess audiologic and/or neurologic function. ABR recordings are interpreted in an effort to predict behavioral hearing thresholds in infants, children, and adults who cannot or will not participate in a behavioral hearing evaluation.
    Assessment requires that the patient is either asleep or in a quiet, relaxed state. A series of clicks or frequency-specific tone bursts is delivered to the patient's ear through an earphone or bone conduction oscillator placed on the mastoid. When the acoustic signal stimulates the auditory system, a series of small electrical potentials is produced along the peripheral and central auditory pathways up to the level of the brainstem. This electrical activity is detected by scalp electrodes, amplified, and averaged using a computer.
    The electrical activity is displayed as a waveform with five peaks. Each peak occurs at a specific latency (millisecond) and corresponds to a site in the auditory pathway. By decreasing the intensity of the sound stimulus to a level not detected by the auditory system, the peaks of the waveform disappear, yielding a flat line that indicates no response to the stimulus.

25. **How do you interpret an auditory brainstem response?**
    The mnemonic E. COLI will help you remember which structure corresponds to each waveform of the ABR.
    Wave I **E**ighth nerve action potential
    Wave II **C**ochlear nucleus
    Wave III **O**livary complex (superior)
    Wave IV **L**ateral lemniscus
    Wave V **I**nferior colliculus
    Audiologists identify the waves and obtain information on interwave intervals and absolute peak latencies at various intensities. Type, degree, and configuration of hearing loss can be estimated using ABR assessment. Additionally, click ABR is the gold standard for diagnosing auditory neuropathy spectrum disorder, a rare auditory disorder diagnosed by the presence of a cochlear microphonic (outer hair cell function), absent or abnormal ABR waveforms, present otoacoustic emissions (OAEs), and absent acoustic reflexes.

26. **What is an auditory steady-state response?**
    Like an ABR, an auditory steady-state response (ASSR) is an AEP used to estimate behavioral hearing thresholds. Unlike click ABR, which provides a single estimate of behavioral hearing thresholds in the mid- to high-frequency region, ASSR uses frequency-specific tonal stimuli. It assesses whether the auditory response and neurologic integrity of the auditory system are phase-locked to the stimulus. Because ASSR utilizes pure-tone stimuli, the presentation intensity can be louder than with an ABR. It is used to estimate hearing thresholds at specific frequencies as well as differentiate degrees of hearing loss. It cannot be used to assess neurologic function.

27. **What are otoacoustic emissions?**
    Otoacoustic emissions (OAEs) are an objective measure of cochlear outer hair cell function. Evoked OAEs are low-level sounds produced by the cochlea following acoustic stimulation. Transient Evoked otoacoustic emissions (TEOAEs) and Distortion Product otoacoustic emissions (DPOAEs) are the two types of OAEs used clinically. OAEs are most often described as present, reduced, or absent in various test frequency regions. Reduced or absent OAEs are an indication of ear pathology. OAEs will be reduced or absent if outer or middle ear

pathology prevents signal transmission through the auditory system or inner ear pathology prevents production of the OAEs such as sensorineural hearing loss. Of note, it is possible for OAEs to be present with mild or even moderate hearing loss. OAEs are present in patients with auditory neuropathy because OAEs are not a measure of neural function.

28. **What is pseudohypacusis (also known as nonorganic or functional hearing loss)?**
A number of factors may lead a person to feign or exaggerate a hearing loss, including psychological factors or potential monetary gain. Certain inconsistencies during a hearing evaluation might indicate pseudohypacusis or malingering. Based on the cross-check principle, all components of the hearing evaluation should be consistent. Specifically, there should be agreement between the PTA and the SRT/SAT, that is the PTA should be within ±7 dB of the SRT/SAT. Test-retest reliability should be good. Another way to determine whether hearing loss truly exists when a patient presents with unilateral or asymmetric hearing loss is the Stenger test. The Stenger test can be done when there is at least a 20 dB threshold difference between ears. It is conducted at any frequency where the threshold difference between ears is ≥20 dB by presenting a tone 10 dB above the threshold in the better ear while simultaneously presenting a tone 10 dB below the threshold in the poorer ear. The patient should respond if the hearing loss is genuine, and this is reported as a *negative* Stenger test. However, patients with nonorganic hearing loss will not respond, and this is reported as a *positive* Stenger test. Additional measures such as ABR, OAEs, and ART can assist in teasing out presence or absence of hearing loss.

CONTROVERSY

29. **When should a primary care physician be concerned about a patient's hearing complaint?**
Always. All patients who suspect hearing loss or who report difficulty with speech understanding need further evaluation. Often, patients with CHL are successfully treated by medical or surgical means. Patients with SNHL need to be medically evaluated prior to being fit with hearing aids. Patients with a history of sudden-onset hearing loss, trauma, infection associated with the loss, or asymmetric hearing loss should have thorough audiologic and otolaryngologic evaluations. Symptoms of tinnitus, aural fullness/pressure, vertigo, or ear drainage also necessitate complete otolaryngologic evaluation.

BIBLIOGRAPHY

Brown DK, Dort JC: Auditory neuropathy: when test results conflict, *J Otolaryngol* 30:46–51, 2001.
Clark JG: Uses and abuses of hearing loss classification, *ASHA* 23:493–500, 1981.
Griffiths TD: Central auditory pathologies, *Br Med Bull* 63:107–120, 2002.
Jerger J, Hayes D: The cross-check principle in pediatric audiometry, *Arch Otolaryngol* 102:614–620, 1976.
Johnson KC: Audiologic assessment of children with suspected hearing loss, *Otol aryngol Clin North Am* 35:711–732, 2002.
Lemkens N, Vermeire K, Brokx JP, et al: Interpretation of pure-tone thresholds in sensorineural hearing loss (SNHL): a review of measurement variability and age-specific references, *Acta Otorhinolaryngol Belg* 56:341–352, 2002.
Martin FN, Clack JG: *Introduction to Audiology*, 8th ed, 2003, Allyn and Bacon.
Meurer J, Malloy M, Kolb M, et al: Newborn hearing testing at Wisconsin hospitals: a review of the need for universal screening, *WMJ* 99:43–46, 2000.
Murphy MR, Selesnick SH: Cost-effective diagnosis of acoustic neuromas: a philosophical, macroeconomic, and technological decision, *Otolaryngol Head Neck Surg* 127:253–259, 2002.
Pichora-Fuller MK, Souza PE: Effects of aging on auditory processing of speech, *Int J Audiol* 42(Suppl 2):2S11–12S, 2003.
Rapin I, Gravel J: Auditory neuropathy: physiologic and pathologic evidence calls for more diagnostic specificity, *Int J Pediatr Otorhinolaryngol* 67:707–728, 2003.
Rosenhall U: The influence of aging on noise-induced hearing loss, *Noise Health* 5:47–53, 2003.
Sininger YS: Audiologic assessment in infants, *Curr Opin Otolaryngol Head Neck Surg* 11:378–382, 2003.
Sininger YS, Hunter LL, Hayes D, Roush PA, Uhler KM: Evaluation of speed and accuracy of next-generation auditory steady state response and auditory brainstem response audiometry in children with normal hearing and hearing loss, *Ear Hear* 39(6):1207–1223, 2018.
Stewart MG: Outcomes and patient-based hearing status in conductive hearing loss, *Laryngoscope* 111(11 Pt 2):1–21, 2001.
Thornton AR, Raffin MJM: Speech-discrimination scores modeled as a binomial variable, *J Speech Hear Res* 21:507–518, 1978.
Vermeire K, Brokx JP, Lemkens N, et al: Speech recognition tests in sensorineural hearing loss, *Acta Otorhinolaryngol Belg* 57:169–175, 2003.
Watkin PM: Neonatal screening for hearing impairment, *Semin Neonatol* 6:501–509, 2001.
Zadeh MH, Selesnick SH: Evaluation of hearing impairment, *Compr Ther* 27:302–310, 2001.

CHAPTER 34

HEARING LOSS AND OTOTOXICITY

Cristina Cabrera-Muffly, MD, FACS

KEY POINTS

1. When evaluating a patient with hearing loss, perform tuning fork tests (Weber and Rinne) to help determine the type of hearing loss. If this does not agree with the audiogram, discuss with the audiologist.
2. It is important to workup speech delay in children with audiometry and a comprehensive ear exam.
3. Medical clearance for hearing aids should be performed in every patient prior to hearing aid fitting. This includes a thorough history and physical exam to rule out other causes besides the most common presbycusis.
4. Common ototoxic medications include aminoglycoside antibiotics, platinum-based chemotherapeutic medications, loop diuretics, and salicylates.
5. If a patient has prolonged unilateral otitis media with effusion, perform nasopharyngoscopy to rule out mass obstruction of the eustachian tube opening.

Pearls

1. Top causes of conductive hearing loss (CHL)
   - Cerumen impaction
   - Otitis media with effusion (most common cause in children)
   - Tympanic membrane perforation
   - Otosclerosis
2. Top causes of sensorineural hearing loss (SNHL)
   - Presbycusis
   - Noise exposure
   - Hereditary
3. Treatment for sudden SNHL
   - Confirm with audiogram
   - High-dose oral steroid burst and taper or transtympanic steroid injection
   - Magnetic resonance imaging (MRI) internal auditory canals (IACs) to evaluate for acoustic neuroma
4. When to obtain imaging for hearing loss
   - Temporal bone trauma
   - Suspected cholesteatoma
   - Suspected tumor (acoustic neuroma, glomus tumor, etc.)
   - In children (especially prior to any surgical intervention beyond pressure equalization (PE) tubes)
5. The most common radiographic finding in pediatric SNHL is enlarged vestibular aqueduct.

QUESTIONS

1. **What should the history include when evaluating hearing loss?**
   When evaluating any type of hearing loss, it is important to ask about laterality, duration, progression, current severity, associated factors (such as otalgia, otorrhea, tinnitus, vertigo, and aural fullness), ototoxic medication use, head trauma, family history (to assess for genetic factors), autoimmune disease, and prior otologic surgery.

2. **What should the physical exam include when evaluating a patient with hearing loss?**
   A complete head and neck exam should be performed, with a focus on otologic and neurologic exams. The otologic exam should include examination of the pinna, external auditory canal, tympanic membrane, and middle ear. Tuning fork tests (Weber and Rinne) and pneumatic otoscopy should also be routinely performed.

3. **How can you differentiate between SNHL and CHL on an audiogram?**
   The two main ways to differentiate between SNHL and CHL on an audiogram include the presence of an air–bone gap and abnormal tympanogram. An air–bone gap (Fig. 34.1) is present during conductive or mixed (both SNHL and CHL) hearing losses and is caused by differences in air-conducted and bone-conducted stimuli. During the vibratory portion of the audiogram, a patient with CHL will be better able to hear the stimulus because the transmission of sound through the mastoid bone is bypassing the site of blockage in the external or middle ear.

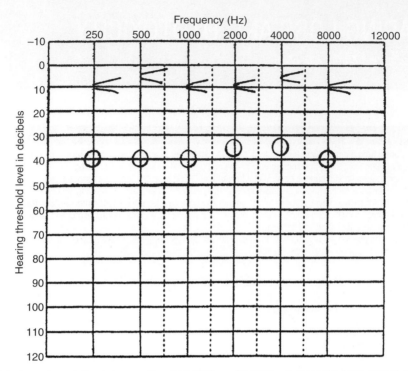

Fig. 34.1 Audiogram demonstrating air–bone gap. (From Jafek BW, Murrow BW: *ENT Secrets*, 3rd ed, Philadelphia, 2005, Mosby.)

The tympanogram measures the compliance of the tympanic membrane. Increased compliance (type A$_d$) can indicate ossicular chain discontinuity, whereas decreased compliance (type A$_s$) can indicate otosclerosis, both of which can cause conductive hearing loss. Poor compliance (type B) on a tympanogram can indicate a tympanic membrane perforation or middle ear effusion.

4. **What are the common causes of SNHL?**
   The most common causes of SNHL are presbycusis, noise exposure (i.e., machinery, artillery, loud music), and heredity. Less common causes are acoustic trauma, ototoxicity, sudden idiopathic hearing loss, autoimmune hearing loss, Meniere's disease, tumors, and infections (i.e., meningitis, viral labyrinthitis).

5. **What is presbycusis?**
   Presbycusis is age-related hearing loss. This is the most common type of hearing loss in adults, encompassing the great majority of adult-onset hearing loss. Presbycusis is bilateral, symmetric, and slowly progressive high-frequency loss. Onset is in adults over 60 years of age, and the exact cause is unknown. Hearing aids are the most effective treatment.

6. **What guidelines are in place for newborn hearing screening?**
   The US federal government mandates newborn hearing screening, although programs are state regulated. The most commonly used is the otoacoustic emissions test, which examines the outer hair cell response to acoustic stimulation. The other common test is the auditory brainstem response test, in which the eighth nerve and central nervous system produce sounds in response to acoustic stimulation. In either case, if the results are abnormal, the newborn is referred for further testing.

7. **What is the incidence of congenital hearing loss?**
   One to three infants per 1000.

8. **What risk factors predispose children to hearing loss?**
   Risk factors that have been correlated with congenital hearing loss are (per the Joint Committee on Infant Hearing):
   - Family history of childhood onset permanent hearing loss
   - In utero infections (ToRCH = toxoplasmosis, other [syphilis, parvovirus, varicella], rubella, cytomegalovirus, herpes)

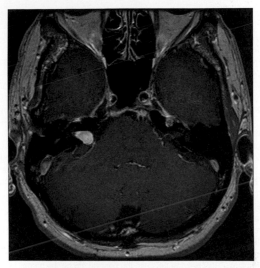

Fig. 34.2 Imaging: acoustic neuroma T1-weighted axial MRI with contrast of a right-sided acoustic neuroma. (Courtesy of Stephen Cass, MD, Department of Otolaryngology Head and Neck Surgery, University of Colorado.)

- Illness requiring Neonatal Intensive Care Unit admission for more than 48 hours
- Craniofacial anomalies, especially involving the pinna or external auditory canal
- Characteristic signs of syndromes known to cause hearing loss

     Other factors associated with increased rates of congenital hearing loss in the literature:
- Low birth weight (less than 1500 g)
- Hypoxia
- Hyperbilirubinemia
- Low Apgar scores
- Head trauma
- Ototoxic medications

9. **What are the developmental milestones for pediatric speech and hearing?**
   0 to 3 months: startled by loud sounds, calmed by familiar voices
   6 months: localize sounds
   9 months: respond to name and can mimic sounds
   12 months: say first words
   18 months: can follow simple commands
   2 years: say 20 or more words and put together two-word sentences

10. **When should SNHL be evaluated with imaging?**
    In children, MRIs or computed tomography (CT) scans of the temporal bones are usually performed for all SNHL, although the majority of these scans will be normal. The most common finding in pediatric SNHL is enlarged vestibular aqueduct. In adults, MRI of the IACs with contrast is performed for asymmetric SNHL or sudden SNHL to evaluate for acoustic neuroma (Fig. 34.2) and other cerebellopontine angle tumors.

11. **Which medications can cause ototoxicity?**
    - Antibiotics (specifically aminoglycosides and vancomycin)
    - Chemotherapy drugs (cisplatin)
    - Loop diuretics (furosemide, ethacrynic acid)
    - NSAIDs and salicylates (aspirin)

12. **How do ototoxic medications cause hearing loss?**
    Aminoglycosides damage both vestibular and cochlear hair cells. Streptomycin and gentamycin affect vestibular function more than hearing function, and the opposite is true for neomycin and tobramycin. Vancomycin potentiates the ototoxic effect of aminoglycosides but does not appear to be ototoxic alone. Cisplatin damages outer hair cells. Loop diuretics damage the stria vascularis (which maintains the endocochlear potential). NSAIDs and salicylates cause damage to the cochlea, only occurring with high doses, which is almost always completely

reversible with discontinuation of the drug. Since most ototoxic medications are excreted by the renal system, renal impairment can lead to higher rates of ototoxicity.

13. **How does ototoxicity present?**
The first symptom is usually tinnitus, followed by perception of hearing loss. Hearing loss is usually symmetric and affects the high frequencies first. With continued exposure, the lower frequencies are affected. The American Academy of Audiology recommends ototoxicity audiology protocols that include pure tone and distortion product otoacoustic emission (a type of otoacoustic emission) testing at ultra-high frequencies (8 kHz to 20 kHz) because the earliest changes occur at frequencies greater than 8 kHz.

14. **Which cause of SNHL is preventable?**
Noise exposure–associated hearing loss is the only preventable cause of hearing loss. Common situations causing noise exposure hearing loss are exposure to industrial machinery, military or other exposure to gunfire, repeated loud music exposure, and acoustic trauma. Acoustic trauma is a single event of very loud noise that causes a permanent change in hearing (such as an explosion). Prevention includes both avoidance and use of hearing protection.

15. **What treatments are available for SNHL?**
Bilateral mild to severe SNHL is usually treated with hearing aids. Profound bilateral SNHL can be treated with a cochlear implant, which converts sound energy into electrical energy, directly stimulating the hearing nerve. Unilateral SNHL can be treated with a regular hearing aid, a contralateral routing of signals (CROS) hearing aid, or a bone conduction implant. CROS hearing aids use the hearing aid on the poorer hearing ear as a microphone, transmitting the sound to the better hearing ear. A bone conduction implant is a hearing aid that turns sound energy into vibrational energy. An abutment is surgically implanted in the skull, to which the patient attaches a hearing aid. The vibration transmits through the skull to the better hearing ear. In cases of acoustic neuroma, surgery or radiation can sometimes improve hearing. For sudden idiopathic and immune-mediated SNHL, steroid therapy can be effective in improving the amount of hearing loss.

16. **What are the causes of sudden SNHL?**
Most cases of sudden SNHL are considered idiopathic because a cause is never identified. Sudden SNHL can rarely be caused by an acoustic neuroma, which is why an MRI of the internal auditory canals is recommended during workup. Other rare causes are syphilis, Lyme disease, vascular disease, or autoimmune disease.

17. **How should sudden SNHL be treated?**
Per the 2019 clinical practice guideline on sudden hearing loss, the mainstay of therapy for sudden SNHL is steroids. This is usually given as an oral burst and taper of prednisone for 10 to 14 days, with a maximal dose of 60 mg daily. For patients who cannot tolerate oral steroids (for example, patients with brittle diabetes or those in whom steroids exacerbate psychiatric disease), an alternative is transtympanic steroid injection. This procedure involves filling the middle ear space with a concentrated steroid solution. Antivirals are not recommended.

18. **Describe immune-mediated SNHL.**
Immune-mediated SNHL is usually bilateral and rapidly progressive. Many patients have roaring tinnitus. The most common treatment is high-dose steroid therapy, usually with a maximum dose of 60 mg for 4 weeks, followed by a taper. If the hearing loss returns after the steroids are weaned, other long-term immunosuppressant medications (such as methotrexate) may be used.

19. **Which types of trauma can cause hearing loss?**
Acoustic trauma occurs due to exposure to a very loud noise. This can cause either a temporary threshold shift, which will resolve over time, or a permanent threshold shift, which does not resolve with time. Barometric trauma most commonly manifests as pain due to increased pressure in the middle ear, which can lead, in severe cases, to tympanic membrane rupture. More rarely, pressure changes in the inner ear can lead to SNHL. Finally, head trauma can lead to either CHL or SNHL. Temporal bone fractures through the cochlea lead to SNHL, whereas fractures of the ossicles or tympanic membrane injury lead to CHL. Concussive injuries can also cause hearing loss, although this is less common.

20. **What are the common causes of CHL?**
The most common causes of CHL are cerumen impaction, foreign body in the canal, tympanic membrane perforation, middle ear effusion, and ossicular chain abnormalities (such as otosclerosis).

21. **What is otosclerosis?**
Otosclerosis is fixation of the stapes footplate in the oval window caused by abnormal remodeling of bone in this area. Otosclerosis causes either unilateral or bilateral conductive hearing loss that can have a Carhart notch

pattern (artificial 10 to 15 dB decrease in bone conduction at 2000 Hz). Many cases of otosclerosis are hereditary. Treatment includes either stapedectomy or a hearing aid.

22. **How much conductive hearing loss does ossicular chain disruption produce?**
While the amount of loss for other causes of CHL is variable, ossicular chain disruption usually causes a greater than 50 dB hearing loss. "Maximal" CHL is 60 dB.

23. **What is cholesteatoma?**
Cholesteatoma is accumulation of keratin debris in the middle ear or external auditory canal. If left untreated, the debris continues to accumulate and can cause erosion into surrounding tissues, leading to tympanic membrane perforation, damage to the ossicular chain, and even perilymphatic fistulas or tegmen defects. Cholesteatomas can become infected and can lead to recurrent otorrhea.

24. **When should nasopharyngoscopy be performed in the evaluation of CHL?**
Unilateral serous effusion lasting more than 3 months or without a preceding history of acute otitis media should be evaluated with a nasopharyngoscopy to assess for obstruction of the eustachian tube opening. Also, any serous effusion associated with recurrent epistaxis, headache, vision changes, or a painless neck mass should be evaluated with a nasopharyngoscopy to assess for nasopharyngeal carcinoma.

25. **When should CHL be evaluated with imaging?**
CHL after head trauma should be evaluated with temporal bone CT scan. Suspicion for cholesteatoma or middle ear mass (such as glomus tumor) should also be evaluated with a temporal bone CT. Prior to surgical correction of CHL in children, imaging is often performed to check for abnormalities of the inner ear such as enlarged vestibular aqueduct.

26. **What surgical therapies are used to address CHL?**
Perforated tympanic membrane can be repaired with tympanoplasty. Middle ear effusion can be treated by myringotomy with or without an ear tube. Stapedectomy can be done for otosclerosis, in which the stapes is replaced with a prosthesis. Cholesteatoma is treated with mastoidectomy to remove all of the squamous and keratinous debris. If the ossicular chain is disrupted, either a partial or total reconstruction prosthesis can be used to reconstruct the chain.

27. **What are the indications for placement of pressure equalization tubes in children?**
Per the 2013 clinical practice guidelines on tympanostomy tubes in children, tubes should be placed in children who have both persistent middle ear effusion for more than 3 months and documented evidence of hearing difficulty, vestibular problems, or ear discomfort or are at high risk for speech delay. Tubes should also be placed in children with recurrent acute otitis media if persistent effusion is present when the child is evaluated in the office.

28. **What is semicircular canal dehiscence and how does it cause hearing loss?**
This condition, also called labyrinthine fistula, can cause CHL by creating a third window into the inner ear (the first two are the oval and round windows). This is most commonly caused by a dehiscence of bone along the superior semicircular canal next to the dura. CHL occurs because sound energy is lost through the fistula. Tullio sign (dizziness or nystagmus after a loud sound) and Hennebert sign (dizziness or nystagmus after Valsalva maneuver or pneumatic otoscopy) are usually positive if a fistula is present.

BIBLIOGRAPHY

American Speech-Language-Hearing Association, Noise. Available at http://www.asha.org/public/hearing/Noise.

Ashad S, Bojrab DI, Burgio DL, et al: Otology and neurotology. In Pasha R, ed: *Otolaryngology Head and Neck Surgery: Clinical Reference Guide*, 2006, Plural Publishing, pp. 295–390.

Brockenbrough JM, Rybak LP, Matz GJ: Ototoxicity. In Bailey B, ed: *Head and Neck Surgery – Otolaryngology*, Lippincott Williams & Wilkins, pp. 1893–1899.

Chandrasekhar SS, Tsai Do BS, Schwartz SR, et al: Clinical practice guideline: sudden hearing loss (update), *Otolaryngol Head Neck Surg* 161(Suppl 1):S1–S45, 2019.

Durrant JD, Campbell K, Fausti S, et al: *Ototoxicity Monitoring*, 2009, American Academy of Audiology.

Joint Committee on Infant Hearing; American Academy of Audiology: American Academy of Pediatrics; American Speech-Language-Hearing Association; Directors of Speech and Hearing Programs in State Health and Welfare Agencies: Year 2000 position statement: principles and guidelines for early hearing detection and intervention programs, *Pediatrics* 106(4):798–817, 2000.

Rosenfeld RM, Schwartz SR, Pynnonen MA, et al: Clinical practice guideline: tympanostomy tubes in children, *Otolaryngol Head Neck Surg* 149(Suppl 1):S1–S35, 2013.

Ryan AF, Harris JP, Keithley EM: Immune-mediated hearing loss: basic mechanisms and options for therapy, *Acta Otolaryngol Suppl.* (548):38–43, 2002.

Stachler RJ, Chandrasekhar SS, Archer SM, et al: Clinical practice guideline: sudden hearing loss, *Otolaryngol Head Neck Surg* 146(Suppl 3):S1–S35, 2012.

CHAPTER 35

TINNITUS AND HYPERACUSIS

Renee Banakis Hartl, MD, AuD

KEY POINTS

1. Tinnitus is a relatively common disorder, with up to 15% of the population suffering from some degree of abnormal perception.
2. Most subjective tinnitus is hypothesized to result from changes in peripheral auditory function leading to central neural hyperexcitability and cortical reorganization.
3. Though most patients with tinnitus have hearing loss, up to 10% may show no changes in hearing sensitivity on standard audiometric evaluation.
4. Most therapy for subjective tinnitus focuses on integrating principles of sound masking, counseling, and/or psychotherapy.
5. The role of surgery for management of most tinnitus is limited.

Pearls

1. Pulsatile tinnitus may suggest a vascular malformation or neoplasm and indicate a need for radiologic evaluation.
2. MRI with gadolinium contrast and steady-state gradient-echo sequencing is the imaging study of choice for evaluation of asymmetric nonpulsatile tinnitus to test for the presence of a schwannoma of the vestibulocochlear nerve.
3. Palatal or stapedial myoclonus may cause a clicking tinnitus perception and can be associated with systemic disease, requiring additional evaluation.
4. High-dose salicylates are a known cause of reversible mild to moderate flat sensorineural hearing loss and tinnitus.
5. Cochlear implants are an emerging treatment for single-sided deafness that has demonstrated some success in improving the unilateral tinnitus that frequently accompanies this hearing loss.

QUESTIONS

1. **What is tinnitus?**

   Tinnitus is an involuntary perception of sound that originates in the head and is not attributable to a perceivable external source. The word *tinnitus* is derived from the Latin *tinnire*, which means "to ring". Tinnitus is often described as a "ringing" sound in the ear but also includes descriptions such as buzzing, humming, roaring, hissing, and chirping. Tinnitus is a symptom and not a disease in itself.

2. **What is the prevalence of tinnitus?**

   It is generally accepted that approximately 10% to 15% of the population suffers from some degree of tinnitus, and 1% to 2% report that tinnitus has a severely negative impact on quality of life.

3. **How can tinnitus be classified?**

   Tinnitus has historically been classified as either objective (audible to an observer other than the patient) or subjective (perceptible by the patient alone). More useful classification includes description of tinnitus as either pulsatile or nonpulsatile, or categorization by location of injury or generation (external ear, middle ear, sensorineural, or central).

4. **What are somatosounds?**

   A more specific term for many forms of objective tinnitus, somatosounds are objective sounds that are created by the body and potentially audible to the examiner. Examples of somatosounds include perception of myoclonic contractions of the tensor tympani or pulsatile variations in blood flow in vessels near the ear.

5. **What are the proposed mechanisms to explain subjective tinnitus?**

   Both central and peripheral mechanisms have been proposed to explain the origin of tinnitus, but the exact cause remains unclear. Most tinnitus is associated with a cochlear abnormality, although not all patients with tinnitus have associated measurable changes in hearing. It has been proposed that sensory deprivation at the periphery leads to alterations in neural function at higher levels and persistence of these neural changes may contribute to the subjective perceptions of tinnitus. Tonotopic maps in the auditory cortex have been shown to reorganize in animal studies after sensory deprivation in a manner similar to somatosensory cortical organization changes after amputation, leading to the description of tinnitus as a "phantom limb" perception of the auditory cortex.

6. **How is tinnitus evaluated?**
   No objective test is available to definitively verify tinnitus or identify its cause in most cases. An evaluation of tinnitus consists of a thorough case history, complete otologic exam, and an audiometric evaluation. Evaluation may also consist of administration of one of several validated questionnaires, such as the Tinnitus Handicap Inventory, the Tinnitus Handicap Questionnaire, or the Tinnitus Severity Index. Though these surveys provide little objective data, they can help to quantify the severity of impact on quality of life and may be used to track changes in tinnitus perception across various therapy modalities. Additional studies, such as imaging or vestibular evaluation, may be indicated depending on the initial presentation and differential diagnosis.

7. **What is tinnitus matching and what is its value in the assessment and treatment of subjective tinnitus?**
   Tinnitus matching is an audiometric evaluation that generally consists of pitch matching, loudness matching, and minimal suppression level (the amount of masking required to subjectively mask an individual's tinnitus). These objective measures of tinnitus have little validity or clinical application, as tinnitus loudness, pitch, and maskability typically bear no relationship to the severity of the patient's experience or ability to benefit from treatment. Some treatment modalities, including individualized sound stimulation devices, may rely on pitch matching or minimum suppression levels to create customized listening programs targeted at masking an individual's tinnitus.

8. **What signs or symptoms are suggestive of a vascular cause of tinnitus?**
   A pulsatile or throbbing quality that parallels the heartbeat should raise the index of suspicion. A reddish or blue mass behind the tympanic membrane may indicate a glomus tumor arising within the middle ear or a dehiscence of the jugular bulb or carotid artery. Arteriovenous malformations are uncommon but may occur between the occipital artery (passing medial to the mastoid process) and the transverse sinus. A venous hum may represent one of the more common causes of vascular tinnitus. It may signify impingement of the jugular vein by the second cervical vertebrae or suggest an underlying high-output cardiac condition, such as anemia, exercise, pregnancy, or thyrotoxicosis.

9. **What is the imaging study of choice for nonpulsatile tinnitus?**
   MRI with gadolinium is the study of choice to exclude a vestibular schwannoma or other neoplasm of the cerebellopontine angle. Steady-state gradient echo sequences (such as CISS or FIESTA) are also helpful in the workup for vestibular schwannoma. This type of sequence emphasizes T2 signals, making it useful for the evaluation of small structures that are surrounded by cerebrospinal fluid such as cranial nerves.

10. **What is the imaging study of choice for pulsatile tinnitus?**
    Pulsatile tinnitus suggests a vascular neoplasm, vascular anomaly, or vascular malformation (although the cause may be as simple as transient otitis media). Glomus tumors are the most common type of vascular neoplasm. Most neoplasms and anomalies are best seen on bone windows of computed tomography (CT) studies. Dural vascular malformations are often elusive on all cross-sectional imaging studies, and conventional angiography may be necessary to make this diagnosis. Flow-sensitive MR images show vascular loops compressing the eighth cranial nerve. Carotid dissections, aneurysms, atherosclerosis, and fibromuscular dysplasia can be identified on both magnetic resonance (MR)/MR-angiographic studies and CT/CT-angiographic studies.
    Other causes, such as superior semicircular canal dehiscence, otosclerosis, and Paget's disease, may be seen on CT scan. Idiopathic intracranial hypertension often shows characteristic findings of empty sella, thinning of the bony skull base, and prominent arachnoid pits. Multiple sclerosis is a rare cause of pulsatile tinnitus and is best seen on MR studies.

11. **What causes of tinnitus are associated with pathology of the external ear canal?**
    Foreign bodies and cerumen accumulation often cause tinnitus. Hair, insects, and other small objects may come in contact with the tympanic membrane and motion may cause the perception of sound. The mandibular condyle is in close proximity with the external ear canal and disorder of the temporomandibular joint may result in a somatosound perception. Thorough case history and a careful examination are important to help rule out these causes, which often may be easily treated.

12. **What is palatal myoclonus?**
    Palatal myoclonus is the regular, rhythmic contraction of the soft palate and pharyngeal musculature. The muscles involved are the tensor veli palatine, levator veli palatine, salpingopharyngeus, and superficial pharyngeal constrictor.

13. **How can palatal myoclonus be evaluated?**
    The best way to detect palatal myoclonus is by using flexible nasopharyngoscopy in the awake patient to visualize the palate from a superior perch in the nasopharynx. Examining the palate from an oral cavity approach may lead to temporary extermination of the myoclonus while the mouth is stretched open. From a practical approach, both methods of examination should be used.

14. **What is stapedial myoclonus?**
    The rhythmic contractions of the stapedius muscle of the middle ear are known to cause a clicking tinnitus. The tensor tympani may also demonstrate a similar middle ear myoclonus.

15. **How can stapedial myoclonus be evaluated?**
    Myoclonus of the stapedius or tensor tympani musculature is best detected using audiometric immittance testing. Changes in middle ear impedance can be objectively measured in the absence of external stimuli and often correlated subjectively by the patient with the perception of clicking.

16. **Which systemic diseases are associated with myoclonus?**
    Multiple sclerosis, cerebrovascular accidents, intracranial neoplasms, trauma, syphilis, malaria, various psychogenic causes, and other degenerative processes.

17. **Describe the relationship between hearing loss and tinnitus.**
    Most patients with tinnitus (approximately 85%) present with some degree of hearing loss, though not all patients with hearing loss develop tinnitus and all patients with tinnitus do not have abnormal hearing. Approximately 10% of patients with tinnitus present with normal hearing.

18. **What objective changes in otologic function have been found in patients with tinnitus and clinically "normal" hearing?**
    Recent studies have found that patients with tinnitus with hearing thresholds within audiometrically normal limits demonstrate significantly smaller amplitudes of wave I of the ABR than individuals with similar thresholds who do not have tinnitus (Schaette, 2013). This suggests that possible early cochlear damage causing reduced neuronal input may be a contributing factor to the development of tinnitus, even in patients with clinically normal hearing.

19. **What is the relationship between noise exposure and tinnitus?**
    With brief, isolated exposure to loud noise, most individuals experience temporary partial loss in hearing sensitivity and tinnitus that disappears within hours or days of the exposure. Repetitive excessive exposure to noise increases the risk of these changes becoming permanent.

20. **What is hyperacusis? What is the relationship between hyperacusis and tinnitus?**
    Hyperacusis is decreased tolerance to sound stimuli of normally comfortable sound level and pitch. Individuals who suffer from hyperacusis often report that typically tolerable stimuli or sounds of a certain pitch are unbearable or painful. Some researchers believe that tinnitus and hyperacusis are two manifestations of the same alterations in central auditory processing associated with decreased cochlear input and that almost all patients with hyperacusis eventually experience tinnitus.

21. **What is recruitment? What is the relationship between hyperacusis and recruitment?**
    Recruitment is the abnormal loudness growth experienced by many individuals with sensorineural hearing loss in which a small increase in sound intensity level may be perceived as rapidly loud and uncomfortable. The neurophysiologic mechanism underlying recruitment is proposed to relate to broadening of basilar membrane tuning curves, leading to faster activation of a spatial population of auditory nerve fibers. Recruitment can be considered as a peripheral phenomenon secondary to the hair cell loss associated with cochlear pathology, and hyperacusis is considered to be a central phenomenon that can occur in the absence of peripheral injury. While recruitment only occurs in the setting of cochlear hearing loss, hyperacusis is independent of peripheral pathology and can occur with or without hearing loss.

22. **Which medications commonly cause tinnitus?**
    Tinnitus is a known potential side effect of many medications (for a complete list, see Table 35.1). The medications more commonly associated with tinnitus as a side effect are salicylates and aminoglycosides.

23. **What are the effects of high-dose salicylates on tinnitus and hearing?**
    High serum concentrations of salicylates and some nonsteroidal anti-inflammatory drugs (NSAIDs) cause a flat, bilateral hearing loss and tinnitus. The hearing loss is a mild to moderate sensorineural hearing loss of approximately 20 to 40 dB. The incidence rate of salicylate-induced ototoxicity is less than 1%. Salicylates act as competitive inhibitors of chloride at the anion binding site of prestin, the motor protein of the outer hair cell,

Table 35.1 Common Medications That Can Cause Tinnitus

CLASS	EXAMPLES
ACE inhibitor	Enalapril, fosinopril (Monopril)
Anesthetic	Dyclonine, bupivacaine (Marcaine, Sensorcaine), lidocaine
Antibiotic	Aztreonam, ciprofloxacin, erythromycin estolate, erythromycin ethyl succinate/sulfisoxazole (Pediazole), gentamicin (Garamycin), imipenem-cilastatin (Primaxin), sulfisoxazole, trimethoprim/sulfamethoxazole, vancomycin
Antidepressant	Alprazolam (Xanax), amitriptyline (Elavil), desipramine, doxepin, fluoxetine (Prozac), imipramine, maprotiline (Ludiomil), nortriptyline (Pamelor)
Antihistamine	Aspirin-promethazine-pseudoephedrine (Phenergan), chlorpheniramine-phenylpropanolamine (Triaminic), clemastine (Tavist), pseudoephedrine-chlorpheniramine (Deconamine), pseudoephedrine-triprolidine (Actifed)
Antimalarial	Chloroquine, pyrimethamine-sulfadoxine (Fansidar)
Beta blocker	Betaxolol (Kerlone), carteolol (Cartrol), metoprolol (Lopressor), nadolol (Corgard), timolol (Timoptic)
Calcium channel blocker	Diltiazem (Cardizem), nicardipine (Cardene), nifedipine (Procardia)
Diuretic	Acetazolamide (Diamox), amiloride, ethacrynic acid
Narcotic	Dezocine (Dalgan), pentazocine (Talwin)
NSAID	Diclofenac (Voltaren), diflunisal (Dolobid), flurbiprofen (Ansaid), ibuprofen, indomethacin, meclofenamate (Meclomen), naproxen (Naprosyn), sulindac (Clinoril), tolmetin (Tolectin)
Sedative/hypnotic/anxiolytic	Azatadine (Optimine), buspirone (BuSpar), chlorpheniramine phenylpropanolamine (Ornade)
Miscellaneous	Albuterol (Proventil), allopurinol, bismuth subsalicylate (Pepto-Bismol), carbamazepine (Tegretol), cyclobenzaprine (Flexeril), cyclosporine, diphenhydramine (Benadryl), flecainide, hydroxychloroquine (Plaquenil), iohexol (Omnipaque), isotretinoin (Accutane), lithium, methylergonovine (Methergine), nicotine polacrilex (Nicorette), prazosin, omeprazole (Prilosec), quinidine, recombinant hepatitis B vaccine (Recombivax), salicylates, sodium nitroprusside (Nipride), sulfasalazine (Azulfidine), tocainide

ACE, angiotensin-converting enzyme; NSAID, nonsteroidal anti-inflammatory drug.

resulting in reversible alteration in outer hair cell function. Both hearing loss and tinnitus are reversible within 24 to 72 hours of discontinuation of the offending medication.

24. **What percentage of patients with acoustic neuromas have tinnitus as the presenting symptom?**
Ten percent of patients with acoustic neuromas present with tinnitus; however, more than 80% have tinnitus at some point during the course of the disease.

25. **How is auditory stimulation used in the treatment of tinnitus?**
Various methods of treatment involve the use of auditory stimulation. Most early forms of treatment relied on tinnitus masking or the use of external sound stimuli to cover up or mask the tinnitus. Environmental sound generators, radios, televisions, fans, and custom devices worn like hearing aids with broadband masking generators have all been used with varying degrees of success. Hearing aids have also been shown to aid in tinnitus reduction when the pitch of the tinnitus is within the amplification range of the device. Individualized sound stimulation devices focus on providing an enriched acoustic environment to compensate for hearing loss with musical stimuli of a customized frequency spectrum.

26. **What is tinnitus retraining therapy?**
Tinnitus retraining therapy (TRT) is a treatment modality composed of specific counseling strategies and sound therapy. The counseling aspect of TRT focuses on education regarding the neurophysiologic basis of tinnitus and decoupling of tinnitus perception from emotional, stress-based responses. Concurrent sound therapy attempts to reduce the strength of the tinnitus signal through gradual habituation. By reclassifying tinnitus and disengaging the emotionally driven responses, TRT seeks not to physiologically alter tinnitus but rather to decrease the negative impact on quality of life.

27. **Which pharmacologic agents have been used as adjuvant therapy for tinnitus?**
No pharmacologic agent has been demonstrated to show any long-term reduction in tinnitus greater than that of a placebo. Though the role of medication is limited in affecting an individual's perception of tinnitus, several drugs can be used to mediate the stress and anxiety that frequently accompany tinnitus. Tricyclic antidepressants and SSRIs have been used with moderate success in treating associated depression. Benzodiazepines are appropriate therapy to try in patients with severe stress from tinnitus, though they should be used with caution. Interestingly, IV lidocaine has been shown to decrease tinnitus, but its administration and side effects make this therapy impractical. For tinnitus caused by myoclonus, botulinum toxin has been used to temporarily paralyze the causative muscles.

28. **Describe the mechanism of action of lidocaine in tinnitus treatment.**
Lidocaine and several related anesthetics act as central nervous system depressants by inhibiting the influx of sodium and therefore reducing the number of action potentials. One theory to explain tinnitus pertains to the high basal firing rate of the normal auditory system and the loss of its natural inhibitors. Anesthetics are thought to augment or replace this natural inhibition process, holding tinnitus in check. At present, intravenous lidocaine is the only medication that can reliably stop tinnitus in many patients. However, it is impractical because of the short duration of action and need for intravenous administration.

29. **What is the role of complementary and alternative medicine in tinnitus treatment?**
No treatments available through complementary or alternative medicine have been shown to be effective at reducing tinnitus perception in randomized controlled trials. Meditation, acupuncture, controlled breathing, biofeedback, and hypnotherapy have not demonstrated reduction in tinnitus, but relaxation techniques are often beneficial in managing stress-related side effects of tinnitus. Relaxation techniques are often incorporated into cognitive behavioral therapy (CBT), which seeks to methodically identify and modify maladaptive behaviors associated with abnormal tinnitus perception.

30. **What surgical treatments are available for tinnitus management?**
The role of surgery in the management of tinnitus is limited. Surgical management of pathologic conditions often associated with tinnitus, such as vascular malformations, otosclerosis, acoustic neuromas, and temporomandibular joint disorder, may improve subjective perceptions, but the majority of patients with tinnitus do not have an identifiable pathology. Cochlear implantation in patients with bilateral profound hearing loss has been demonstrated to reduce or completely eliminate tinnitus in up to 86% of patients, though small percentages report a worsening or development of new tinnitus after surgery. More recently, cochlear implantation has been approved by the U.S. Food and Drug Administration for treatment of single-sided deafness (SSD), in which patients meet candidacy for implantation in one ear but retain normal hearing sensitivity in the other ear. Across several large reviews, patients with SSD who have undergone cochlear implantation have reported high levels of subjective relief from tinnitus when using the device. For tinnitus related to palatal myoclonus, injection of botulinum toxin into the palatoglossus muscle has proven to effectively reduce the perception. Stapedial or tensor tympani myoclonus has been successfully treated with lysis of the tendons via a surgical middle ear exploration.

BIBLIOGRAPHY

Andersson G, Vretblad P, Larsen HC, et al: Longitudinal follow-up of tinnitus complaints, *Arch Otolaryngol Head Neck Surg* 127:175–179, 2001.
Baguley D, McFerran D, Hall D: Tinnitus, *Lancet* 382:1600–1607, 2013.
Berry JA, Gold SL, Frederick EA, et al: Patient-based outcomes in patients with primary tinnitus undergoing tinnitus retraining therapy, *Arch Otolaryngol Head Neck Surg* 128:1153–1157, 2002.
Dauman R, Bouscau-Faure F: Assessment and amelioration of hyperacusis in tinnitus patients, *Acta Otolaryngol* 125(5):503–509, 2005.
Eggermont JJ, Roberts LE: The neuroscience of tinnitus, *Trends Neurosci* 27(11):676–682, 2004.
Folmer RL, Griest SE: Chronic tinnitus resulting from head or neck injuries, *Laryngoscope* 113:821–827, 2003.
Isaacson JE, Moyer MT, Schuler HG, et al: Clinical associations between tinnitus and chronic pain, *Otolaryngol Head Neck Surg* 128:706–710, 2003.
Jastreboff PJ: Phantom auditory perception (tinnitus): mechanisms of generation and perception, *Neurosci Res* 8:221–254, 1990.
Jastreboff PJ, Hazell JWP: *Tinnitus Retraining Therapy: Implementing the Neurophysiologic Model*, 2004, Cambridge University Press.
Langguth B, Kreuzer PM, Kleinjung T, et al: Tinnitus: causes and clinical management, *Lancet Neurol* 12:920–930, 2013.
Lockwood AH, Salvi RJ, Burkard RF: Tinnitus, *N Engl J Med* 347:904–910, 2002.
Nelson JJ, Chen K: The relationship of tinnitus, hyperacusis, and hearing loss, *Ear Nose Throat J* 83(7):472–476, 2004.
Schaette R: Tinnitus in men, mice (as well as other rodents), and machines, *Hear Res* 311:63–71, 2014.
Tyler RS: *Tinnitus Treatment*, 2006, Thieme.
Weissman JL, Hirsch BE: Imaging of tinnitus: a review, *Radiology* 216:342–349, 2000.

CHAPTER 36

EVALUATION OF THE VESTIBULAR SYSTEM AND VESTIBULAR DISORDERS

Carol A. Foster, MD

KEY POINTS

1. **Characteristics of Nystagmus in Benign Paroxysmal Positional Vertigo (BPPV):** nystagmus in posterior canal BPPV is a torsional, up-beating positional nystagmus triggered by the Dix-Hallpike test with the affected ear down. It has a paroxysmal quality, building to a peak and then disappearing over several more seconds. There is a latency of a few seconds before it appears, and it fatigues with repeated Dix-Hallpike maneuvers.
2. **Vestibular Migraine:** history of recurrent, severe, nauseating headaches or recurrent auras with vertiginous episodes. Vertigo spells vary in duration, from seconds or minutes up to hours or days. It is common in people <50 years of age, and there is an increased risk of BPPV, sleep apnea, and Ménière's disease in this group.
3. **Ménière's Triad:** 1. Hearing loss that fluctuates, worsens during vertigo spells, and is associated with a sensation of fullness or pressure in the ear. 2. Tinnitus that fluctuates, can have a roaring quality, and is louder during vertigo spells. 3. Vertigo is usually hours in duration, severe, and associated with vomiting.
4. **Characteristics of the Normal Caloric Response:** cold water irrigation causes nystagmus beating away from the irrigated ear, whereas warm water irrigation causes nystagmus beating toward the irrigated ear. A useful mnemonic for nystagmus direction is **COWS** (**C**old **O**pposite, **W**arm **S**ame). The ear with the weakest response is the damaged ear.
5. **How to Test Each Inner Ear Sensory Organ**
   a. Horizontal semicircular canal: horizontal head impulse test, caloric examination, rotational chair tests
   b. Anterior semicircular canal: vertical head impulse test, Dix-Hallpike test
   c. Posterior semicircular canal: vertical head impulse test, Dix-Hallpike test
   d. Utricle: ocular VEMP
   e. Saccule: cervical VEMP

Pearls
1. Peripheral nystagmus becomes faster and more apparent when the patient gazes in the direction of the fast phase; for example, a right-beating nystagmus worsens on right gaze. This is called **Alexander's law**.
2. Multisensory imbalance can be improved using walking aids. Trekking poles are helpful early in the disorder, but as the disease progresses, a rolling walker with handbrakes is the most effective treatment.
3. Patients with headaches and vertigo should be questioned about snoring. Sleep apnea is associated with morning headaches and worsened migraine and can be associated with recurrent brief dizziness and progressive inner ear disorders such as Ménière's disease.
4. Peripheral vestibular losses of less than 50% are usually hard to detect by impulse testing. Caloric testing is better able to detect these mild to moderate deficits.

QUESTIONS

1. **When you evaluate a dizzy patient, what should your examination include?**
   Careful observation for nystagmus; examination of the ears and hearing assessment are always required. The neurologic examination should include an evaluation of cranial nerves and examination of cerebellar function by testing coordination, gait, and balance. The neck should be evaluated for carotid artery bruits. Examination of the legs and feet for sensory lesions or range-of-motion restrictions is important. At the end of the exam, you should always perform a Dix-Hallpike maneuver (Fig. 36.1) to rule out BPPV and head impulse testing to rule out vestibular loss.

2. **How do you properly examine a patient for nystagmus?**
   Nystagmus has slow and quick components. The slow component is generated by the vestibular system and causes the eye to smoothly rotate. The fast phase represents a corrective response, a saccade that quickly returns the eyes to their original position. By convention, the direction of the nystagmus is named by its fast component,

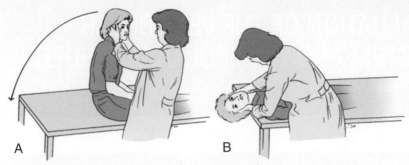

A B

Fig. 36.1 The Dix-Hallpike test. The Dix-Hallpike maneuver for the right ear. **(A)** With the examiner on the seated patient's right side, the head is rotated 45 degrees toward the right shoulder. **(B)** The patient is reclined rapidly into the supine position with the head turned toward the right. The position should be maintained for 15–30 seconds while the eyes are observed for nystagmus. (Reprinted from Crane BW, et al: Peripheral vestibular disorders. In Flint PW, et al, *Cummings Otolaryngology: Head & Neck Surgery*, 5th ed, Philadelphia, 2011, Mosby/Elsevier.)

since to the observer the eyes appear to be "beating" in the direction of the saccades. You should evaluate for spontaneous nystagmus by viewing the patient's eyes with the eyes centered and then focused to the left and right. Direct the patient to focus the eyes upward and then downward. Note the direction of nystagmus for each eye position.

3. **How is the Dix-Hallpike maneuver performed?**
   The Dix-Hallpike maneuver is a test for BPPV (Fig. 36.1). The patient is seated on the examination table with the examiner on the side to be tested. Emphasize to the patient that the eyes should be kept open throughout the maneuver, so that you can observe nystagmus. To test the right ear, hold the patient's head turned 45 degrees to the right and then swiftly move the patient into the supine position until the head overhangs the table edge. Continue to support the patient's head throughout the test. After at least 30 seconds, assist the patient in reassuming the sitting position. The test is then repeated on the left. If the patient is elderly or frail or has neck problems, the test can be done by lowering the head onto the table instead of allowing the head to overhang the edge of the table.

4. **What constitutes an abnormal Dix-Hallpike maneuver?**
   Although this test has many implications, it is most commonly used to diagnose posterior semicircular canal BPPV. A rotatory nystagmus and sensation of vertigo that begins a few seconds after assuming the head-hanging position is characteristic of BPPV. The nystagmus fades in less than 1 minute, reverses direction upon sitting and "fatigues" or decreases in intensity with repeated testing. For example, if the patient has a left pathologic ear, he or she will manifest a mixed vertical and rotatory nystagmus when positioned with the left ear down, and the upper poles of the eyes will appear to you as if they are beating toward the floor.

5. **Can BPPV also affect the horizontal or anterior semicircular canals?**
   Yes, horizontal canal BPPV causes a violent, purely horizontal paroxysm of nystagmus on Dix-Hallpike testing that can last for as long as a minute and often causes vomiting. Anterior canal BPPV causes a fine downbeating nystagmus that can be persistent for a few minutes on Dix-Hallpike testing. Repeating the Dix-Hallpike test immediately after a BPPV treatment maneuver can cause particles to fall into the horizontal semicircular canal. Anterior canal BPPV is also more likely to appear in patients who have been recently treated with in-office or home maneuvers for posterior canal BPPV.

6. **Do other disorders cause nystagmus with the Dix-Hallpike maneuver?**
   Other disorders of central or peripheral vestibular pathways may cause pathologic positional nystagmus. This kind of nystagmus usually does not fade away while the head remains in the hanging position, nor does it fatigue on repeated testing. It can appear when the patient is slowly brought to the supine position and does not require a quick movement like the Dix-Hallpike test to bring it out.

7. **What are the usual symptoms of BPPV?**
   Typically, sudden episodes of vertigo are precipitated by specific head movements, usually in bed at night. For example, the patient may complain of vertigo precipitated by rolling over in bed, lying down into bed, or arising quickly. These episodes are brief, lasting less than a minute. A change in hearing or tinnitus is not typical. Although BPPV becomes more frequent with age, it can occur in patients of any age group. This condition usually resolves spontaneously over a period of weeks to months. Failure to respond to treatment maneuvers is an indicator for formal vestibular testing.

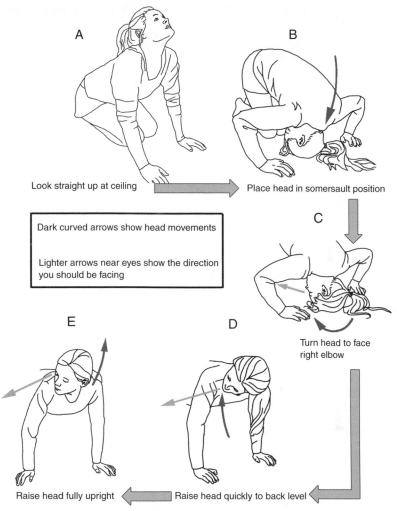

A — Look straight up at ceiling

B — Place head in somersault position

Dark curved arrows show head movements

Lighter arrows near eyes show the direction you should be facing

C — Turn head to face right elbow

E — Raise head fully upright

D — Raise head quickly to back level

Fig. 36.2 The half somersault maneuver. (A) The head is rapidly tipped upward to face the ceiling. **(B)** The head is then placed upside down on the floor. **(C)** The head is rotated to face the elbow on the affected side and is maintained in this turned position (Ex: R elbow for R posterior canal BPPV). **(D)** The turned head is quickly lifted to back level. **(E)** The turned head is then briskly raised to the fully upright position. Each position is held until the dizziness pauses or 30 seconds has elapsed. (Reprinted from Foster CA, et al: Canal conversion and re-entry: a risk of Dix-Hallpike during canalith repositioning procedures, *Otol Neurotol* 33:199–203, 2012.)

8. **How is BPPV treated?**

   This disorder usually disappears without treatment over several weeks, but the course can be shortened dramatically by using therapeutic head maneuvers designed to rotate the particles out of the affected canal. The Epley maneuver, also called the canalith repositioning procedure, has proven very useful, with a success rate near 90%. Other liberatory maneuvers have also been described.

9. **A patient returns after a third episode of BPPV. Is there a home exercise for this condition?**

   The half somersault maneuver has been shown to be a useful home exercise (Fig. 36.2). The head is inverted in the somersault position, turned to face the elbow on the affected side, and then raised first to back level and then fully upright, pausing for 30 seconds in each position. Patients who cannot perform the half somersault can use the Epley maneuver or the Semont maneuver at home but will usually require an assistant to help. It is best to wait 15 minutes between repetitions of maneuvers to avoid displacing newly removed particles back into the semicircular canals.

10. **You suspect that a patient's vestibular symptoms are due to migraine. On what grounds do you base your diagnosis?**

Migraine-associated dizziness is the most common cause of chronic dizziness in children and young adults. Although this disorder often has a benign course between attacks, it can cause serious debility. Migraine is believed to be genetic in origin. Vertigo may occur as part of an aura, as part of the headache phase, or between the headaches, and it varies in duration from seconds to days. Typically the headaches are moderate to severe, last for hours, and are associated with nausea, photophobia, or phonophobia. Headaches may be accompanied by an aura, often consisting of visual illusions such as a scintillating scotoma, or they may occur without aura. There is an association between migraine and other more serious vertigo disorders, particularly Ménière's disease. Migraines in children may not present like adult migraines and are characterized by orbital or frontal headaches that have shorter duration.

11. **How is migraine-associated dizziness treated?**

Migraine with vertigo can be treated with suppressants such as meclizine or promethazine if attacks are infrequent. However, prophylactic treatment is necessary if attacks are occurring more than once every few weeks. Tricyclic antidepressants such as amitriptyline are a good first-line choice; beta blockers, calcium channel blockers, topiramate, divalproex, and acetazolamide are also effective in some individuals. Medications should be tried for at least 1 month before another type is tried because the effect often builds over several weeks. Newer migraine treatments aimed at the headache phase, such as triptans, are generally not effective for migraine-associated vertigo spells.

12. **What is the relationship between sleep apnea and dizziness?**

Dizziness is a symptom of sleep apnea. Pauses in breathing during sleep can cause endothelial dysfunction resulting in a heightened risk for ischemia affecting the brain and inner ears. The daytime somnolence can result in microsleep episodes, and patients often report brief sudden spells of dizziness during the day. Ménière's disease and migraine are more common in patients with sleep apnea, so a history of snoring should be sought in all dizzy patients.

13. **Why do the elderly develop imbalance?**

Normal balance depends on a normal vestibular system, normal vision and visual tracking, and normal sensation and proprioception in the lower extremities. Usually vision, visual tracking, and sensation in the feet become impaired with age. When coupled with any vestibular disorder, or with a gradual age-related decline in vestibular function, multisensory imbalance occurs. Affected people usually feel dizzy only when ambulating, and their dizziness is relieved when using a grocery store cart, for example.

14. **What is the typical course of viral infections of the eighth nerve?**

This acute unilateral vestibulopathy can be preceded by a nonspecific viral illness. Within hours to days, the patient experiences the sudden onset of vertigo. The vertigo reaches a peak rapidly and then gradually declines over a few days to weeks. Cochlear symptoms vary, ranging from normal hearing to a mild high-frequency hearing loss to sudden profound deafness in one ear. If there is no hearing loss, the disease is called *vestibular neuritis*. Total destruction of all auditory and vestibular function in one ear can occur with certain viral infections, such as measles, mumps, or herpes zoster. After the severe symptoms have subsided, the patient may experience mild light-headedness with sudden movement that can persist for months. With time, however, the patient's vestibular system compensates and the dizziness usually clears.

15. **How are viral inner ear infections treated?**

A brief course of steroids should be initiated within the first few days if possible. Vestibular suppressant medication, such as meclizine, diazepam, or promethazine, is used to control vomiting. Suppressants should be discontinued after a week because they interfere with the normal process of compensation to vestibular injuries. Patients who are still symptomatic at that time are good candidates for vestibular rehabilitation.

16. **Describe the head impulse test.**

This test of the vestibular system, also called the "head thrust test" (in awake patients) or the "doll's eye test" (in comatose patients) uses quick head rotation to demonstrate high-grade vestibular lesions in disorders such as vestibular neuritis. Awake patients should be asked to stare into your eyes during the test (Fig. 36.3). Face the patient while holding the patient's head and then briskly turn the head to the right and to the left. Normally, the patient's gaze remains "locked" straight ahead on your eyes. The test is abnormal if the patient's gaze can be jerked away from yours by the quick head turn. In patients with peripheral vestibular loss, a series of "catch-up" or refixation saccades (Halmagyi's sign) may occur as the eyes attempt to regain focus on you. If the test results are abnormal with a right head turn, the patient has right vestibular injury; if abnormal to the left, the left ear is injured.

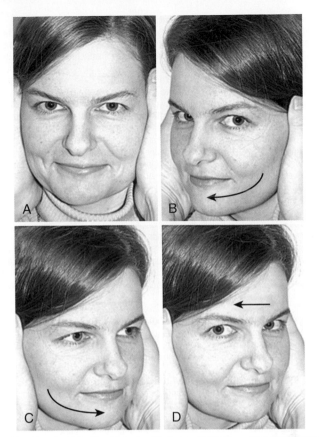

Fig. 36.3 The horizontal head impulse test with unilateral vestibular loss. (A) Starting position; **(B)** when the head is turned rapidly toward the normal right ear, the eyes remained fixed on the examiner's; **(C)** when the head is turned rapidly toward the abnormal left ear, the eyes move with the head and lose fixation with the examiner's; **(D)** the eyes then return in a rightward refixation saccade to regain focus on the examiner's eyes. (Reprinted from Hullar TE, et al: Approach to the patient with dizziness. In Flint PW, et al, *Cummings Otolaryngology: Head & Neck Surgery*, 5th ed, Philadelphia, 2010, Mosby/Elsevier.)

17. Which studies should be performed on patients with suspected inner ear disorders other than BPPV?

Initially, an audiogram and a videonystagmogram (VNG) should be obtained. Vestibular evoked myogenic potentials (VEMP) can be used to assess the function of the otolith organs. If these tests or the neurologic examination show an asymmetric or localizing finding, further studies are indicated. At this point, you should perform magnetic resonance imaging with gadolinium contrast to include the posterior fossa and internal auditory canals. If a congenital malformation of the temporal bone is suspected, an enhanced fine-cut computed tomographic scan without contrast would be the most useful study. If the patient has long (more than 1 hour) spells of vertigo, laboratory studies may be beneficial, including a complete blood count, sedimentation rate, and antinuclear antibody testing. Tests to rule out HIV, syphilis, diabetes, clotting disorders, and lipid abnormalities may be useful if dictated by patient history.

18. What is Ménière's disease?

This is a set of symptoms associated with a chronically progressive, destructive disorder involving both the cochlea and labyrinth, resulting in permanent hearing loss and vestibular injury over time. It can affect one or both ears and follows a relapsing and remitting course. Spells typically last from 30 minutes to several hours. A number of disorders, such as autoimmune disease, HIV infection, and syphilis, can cause identical symptoms, so the term Ménière's disease is used only for cases in which the cause is unknown. The term is often used interchangeably with its pathologic description, *endolymphatic hydrops*. Patients with recurrent vertigo but without evidence of progressive hearing loss or permanent vestibular injury do not meet diagnostic criteria for this disorder.

19. **What history should I obtain in patients with Ménière's disease?**
Patients under the age of 50 years should be asked about migraine headaches, since these are commonly associated with Ménière's disease in this age group. All patients should be questioned about snoring because there is an association with sleep apnea. Vascular risk factors, such as a history of smoking, diabetes, vasculitis, MI, or stroke, are also associated.

20. **Describe the uses and limitations of caloric testing.**
Caloric tests reveal abnormalities by comparing the two ears to each other. Caloric tests examine only the function of the horizontal semicircular canals. Each ear is irrigated twice, using cold water and warm water, and the resulting nystagmus slow-phase velocities are measured. The symmetry of the paired responses is then calculated, giving two results, both expressed as a percentage: (1) canal paresis or unilateral weakness, describing the side and extent of a peripheral vestibular impairment, and (2) directional preponderance, suggesting an underlying tendency toward nystagmus. If both ears have identical impairments or if the impairments affect only the vertical canals or the otolith organs, a false negative result may occur.

21. **How can the otolith organs be tested?**
Vestibular evoked myogenic potential (VEMP) testing is able to assess the function of the otolith organs, the utricle and saccule. Electrodes over the sternocleidomastoid muscles are able to detect electromyographic waveforms that result when the saccule is stimulated by loud sounds (cervical or cVEMP). Absence of the waveform on one side is a significant abnormality. However, the test is less reliable in patients over the age of 60 years and in those with neck pain, stiffness, or weakness. Delays in the response can indicate a retrocochlear lesion on the affected side, and a lowered sound threshold for the response can be a sign of semicircular canal dehiscence. Electrodes positioned below the eyes can detect waveforms resulting from sound stimulation of the utricle (ocular VEMP or oVEMP).

22. **What are the symptoms of superior semicircular canal dehiscence?**
Patients typically report torsional vertigo that is triggered by loud sounds. Blowing the nose, sneezing, or straining can set off spells. Some also report hearing internal bodily sounds, like their pulse or chewing, magnified in one ear. Others report a brief tinnitus brought on when the eyes move from side to side.

23. **Are there tests to evaluate the function of the vertical semicircular canals?**
Head impulse tests performed in the plane of the anterior or posterior semicircular canals can reveal refixation saccades if there is a loss of function in the tested canal. The head must be turned to one side and then tipped briskly upward or downward for these tests. You can sometimes see refixation saccades by looking at the eyes as you perform the test, but there are commercial systems that are better able to detect and record these high-acceleration responses.

BIBLIOGRAPHY

Dix MR, Hallpike CS: The pathology, symptomatology, and diagnosis of certain common disorders of the vestibular system, *Proc R Soc Med* 45:341–534, 1952.
Foster CA: *Overcoming Positional Vertigo*, 2019, Bull Publishing.
Foster CA, Ponnappan A, Zaccaro K, et al: A comparison of two home exercises for benign positional vertigo: half somersault vs. Epley maneuver. *Audiol Neurotol Extra*. 2:16–23, 2012.
Foster CA, Zaccaro K, Strong D: Canal conversion and re-entry: a risk of Dix-Hallpike during canalith repositioning procedures, *Otol Neurotol* 33:199–203, 2012.
Halmagyi GM: Diagnosis and management of vertigo, *Clin Med* 5:159–165, 2005.
Halmagyi GM, Curthoys IS: A clinical sign of canal paresis, *Arch Neurol* 45:737–739, 1988.
Halmagyi GM, Weber KP, Aw ST, et al: Impulsive testing of semicircular canal function, *Prog Brain Res* 171:187–194, 2008.
Jacobson G, Shepherd N: *Balance Function Assessment and Management*, 2008, Plural Publishing.
Kerber KA, Baloh RW: The evaluation of a patient with dizziness, *Neurol Clin Pract* 1:24–33, 2011.
Rosengren SM, Kingma H: New perspectives on vestibular evoked myogenic potentials, *Curr Opin Neurol* 26:74–80, 2013.
Serra A, Leigh RJ: Diagnostic value of nystagmus: spontaneous and induced ocular oscillations, *J Neurol Neurosurg Psychiatry* 73:615–618, 2002.

CHAPTER 37

HEARING AIDS AND IMPLANTABLE DEVICES

Cory Portnuff, AuD PhD, Samuel P. Gubbels, MD and Allison Ramakrishnan, AuD, MS

KEY POINTS

1. A hearing aid consultation with an audiologist is recommended for any patient who exhibits hearing loss and complains of difficulty communicating.
2. The patient's type, configuration, and severity of hearing loss, their communication needs, and lifestyle all contribute to determining the best individualized amplification option.
3. Indications for a bone conduction hearing aid include conductive or mixed hearing loss, chronically draining ear, or single-sided deafness.
4. Fitting hearing aids on children requires careful verification of function and validation of benefit. Children are best served by an interdisciplinary team of professionals including audiologists, otologists, speech-language pathologists, early interventionists, educators, and others.
5. Two hearing ears are better than one: using either two hearing aids, a hearing aid and a cochlear implant, or two cochlear implants.

Pearls
1. Hearing aids are widely used devices that can be helpful tools for ameliorating the effects of hearing loss. Patients who wear hearing aids consistently gain more benefit from their devices than patients who wear hearing aids intermittently.
2. Acoustic feedback occurs when amplified sound leaks out of the receiver back into the microphone and usually occurs with poorly fitting hearing aids or cerumen impaction.
3. There are several treatment options available for single-sided deafness, including contralateral routing of signals (CROS)/bilateral CROS (BiCROS) devices, bone conduction hearing aids worn on a headband, transcutaneous/percutaneous bone-anchored hearing aids, and bone conduction hearing aids anchored by adhesive to the mastoid.
4. MRIs are contraindicated for patients with implanted hearing devices because they have implanted magnets.

QUESTIONS

1. **What are the major components of a digital hearing aid and how does each contribute to the function of the device?**
   Broadly speaking, the digital hearing aid has five major components: microphone, analog-to-digital converter, digital signal processor (microprocessor), digital-to-analog converter, and receiver. The microphone on the outside of the hearing aid picks up sound and converts sound pressure into an electrical signal. This signal is then passed through an analog-to-digital converter and sent to the microprocessor, which is essentially a tiny computer chip. The microchip filters the signal into frequency channels and amplifies the sound according to the programming of the device (according to the user's hearing loss). The manipulated signal is converted back to an analog electrical signal through the digital-to-analog converter. The analog electrical signal is sent to the receiver where it is converted back to an acoustic signal that the patient hears.

2. **When should a patient be referred to audiology for a hearing aid consultation?**
   A hearing aid consultation should be recommended for patients who exhibit hearing loss and report a disruption in communication with others. With the improved hearing aid technology available today, hearing aids can enhance the quality of life for almost any patient with hearing loss, regardless of the type, severity, or configuration. Emerging data over the last decade have demonstrated that hearing loss is associated with a higher risk for the development of dementia, with some evidence that auditory rehabilitation with hearing aids can return this risk level to baseline. As such, hearing loss is emerging as one of the most modifiable risk factors for the development of dementia. Hearing aids can be fitted on children of any age and are commonly used for children with congenital hearing losses as early as 3 months of age.

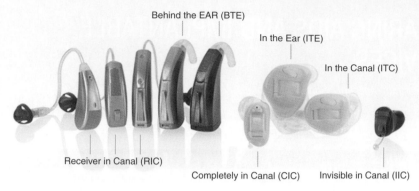

Behind the EAR (BTE)

In the Ear (ITE)

In the Canal (ITC)

Receiver in Canal (RIC)

Completely in Canal (CIC)

Invisible in Canal (IIC)

Fig. 37.1 Different styles of hearing aids.

3. **Name the most common styles of hearing aids (Fig. 37.1).**
   - Behind the ear (BTE)
   - Receiver in the canal (RIC)
   - In the ear (ITE)
   - In the canal (ITC)
   - Completely in the canal (CIC)
   - Invisible in the canal (IIC)
   - CROS and BiCROS

4. **What is acoustic feedback and what causes it?**
   Acoustic feedback occurs when the acoustic signal leaks out from the receiver of the hearing aid and is picked up again by the microphone and amplified. This amplification loop results in an unpleasant, high-pitched squealing sound. Feedback occurs most often in high-power hearing aids and hearing aids used in conjunction with a vented earmold or open-fit configuration. Feedback is most typically an indication that the patient's earmolds are not inserted properly or are a poor fit or the patient has outgrown the molds. Feedback can also be caused by cerumen impaction.

5. **What is reduced dynamic range and how does this impact the fitting of hearing aids?**
   Patients with sensorineural hearing loss (SNHL) experience a reduced dynamic range compared to individuals with normal hearing sensitivity. With SNHL, patients lose the perceived soft sounds at a higher absolute level than individuals with normal hearing, although the loudest tolerable sound is similar between the groups. Some with SNHL experience "recruitment" of loudness, where the growth rate of perceived loudness increases abnormally rapidly with increasing sound level. One theory of recruitment is that as the hair cells in the cochlea become damaged, normal adjacent hair cells are "recruited" to help hear the frequency of the damaged hair cell in addition to their own frequency, especially for high-level inputs. This increases the signal from the good hair cell and perceived loudness at the brain rapidly increases, causing discomfort. Clinically, dynamic range can be assessed by calculating the difference between the maximum tolerable loudness for speech (uncomfortable loudness level or UCL) and the speech reception threshold (SRT). Patients with SNHL commonly complain of recruitment and often describe this as "I have difficulty understanding soft speech, but it feels like loud sounds are uncomfortable."
   One way to address recruitment in the hearing aid fitting is through the use of wide dynamic range compression (WDRC). WDRC increases the audibility of soft sounds and reduces discomfort of loud sounds by applying more gain to low-level inputs and less gain to high-level inputs. Additionally, the maximum power output of hearing aids can be limited for patients who experience recruitment.

6. **What advancements in hearing aid technology have we seen in the last decade?**
   Hearing aid technology is now close to completely digital. The most significant advancements lie in signal processing. Digital signal processing improvements have allowed hearing aids to make changes to several features in response to environmental changes, including the directionality of the microphones, gain settings (amount of amplification applied), compression (nonlinear amplification), advanced digital noise reduction, digital speech enhancement, and acoustic feedback reduction. All of these features work together to improve the user's ability to understand speech in varied environments. Binaurally integrated hearing systems use wireless connectivity to exchange information between the right and left hearing aids and adjust the settings based on the user's listening environment. Additionally, hearing aids have improved connectivity, allowing hearing devices to connect to other sound sources including cell phones, landline phones, and televisions.

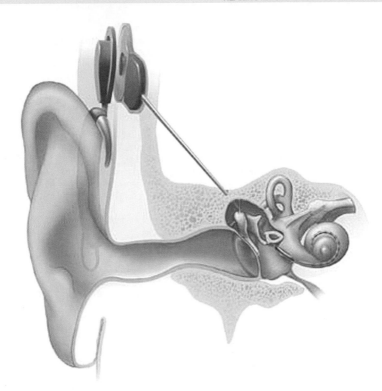

Fig. 37.2 Schematic of a cochlear implant.

7. **How are hearing aids connected to other devices?**
Wireless connectivity available in today's digital hearing aids allows for wireless communication between hearing aids and numerous forms of media devices. Individuals are now able to stream television, music, and phone calls wirelessly to their hearing aids. This allows for a gateway to media connectivity and greater convenience in communication that was once not available to hearing aid users. Many hearing aids can also use smart phones as remote control devices or for streaming audio from smart phones. Telecoils can be used to connect to landline phones or hearing loops (an induction loop connected to a public address system in a public place such as an auditorium or house of worship).

8. **How can hearing aid users enhance hearing aid function in challenging environments?**
In addition to wireless connectivity to media devices, many hearing aids can use remote microphone, digital microphone, or FM microphone technologies to allow for improved signal-to-noise ratios. In these systems, a speaker can wear a microphone that transmits their voice directly to the listener's hearing aids. These systems can help individuals with more severe hearing loss to hear better in noisy environments.

9. **How are hearing aids fit for individuals?**
An audiologist programs a hearing aid using proprietary software based on the patient's hearing loss using a pre-scriptive fitting algorithm. The output of the hearing aid should be verified using an independent testing system, such as probe microphone measures in the ear canal ("real ear measures") or measurements in an acoustically treated test box. Hearing aids fitted without verification of proper sound levels may not provide adequate audibility of sound for the patient.

10. **How do we evaluate how much benefit a patient receives from a hearing aid?**
Patients should undergo hearing aid validation testing, including evaluations of speech understanding in quiet and noise with the hearing aids on and off to assess functional benefit from hearing devices. Aided testing can also be used as an assessment prior to fitting personal hearing aids to determine whether a patient will benefit from the devices.

11. **What are indications for a bone conduction hearing device?**
    - Conductive or mixed hearing loss due to congenital malformations of the external (e.g., microtia/atresia) and/or middle ear (e.g., congenital ossicular fixation) or acquired defects of conduction (e.g., ossicular chain abnormalities secondary to middle ear surgery).
    - Chronically draining ear (e.g., from chronic otitis media or mastoiditis).
    - Single-sided deafness.
    - As an option for patients who cannot wear conventional hearing aids or are dissatisfied with outcomes, when appropriate for the hearing loss.

12. **What types of bone conduction hearing devices are available?**
    Bone conduction hearing devices are available in several styles, including bone conduction hearing aids set on a headband or adhesive pad on the mastoid or surgically implanted devices. Bone conducting implants can attach to the underlying bone through use of titanium screws or through implantation of an abutment that osseointegrates the surrounding bone into its threads. Bone conduction implants are generally categorized into the following:
    - Percutaneous devices that attach a vibrating sound processor to a surgically implanted abutment that protrudes through the skin.
    - Transcutaneous devices that connect a vibrating sound processor magnetically to an implanted abutment with an internal magnet. The skin is closed between the magnets.
    - Transcutaneous active implants, where the vibrating stimulator is implanted in the temporal bone under the skin, while the external sound processor does not vibrate. The implanted vibrating stimulator in these types of devices can be based upon a piezoelectric or electromechanical oscillator.

13. **What are the challenges associated with percutaneous bone conduction implants and are nonsurgical bone conduction hearing aid options available?**
    The rate of postoperative complications associated with percutaneous bone-anchored hearing aids ranges from 8% to 59%. The two most common postoperative complications include infection or inflammation at the implant site and failure of the device to osseointegrate. Skin reactions to percutaneous bone conduction implants occur more commonly in children and are commonly rated in severity using the Holger scale. Longevity and health of the device are highly dependent on patient hygiene and at-home care of the implant. Transcutaneous devices have lower complication rates, though magnetic coupling does include risk of skin breakdown and alopecia due to the force of the magnetic attraction. When surgery is not an option, several bone conduction devices can be fitted on a headband.

14. **What are the most common devices used to treat single-sided deafness (SSD)?**
    A common treatment approach to SSD is the fitting of contralateral routing of sound (CROS) or bilateral CROS (BiCROS) amplification. Individuals who use a CROS system have normal or near-normal hearing in the better ear and no useable hearing in the poorer ear. A transmitting device with a microphone is placed on the poorer ear and a receiving instrument is placed on the better ear. Sound picked up by the transmitting device's microphone is sent wirelessly to the receiving hearing instrument on the better ear. A BiCROS system is appropriate for those patients who exhibit some hearing loss in the better ear. In addition to the CROS, it has a second microphone located on the receiving hearing instrument that picks up and amplifies sound. Historically, patients using CROS or BiCROS systems have been dissatisfied with sound quality and cosmetic appearance, but advancements in hearing aid technology have improved these systems significantly. A second common treatment option for SSD is using a bone conduction hearing device on the worse side to stimulate the contralateral ear. One cochlear implant is currently labeled for limited use for SSD and asymmetric hearing loss, though insurance reimbursement is challenging. The use of cochlear implants for SSD is common practice in some parts of the world but is uncommon in the United States. As insurance reimbursement changes, it is likely that cochlear implants will be more commonly recommended for SSD.

15. **How should a patient be evaluated for SSD device candidacy?**
    As a part of the candidacy evaluation for different devices to manage SSD, patients should be allowed to test devices as much as possible. Patients should be tested with devices on and off in simulated noisy environments using speech-in-noise tests. Gaining as much information about projected outcomes is beneficial to both the patient and provider in making choices about surgical and nonsurgical options.

16. **What is an implantable hearing aid?**
    An implantable hearing aid is designed for those individuals with mild to severe hearing loss who are unable to wear or do not wish to wear a conventional hearing aid. There is currently one FDA-approved, fully implantable hearing device on the market. This device consists of three implantable components: the sound processor, a sensor, and a driver. Implantation of the device requires disruption of the ossicular chain, and the device then vibrates the ossicular chain directly.

17. **What are the challenges associated with implantable hearing aids?**
    - Capacity and recharging ability of batteries required to power the device.
    - Adequate middle ear space necessary to house the device. Inadequate space can limit the amount of gain the device can provide, making it challenging to aid more severe degrees of hearing loss.
    - Cost is significantly more than conventional hearing aids.
    - Insurance coverage may be limited.
    - MRI contraindicated.

18. **What special considerations are required for fitting children with hearing aids?**
    For children, audiologists often consider a mild hearing loss to be educationally significant and should consider the use of amplification. Pediatric audiologists work closely with parents, schools, speech-language pathologists, early interventionists, and teachers of children who are deaf/hard-of-hearing to ensure that children receive the proper (re)habilitative services to develop speech, language, and learning skills. Children require more regular follow-up for amplification services, including remaking earmolds due to growth, close monitoring of hearing thresholds for progression, and repeated aided hearing testing to ensure that amplification devices are appropriately functional for a child. For children, verification of hearing aids using probe microphone measures is critical to ensuring that speech sounds are audible.

CONTROVERSIES

Over-the-counter hearing aids

An emerging market for hearing aids is being created in the United States, where hearing aids for mild to moderate hearing losses could be purchased over the counter (OTC). At present, it is unclear how OTC hearing aids will function or what they will look like. While these devices may be advantageous for some users, research in hearing aids suggests that the primary factor that makes individuals successful with hearing devices is how they are fitted and verified. Hearing aids fitted without verification of appropriate fit, as OTC devices would be, may result in inadequate audibility of speech for users. OTC hearing aids will not be appropriate for children.

BIBLIOGRAPHY

Azadarmaki R, Tubbs R, Chen DA, et al: MRI information for commonly used otologic implants: review and update, *Otolaryngol Head Neck Surg* 150(4):512–519, 2014.

Badrana K, Arya AK, Bunstone D, et al: Long-term complications of bone-anchored hearing aids: a 14-year experience, *J Laryngol Otol* 123(2):170–176, 2009.

Doshi J, Sheehan P, McDermott AL: Bone anchored hearing aids in children: an update, *Int J Pediatr Otorhinolaryngol* 76(5):618–622, 2012.

Firszt JB, Holden LK, Reeder RM, et al: Auditory abilities after cochlear implantation in adults with unilateral deafness: a pilot study, *Otol Neurotol* 33(8):1339–1346, 2012.

Hobson JC, Roper AJ, Andrew R, et al: Complications of bone-anchored hearing aid implantation, *J Laryngol Otol* 124(2):132–136, 2010.

Kraus EM, Shohet JA, Catalano PJ: Envoy Esteem Totally Implantable Hearing System: phase 2 trial, 1-year hearing results, *Otolaryngol Head Neck Surg* 145(1):100–109, 2011.

Siegert R, Kanderske J: A new semi-implantable transcutaneous bone conduction device: clinical, surgical, and audiologic outcomes in patients with congenital ear canal atresia, *Otol Neurotol* 34(5):927–934, 2013.

Syms MJ, Hernandez KE: Bone conduction hearing: device auditory capability to aid in device selection, *Otolaryngol Head Neck Surg* 150(5):866–871, 2014.

CHAPTER 38

COCHLEAR IMPLANTS

Nathan D. Cass, MD and Samuel P. Gubbels, MD, FACS

KEY POINTS

1. Younger patients with post-lingual deafness and a shorter duration of severe to profound hearing loss have a greater likelihood of detecting speech after cochlear implantation.
2. Broadly speaking, individuals who have significant hearing loss and limited benefit from hearing aids are candidates for cochlear implantation. In addition, they should have a cochlear nerve, no significant middle ear pathology, and be healthy enough to undergo surgery, and they or their family (in the case of children) should have reasonable expectations and understand the long-term follow-up commitment.
3. To preserve residual hearing during cochlear implant surgery, techniques to avoid unnecessary trauma should be attempted, including preservation of perilymph by inserting the implant into the cochlea "underwater" (with saline or hyaluronic acid), using slow insertion speeds of the electrode array, and the administration of some type of perioperative corticosteroid.

Pearls

1. Preoperative imaging is useful for two purposes: to ensure that a cochlear nerve exists (especially in children with profound hearing loss or ANSD) and to evaluate the mastoid anatomy in preparation for a mastoidectomy and facial recess.
2. Bacterial meningitis is slightly more likely after cochlear implantation, and all implantees should undergo pneumococcal vaccination prior to implantation according to CDC guidelines.
3. Cochlear anomalies are more commonly encountered in pediatric cochlear implantation.

QUESTIONS

1. **Why were cochlear implants developed?**
   Bilateral hearing loss is present in 12.7% of U.S. adults, and severe to profound loss in 0.26% to 0.7% of adults, leading to significant difficulty with verbal communication. The enormous problem of irreversible sensorineural hearing loss prompted multiple researchers to develop, collaborate, and compete to create the world's most successful neural implant.

2. **Who created cochlear implants?**
   In 1957 a surgeon in France temporarily implanted an electrode near cranial nerve VIII within the internal auditory canal (IAC) while operating on a patient deafened by temporal bone resection. The first implantation of an electrode into the cochlea was performed by Dr. William House (neurotologist) and Dr. John Doyle (neurosurgeon) in 1961. Over the course of the 1960s and the 1970s, the development of single- and multi-channel implants was pioneered by teams in the United States, France, and Australia. By the late 1980s, cochlear implantation was a scientifically and commercially accepted method of enabling sound awareness and verbal communication in THE profoundly deaf.

3. **What are the components of a cochlear implant?**
   A cochlear implant consists of an internally implanted portion and an externally worn portion that is taken off and on like a hearing aid (Fig. 38.1). The microphone, which detects the ambient sound waves intended to be transmitted to the user, and the speech processor, a computer that deconstructs the sound waves into electrical signals, sit behind the ear. These components are coupled, either within the same component or via a cord, to the transmitter which is a coiled wire that transmits electrical signals to the internal device via radiofrequency waves.

   Implanted under the scalp is the receiver-stimulator, which has a matching coiled wire to receive electrical impulses from the transmitter. The transmitter and the receiver-stimulator both contain a magnet to facilitate colocalization (and accurate transmission of impulses) when the external portion is placed on the scalp. The receiver-stimulator is connected to an electrode array that is placed within the cochlea and transmits electrical signals to the appropriate portions of the acoustic nerve within Rosenthal's canal. Some cochlear implants feature a separate ground electrode, while others contain the ground within the electrode array.

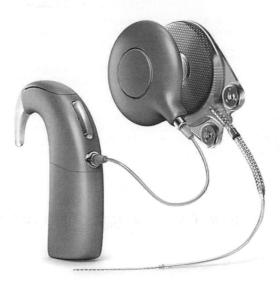

Fig. 38.1 Cochlear implant components. (Source: https://www.oticonmedical.com/cochlear-implants/solutions/systems)

4. **How do cochlear implants enable the perception of sound in users?**
   The speech processor is designed to encode sound in the same way that the normal-hearing cochlea does: signal location and signal timing. As the basilar membrane ascends from the base to the apex, the hair cells are tuned to gradually decreasing characteristic frequencies. Cochlear implants take advantage of the physical layout of this tonotopic map to deliver electrical impulses derived from high-frequency sounds to the basal electrodes and those from low-frequency sounds to the apical electrodes. As hair cells normally transmit an increasing frequency of actional potentials with increasing frequency of tones, the processor encodes the electrical impulses in the same way.

5. **Do cochlear implant users experience sound the same way as normal hearers?**
   In a normally functioning cochlea, the 3000 to 3500 inner hair cells with unique characteristic frequencies allow fine-tuning of the place coding provided to the auditory nerve. The lesser number of electrodes (up to 22) in a cochlear implant require the same electrical information to be bundled in larger packets, reducing the dynamic range of sounds perceived by the brain. Due to this and other factors, implants are unable to convey the full tonal richness of language and music. In addition, bypassing the hair cells to directly stimulate the spiral ganglion neurons sometimes results in users experiencing sound perceptions such as hissing, buzzing, or an electronic or robotic quality, especially when the implant is first activated. However, with time, cochlear implant users become adept at utilizing this electrical signal to enable greatly improved speech and environmental sound perception.

6. **How well do cochlear implants work?**
   Many factors impact how well an implant helps a particular user to achieve verbal communication. Younger patients with post-lingual deafness and a shorter duration of severe to profound hearing loss have a greater likelihood of detecting speech after implantation. The surgical technique also plays a role in outcomes. Patients in whom the implant's final location lies entirely within the scala tympani demonstrate better performance, on average, than those whose electrode translocates through the basilar membrane into the scala vestibuli. However, even when taking all of the above factors into account, there is still significant variability in individual outcomes. In other words, despite overall favorable prospects, we cannot accurately predict whether a given candidate will achieve open-set word recognition after cochlear implantation, although, on the whole, most implantees will.

7. **Who is a candidate for cochlear implantation?**
   Broadly speaking, individuals with significant hearing loss and limited benefit from hearing aids are candidates for cochlear implantation. In addition, they should have a cochlear nerve, no significant middle ear pathology, and be healthy enough to undergo surgery, and they or their family (in the case of children) should have reasonable expectations and understand the long-term follow-up commitment. Both adults and children may be implanted. Pediatric criteria require bilateral moderate-to-severe hearing loss with limited benefit from hearing aids. Adult criteria include not only bilateral moderate to severe hearing loss but also those with some residual low-frequency hearing who are candidates for hybrid cochlear implant systems. Furthermore, one cochlear implant manufacturer

(Med-El Corporation, Innsbruck, Austria) recently received FDA approval for the implantation of individuals aged 5 years and older with single-sided deafness or asymmetrical sensorineural hearing loss.

8. **How is candidacy determined audiologically?**
Candidacy in older children and adults is determined by testing their ability to understand (usually sentence-level) speech in the patient's best aided condition; this includes wearing hearing aids during the test. A variety of open-set tests are used to ascertain an individual's ability to understand speech. The Consonant-Nucleus-Consonant (CNC) is delivered as a list of 50 monosyllabic words, the Hearing in Noise Test (HINT) as 10 sentences, and the Arizona Bioindustry Association (AzBio) test as 20 sentences. The Food and Drug Administration (FDA) requires potential adult candidates to score <50% on these tests in the best aided condition for the planned implant ear and <60% for the nonimplant ear. The Centers for Medicare & Medicaid Services (CMS) require scoring <40% for the planned implant ear. As the FDA does not mandate the circumstances in which the tests are given, they are left up to the provider or the center to determine for themselves. Some centers administer speech battery tests under quiet conditions and others with background noise, usually between +10 and +5 speech-to-noise ratio (SNR). The difficulty of the test determines the relative number of patients who will be labeled as candidates. If the tests are too easy, some individuals who might have benefited from implantation will not score poorly enough to qualify. However, if the tests are too difficult, some high-functioning individuals may inappropriately qualify for implantation when they might perform worse with the implant than with their hearing aids.

9. **What about individuals who have unilateral hearing loss?**
Cochlear implantation in single-sided deafness (SSD) is an area of active research. Implantation appears to provide meaningful improvement for individuals affected by SSD. The FDA approved one implant for an indication of SSD in 2019.

10. **Who is not a candidate for cochlear implantation?**
Care must be taken when determining when implantation should be avoided, even in patients who meet the audiologic criteria. Cochlear implants were developed for those with hearing loss of cochlear origin, as they require at least some function of the spiral ganglion neurons; thus patients with primary auditory nerve-based hearing loss may not be good candidates. Surgeons should be wary of implanting those who have lost hearing after surgery of the brainstem, cerebellopontine angle, or IAC, unless rigorous testing (such as promontory stimulation) is first undertaken and/or an intact status of the auditory nerve was confirmed at the end of the prior surgery. Patients with auditory neuropathy spectrum disorder—healthy cochlear function with some degree of auditory nerve dysfunction—demonstrate variable results after implantation, although many perform much better with cochlear implants than with hearing aids. Finally, the FDA does not currently approve of implanting patients under 12 months of age and thus insurance companies may deny coverage for such patients. However, in many cases of severe to profound hearing loss, the earlier the child is implanted the better, as central nervous system plasticity makes a child's early months of life critical for auditory development. In addition, in special circumstances such as meningitis-induced hearing loss with impending labyrinthitis ossificans, earlier implantation provides the child with the best possible chance of achieving successful implantation and developing verbal communication.

11. **What is an auditory brainstem implant (ABI)?**
As noted above, in some situations, the auditory nerve itself is compromised, making a cochlear implant inappropriate. For patients such as this—primarily those with neurofibromatosis type 2 (NF2)—the ABI was developed. An ABI is an internally implanted device in which the brainstem's cochlear nucleus is stimulated at the lateral recess of the fourth ventricle, bypassing the cochlea and auditory nerve. The tonotopic map of the cochlear nucleus is not as anatomically organized as that of the cochlea and does not lend itself to implantation with a linear device. In addition, auditory information is already starting to be processed at this level in the pathway; thus the raw sound information input usually generates a decreased signal quality perception by the patient compared to a cochlear implant.

12. **What is a hybrid cochlear implant?**
Many patients experience significant high-frequency hearing loss with preservation of low-frequency acoustic hearing ("ski slope" hearing loss). Hybrid cochlear implants were designed to be of shorter length, sitting only within the basal turn of the cochlea and delivering electric signals to the portions tuned to higher characteristic frequencies, and concomitantly avoiding trauma to the cochlea, which may come with increased angle of insertion depth and larger electrodes. This design theoretically allows patients to use electric acoustic stimulation (EAS) in the form of both a cochlear implant and a hearing aid in the same ear. Implantation with a hybrid implant requires a speech battery test score of 10% to 60% in the planned implant ear and <80% in the non implant ear.

13. **Does a cochlear implant affect tinnitus?**
Although cochlear implants were primarily developed to treat severe to profound hearing loss, they often have an effect on the tinnitus that commonly accompanies such loss. In many cases, using an implant improves tinnitus and tinnitus-related quality of life. Tinnitus, however, is not an approved indication for cochlear implantation.

14. **When planning cochlear implantation, what other considerations exist for the surgeon?**

    A surgeon planning cochlear implantation should take precautions to ensure a safe and successful implantation, as well as a reasonable likelihood that the user will obtain good speech recognition. Preoperative imaging is useful for two purposes: to ensure that a cochlear nerve exists (especially in children with profound hearing loss or ANSD) and to evaluate the mastoid anatomy in preparation for a mastoidectomy and facial recess. MRI best assesses the former, while CT is superior for the latter. Some practitioners obtain one, some both, and some none; the clinical situation of each case should dictate the most appropriate strategy. In patients who have had meningitis or surgery involving the inner ear, imaging (generally T2-weighted MRI) is used to rule out labyrinthitis ossificans, which demonstrates a fibrous inflammatory reaction within the cochlea and labyrinth, followed by a bony reaction that complicates electrode insertion. When planning any surgery, comorbidities should be explored and the patient evaluated by the anesthesiologist, if appropriate, prior to surgery. Finally, as bacterial meningitis is slightly more likely after cochlear implantation, all implantees should undergo pneumococcal vaccination prior to implantation according to the CDC guidelines.

15. **How is cochlear implantation performed?**

    Patients are usually given general anesthesia, although local anesthesia alone may be used in select cases. Facial nerve monitoring is applied, and neuromuscular blockade is avoided. With the patient in a supine position, the head is rotated to the side in preparation for a postauricular approach. A mastoidectomy and facial recess/posterior tympanotomy is performed and a subperiosteal pocket is created posteriorly for the receiver-stimulator to reside. Two methods may be used to access the scala tympani. Some surgeons drill a cochleostomy anterior and inferior to the round window; more often, a round window (RW) approach is utilized by drilling away the overhang of the RW niche and incising the RW membrane itself. The electrode array is then carefully and slowly inserted into the cochlea to the desired depth. The round window is often packed with endogenous tissue to reduce potential movement of the electrode and risk of meningitis and the incision is then closed.

16. **How does one know whether the electrode array was inserted correctly and that the implant will work?**

    Various tests may be used to ensure proper insertion. A simple intraoperative x-ray will provide information about tip fold over or extra cochlear insertion. More advanced imaging such as flat-panel CT scan may be able to determine whether the electrode lies within the scala tympani for its entire length without translocation. In the early days of cochlear implantation, due to less reliable manufacturing, "hard failure" (device hardware malfunction upon delivery) was more common than with current implants. Thus impedance testing was performed on all implants immediately after insertion to test the integrity of the electrical system; if the electrical system is faulty *or* if the electrode is surrounded by air rather than fluid, then impedances will be very high. This does not protect against all misplaced electrodes; all misplaced electrodes, however: if the electrode lies within an infracochlear air cell tract surrounded by blood, impedances will still be low. This type of testing may also be useful postoperatively to test whether electrodes on the array have extruded over time: any basal electrodes found to have high impedances will likely demonstrate extrusion on CT scan.

    The final type of testing is known as neural response telemetry (NRT), neural response imaging (NRI), or auditory nerve response telemetry (ART), depending on which manufacturer's implant is being used. This test is essentially of an auditory brainstem response (ABR) where, instead of an acoustic stimulus, an electrical stimulus is delivered by the implant itself to the auditory nerve and the resultant brainwave is recorded. Neural testing can provide an estimation of the integrity of the auditory system and, in the case of children who are unable to perform behavioral audiometry, may give the audiologist an approximation of the electrical thresholds at which to start when programming the implant.

17. **What anomalous anatomy may be encountered in cochlear implantation?**

    Cochlear anomalies are more commonly encountered during pediatric cochlear implantation. Less severe anomalies in which the basic structure of the cochlea remains intact, such as incomplete partition type II (Mondini deformity) and I and mild cochlear hypoplasia, do not require special techniques, although cerebrospinal fluid gusher may be more commonly encountered. More severe anomalies, such as common cavity, may herald an anomalous course of the facial nerve, requiring more complex surgical approaches. Middle ear and mastoid anomalies may require more creative approaches on the part of the surgeon. Canal wall-down mastoidectomy cavities and a middle ear with prior cholesteatoma both require extra caution and care during the approach to the cochlea, consideration of electrode placement, and follow-up care and monitoring.

18. **What is the impact of cochlear implantation on residual hearing, if present?**

    When first pioneered, cochlear implantation was performed only on the profoundly deaf. It was also standard practice during implantation to suction all of the perilymph from the cochlea before the electrode was inserted. As a result, what little residual hearing existed in early implantees was expected to be fully lost. In the mid-1990s the concept of "soft surgery" for preservation of residual hearing after cochlear implantation emerged. Studies examining the factors that affect hearing preservation are mostly retrospective, but a few features seem consistent. The preservation of perilymph and insertion of the implant into the cochlea "underwater" (with saline or hyaluronic acid) is vital for maintaining residual hearing. Avoiding direct trauma to the cochlea using slow insertion speeds also seems to be protective, as does administration of some sort of perioperative corticosteroid. Conflicting data exist regarding the effects of approach (cochleostomy vs. RW) and electrode type on hearing preservation. With regard to some factors, acoustic hearing preservation is at odds with maximal benefit from the implant; increasing the angle of insertion decreases residual hearing but increases open-set word recognition in implant users.

19. **What different types of electrode arrays are available for cochlear implantation?**
Three basic shapes of array have been designed: lateral wall, midmodiolar, and perimodiolar. Lateral wall arrays are intended to slide along the lateral wall of the scala tympani as they ascend from the base to the apex. Midmodiolar arrays are designed to remain roughly within the center of the scala tympani and not in contact with either the lateral or modiolar wall. Perimodiolar arrays are intended to hug the modiolus and contain a mechanism, either an inner stylet or an outer sheath, to facilitate this curving during insertion. Thin lateral wall arrays are usually easier to insert and may cause less damage to the cochlea but are slightly more prone to extrusion. Due to their close proximity to the spiral ganglion neurons, perimodiolar arrays may require less energy to transmit electric signals and may enable more precise activation of certain neural bundles, although some studies note greater damage with less hearing preservation (controversial). A hybrid implant refers to a shorter, lateral wall array, which is only inserted into the basal turn of the cochlea and causes less trauma, attempting to preserve the apical (low-frequency) acoustic hearing while electrically stimulating the areas with more cochlear hearing loss. A double array contains two separate arrays: one is implanted in the basal turn and one in the middle turn. This implant was designed for patients with hearing loss due to labyrinthitis ossificans, in whom the cochlea must be drilled out to varying degrees to accommodate electrode placement.

20. **Who makes cochlear implants?**
The current US market is dominated by three manufacturers: MED-EL, Advanced Bionics, and Cochlear Corporation. MED-EL, based in Austria, arose from work at the University of Vienna and now makes middle ear and bone conduction implants, in addition to cochlear implants. The technology utilized by Southern California–based Advanced Bionics was developed at UCSF, and the company is now a subsidiary of a company that also owns Phonak, the world market share leader in hearing aids. Cochlear Corporation was formed in Australia based on the work of Dr. Graeme Clark, an early pioneer in cochlear implants as well as bone conduction implants.

21. **Are there any implications of having a permanently implanted magnet?**
MRI incompatibility remains the greatest challenge regarding the magnet component of cochlear implants. The function of the magnet is to maintain the transmitter immediately adjacent to the receiver-stimulator, to facilitate precise positioning and ensure accurate transmission of radio-frequency signals. However, magnets are subjected to immense forces when brought into the powerful magnetic field of an MRI machine, unless they are aligned with the field. For most of the history of cochlear implantation, MRI has been contraindicated in implantees. Over time, various manufacturers have modified the internal implant casings to include a semiopen silicone gasket to house the magnet, enabling its surgical removal when an MRI is required (with surgical reimplantation afterward). Some models are also able to undergo 1.5T MRI with little movement when a tight head wrap is applied, although numerous complications can arise in these situations. The magnet may flip or partially extrude from the casing, leading to pain and local tissue inflammation. Recently, implants have been developed with freely rotatable internal magnets that can align with the magnetic field of MRI, enabling a safe environment without the need for head wrap or surgical magnet removal. It should be noted, however, that the internal magnet will always create an artifact within the MRI image, which may obscure the region of interest if it lies within the ipsilateral cranial vault.

BIBLIOGRAPHY

Balkany TJ, et al: Conservation of residual acoustic hearing after cochlear implantation, *Otol Neurotol* 27(8):1083–1088, 2006.
Blanchfield BB, et al: The severely to profoundly hearing-impaired population in the United States: prevalence estimates and demographics, *J Am Acad Audiol* 12(4):183–189, 2001.
Cass ND, et al: First MRI With New Cochlear Implant With Rotatable Internal Magnet System and Proposal for Standardization of Reporting Magnet-Related Artifact Size, *Otol Neurotol* 40(7):883–891, 2019.
Causon A, Verschuur C, Newman TA: A Retrospective Analysis of the Contribution of Reported Factors in Cochlear Implantation on Hearing Preservation Outcomes, *Otol Neurotol* 36(7):1137–1145, 2015.
Hodges AV, Schloffman J, Balkany T: Conservation of residual hearing with cochlear implantation, *Am J Otol* 18(2):179–183, 1997.
Holden LK, et al: Factors affecting open-set word recognition in adults with cochlear implants, *Ear Hear* 34(3):342–360, 2013.
Lin FR, Niparko JK, Ferrucci L: Hearing loss prevalence in the United States, *Arch Intern Med* 171(20):1851–1852, 2011.
Mudry A, Mills M: The early history of the cochlear implant: a retrospective, *JAMA Otolaryngol Head Neck Surg* 139(5):446–453, 2013.
O'Connell BP, et al: Electrode Location and Angular Insertion Depth Are Predictors of Audiologic Outcomes in Cochlear Implantation, *Otol Neurotol* 37(8):1016–1023, 2016.
Olze H, et al: The impact of cochlear implantation on tinnitus, stress and quality of life in postlingually deafened patients, *Audiol Neurootol* 17(1):2–11, 2012.
Pujol, R., M. Lenoir, and S. Irving, Inner Hair Cells: An Overview. 2016.

Rajan GP, Kontorinis G, Kuthubutheen J: The effects of insertion speed on inner ear function during cochlear implantation: a comparison study, *Audiol Neurootol* 18(1):17–22, 2013.

Schuman TA, et al: Anatomic verification of a novel method for precise intrascalar localization of cochlear implant electrodes in adult temporal bones using clinically available computed tomography, *Laryngoscope* 120(11):2277–2283, 2010.

Sullivan CB, et al: Long-term audiologic outcomes after cochlear implantation for single-sided deafness, *Laryngoscope*, 2019.

Turton L, Smith P: Prevalence & characteristics of severe and profound hearing loss in adults in a UK National Health Service clinic, *Int J Audiol* 52(2):92–97, 2013.

Welch C, Dillon MT, Pillsbury HC: Electric and Acoustic Stimulation in Cochlear Implant Recipients with Hearing Preservation, *Semin Hear* 39(4):414–427, 2018.

CHAPTER 39

INFECTIONS OF THE EAR

Melissa A. Scholes, MD

KEY POINTS

Essentials of diagnosis of otitis media:
- Middle ear effusion must be present as diagnosed by pneumatic otoscopy or tympanometry with
- Moderate to severe bulging of the tympanic membrane or new otorrhea not associated with otitis externa or
- Mild bulging of the tympanic membrane and less than 48 hours of otalgia or erythema of the tympanic membrane

Pearls
1. For a diagnosis of acute otitis externa, there must be a rapid onset (usually within 48 hours) of symptoms and signs of ear canal inflammation.
2. The most common bacterial pathogens contributing to acute otitis media are *Streptococcus pneumoniae* (35% to 40%), *Haemophilus influenzae* (30% to 35%), and *Moraxella catarrhalis* (15% to 25%).
3. Amoxicillin remains the first-line therapy for acute otitis media because approximately 80% of bacterial isolates remain susceptible. Pain is an important symptom of otitis externa and otitis media and needs to be treated appropriately.
4. Acute otitis media in children less than 6 months of age or with severe symptoms and/or bilateral ear involvement from 6 months to 23 months of age should be treated with antibiotics. Asymptomatic children over 2 years of age may be observed without antibiotic therapy.
5. The American Academy of Pediatrics recommends pneumococcal conjugate vaccines and annual influenza vaccines according to the Advisory Committee on Immunization Practices in order to reduce episodes of otitis media related to these pathogens.

QUESTIONS

1. **What is otitis externa (OE)?**
   Otitis externa is diffuse inflammation of the skin of the external auditory canal (EAC), which can extend to surrounding structures such as the pinna, tragus, tympanic membrane, and regional lymph nodes.

2. **What is the pathogenesis of OE?**
   OE occurs when the protective mechanisms of the ear canal are disrupted. Cerumen, produced by glands in the cartilaginous ear canal, is bacteriostatic and protects the ear canal by acting as a barrier to moisture. Cerumen is also slightly acidic, which aids in inhibiting infection. If this cerumen layer is disrupted and the skin of the ear canal is traumatized with a cotton swab, fingernail, or other foreign body, an infection may occur. Moist and humid environments also contribute to infections by weakening skin barriers. Almost all AOE is bacterial and *Staphylococcus aureus* and *Pseudomonas aeruginosa* are the most common causative organisms.

3. **What are the risk factors for acute otitis externa (AOE)? How do you prevent AOE?**
   Water exposure is the most common culprit associated with AOE as seen in warmer, humid climates or from direct contact with water while bathing or swimming (so-called "swimmer's ear"). There is a relationship between the bacterial load of water and the development of AOE. There also may be a genetic basis to the development of AOE such as Type A blood group. AOE can be prevented by reducing water exposure in the ear canal. Preventative measures include acidifying ear drops, removal of obstructing cerumen, drying the ear canal with a hair dryer (on a cool setting), ear plug use, and avoidance of direct ear canal trauma.

4. **What are the signs and symptoms of AOE?**
   AOE usually presents as a rapid onset (usually less than 48 hours) of intense ear pain. The pain is often out of proportion to the examination and is exacerbated by palpation of the tragus and pinna. Signs of ear canal inflammation such as erythema, edema, and drainage must also be present. Additional symptoms include purulent ear drainage, otalgia (ear pain), plugged feeling in the affected ear, and debris in the ear canal.

5. **What is chronic otitis externa (COE)?**
Chronic otitis externa is inflammation of the skin of the EAC lasting more than 6 weeks and can be related to bacterial infection, skin disorders such as eczema, fungus, allergy, chronic otorrhea, or chronic irritation. The pain is often not as severe as acute OE. COE may occur after inadequate treatment of AOE.

6. **What is malignant otitis externa? What are other complications of OE?**
Malignant otitis externa is an infection of the skull base that can occur after acute or chronic OE. It is most often seen in elderly patients with diabetes and the immunocompromised. The infection can spread intracranially, causing cranial nerve deficits, and is a life-threatening condition requiring intravenous antibiotic therapy and correction of the underlying immunocompromise. Other symptoms of malignant otitis media include a deep stabbing ear pain that worsens with head motion, otorrhea, fever, loss of voice, dysphagia, and facial weakness. Less seriously, OE can spread and cause facial cellulitis.

7. **What are other causes of ear pain or otorrhea that may be confused for acute otitis externa?**
An infected hair follicle (furunculosis), viral infections, temporomandibular joint syndrome, dental abnormalities, or referred pain from aerodigestive processes can cause otalgia and must be considered when the history and physical examination are not convincing of AOE.

8. **How do you treat OE?**
OE is best treated by debriding the ear of desquamated skin and cerumen, restoring the normal pH, topical antimicrobial therapy, and removal of causative agents. Fluoroquinolone drops are first-line therapy. Oral antibiotics are not indicated unless infection has spread outside the ear canal. If patients are predisposed to recurrent OE, two to three drops of a 1:1 solution of white vinegar and 70% ethyl alcohol can be instilled into the ear before and after swimming. Physicians should be sure to address pain management as well as counsel patients on how to administer drops to themselves or children to promote adherence to therapy.

9. **What is bullous myringitis?**
Bullous myringitis is the formation of serous or hemorrhagic bullae on the tympanic membrane. It is associated with viral, *Streptococcus pneumoniae*, or staphylococcal infections. It is often very painful and may cause conductive hearing loss. Drainage may occur if the bullae ruptures. Supportive treatment is indicated including analgesics and anti-inflammatory medications. If signs of bacterial infection are present, topical or oral antibiotics are appropriate.

10. **What is otitis media (OM)? What are the predisposing factors for OM?**
Otitis media (OM) is inflammation of the middle ear space. It is common in younger children secondary to an immature immune system, eustachian tube dysfunction, and unfavorable anatomy. Other predisposing factors include colonization of the nasopharynx with otitis pathogens, upper respiratory infection, smoke exposure, bottle feeding, time of year, daycare attendance, and genetic susceptibility.

11. **What role does the eustachian tube play in OM?**
The eustachian tube (ET) runs from the anterior middle ear to the nasopharynx and equalizes the pressure in the middle ear space. It is bony in its proximal portion and cartilaginous in its distal portion and is associated with four muscles: salpingopharyngeus, tensor veli palatini, tensor tympani, and levator veli palatine. The ET intermittently opens in response to different actions on these muscles, including yawning, talking, and performing a Valsalva maneuver. The middle ear space is under constant negative pressure, and equalization by the ET prevents buildup of fluid. If the ET is dysfunctional for any reason, then fluid buildup occurs, causing a middle ear effusion. Common causes for ET dysfunction include anatomic variants and viral infections with concomitant swelling. In children, the eustachian tube is flatter and less rigid, which can contribute to dysfunction (Fig. 39.1). The fluid can then become infected from exposure to pathogens that are found in the nasopharynx.

12. **What are the most common bacterial pathogens found in OM? What are the most common organisms found in mastoiditis?**
Classically, the most common bacterial pathogens contributing to OM are *Streptococcus pneumoniae* (35% to 40%), *Haemophilus influenzae* (30% to 35%), and *Moraxella catarrhalis* (15% to 25%). *Streptococcus pyogenes* and *S. pneumoniae* are the most common pathogens found in mastoiditis. With the advent of the pneumococcal vaccine there has been a decrease in the number of infections from *S. pneumoniae* but an increase in infections from other bacteria such as *Staphylococcus aureus* and *H. influenzae*. There is a trend for an overall decrease in OM by approximately 6% to 7% since vaccinations were introduced.

13. **What are biofilms and what is their role in OM?**
Biofilms are groups of microorganisms that reside in an extracellular matrix. The extracellular matrix is resistant to antibiotic penetration. Additionally, different bacteria in the biofilm can share host defense mechanisms and

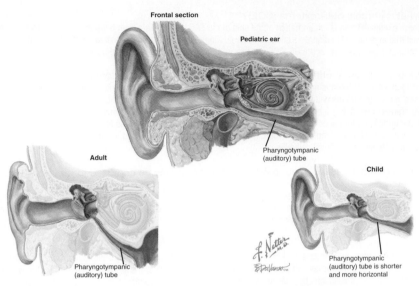

Fig. 39.1 Eustachian tube anatomy. (From Jong EC, Stevens DL: *Netter's Infectious Diseases*, Philadelphia, 2011, Saunders.)

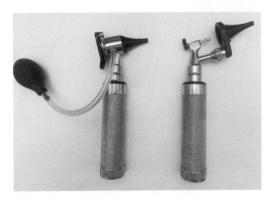

Fig. 39.2 Closed and open head otoscopes.

resistant genes. Biofilms have been found in the middle ear and nasopharynx of children with otitis media. It is thought that biofilms contribute to OM by shedding planktonic bacteria, inducing mucosal inflammation, and allowing bacteria to escape immune responses.

14. **What examination techniques are used in the diagnosis of OM?**
Any obstructing cerumen should be cleared from the ear canal to see the tympanic membrane. This can be done with an open operating otoscope (Fig. 39.2) or under a microscope. Irrigation of the ear canals should be used with caution in case there is an unrecognized tympanic membrane perforation. The tympanic membrane is examined for color, thickness, bulging, loss of landmarks, and presence of effusion. Loss of the light reflex is not specific for otitis media. Next, pneumatic otoscopy is performed with an insufflator bulb attached to a closed head otoscope. Gentle pressure is applied, which will cause a pressure change in the canal. If an effusion is present the eardrum will not move; in the absence of an effusion the eardrum will move. Only gentle pressure is needed. Too much pressure can cause pain. If pneumatic otoscopy cannot be performed, then tympanometry can be used to establish presence of an effusion.

15. **What tips for pneumotoscopy will help you perform an ear examination?**
    • Choose the largest ear speculum to ensure a tight seal.
    • Insert the speculum into only the outer one third of the external canal to avoid pain from pressure on the bony canal.

- Insert the speculum after compressing the bulb slightly and then release to check for movement. This helps avoid discomfort and can diagnose negative ear pressure.
- Use only gentle pressure to minimally flutter the tympanic membrane.

16. **What antibiotics are used in the treatment of OM?**
Amoxicillin remains the first-line therapy because the majority of bacterial isolates remain susceptible. Amoxicillin with clavulanic acid is used when the patient has failed clinically after 48 to 72 hours or has had amoxicillin in the last 30 days. In patients with penicillin sensitivity without severe reactions, cephalosporins are used. For children with IgE-mediated allergic reactions, trimethoprim-sulfamethoxazole, clindamycin, or a macrolide is used. Intramuscular ceftriaxone is usually reserved for failures of oral therapies (Tables 39.1 and 39.2).

17. **Are there other options besides antibiotics to treat OM?**
Patients over 6 months of age with minimal symptoms can be observed for 48 to 72 hours. However, a plan should be in place if failure occurs, such as a "wait and see" prescription or an additional ear examination to ensure improvement.

18. **Is there any way to prevent OM?**
Most episodes of otitis media occur in children because of anatomic issues as well as immaturity of the immune system. These factors cannot be changed. Avoidance of daycare centers and cigarette smoke and bottle propping can help. Breastfeeding has a protective effect by providing maternal antibodies. One study reported that pacifier use might help to decrease episodes of AOM. If a child has additional infections, such as pneumonia, an immune evaluation may be prudent. Antibiotic prophylaxis is not recommended because it contributes to resistance, can have side effects, and is not effective in the long term.

19. **What is otitis media with effusion (OME)? When does it become chronic otitis media with effusion (COME)?**
OME is the presence of an effusion in the middle ear without signs of acute inflammation. This can occur primarily from negative middle ear pressure from eustachian tube blockage as seen with adenoid hypertrophy, upper

---

Table 39.1 Treatment of Acute Otitis Media in an Era of Drug Resistance; Initial Immediate or Delayed Antibiotic Treatment

FIRST-LINE TREATMENT	ALTERNATIVE TREATMENT (IF PENICILLIN ALLERGIC)
1. Amoxicillin (80–90 mg/kg/day in two divided doses) • For children aged <2 years or children of all ages with severe symptoms, treat for 10 days • Aged 2–6 years with mild-moderate symptoms, treat for 7 days • Aged >6 years with mild-moderate symptoms, treat for 5 days. or 2. Amoxicillin-clavulanate (90 mg/kg/day or amoxicillin, with 6.4 mg/kg/day of clavulanate in two divided doses) • For patients who have received amoxicillin in the previous 30 days or who have otitis-conjunctivitis syndrome.	1. Cefdinir (14 mg/kg/day in one or two doses) 2. Cefuroxime (30 mg/kg/day divided BID) 3. Cefpodoxime (10 mg/kg/day in two divided doses) 4. Ceftriaxone (50 mg IM or IV per day for 1 or 3 days) 5. If unable to take oral medications 6. For children with severe penicillin allergies (IgE-mediated events): • Trimethoprim-sulfamethoxazole • Macrolide • Clindamycin (30–40 mg/kg/day, divided TID)

Table 39.2 Antibiotic Treatment After 48–72 Hours of Failure of Initial Antibiotic

RECOMMENDED FIRST-LINE TREATMENT	ALTERNATIVE TREATMENT
1. Amoxicillin-clavulanate (90 mg/kg/day or amoxicillin, with 6.4 mg/kg/day of clavulanate in two divided doses) • For patients who have received amoxicillin in the previous 30 days or who have otitis-conjunctivitis syndrome or 2. Ceftriaxone (50 mg IM or IV per day for 3 days)	1. Ceftriaxone (50 mg IM or IV per day for 3 days) 2. Clindamycin (30–40 mg/kg/day, divided TID) with or without a third-generation cephalosporin 3. Consider tympanocentesis • Consult specialist 4. Recurrence >4 weeks after initial episode: • A new pathogen is likely, so restart first-line therapy. • Be sure diagnosis is not OME, which may be observed for 3–6 months without treatment.

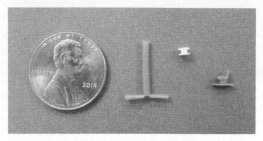

Fig. 39.3 Different types of ear tubes.

respiratory infection, or some other dysfunction. It can also be seen following an episode of acute otitis media after the inflammation has subsided. An effusion after AOM can be present for several weeks with 90% resolution by 3 months. After 3 months it is considered COME. OME must be differentiated from AOM because OME does not benefit from treatment with antibiotics.

20. **What is the medical treatment of OME?**
OME is not improved by administration of antibiotics, steroids, antihistamines, or decongestants. A patient with an effusion lasting for more than 3 months should undergo testing of their hearing unless this is a child with risk factors for language delay, in which case they should be tested sooner. If a middle ear effusion is present for more than 3 months and there is hearing loss, then tympanostomy tubes are often recommended.

21. **What are tympanostomy tubes? How do tympanostomy tubes help OME and AOM?**
Tympanostomy tube placement is the most common ambulatory surgery performed in the United States. The tubes are small cylinders, usually with a flange or collar that sits in the tympanic membrane (Fig. 39.3). The role of the tube is to drain fluid and equalize middle ear pressure. In children with acute otitis media, they prevent a buildup of middle ear fluid and subsequent inflammation and infection. In otitis media with effusion, they remove the effusion, allowing for improvement in hearing. On average the tubes last for 6 months to a year. They are pushed out of the ear-drum by the natural desquamation of the epithelial layer of the tympanic membrane. Tympanostomy tubes are the main surgical treatment for recurrent otitis media and otitis media with effusion. There are specific surgical indications for each disease process.

22. **What is chronic suppurative otitis media?**
Chronic suppurative otitis media is otorrhea from a perforated tympanic membrane or open myringotomy tube that lasts more than 3 months. The perforation can occur from an acute otitis media or chronic middle ear effusion. Otorrhea can be the result of secretions entering the middle ear from the eustachian tube or from water exposure of the middle ear mucosa.

23. **How is chronic suppurative otitis media treated?**
The first step is to clean the ear canal and secretions to evaluate the middle ear. You must rule out a cholesteatoma, which can also lead to chronic ear drainage. In the absence of cholesteatoma, the ear is treated with topical antibiotic ear drops, usually ofloxacin. The patient is put on dry ear precautions to avoid any water exposure of the middle ear. If there are allergy issues or enlarged adenoids, these may need to be addressed to reduce secretions from the eustachian tube. A culture can be obtained to help direct antibiotic coverage in cases of recalcitrant drainage.

BIBLIOGRAPHY

Bluestone CD, Simons JP, Healy GB, et al: *Pediatric Otolaryngology* (Vol 1), 5th ed, 2014, People's Medical Publishing House.
Hay WW, Deterding RR, Levin MJ, et al: *Current Diagnosis and Treatment Pediatrics*, 24th ed, 2018, McGraw-Hill Medical.
Liberthal AS, Carroll AE, Chonmaitree T, et al: The diagnosis and management of acute otitis media, *Pediatrics* 131(3):e964–e999, 2013.
Rosenfeld RM, Schwartz SR, Cannon CR, et al: Clinical practice guideline: acute otitis externa, *Otolaryngol Head Neck Surg* 150(1 Suppl):S1–S24, 2014.
Shirai N, Preciado D: Otitis media: what is new? *Curr Opin Otolaryngol Head Neck Surg* 27(6):495–498, 2019.

CHAPTER 40

COMPLICATIONS OF OTITIS MEDIA

Jameson K. Mattingly, MD and Kenny H. Chan, MD

KEY POINTS

Pathophysiology and etiology of the complications of otitis media (OM)
- OM results in complications by different mechanisms.
- Preformed pathways increase the risk of spread of infection from the middle ear and mastoid to other areas.
- The three main routes of spread of OM are hematogenous, direct extension, and thrombophlebitis.
- Most common pathogens associated with complications in AOM are *S. pneumonia, H. influenzae*, and *M. catarrhalis*.
- Complicated OM (COM) is associated with increased bacterial resistance including strains of *S. aureus, P. aeruginosa, K. pneumoniae*, anaerobes, and, frequently, polymicrobial infections.

Pearls

Management of the complications of OM
1. Most complications will involve at minimum antibiotic therapy and myringotomy and ventilation tube insertion.
2. Initial antibiotic regimens should be broad-spectrum, and degree of CSF penetration should be considered.
3. Surgical intervention is warranted with no improvement on medical therapy, development of complications, or presentation with intracranial complications.
4. Culture-directed antibiotic treatment should be instituted once available.
5. Certain complications have additional treatments and can be controversial (e.g., sigmoid sinus thrombosis).

QUESTIONS

1. **Describe the pathophysiology of complications related to acute otitis media (AOM).**
   The pathophysiology of complications of otitis media (OM) depends on whether it arises in the setting of acute otitis media (AOM) or chronic suppurative otitis media (CSOM). AOM frequently develops in previously nondiseased ears and is characterized by mucosal edema, fluid exudation, bacterial proliferation, and pus formation. Infection then spreads contiguously into the mastoid through direct extension via preformed pathways or hematogenously.

2. **Describe the pathophysiology of complications related to CSOM.**
   CSOM reflects persistent (e.g., several weeks) mastoid and middle ear inflammation and infection. This process can occur with or without cholesteatoma, although the suspicion for cholesteatoma should be high. When infection and inflammation persist, mucosal edema blocks normal aeration between the mastoid and middle ear. Continued inflammation results in bony destruction and granulation tissue formation. Infection subsequently spreads through direct extension via bony erosion from cholesteatoma or osteitis or possibly through preformed pathways.

3. **What are the three pathways for OM to develop into complications?**
   The three main pathways for OM that result in complications are hematogenous spread, direct extension through bony erosion or preformed pathways, and thrombophlebitis of local perforating (diploic) veins. An example of thrombophlebitis of local perforating blood vessels is the mastoid emissary veins.

4. **What is an example of *hematogenous* spread of infection with OM?**
   Meningitis is an example of hematogenous spread. Symptoms of meningitis include headache, nausea, nuchal rigidity, photophobia, altered mental status, and fever. Cerebrospinal fluid examination is critical, and computed tomography (CT) is often performed to rule out other intracranial complications (e.g., abscess) and mass lesions.

5. **What are examples of *direct extension*?**
   Direct extension results in various complications depending on the direction of the spread. Complications such as postauricular abscess, Bezold abscess, sigmoid sinus thrombosis, epidural abscess, and subdural empyema can all result from direct extension (Fig. 40.1).

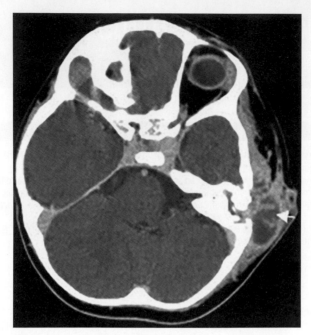

Fig. 40.1 Axial CT scan with contrast demonstrating a postauricular abscess.

6. **What are some examples of *preformed pathways*?**
Examples of preformed pathways are Mondini's malformation, enlarged vestibular aqueduct, iatrogenic (e.g., previous surgery), congenital stapes footplate abnormalities, tegmen defects, or temporal bone fractures. These pathways increase the risk of direct extension of infection in the middle ear and mastoid. Recurrent intracranial complications (e.g., meningitis) should prompt investigation for these preformed pathways.

7. **What are the etiologic agents for OM?**
The most common organisms resulting in AOM are *S. pneumoniae, H. influenzae*, and *M. catarrhalis*. Smaller proportions are due to *S. pyogenes and S. aureus*.
    COM characteristically has an increase in resistant organisms and is often polymicrobial. Frequently cultured organisms include *P. aeruginosa, S. aureus* including methicillin-resistant strains, *S. pyogenes, K. pneumoniae, P. acnes*, and *Bacteroides* species.

8. **What is the epidemiology of complications associated with OM?**
Incidence varies among studies, but most reports show that 60% to 80% of complications occur in the first two decades of life. Vaccinations to *H. influenzae* and *S. pneumococcus* have resulted in a decline in certain complications such as meningitis.

9. **What is the most common complication of OM?**
The most common complication of OM is otitis media with effusion (OME). This entity is defined as middle ear effusion without signs of acute infection or inflammation. This is a relatively benign process compared with infectious complications but can be a substantial contributor to hearing loss and an indication for ventilation tubes.

10. **What is the classification schema for complications of OM?**
Complications can be divided into intracranial or extracranial/intratemporal (Table 40.1).

11. **What are important presenting symptoms of complications of OM?**
The signs and symptoms of OM and its associated complications are quite broad. Symptoms typically begin with otalgia, irritability, and fever. CSOM may be initially more subtle, presenting with persistent purulent otorrhea only. Patients can progress to postauricular pain, erythema, edema, and otorrhea.
    In addition, a patient's level of consciousness with intracranial complications may be altered. The time period of mental status change varies based on the specific type of intracranial complication. For example, an

Table 40.1 Classification Schema for the Complications of OM

EXTRACRANIAL/INTRATEMPORAL	INTRACRANIAL
Acute mastoiditis	Meningitis
Coalescent mastoiditis	Brain abscess
Chronic mastoiditis	Subdural empyema
Postauricular abscess	Epidural abscess
Bezold abscess	Lateral sinus thrombosis
Temporal abscess	Otitic hydrocephalus
Petrous apicitis	
Labyrinthine fistula	
Facial paralysis	
Acute suppurative labyrinthitis	
Encephalocele	
CSF leak	
Hearing loss (conductive and sensorineural)	

intracranial abscess may present more subtly, while rapid and severe neurologic deterioration may occur with meningitis or subdural empyema. Patients may also have papilledema, cranial nerve palsies, nuchal rigidity, or other neurologic findings.

DIAGNOSIS

12. **How does imaging play a role in the diagnosis of complications of OM?**
    CT is the mainstay of the initial radiologic evaluation of patients suspected of having complications associated with OM. Since the middle ear is connected to the mastoid air cell system, imaging of any acute OM will likely show mastoid opacification and thus may be interpreted as mastoiditis. It should be noted that the diagnosis of mastoiditis is made by taking the complete clinical picture into account (e.g., examination, labs, vital signs), but findings such as coalescence of mastoid air cells, abscess, or meningeal enhancement can support the diagnosis.

    CT should be performed with contrast to assess for soft tissue and intracranial abscesses, inflammation, and flow voids in vessels. CT also allows evaluation of the osteology of the temporal bone, specifically related to aeration of the middle ear and mastoid, bony dehiscence or erosions, and evidence supporting cholesteatoma. Additionally, CT is a much quicker alternative than magnetic resonance imaging (MRI) in patients who are unstable or have altered mental status.

    Although CT offers excellent initial evaluation of suspected complications of OM, MRI is more sensitive for the diagnosis of intracranial complications and is complementary to CT. MRI detects cerebral edema, dural enhancement, abscess, and vessel lumen patency earlier than CT.

13. **What are the important physical exam findings?**
    A complete head and neck and neurologic exam should be completed with any suspicion of OM complications. The otologic exam may reveal signs of acute infection, such as an erythematous, bulging, and opaque tympanic membrane or perforation with purulent otorrhea, granulation tissue, or signs of cholesteatoma. Postauricular abscesses may have pain with palpation, erythema, fluctuance, and proptosis of the pinna. Vestibular symptoms may be present in certain cases with periods of imbalance, dysequilibrium, and vertigo.

    A complete cranial nerve examination should also be performed. Intracranial complications may present with papilledema, abducens nerve palsy, nuchal rigidity, meningeal signs, and altered mental status. Petrous apicitis may present with abducens nerve palsy.

14. **What are some eponyms that your attending might quiz you on?**
    - *Queckenstedt's sign* is a test to determine whether cerebrospinal fluid (CSF) flow is obstructed in the spinal canal and is performed by applying bilateral pressure on the internal jugular veins during lumbar puncture. No rise in pressure during this maneuver indicates an obstruction of CSF flow.
    - *Gradenigo syndrome* is a triad of symptoms associated with petrous apicitis, including retroorbital pain, abducens nerve palsy, and otorrhea.

- *Bezold's abscess* is a cervical infection on the medial side of the mastoid deep to the digastric ridge that develops into an abscess.
- *Citelli's abscess* is an extratemporal abscess that forms from extension of a mastoid infection down the posterior belly of the digastric muscle into the occipital and cervical regions.

TREATMENT

15. **What is the general treatment for complications associated with AOM?**
Determining the status of the middle ear prior to infection is crucial for the development of a treatment algorithm. Given that AOM develops in a previously normal ear, medical treatment with antibiotics is usually adequate to treat the otitis, and ventilation tubes and/or mastoidectomy may not be needed. Watchful waiting for asymptomatic AOM is increasingly recommended in the age of increasing antimicrobial resistance.

16. **What is the general treatment for complications associated with COM?**
In CSOM, complications frequently occur with bone erosion, granulation tissue formation, or cholesteatoma. In addition to bony erosion or cholesteatoma, infection can gain access to local structures through direct extension and less frequently from preformed pathways. Infection may also propagate along veins from the mastoid to adjacent structures. In contrast to AOM, CSOM frequently necessitates the combination of antibiotics and surgery for management.

17. **What is the role of medical therapy in treating complications of OM?**
Antibiotic therapy is the mainstay of treatment, with complications associated with both AOM and CSOM. In almost all cases, intravenous (IV) antibiotics will be administered with initial broad-spectrum activity against aerobes and anaerobes. Initial regimens are meant to be broad and commonly involve a combination of antibiotics such as vancomycin, β-lactam with a β-lactamase inhibitor (e.g., ampicillin-sulbactam), cephalosporins (e.g., ceftriaxone, cefepime, cefotaxime), and/or metronidazole. It should also be noted that there may be significant institutional variability among antibiotics of choice. Providers from Infectious Disease may be invaluable for determining specific antibiotic choices, length of treatment, and monitoring of complications associated with prolonged antibiotic use (e.g., renal dysfunction, *C. difficile* colitis). Cerebrospinal fluid penetration should also be considered when intracranial complications are suspected. Culture-directed treatment should be initiated as soon as possible.

18. **What is the role of anticoagulation with sigmoid sinus thrombosis due to OM?**
Sigmoid sinus thrombosis is an intracranial complication of OM. This may occur through local inflammation/infection that eventually involves the sinus wall or through thrombophlebitic extension from local vessels. Surgery and antibiotics are well-established treatments with anticoagulation as a possible adjunct. Although controversial, anticoagulation may be beneficial in preventing clot extension and embolization, although the current literature is inconclusive regarding its use.

19. **What is the role of surgical intervention?**
It should be stressed that Table 40.2 represents general treatment guidelines for complications of OM, and complications may occur in concert with one another. Medical therapy alone without surgery may be warranted initially, especially in uncomplicated cases of acute mastoiditis. Surgery is usually recommended with failure to improve on medical therapy, development of complications, or presentation with intracranial complications.
Special consideration must be given to complications associated with cholesteatoma, as the need for extirpation must be emphasized for adequate treatment. One should also consider the role of neurosurgery in both medical and surgical management of the indicated complications.

Table 40.2 General Treatment Strategies for the Complications of OM Including Surgical Options

COMPLICATION	MEDICAL TREATMENT	SURGICAL TREATMENT
Acute mastoiditis	IV antibiotics	+/- myringotomy and ventilation tube, +/- mastoidectomy
Coalescent mastoiditis	IV antibiotics	Ventilation tube and mastoidectomy
Postauricular abscess	IV antibiotics	Ventilation tube, incision and drainage, mastoidectomy
Bezold abscess	IV antibiotics	Ventilation tube, incision and drainage, mastoidectomy
Temporal abscess	IV antibiotics	Ventilation tube, incision and drainage, mastoidectomy

(Continued)

Table 40.2 General Treatment Strategies for the Complications of OM Including Surgical Options (*Cont.*)

COMPLICATION	MEDICAL TREATMENT	SURGICAL TREATMENT
Petrous apicitis	IV antibiotics, +/- steroids	Ventilation tube, +/- mastoidectomy, +/- petrous apex drainage
Labyrinthine fistula	+/- IV antibiotics	Removal of cholesteatoma, +/- fistula repair
Facial nerve paralysis	+/- IV antibiotics, +/- steroids	+/- tympanocentesis, +/- removal of cholesteatoma
Acute suppurative labyrinthitis	IV antibiotics, +/- steroids, physical therapy	+/- mastoidectomy
Encephalocele, CSF leak	No antibiotics	Mastoid or middle fossa approach repair
Meningitis	IV antibiotics, +/- steroids	Ventilation tube, +/- mastoidectomy
Intraparenchymal brain abscess	IV antibiotics	Ventilation tube, mastoidectomy, +/- incision and drainage
Subdural empyema	IV antibiotics	Ventilation tube, mastoidectomy, incision and drainage
Epidural abscess	IV antibiotics	Ventilation tube, mastoidectomy, +/- incision and drainage
Sigmoid sinus thrombosis	IV antibiotics, +/- anti-coagulation	Ventilation tube, mastoidectomy, +/- clot/abscess removal
Otitic hydrocephalus	IV antibiotics, +/- steroids, +/- diuretics, +/- anti-coagulation	Ventilation tube, mastoidectomy, +/- clot removal, +/- serial lumbar punctures

BIBLIOGRAPHY

Budenz C, El-Kashlan H, Shelton C, Aygun N, Niparko J: Complications of temporal bone infections. In: Flint P, et al, ed: *Cummings Otolaryngology Head and Neck Surgery*, 6th ed, Philadelphia, 2015, Elsevier Saunders, pp 2156–2176.

Casselbrant M, Mandel E: Acute otitis media and otitis media with effusion. In: Flint P, et al, ed: *Cummings Otolaryngology Head and Neck Surgery*, 6th ed, Philadelphia, 2015, Elsevier Saunders, pp 3019–3037.

Chole R: Chronic otitis media, mastoiditis, and petrositis. In: Flint P, et al, editor: *Cummings Otolaryngology Head and Neck Surgery*, 6th ed, Philadelphia, 2015, Elsevier Saunders, pp 2139–2155.

Isaccson B, Mirabal C, Kutz W, Lee K, Roland P: Pediatric otogenic intra-cranial abscesses, *Otolaryngol Head Neck Surg* 142:434–437, 2010.

Loh R, Phua M, Shaw C: Management of pediatric acute mastoiditis: systematic review, *J Laryngol Otol* 132(2):96–104, 2018.

Osma U, Cureoglu S, Hosgoglu S: The complications of chronic otitis media: report of 93 cases, *J Laryngol Otol* 114:97–100, 2000.

Psarommatis IM, Voudouris C, Douros K, Giannakopoulos P, Bairamis T, Carabinos C: Algorithmic management of pediatric acute mastoiditis, *Int J Pediatr Otorhinolaryngol* 76(6):791–796, 2012.

Sitton MS, Chun R: Pediatric otogenic lateral sinus thrombosis: role of anti-coagulation and surgery, *Int J Pediatr Otorhinolaryngol* 76:428–432, 2012.

Yorgancilar E, Yildrum M, Gun R, et al: Complications of chronic suppurative otitis media: a retrospective review, *Eur Arch Otorhinolaryngol* 270:69–76, 2013.

CHAPTER 41

TYMPANOMASTOIDECTOMY AND OSSICULAR CHAIN RECONSTRUCTION

Brianne Barnett Roby, MD and Patricia J. Yoon, MD

KEY POINTS

1. Key landmarks for a mastoidectomy are the tegmen, sigmoid sinus, lateral semicircular canal, incus, and posterior canal wall.
2. A mastoidectomy is the surgical removal of mastoid air cells. It is indicated for certain types of infection, cholesteatoma, and approaches to other landmarks in the temporal bone.
3. Different types of mastoidectomies are performed based on the extent of the ear disease and include a canal wall up mastoidectomy and canal wall down mastoidectomy.
4. Ossicular chain reconstruction is performed when there is a disruption between any of the ossicles.

Pearls
1. A canal wall down mastoidectomy is indicated when there is a semicircular canal fistula or posterior canal wall damage due to cholesteatoma, a sclerotic mastoid prevents adequate visualization with a wall up mastoidectomy, or the patient is unable to follow up or undergo additional surgeries for proper monitoring of recurrent cholesteatoma.
2. A second-look procedure is indicated in a canal wall up mastoidectomy for cholesteatoma and is performed 6 to 12 months after initial surgery to look for recurrence of cholesteatoma.
3. The facial recess is bordered anteriorly by the chorda tympani, posteriorly by the facial nerve, and superiorly by the incus buttress.
4. A partial ossicular chain prosthesis (PORP) is indicated when the stapes suprastructure is present, whereas a total ossicular chain prosthesis (TORP) is indicated when the stapes suprastructure is not present.

QUESTIONS

1. **What is a mastoidectomy? What is a tympanomastoidectomy?**
   The mastoid is a portion of the temporal bone that houses air cells connected to the middle ear space. A mastoidectomy is a surgical procedure in which mastoid bone and air cells are removed. A tympanomastoidectomy is a tympanoplasty plus mastoidectomy. This procedure is commonly used to address chronic ear disease in the mastoid bone as well as a tympanic membrane that is perforated, severely retracted, or involved with cholesteatoma.

2. **What are the main types of mastoidectomy?**
   There are a number of different types of mastoidectomy surgery, broadly grouped into canal wall up (CWU) and canal wall down (CWD) procedures.

   In a CWU mastoidectomy, the mastoid air cells are removed, leaving the posterior external auditory canal wall intact. The borders of a complete mastoidectomy are the tegmen superiorly, the sigmoid sinus posteriorly, and the posterior canal wall anteriorly.

   A CWD mastoidectomy is one in which the mastoid air cells are removed along with the posterior wall of the external auditory canal. This creates a mastoid cavity or "bowl." With this procedure, a meatoplasty is also usually performed, which widens the opening of the outer ear canal in order to improve visualization and access to the mastoid bowl. A canal wall down mastoidectomy effectively "exteriorizes" the mastoid.

   In a modified radical mastoidectomy the canal wall is taken down and the epitympanum, mastoid antrum, and external auditory canal are converted into a common cavity. The middle ear space, tympanic membrane, and ossicles are preserved. This procedure is sometimes called the Bondy modified radical mastoidectomy.

   In a radical mastoidectomy, a CWD mastoidectomy is performed and the tympanic membrane and ossicles, except for the stapes, are also permanently removed. These structures are not reconstructed.

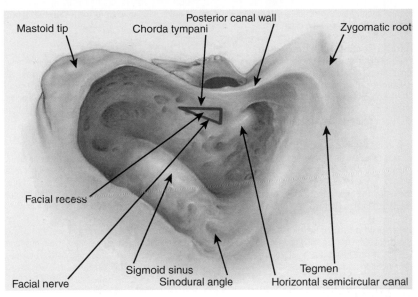

Fig. 41.1 Landmarks in mastoidectomy surgery. (From Nelson RA: *Temporal Bone Surgical Dissection Manual from the House Ear Institute, Los Angeles,* 3rd ed.)

3. **What are the indications for a mastoidectomy?**
The most common indication for a mastoidectomy is chronic disease such as cholesteatoma or mastoiditis. A mastoidectomy is also indicated for some complications of acute otitis media, such as acute mastoiditis or a subperiosteal abscess.
A mastoidectomy is a key portion of the approach for cochlear implantation or facial nerve decompression. A mastoidectomy may be performed as part of a transmastoid approach for excision of temporal bone tumors, such as vestibular schwannoma, glomus tumor, or meningioma. In unusual cases, a mastoidectomy may be required for repair of a cerebrospinal fluid leak.

4. **What are the important landmarks in mastoidectomy surgery? (Fig. 41.1)**
The superior border of a mastoidectomy is the tegmen, which is the thin bone layer separating the middle cranial fossa from the ear. The posterior border is the sigmoid sinus. The anterior border is the posterior wall of the external auditory canal. The deep (medial) border is the lateral semicircular canal and incus, which are found in the aditus ad antrum, the connection between the mastoid cavity and the middle ear space. Another key landmark is the facial nerve.

5. **When is a canal wall down procedure indicated?**
A canal wall down procedure is indicated in the following situations:
- Cholesteatoma involving the sinus tympani area, not accessible transcanally or through the facial recess
- Semicircular canal fistula with adherent cholesteatoma matrix
- The posterior canal wall is extensively damaged by disease
- The mastoid is contracted and sclerotic, preventing adequate visualization and access via a CWU approach
- Unresectable cholesteatoma matrix on the dura or posterior cranial fossa
- Attic or mastoid cholesteatoma in a patient unable to maintain follow-up or unable to safely tolerate further surgery

6. **What are the disadvantages of a CWD mastoidectomy?**
The mastoid bowl often fills with cerumen and requires periodic debridement to prevent infection. Although not necessarily unsightly, the meatoplasty is often visible. Hearing outcomes may be slightly diminished due to the change in the acoustic properties of the ear canal. Water restrictions are recommended due to risk of mastoid bowl infection.

7. **What are the disadvantages of a CWU procedure?**
There is a higher chance of recurrent or residual cholesteatoma, as exposure of the attic, antrum, and facial recess is more limited if the canal wall is left intact. Patients who have had a CWU procedure are more likely to

require a "second-look" procedure in the operating room, whereas patients undergoing a CWD mastoidectomy can often be monitored in the clinic.

8. **What is a second-look procedure?**

   For patients who have had cholesteatoma removed using the CWU technique, a second-look surgery may be performed several months later (typically 6 to 12 months) to determine whether there is recurrent or residual disease that was not visible at the time of the previous surgery and could not be detected on office examination.

   The procedure is performed several months later to allow time for any microscopic residual disease to grow large enough to be visualized. However, one should not wait too long, as residual or recurrent cholesteatoma may grow large enough to cause damage to ear structures.

9. **What is a facial recess approach? What are the borders of the facial recess?**

   The facial recess is an area within the mastoid that frequently contains air cells and is a pathway to the middle ear space. The facial recess is bordered anteriorly by the chorda tympani, posteriorly by the facial nerve, and superiorly by the incus buttress. The facial recess air cells are at the same level as the tip of the short process of the incus. The facial recess may be opened up to help eradicate cholesteatoma and is also used in cochlear implantation to allow introduction of the electrode through the middle ear space into the round window.

10. **How should a lateral semicircular canal fistula be managed?**

    This is most often managed by performing a CWD mastoidectomy and leaving a portion of squamous matrix over the fistula. In rare cases, the cholesteatoma may be removed in its entirety and the fistula patched with a graft. Suctioning of the area should be avoided to preserve the endolymph within the canal.

11. **What are the potential complications of a mastoidectomy?**

    Major complications include facial nerve injury, sensorineural hearing loss, cerebrospinal fluid leak, and dural venous sinus injury.

    Minor complications include temporary change in taste sensation from manipulation of the chorda tympani, vertigo, and tympanic membrane perforation.

12. **What is a Bondy atticotomy?**

    This procedure involves a limited approach to an attic cholesteatoma. An endaural incision is used and then a small atticoantrostomy is performed. The bone overlying the attic is then taken down to inferior to the level of the disease. The pars tensa and the ossicular chain are left intact.

13. **What is an "inside-out" mastoidectomy?**

    An "inside-out" approach usually begins endaurally by raising a tympanomeatal flap and drilling an atticotomy. The mastoid air cells are drilled starting from the atticotomy and posterior canal wall, rather than starting from the mastoid cortex as with a traditional mastoidectomy. This approach can be useful when there is a very low-lying tegmen or anteriorly placed sigmoid sinus, which can limit the approach for a typical atticoantrostomy.

14. **What are the indications for an ossicular chain reconstruction?**

    The ossicular chain is composed of the three bones of the middle ear: the malleus, incus, and stapes (Fig. 41.2). Ossicular chain reconstruction is performed when conductive hearing loss is due to a disruption or abnormality of

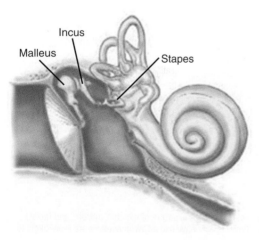

Incus
Malleus
Stapes

Fig. 41.2 Ossicular chain. (Modified from *Dorland's Illustrated Medical Dictionary,* 32nd ed, Philadelphia, 2011, Saunders.)

these bones. The disruption may be due to trauma, congenital abnormalities, chronic ear disease, cholesteatoma, or surgery. Osteoclastic properties of cholesteatoma often erode the ossicular chain. Ossicular chain reconstruction is undertaken when the ear is felt to be free of disease, which is often not until a second-look or subsequent procedure.

15. **What are contraindications for an ossicular chain reconstruction?**
    Acute otitis media at time of reconstruction is an absolute contraindication. Relative contraindications include persistent middle ear disease such as cholesteatoma, dehiscent facial nerve overlying the oval window, or an only hearing ear.

16. **What are some of the different prostheses that may be used in ossicular chain reconstruction and their specific indications?**
    Two broad categories exist: PORPs and TORPs. A PORP is used when the stapes suprastructure is present where the PORP can sit on the stapes head and then connect the tympanic membrane. A TORP sits on the stapes footplate and extends to contact the tympanic membrane. A cartilage graft is placed on the head of the prosthesis to help prevent extrusion through the tympanic membrane.
    TORPs and PORPs are made of different materials, commonly titanium and hydroxyapatite-polyethylene.
    Bone cement is useful in certain situations, such as reconstructing the long process of the incus and stabilizing prostheses.

17. **What is an incus interposition graft?**
    An incus interposition graft can be used when there are abnormalities of either the incudomalleal joint or the incudostapedial joint but with normal malleus and stapes. The incus is removed and sculpted with a groove to accommodate the malleus and a cup to hold the stapes capitulum. The carved incus is then placed back between the malleus and stapes, making sure that it makes proper contact with both.

18. **What are the expected outcomes for ossicular reconstruction surgery?**
    It is important to set realistic expectations for patients undergoing ossicular reconstruction. Results are quantified based on the postoperative air–bone gap achieved and are stratified as follows: excellent (<10 dB), good (11 to 20 dB), and fair (21 to 30 dB). Success is dependent on multiple factors, including absence or presence of a mobile stapes superstructure, eustachian tube function and middle ear status, and presence or absence of the canal wall. Hearing outcomes are generally more successful with PORPs than with TORPs.

19. **What are potential complications of ossicular reconstruction surgery?**
    Complications include perilymphatic fistula resulting in sensorineural hearing loss and vertigo, extrusion or displacement of the prosthesis, tympanic membrane perforation, facial nerve injury, and change in taste sensation.

20. **What is endoscopic ear surgery and what are its advantages?**
    Traditional ear surgery is performed under a microscope and the field of view via a transcanal approach is limited by the narrowest portion of the ear canal. A mastoidectomy is therefore often required even when the mastoid is free of disease in order to gain visualization and access to the attic, facial recess, and hypotympanum. In recent years, the use of rigid surgical endoscopes for cholesteatoma surgery has increased in popularity. Both 0-degree and angled rigid endoscopes through the ear canal allow for a wider field of view within the middle ear and allow visualization of areas that cannot be seen using the microscope. With the use of endoscopes and specially designed endoscopic ear surgery instruments, surgery for cholesteatoma and other middle ear problems is now possible in many cases through much smaller postauricular or even transcanal incisions, with significantly improved visualization.

BIBLIOGRAPHY

Brackmann DE, Shelton C, Arriaga MA, eds: *Otologic Surgery*, 4th ed, 2015, Elsevier.
Coker NJ, Jenkins HA, eds: *Atlas of Otologic Surgery*, 2001, W. B. Saunders.
Gopen Q, ed: *Fundamental Otology Pediatric and Adult Practice*, 2013, Jaypee Medical Publishers.
In: Hathiram BT, Khattar VS, eds: *Atlas of Operative Otorhinolaryngology, Head, Neck Surgery*, 2012, Jaypee Medical Publishers, pp. 112–123.
Johnson J, Rosen C, eds: *Bailey's Head and Neck Surgery: Otolaryngology*, 5th ed, 2013, Lippincott Williams and Wilkins, pp. 2447–2486.
Kiringoda R, Kozin ED, Lee DJ: Outcomes in endoscopic ear surgery, *Otolaryngol Clin North Am* 49(5):1271–1290, 2016.
Lalwani A, ed: *Current Diagnosis, Treatment in Otolaryngology Head, Neck Surgery*, 3rd ed, 2012, McGraw Hill Medical.
Myers EN, ed: *Operative Otolaryngology*, 3rd ed, 2017, Elsevier.

CHAPTER 42

OTOSCLEROSIS

Jameson K. Mattingly, MD and Herman Jenkins, MD

KEY POINTS

Pathophysiology of otosclerosis
1. Otosclerosis involves the otic capsule.
2. Originates from altered bony metabolism with ongoing resorption and deposition of disorganized bone.
3. Results in fixation of the ossicular chain, typically the stapes, producing conductive hearing loss.
4. Can also rarely involve the cochlea, resulting in "cochlear otosclerosis".
5. Possible contributing factors include genetics, measles infection, autoimmunity, multiple endocrine abnormalities, and low fluoride consumption.

Pearls

Otosclerosis
1. The ear frequently appears normal on physical exam.
2. The most common presentation is progressive conductive hearing loss with absent acoustic reflexes ipsilateral to the affected ear.
3. Although not required for diagnosis, many patients will have a positive family history; frequently bilateral.
4. Stapes surgery has a high success rate for improvement of hearing.
5. Medical therapies, including sodium fluoride and bisphosphonates, are controversial in their clinical effectiveness.

QUESTIONS

1. **Define otosclerosis.**
   Otosclerosis is derived from the Greek word for "hardening of the ear." It is characterized by altered bony metabolism of the otic capsule with ongoing resorption and deposition of bone. This metabolic process frequently results in fixation of the ossicular chain, most commonly the stapes, and resultant conductive hearing loss (CHL).

2. **Describe the epidemiology of otosclerosis.**
   Otosclerosis most commonly occurs in Caucasians between the second and fifth decades of life, with a female-to-male ratio of 2:1. Bilateral disease occurs in 70% to 80% of patients, and approximately 20% to 30% develop sensorineural hearing loss (SNHL).

3. **What is the pathophysiology of otosclerosis?**
   In the normal state, endochondral calcification is usually complete in the otic capsule during the first year of life, with little remodeling thereafter. Otosclerosis, however, causes bone remodeling in and around the otic capsule by osteoblasts and osteoclasts. This abnormal process results in poorly organized bone that becomes active, well vascularized (spongiotic), and/or densely mineralized (sclerotic) (see Fig. 42.1). The end result in classic otosclerosis is fixation of the stapes footplate, usually beginning anteriorly at the fissula ante fenestram with progression to complete footplate involvement.

4. **What are the initial symptoms of otosclerosis?**
   The characteristic presentation of otosclerosis is adult-onset progressive unilateral or bilateral conductive hearing loss. Although less likely, otosclerosis can present with SNHL due to "cochlear otosclerosis." Some patients report improved hearing in a noisy environment, which is referred to as the paracusis of Willis, but this symptom is unreliable in the diagnosis. The second most common complaint is tinnitus, and vestibular symptoms are rarely reported.

5. **Does genetics play a role in the development of otosclerosis?**
   Studies in families with otosclerosis have supported an autosomal dominant pattern of inheritance with incomplete penetrance. Within these groups, multiple genes have been implicated, although there is significant heterogeneity in the genetic pattern. Although genetic factors likely influence the development of otosclerosis, many cases arise without a positive family history.

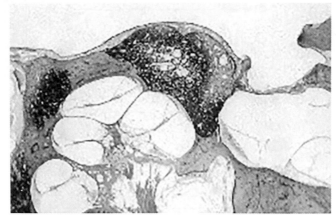

Fig. 42.1 Multiple otosclerotic lesions around the cochlea and anterior to the stapes footplate.

6. **What other factors may be causative in the development of otosclerosis?**
Although literature supporting various etiologies is limited, genetics, persistent measles infection, autoimmunity, multiple endocrine factors, and low fluoride consumption have been implicated in the development of otosclerosis.

7. **What is Schwartze sign?**
Schwartze sign is a reddish hue seen though the tympanic membrane reflecting the increased vascularity of the bone over the promontory. Although this may be seen early in the disease process, this finding is not observed in all cases.

8. **What physical exam findings are expected in patients with otosclerosis?**
The physical examination findings of patients with otosclerosis are limited. Most patients present with a normal external auditory canal and tympanic membrane, with an occasional Schwartze sign. Rinne and Weber tuning fork examinations will typically reveal bone conduction to be greater than air conduction and lateralization to the affected side, respectively, although these findings are not specific. Negative Rinne testing (bone conduction greater than air conduction) indicates an air-bone gap of at least 15 to 20 dB. Many surgeons will not perform surgery for otosclerosis in patients if the Rinne test does not reveal this finding.

9. **What are the expected audiogram findings of otosclerosis?**
Audiometric studies typically show a CHL worse at low frequencies with absent stapedial reflexes ipsilateral to the affected ear. The Carhart notch is characteristic of otosclerosis, showing an apparent SNHL at 2000 Hz (see Fig. 42.2).

10. **What role does acoustic immittance testing play in diagnosis of otosclerosis?**
Tympanometry will typically be normal or show an A_s configuration reflecting normal middle ear pressure but decreased amplitude, indicative of some degree of ossicular chain fixation. The stapedial reflex may be present in the early stages of the disease process but may show abnormalities including biphasic reflexes. Reflexes become absent with progression of the disease to stapes fixation. Absent reflexes are key to ensuring that hearing loss is a middle ear process and not due to other diseases that can mimic otosclerosis (e.g., superior semicircular canal dehiscence).

11. **Does imaging play a role in otosclerosis?**
Imaging modalities for otosclerosis such as computed tomography (CT) and magnetic resonance imaging (MRI) are not routinely needed. However, recent studies have suggested that high-resolution CT, along with physical and audiometric data, is highly sensitive in diagnosing otosclerosis (see Fig. 42.3). In addition to assisting in diagnosis, CT may provide information helpful for surgical planning and prevention of complications.

12. **Does medical treatment play a role in otosclerosis?**
Current medical therapies aim to decrease bone remodeling, specifically targeting osteoclastic activity. Much of this theory was initially based on successful treatment of osteoporosis. Possible medical therapies include bisphosphonates and sodium fluoride. Given the success of surgical treatment, medical therapy is not consistently recommended.
   It should also be mentioned that hearing aids offer a successful nonsurgical alternative for correction of hearing loss associated with otosclerosis, especially in those who are poor surgical candidates.

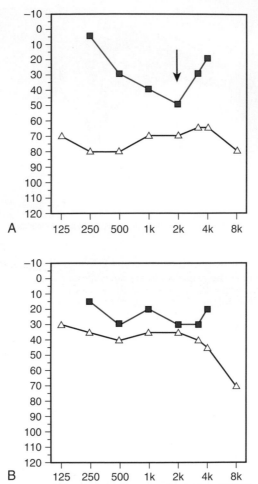

Fig. 42.2 Audiogram with a conductive hearing loss and apparent sensory hearing loss at 2000 Hz representing a Carhart notch.

13. **Describe the surgical treatment of otosclerosis.**

Multiple techniques are currently used for the surgical treatment of otosclerosis. Regardless of variations in technique, the current literature reports successful outcomes in more than 90% of patients as measured by closure of their preoperative air-bone gap. This includes stapedectomy and stapedotomy and the use of a variety of prostheses.

In general, the goal of surgery is to allow the transmission of sound from the tympanic membrane through the ossicular chain to the oval window while bypassing the fixed stapes footplate. This process typically involves some variation in the removal of the arch of the stapes, fenestration, or some degree of removal of the stapes footplate and insertion of a prosthesis connecting the incus to the oval window (see Fig. 42.4). In cases of incus necrosis, a prosthesis connecting the malleus to the oval window can be used, although this surgery is much more technically difficult and has more variability in outcomes.

14. **Are there any special considerations in patients with bilateral otosclerosis?**

Bilateral otosclerosis occurs in approximately 70% to 80% of cases. When electing to operate on a patient with bilateral disease, the poorer hearing ear is generally operated on first, followed by, if successful, the contralateral ear several months later.

15. **What are the risks associated with stapes surgery?**

Risks that should be considered during informed consent include SNHL (including deafness, 1%–2%), vertigo, facial nerve injury, loss or change of taste, continued conductive hearing loss, prosthesis extrusion or displacement, and tympanic membrane perforation.

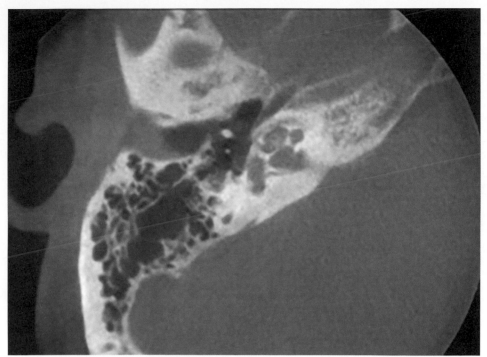

Fig. 42.3 CT showing classic appearance of otosclerosis. Note the halo surrounding the cochlea.

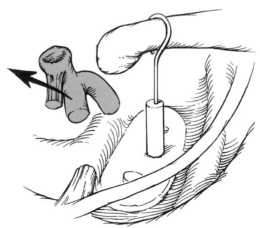

Fig. 42.4 Stapes prosthesis from the incus into the stapedotomy fenestra after removal of the stapes superstructure.

16. **Discuss the important points regarding revision stapes surgery.**
    Despite the success of primary stapes surgery, the need for revision does occur. Common reasons for revision surgery include persistent or recurrent CHL, vertigo, SNHL, and sound distortion. Prior to undergoing revision stapes surgery, other factors for these symptoms should be thoroughly explored. CT scan of the temporal bones is warranted to evaluate the middle ear and prosthesis and to rule out other causes of CHL. In addition to discussing the risks of surgery, special attention should be paid to informed consent regarding decreased success for revision surgery and increased risk of SNHL (including deafness) in comparison with primary surgery.

BIBLIOGRAPHY

Chole RA, McKenna M: Pathophysiology of otosclerosis, *Otol Neurotol* 22:249–257, 2001.

Glasscock M III, Storper I, Haynes D, Bohrer P: Twenty-five years of experience with stapedectomy, *Laryngoscope* 105:899–904, 1995.

House J, Cunningham C: Otosclerosis. In: Flint P, et al, ed: *Cummings Otolaryngology Head and Neck Surgery*, 6th ed, Philadelphia, 2015, Elsevier Saunders, pp 2211–2219.

Jenkins H, McKenna M, Quesnel A: Otosclerosis. In: Snow J, Wackym P, eds: *Ballenger's Otorhinolaryngology Head and Neck Surgery*, 18th ed, Shelton, CT, 2016, People's Medical Publishing House.

Kursten R, Schneider B, Zrunek M: Long-term results after stapedectomy versus stapedotomy, *Am J Otol* 15(6):804–806, 1994.

Lagleyre S, Sorrentino T, Calmels MN, et al: Reliability of high-resolution CT scan in diagnosis of otosclerosis, *Otol Neurotol* 30(8):1152–1159, 2009.

Rudic M, Keogh I, Wagner R, et al: The pathophysiology of otosclerosis: review of current research, *Ear Hearing* 330(Part A):51–56, 2015.

Schrauwen I, Van Camp G: The etiology of otosclerosis: a combination of genes and environment, *Laryngoscope* 120:1195–1202, 2010.

Shea J: Forty years of stapes surgery, *Am J Otol* 19:52–55, 1998.

Ziya Ozuer M, Olgun L, Gultekin G: Revision stapes surgery, *Otolaryngol Head Neck Surg* 146(1):109–113, 2011.

CHAPTER 43

CHOLESTEATOMA

Jameson K. Mattingly, MD and Kenny H. Chan, MD

Pearls

1. Congenital, primary acquired, and secondary acquired are the different types of cholesteatomas.
2. Cholesteatomas characteristically become infected and/or erode bone, resulting in a variety of complications.
3. CT is the most commonly used imaging modality to evaluate cholesteatomas.
4. Surgery is the definitive treatment, with goals geared toward complete eradication of disease, preservation of hearing, and overall improvement of ear hygiene.
5. Second-stage operations or MRI may be used to evaluate residual and recurrent disease, especially with extensive cholesteatomas after the first operation.

QUESTIONS

PATHOPHYSIOLOGY, ETIOLOGY, AND CLASSIFICATION

1. **What is a cholesteatoma?**
   Cholesteatomas are epidermal inclusion cysts of the temporal bone and are composed of squamous epithelium and associated debris. Cholesteatomas enlarge over time and become destructive, commonly with surrounding inflammation and granulation tissue.

   The word cholesteatoma was first used to describe its light color and gross resemblance to cholesterol crystals under microscopy. This observation is a misnomer because of the lack of cholesterol or fat in cholesteatomas.

2. **What are the different types of cholesteatomas?**
   The three main types are congenital, primary acquired, and secondary acquired (Table 43.1).

3. **Briefly describe the different pathogenic mechanisms.**
   Congenital cholesteatomas are thought to originate from the keratinizing squamous epithelium of the middle ear. Although the etiology remains unknown, multiple theories exist to describe the origin of the squamous epithelium. These theories include epidermoid cell rests within the middle ear (most favored theory), squamous metaplasia,

Table 43.1 Various Types of Cholesteatomas and Their Associated Origin

TYPE	ORIGIN
Congenital	Keratinizing epithelium in the middle ear cleft with an intact tympanic membrane; multiple theories exist
Primary acquired	Occurs in the setting of tympanic membrane retraction; multiple theories exist
Secondary acquired	Occurs in the setting of tympanic membrane perforation; multiple theories exist

epithelial migration through tympanic membrane (TM), microperforations, and deposition of desquamated epithelial cells from the amniotic fluid.

Primary acquired cholesteatomas usually arise in the setting of retraction of the TM, usually as a result of otitis media and chronic eustachian tube dysfunction. Although usually arising from the pars flaccida (or epitympanic area), they can also develop in the pars tensa (commonly the mesotympanic area). Alternatively, secondary acquired cholesteatomas arise in the setting of TM perforations. Multiple theories exist to explain the pathogenesis of acquired cholesteatomas, including TM invagination, migration of epithelium through TM perforations, basal cell hyperplasia, squamous metaplasia, and implantation.

4. What is the invagination theory?

Invagination is the most accepted theory of primary acquired cholesteatomas. TM retraction results from negative middle ear pressure due to eustachian tube dysfunction, poor pneumatization of the mastoid, inflammation, and/or TM atrophy. Progressive retraction forms a pocket, resulting in disrupted normal epithelial migration and drainage of keratin debris. As this process progresses, the collection of keratin debris becomes large and a cholesteatoma forms.

5. Why treat cholesteatoma?

Cholesteatomas have a propensity to become recurrently infected and locally destructive. Once infected, eradication of an infection may be very difficult and can result in a variety of intracranial and extracranial complications associated with chronic otitis media. The bacterial flora associated with cholesteatomas are also different from those associated with acute otitis media. Infections associated with cholesteatomas are frequently polymicrobial, with an increase in anaerobes and antibiotic-resistant bacteria.

Local bone destruction can affect various structures in the temporal bone, which can result in hearing loss, vestibular dysfunction, facial nerve injury, and intracranial complications. Bone erosion is thought to be due to an influx of inflammatory mediators due to chronic inflammation and infection.

6. How does a congenital cholesteatoma present?

Congenital cholesteatomas usually present as a white or yellow mass in the anterior superior quadrant of the middle ear (Fig. 43.1). Unlike acquired cholesteatomas, congenital cholesteatomas usually arise in the setting of an intact TM in the absence of otorrhea. They are often asymptomatic and symptoms that do occur vary depending upon the extent of the disease. Presenting symptoms include slowly progressive conductive hearing loss (CHL), vertigo, facial nerve paralysis, and intracranial infection.

7. How do acquired cholesteatomas present?

Acquired cholesteatomas usually present as a posterior or superior retraction pocket at the margin of the TM with surrounding keratin debris. Acquired cholesteatomas may or may not have TM perforations with persistent foul-smelling otorrhea and granulation tissue. Presenting symptoms, as in congenital cholesteatoma, vary with the extent of the disease and can include many of the same features.

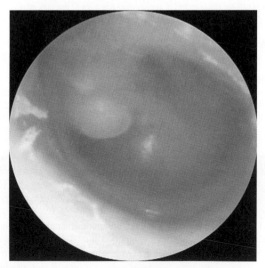

Fig. 43.1 Congenital cholesteatoma behind an intact tympanic membrane.

PRE-OPERATIVE ASSESSMENT

8. **What is the role of imaging in the preoperative assessment?**
Computed tomography (CT) is frequently used to augment physical examination in patients with suspected cholesteatoma. Although not required for uncomplicated cases, CT provides valuable information regarding the extent
of disease, involved structures, and relevant anatomy that assists in preoperative planning. CT may also prove to
be very helpful in revision cases. Magnetic resonance imaging (MRI) is less commonly used preoperatively but is
helpful in evaluating intracranial complications.

9. **What is the one CT finding commonly seen in acquired cholesteatoma that your attending
likely will ask?**
Blunting or erosion of the scutum is a common finding on CT in patients with cholesteatoma (see Fig. 43.2). The
scutum is a bony prominence in the lateral portion of the middle ear and the superior portion of the external
auditory canal.

10. **What is significant about finding cholesteatoma around oval and round windows or eroding
into the lateral semicircular canal?**
Cholesteatoma involving the oval and round windows and with semicircular canal erosion poses an increased
risk of sensorineural hearing loss (SNHL), suppurative labyrinthitis, and perilymphatic fistula. Cholesteatomas can
also frequently erode the fallopian canal, and surgeons must be cautious of facial nerve dehiscence during these
surgeries.

11. **Are audiograms useful in the treatment and management of cholesteatoma?**
Preoperative audiograms are indicated to assess baseline hearing and for long-term follow-up after surgical
removal. They also have both medical and legal implications.

SURGICAL MANAGEMENT

12. **What are the standard surgical approaches?**
Various surgical approaches include atticotomy, tympanomastoidectomy with canal wall-up or-down procedures,
posterior tympanotomy or facial recess approach, and modified radical and radical mastoidectomy. Regardless of
the type of surgery performed, the goal is to completely remove the disease, preserve hearing, prevent residual
or recurrent disease, and improve ear hygiene. The specific surgical approach is mainly determined by the extent
of the disease as well as the surgeon's comfort level. Facial nerve monitoring should be strongly considered,
especially during revision surgery or in cases with extensive disease. Facial nerve monitoring has been shown to
improve the identification of dehiscence and, although small, decrease the rates of nerve injury.
Atticotomy is mainly used when disease is limited lateral to the malleus and incus and is accessible through
a transcanal approach. Tympanomastoidectomy with or without facial recess is used for cholesteatoma extending
medially to the ossicles and into the mastoid through the antrum.

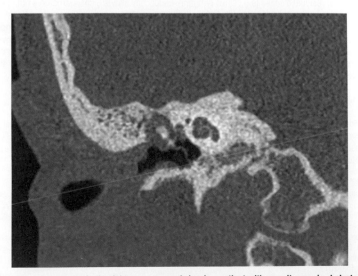

Fig. 43.2 Blunting of the scutum seen in the right ear on coronal view in a patient with an epitympanic cholesteatoma.

The decision of the canal wall-up or wall-down procedure is largely based on the ability to perform complete removal of cholesteatoma. Canal wall-up procedures are preferred because they allow for preserved anatomy and an improved ability for reconstruction, resulting in a more physiologic middle ear with decreased aural care, improved ability to use hearing aids, and no water restriction. Canal wall-down procedures, in contrast, have been shown to provide improved postoperative physical examination and superior intraoperative visualization of disease, specifically in difficult-to-view areas of the middle ear (e.g., sinus tympani).

13. Why are surgeons reluctant to perform canal wall-down mastoidectomy?

Although canal wall-down mastoidectomy procedures provide superior visualization during and after cholesteatoma removal, they often result in difficulty in reconstructing the middle ear, hearing loss, and mastoid cavity problems. Canal wall-down mastoid cavities require lifelong canal cleaning, with an increased risk of infections and persistent otorrhea. They may also result in long-term water restriction and caloric-induced vertigo and impair the use of hearing aids.

14. What are second-stage procedures?

Planned second-stage procedures are performed due to increased rates of recurrence, especially in the pediatric population, and evaluation of residual disease. Recurrent cholesteatomas are thought to be due to recurrent disease, such as eustachian tube dysfunction, creating a new retraction pocket for cholesteatoma formation. Residual disease is also common with extensive cholesteatomas where disease remains inadvertently in hard-to-reach areas or intentionally due to the involvement of critical structures.

Although common, the timing and decision to perform a second-stage procedure are not well established and mainly depend on the surgeon's experience. It should also be mentioned that certain factors, such as the location of disease, have been correlated with a higher risk of recurrence. Some surgeons may also favor a second-stage procedure to perform ossiculoplasty if needed.

15. What is the timing for the second-stage procedure?

The timing of a second-stage procedure is debated but it is typically performed between 6 and 12 months after the original procedure.

16. What are the types of ossicular prostheses?

During surgical removal of cholesteatoma the ossicles can frequently be damaged, most commonly from erosion of the incus, resulting in CHL. Various materials can be used to reconstruct the ossicular chain, including autografts (e.g., bone and cartilage from the patient), homografts (e.g., bone, cartilage from tissue banks), and allografts (e.g., polymers, ceramics, metals). Allografts over recent years have been used more commonly, and depending upon the reconstruction, they are generally used as either partial ossicular replacement prosthesis (PORP) or total ossicular replacement prosthesis (TORP).

17. Describe other techniques used in cholesteatoma surgery.

The use of oto-endoscopy has increased in recent years to allow better visualization of areas known to have a high incidence of residual disease (e.g., sinus tympani). Endoscopy allows hidden structures out of the linear view of a microscope to be viewed and may offer less invasive approaches to second-stage procedures.

Mastoid cavity obliteration is also advocated by some surgeons to prevent future retraction pocket formation and recurrent cholesteatoma. The procedure involves separating the middle ear and mastoid, followed by obliterating the mastoid with materials such as bone dust. This technique allows superior visualization and removal of cholesteatoma associated with a canal wall-down technique but decreases complications such as the need for frequent cleaning, difficulty with hearing aids, and water restriction.

18. What's new in cholesteatoma follow-up?

Historically, second-stage procedures have been commonly used for the evaluation of recurrent and residual cholesteatoma, but new imaging sequences are becoming more popular to prevent needless surgery. MRI has an advantage over CT in differentiating soft tissues and fluid in the middle ear and mastoid. Specifically, non-echo-planar–based diffusion-weighted MRI has been shown to be highly reliable in detecting small cholesteatomas (e.g., greater than 2 millimeters).

BIBLIOGRAPHY

Adams M, El-Kashlan H: Tympanoplasty and ossiculoplasty. In: Flint P, et al, ed: *Cummings Otolaryngology Head and Neck Surgery*, 6th ed, Philadelphia, 2015, Elsevier Saunders, pp 2177–2187.

Chole R: Chronic otitis media, mastoiditis, and petrositis. In: Flint P, et al, ed: *Cummings Otolaryngology Head and Neck Surgery*, 6th ed, Philadelphia, 2015, Elsevier Saunders, pp 2139–2155.

Denoyelle F, Simon F, Chang K, et al: International Pediatric Otolaryngology Group (IPOG) consensus recommendations: congenital cholesteatoma, *Otol Neurotol* 41(3):345–351, 2020.

Han S, Lee D, Chung J, Kim Y: Comparison of endoscopic and microscopic surgery in pediatric patient: a meta-analysis, *Laryngoscope* 129(6):1444–1452, 2019.

Hulka G, McElveen: A randomized, blinded study of canal wall up versus canal wall down mastoidectomy determining the differences in viewing middle ear anatomy and pathology, *Am J Otol* 19:574–578, 1998.

Li P, Linos E, Gurgel R, Fischbein N, Blevins N: Evaluating the utility of non-echo-planar diffusion-weighted imaging in the pre-operative evaluation of cholesteatoma: a meta-analysis, *Laryngoscope* 123(5):1247–1250, 2013.

Noss R, Lalwani A, Yingling C: Facial nerve monitoring in middle ear and mastoid surgery, *Laryngoscope* 111:831–836, 2001.

Prasad S, La Melia C, Medina M, et al: Long-term surgical and functional outcomes of the intact canal wall technique for middle ear cholesteatoma in the paediatric population, *Acta Otorhinolaryngol Ital* 34(5):354–361, 2014.

Schraff S, Strasnick B: Pediatric cholesteatoma: a retrospective review, *Int J Pediatr Otorhinolaryngol* 70(3):385–393, 2006.

Vercruysse J, De Foer B, Somers T, Casselman J, Offeciers E: Mastoid and epitympanic bony obliteration in pediatric cholesteatoma, *Otol Neurotol* 29:953–960, 2008.

CHAPTER 44

FACIAL NERVE

Scott E. Mann, MD and Stephen P. Cass, MD

KEY POINTS

1. In addition to motor fibers, the facial nerve carries visceral motor, general sensory, and special sensory fibers to the following structures:
   - Parasympathetic input to the lacrimal, submandibular, and sublingual glands
   - Taste from the tongue (special sensory)
   - Sensation from ear canal skin (general sensory)
2. The facial nerve is anatomically divided into three segments:
   - Intracranial (pontine, cerebellar-pontine angle, and internal auditory canal); 23 to 24 millimeters in length
   - Intratemporal (known as the fallopian canal); 20 to 30 millimeters in length
   - Extratemporal (from the stylomastoid foramen to the muscles of facial expression, posterior belly of digastric, stylohyoid, and postauricular muscles); 15 to 20 millimeters
3. The extratemporal facial nerve trunk can be found as it exits the temporal bone via the stylomastoid foramen using several anatomic landmarks:
   - Tragal pointer
   - Digastric muscle
   - Tympanomastoid fissure
   - Following a peripheral branch proximally
   - Finding the mastoid segment of the facial nerve by mastoidectomy
4. Though Bell's palsy is the most common cause of facial nerve paralysis, not all facial palsies are Bell's palsy. Consider neoplasm as the etiology rather than Bell's palsy if any of the following are present:
   - Slow, progressive onset of facial weakness
   - Facial spasms
   - Palpable mass in the parotid gland or a mass visible in the middle ear
5. Treatment of Bell's palsy includes:
   - Oral steroids within 72 hours of symptom onset.
   - Oral antivirals should not be used alone for Bell's palsy (no proven benefit) but are an option in combination with oral steroids.
   - Imaging is not required if a patient has a history and physical exam consistent with Bell's palsy.
   - Education on eye care and the importance of physician follow-up until recovery occurs.

Pearls
1. A common mnemonic for the five major motor branches to the facial muscles is: **T**o **Z**anzibar **B**y **M**otor **C**ar (Fig. 44.1).
2. Passive upper eyelid closure can occur by relaxation of the levator palpebrae muscle (innervated by the oculomotor nerve), so upper eyelid motion is not always indicative of an intact facial nerve.
3. The labyrinthine segment of the facial nerve is the narrowest portion of the fallopian canal, making it the area most susceptible to entrapment neuropathy during nerve swelling associated with Bell's palsy.
4. The geniculate ganglion lies at the junction of the labyrinthine and tympanic segments of the facial nerve.
   - The geniculate ganglion contains special sensory ganglion cells serving taste and somatic sensory ganglion cells serving ear canal sensation.
   - The first branch of the facial nerve is the greater superficial petrosal nerve that contains parasympathetic fibers to the lacrimal gland, which exits from the anterior margin of the geniculate ganglion.
5. The marginal mandibular and temporal branches of the facial nerve are the branches most at risk during parotidectomy, rhytidectomy, and repair of mandibular fracture.

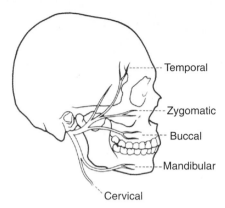

Fig. 44.1 The five major motor branches to the facial muscles. (From May M, Schaitkin B: *The Facial Nerve,* 2nd ed, New York, 2000, Thieme.)

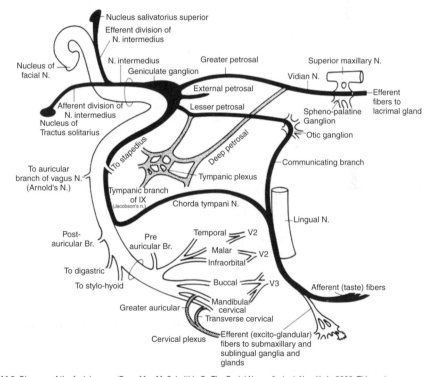

Fig. 44.2 Diagram of the facial nerve. (From May M, Schaitkin B: *The Facial Nerve,* 2nd ed, New York, 2000, Thieme.)

QUESTIONS

1. **What types of nerve fibers are carried by the facial nerve?**
   The facial nerve carries both motor and sensory nerve fibers (Fig. 44.2). These include:
   - Special visceral efferent: motor innervation of the muscles of facial expression, stylohyoid, stapedius, platysma, and posterior belly of the digastric muscle.
   - General visceral efferent: parasympathetic innervation of the lacrimal, submandibular, sublingual, minor salivary, and mucosal glands of the nose and palate.
   - Special sensory afferent: taste from the anterior two thirds of the tongue, palate, and tonsillar fossa.

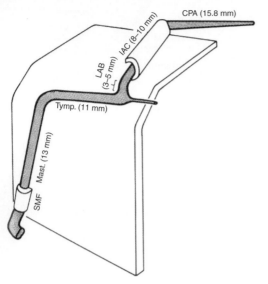

CPA (15.8 mm)

IAC (8–10 mm)

LAB (3–5 mm)

Tymp. (11 mm)

Mast. (13 mm)

SMF

Fig. 44.3 Anatomic segments of the fallopian canal. (From May M, Schaitkin B: *The Facial Nerve,* 2nd ed, New York, 2000, Thieme.)

- Somatic sensory afferent: sensation from the external ear canal and skin of the concha portion of the auricle.
- General visceral afferent sensory: sensation from the nasal mucosa, palate, and pharynx.

2. **Which branchial arch is associated with the facial nerve during development?**
   The second branchial arch. All muscles innervated by the facial nerve are second arch derivatives, as well as the stapes suprastructure, styloid process, stylohyoid ligament, and the lesser cornu of the hyoid.

3. **Name the three anatomic segments of the fallopian canal, their course, and their length (Fig. 44.3).**
   - Labyrinthine segment: from the fundus of the internal auditory canal (meatal foramen) to the geniculate ganglion; 3 to 5 millimeters. The labyrinthine segment represents the narrowest portion of the fallopian canal at 1 millimeters.
   - Tympanic segment: from the geniculate ganglion to the pyramidal process; 8 to 11 millimeters. Begins at the second genu (the first genu is intrapontine). The bony covering of the facial nerve is often dehiscent in this segment. This is the most common site of iatrogenic injury during ear surgery.
   - Mastoid segment: from the pyramidal process to the stylomastoid foramen; 10 to 14 millimeters. The change in direction between the tympanic and mastoid segments represents the last genu before exciting the temporal bone.

4. **What is the nervus intermedius?**
   The nervus intermedius can be thought of as a division of the facial nerve that carries its nonbranchial motor components. It is anatomically adjacent to, but separate from, the main trunk of the facial nerve as it exits the brain stem and then fuses with the facial nerve within the internal auditory canal. The chorda tympani is the terminal extension of the nervus intermedius.

5. **What is the chorda tympani?**
   The chorda tympani carries parasympathetic innervation to both the submandibular and sublingual glands and special sensory afferents from the anterior two thirds of the tongue. It branches off from the mastoid segment of the facial nerve and traverses the middle ear before exiting the tympanic cavity through the petrotympanic fissure to join the lingual branch of the trigeminal nerve. Stretching or cutting of this nerve during middle ear surgery produces taste alteration and tongue numbness that is usually temporary.

6. **What is the pes anserinus?**
   The pes anserinus ("goose's foot") is the first major branching of the extratemporal facial nerve after it leaves the stylomastoid foramen. This branching usually splits the nerve into upper and lower divisions. More distally the branching is variable but normally forms five major branches (see Fig. 44.1):
   - **T**emporal: frontalis, corrugator supercilii, procerus, and upper orbicularis oculi
   - **Z**ygomatic: lower orbicularis oculi
   - **B**uccal: zygomaticus major and minor, levator anguli oris, buccinator, and upper orbicularis oris

- Marginal mandibular: lower orbicularis oris, depressor anguli oris, depressor labii inferioris, and mentalis
- Cervical: platysma

7. **During parotid surgery, what are the landmarks for identifying the facial nerve?**
There are a number of methods to find the main trunk:
- Identify the tragal pointer, which is a triangular extension of the tragal cartilage. The main trunk of cranial nerve (CN) VII typically lies 10 millimeters inferior and 10 millimeters deep to this landmark.
- Follow the posterior belly of the digastric muscle to the styloid process. The stylomastoid foramen lies deep to this structure and is where the nerve exits the temporal bone. Typically it is 25 millimeters deep to the skin's surface. NOTE: In children under the age of 2 years the mastoid is not well developed and the facial nerve lies much closer to the surface of the skin than would otherwise be expected.
- Find the tympanomastoid fissure. The nerve can be found 6 to 8 millimeters inferior to the end of the fissure.
- Identify a peripheral branch (e.g., marginal mandibular) and follow it proximally.
- Perform a mastoidectomy to find the mastoid portion of the nerve and follow it out of the stylomastoid foramen.

8. **What are the three types of nerve injury?**
- **Neuropraxia** results when a lesion stops axoplasm flow within an axon, blocking electrical conduction. Examples include traumatic swelling or pharmacologic blockade. The nerve is viable and returns to normal function when the blockade is corrected. Electrophysiologic testing reveals normal function, except that the electromyogram fails to show voluntary motor action potentials because they are not conducted across the blockade.
- **Axonotmesis** is injury to axons that result in Wallerian degeneration distal to the lesion with preservation of the motor axon endoneural sheaths. Examples include mild crush or stretch injuries. Electrically, the nerve shows rapid and complete degeneration, with loss of voluntary motor units. Regeneration to the motor end plates will occur, as long as the endoneural tubules are intact.
- **Neurotmesis** is characterized by both Wallerian degeneration of axons and loss of endoneural tubules. Electrophysiologic studies yield evidence of complete nerve degeneration. Regeneration is dependent on many factors, including the integrity of the endoneurium, perineurium, and epineurium and the extent of ischemia and scarring around the lesion.

9. **What is synkinesis?**
If a facial nerve lesion results in Wallerian degeneration, subsequent axon regeneration may result in "cross-wiring" in which voluntary movement of one facial muscle group induces involuntary movement of another. For example, after recovering from a facial palsy a patient may have squinting whenever he or she smiles. This is caused in part by aberrant routing of regenerating axons. However, ephaptic transmission (abnormal connections between axons), postsynaptic hyperexcitability, and synaptic reorganization within the facial nucleus also may play roles.

10. **What is facial nerve grading?**
There are several facial nerve grading systems used worldwide. The House-Brackmann grading system is most commonly used in the United States. This grading system is used to classify the degree of function of the facial nerve following its recovery after injury (Table 44.1).

11. **What is Bell's palsy?**
Bell's palsy is the most commonly diagnosed cause of facial paralysis. The etiology is thought to be a viral neuropathy caused by the herpes simplex virus. Most importantly, it is a diagnosis of exclusion with the following minimum diagnostic criteria:
- Paralysis or paresis of all facial muscle groups on one side of the face
- Sudden onset
- Absence of signs of central nervous system disease, ear disease (i.e., otitis media or cholesteatoma), or a parotid mass

  It often follows a viral prodrome with a typical 3- to 5-day duration and a peak in symptoms at 48 hours. The patient may have a widened palpebral fissure, diminished taste, difficulty chewing, hyperesthesia in one or more branches of the fifth cranial nerve, mastoid tip pain, and hyperacusis. In 14% of patients with Bell's palsy, family history is positive. Some 12% of patients may have recurrent facial paralysis, either ipsilateral or contralateral.

  HSV has been shown to be present within the geniculate ganglion of affected individuals, in contrast to the normal population, in which this is rare. It has been proposed that reactivation of this virus in the geniculate ganglion causes swelling and subsequent paralysis. Bell's palsy accounts for roughly 70% of acute facial palsies. However, it is important to remember that this is a diagnosis of exclusion.

12. **List the common etiology categories of facial paralysis.**
- Congenital: Möbius syndrome, congenital unilateral lower lip paralysis, Melkersson-Rosenthal syndrome, dystrophic myotonia.

Table 44.1 House-Brackmann Facial Nerve Grading System

GRADE	GROSS CHARACTERISTICS	MOTION CHARACTERISTICS
I. Normal	Normal facial appearance in all areas	Normal facial function in all areas
II. Mild dysfunction	Slight weakness noticeable only on close inspection. Normal symmetry and tone at rest	Forehead: moderate to good function Eye: complete closure with minimal effort Mouth: slight asymmetry
III. Moderate dysfunction	Obvious but not disfiguring asymmetry. Normal symmetry and tone at rest	Forehead: slight to moderate movement Eye: complete closure with effort Mouth: slightly weak with maximum effort
IV. Moderately severe	Obvious weakness with possible dysfunction	Forehead: none Eye: incomplete closure Mouth: asymmetric with maximum effort
V. Severe dysfunction	Only minimally perceptible motion. Asymmetry at rest	Forehead: none Eye: incomplete closure Mouth: slight movement
VI. Total paralysis	No movement and obvious asymmetry at rest	No movement at any level

- Traumatic: temporal bone fractures, intrauterine compression, birth trauma/forceps delivery, facial contusions or lacerations, penetrating wounds to face or ear, iatrogenic injury (parotid/ear/cranial surgery, embolization for epistaxis, mandibular block anesthesia).
- Infection: Bell's palsy, herpes zoster oticus, otitis media with effusion, acute mastoiditis, malignant otitis externa, tuberculosis, Lyme disease, acquired immunodeficiency syndrome, mononucleosis, influenza, encephalitis, malaria, syphilis, botulism.
- Idiopathic: recurrent facial palsy.
- Neoplasia: cholesteatoma, carcinoma, acoustic neuroma, meningioma, facial nerve schwannoma, glomus jugulare or tympanicum, leukemia, hemangioblastoma, osteopetrosis, histiocytosis, rhabdomyosarcoma.
- Metabolic/systemic: diabetes, hyperthyroidism, pregnancy, autoimmune disorders, sarcoidosis, hypertension.
- Neurologic: Guillain-Barré syndrome, multiple sclerosis, Millard-Gubler syndrome.

13. **What elements of the history and physical examination are important in evaluating a facial paralysis?**
Identifying factors for systemic and/or infectious causes is mandatory. Any palsy with slow progression or without improvement after 3 months should be considered a neoplasm until proven otherwise. Additional signs of possible tumor involvement include facial twitching, other cranial nerve involvement, hearing loss, recurrent episodes of facial paralysis, a mass behind the tympanic membrane or in the parotid gland, unilateral eustachian tube dysfunction, skin lesions suggesting skin cancer, and/or prolonged ear pain.
   Bell's palsy and herpes zoster oticus may also have associated numbness in the middle and lower face, otalgia, hyperacusis, decreased tearing, or altered taste sensation. Lyme disease may have a characteristic rash (bull's-eye) preceding the facial weakness.

14. **How can you distinguish whether the lesion causing facial paralysis is peripheral or central?**
A unilateral central lesion (supranuclear) will spare the upper face, since these muscles receive both crossed and uncrossed fibers. Lesions of the peripheral system involve both the upper and lower face. A central lesion is also suggested by the lack of emotional facial movement as well as decreased lacrimation, taste, and salivation on the ipsilateral side. Cortical lesions are also frequently associated with tongue or hand dysfunction.

15. **Which radiologic studies should be part of the diagnostic workup for a patient with a facial paralysis?**
Routine radiologic tests are not indicated for the assessment of every patient presenting with a facial nerve paralysis. The need for such studies is based on both the clinical history and the course of the paralysis (i.e., if a neoplasm is suspected). If radiologic imaging is deemed necessary, high-resolution computed tomography (CT) and magnetic resonance imaging (MRI) are the studies of choice. MRI scans are superior to CT in imaging the nerve at the cerebellopontine angle and internal auditory canal. Gadolinium-enhanced MRI is the test of choice for facial nerve paralysis secondary to inflammatory, neoplastic, and other nontraumatic etiologies. CT, on the other hand, is preferred for the evaluation of traumatic seventh nerve paralysis and other etiologies involving the temporal bone such as cholesteatoma.

16. **What is Schirmer's test?**

    Schirmer's test is a method to assess parasympathetic innervation to the lacrimal gland via the greater superficial petrosal nerve. The procedure entails placing small filter paper strips in the conjunctival fornix of each eye and measuring lacrimation by comparing the length of paper moistened by tear flow over a 5-minute period. An abnormal Schirmer's test occurs with <15 millimeters lacrimation or a 25% reduction compared to the contralateral eye.

17. **Describe the electrophysiologic tests that are important in evaluating a patient with a facial paralysis?**
    - **Nerve Excitability Test (NET):** In this study, a $1/s^2$ wave pulse, which is 1 millisecond in duration, is applied over both the affected and the unaffected facial nerves. Thresholds for minimal facial muscle response are recorded and compared. A 3- to 4-mA or greater difference is considered significant, suggesting denervation. This test is not accurate during the first 72 hours after onset of paralysis, since it takes 3 days for Wallerian degeneration to occur.
    - **Maximal Stimulation Test (MST):** A variation of the NET, the MST stimulates the ipsilateral and contralateral facial muscles at a level sufficient to depolarize all motor axons underlying the stimulator. Therefore, it utilizes maximal as opposed to minimal stimulation to evaluate muscular response. The results of the test are recorded as a subjective account of the difference in facial muscle movement between the normal and involved sides. Generally, it is thought that the MST becomes abnormal before the NET and is therefore a better prognostic indicator. However, the MST is limited by its lack of objectivity.
    - **Electroneuronography (ENoG):** ENoG measures and compares the amplitudes of the muscle summation potentials that are elicited when a supramaximal level of current is applied over the main trunk of the facial nerve on the affected and unaffected sides. The peak-to-peak amplitude is directly proportional to the number of intact motor axons, thus providing a gauge to assess neuronal degeneration. For example, an evoked summation potential of 5% to 10% indicates 90% degeneration. This test is commonly used to predict who may benefit from a surgical facial nerve decompression. Just like the MST, it is only accurate after Wallerian degeneration has occurred, so it must be performed more than 72 hours after onset of symptoms. To accurately predict which patients may benefit from surgical decompression, ENoG must be performed within 2 weeks of the onset of symptoms.
    - **Electromyography (EMG):** EMG is complementary in the evaluation of acute facial paralysis, helping to eliminate false positive results obtained by NET, MST, and ENoG. The EMG determines the activity of the muscle rather than the activity of the nerve. This test can (1) provide information regarding intact motor units in the acute phase and (2) confirm the integrity of intact axons in the recovery phase, detecting reinnervation potentials 6 to 12 weeks before the return of facial muscle function is clinically evident. However, unlike NET, MST, and ENoG, an EMG cannot assess the degree of degeneration or prognosis for recovery.
    - **Audiometry:** Audiometry should be performed to evaluate for conductive and sensorineural hearing losses. Conductive hearing losses are most consistent with middle ear tumors, cholesteatomas, and other middle ear processes involving the tympanic segment of the facial nerve. Sensorineural hearing losses may indicate neoplastic conditions such as acoustic neuroma, meningioma, and facial nerve neuromas, which affect the nerve in the cerebellopontine angle or internal auditory canal.

18. **What is the most important complication following the onset of facial paralysis?**

    Exposure keratitis in the eye of the affected side can lead to vision loss. It is caused by (1) paralysis with inability to close the eyelid completely, (2) diminished tearing, and (3) loss of corneal sensitivity if there is coexistent trigeminal nerve dysfunction. Evidence for corneal irritation includes redness, itching, foreign body sensation, and visual blurring. Avoidance of this complication involves using artificial tears 4 to 5 times/day. Before sleeping, ophthalmic lubricant should be instilled along with taping the eyelid shut. The eye should be protected from wind, foreign bodies, and drying with glasses and/or moisture chambers. Surgical placement of a gold weight within the eyelid can facilitate full closure in complete paralysis. An ophthalmology consult should be obtained for these patients.

19. **What are crocodile tears?**

    Injuries to the facial nerve may be associated with aberrant nerve regeneration. Fibers that normally innervate the salivary glands may regenerate to innervate the lacrimal gland. This leads to "crying" when the patient eats (gustatory tearing). Similarly, these fibers can regenerate to innervate sweat glands in the skin, leading to gustatory sweating (Frey's syndrome).

20. **How do you treat facial nerve paralysis medically?**
    - If infectious processes are involved, appropriate treatment with antimicrobial and/or antiviral agents, in addition to eradication of the infectious nidus (i.e., mastoidectomy/myringotomy), should be instituted.
    - A course of oral steroids, if initiated within the first 72 hours after onset of symptoms, may improve recovery via decreased inflammation.
    - Electrophysiologic assessment of the extent of nerve damage provides valuable information, particularly in cases in which surgical decompression may be a treatment option.

Table 44.2 Surgical Strategies as Determined by Etiology

CLINICAL SCENARIO	SURGICAL INTERVENTION
Facial paralysis due to trauma	Nerve decompression, anastomosis
Paralysis secondary to acute OM	Myringotomy
Nerve paralysis due to chronic OM	Decompression, mastoidectomy
Iatrogenic injury to facial nerve	Decompression, anastomosis
Complete idiopathic paralysis	Decompression

- Prophylactic eye care to protect against exposure keratitis should be initiated in all patients with a facial nerve paralysis.
- For Bell's palsy specifically, the current recommendation for treatment is (1) oral steroids to begin within 72 hours of onset of symptoms, (2) optional oral acyclovir in addition to steroids if started within 72 hours of onset of symptoms, and (3) eye care.

21. **When is surgical treatment indicated?**
Surgical intervention may take multiple forms depending on the etiology of the facial nerve lesion. Bony decompression of the facial nerve may improve recovery in certain cases where total paralysis is present with evidence of rapid severe nerve degeneration. Serial studies with ENoG have shown that when the number of motor fibers falls to less than 10% of normal (tested prior to day 14 post-onset), the recovery rate of normal function is substantially decreased. It is therefore at this level that surgical exploration/decompression is most likely to be considered. In Bell's palsy, swelling in the labyrinthine segment causes an entrapment neuropathy, which is decompressed via a middle fossa craniotomy.

    Table 44.2 contains a list of possible surgical strategies by etiology.

22. **If the nerve is cut during surgery, can it be fixed?**
Yes. Several techniques may be employed for repairing a transected or partially transected nerve. A common clinical rule of thumb is that if more than 50% of the nerve is transected, it should be repaired.

    Direct anastomosis involves repair of the perineurium with exact end-to-end approximation. An 8-0 monofilament suture is used to approximate the nerve ends together without tension at the anastomosis. Grafting can also be utilized if there is loss of a segment of the nerve; great auricular or sural nerves can be used for interposition grafts. Jump grafts from other CNs (such as CN XII) have also been used successfully to reanimate the facial muscles in cases in which the proximal facial nerve is not present. Cross-nerve grafts connected to the contralateral facial nerve can also be used.

23. **What is the association between facial nerve paralysis and otitis media? Mastoiditis? Cholesteatoma?**
In otitis media (OM), facial palsy can present as a complication of acute suppurative OM, OM with effusion, and chronic OM. The palsy results from an inflammatory reaction or bacterial toxins within the bony fallopian canal. In both mastoiditis and cholesteatoma, compression of the nerve and inflammatory response can result in facial nerve palsy.

    The mainstay of treatment, particularly if the palsy is a complication of OM, is to eradicate the infection with a combination of aggressive antibiotic therapy and surgical drainage via myringotomy or tympanomastoid surgery. Facial palsy secondary to coalescent mastoiditis can be managed surgically with myringotomy followed by a mastoidectomy. The presence of cholesteatoma requires surgical management.

24. **What are the most common facial nerve tumors?**
The two most common facial nerve tumors are facial nerve schwannomas (facial neuromas) and geniculate ganglion hemangiomas. Facial schwannomas arise from the myelin-producing Schwann cells. Hemangiomas of the geniculate ganglion arise from the vascular plexus surrounding the ganglion. These tumors are often observed initially but many will require treatment due to growth and/or progressive facial nerve paralysis.

25. **What are herpes zoster oticus and Ramsay Hunt syndrome?**
Herpes zoster oticus is characterized by intense ear pain and vesicles on the external auditory canal and concha. It is caused by reactivation of the dormant herpes zoster (chickenpox) virus within the afferent sensory neurons of the facial nerve. If this progresses to involve the efferent motor axons of the facial nerve, a facial palsy can result. When both a facial palsy and painful vesicles are present, it is referred to as Ramsay Hunt syndrome. Hearing loss and vertigo may also occur. Treatment includes narcotic analgesics for pain relief, oral corticosteroids to decrease inflammation, and acyclovir to inhibit viral DNA replication. Topical antibiotic drops may also be used if there is

concern for secondary bacterial otitis externa. Additionally, the facial paresis may affect eyelid closure and place the orbit at risk for dryness and excoriation, and possible permanent damage.

BIBLIOGRAPHY

Baugh RF, Basura GJ, Ishii LE, et al: Clinical practice guideline: Bell's palsy, *Otolaryngol Head Neck Surg* 149(Suppl 3):S1–S27, 2013.

Carrasco VN, Zdanski CJ, Logan TC, et al: Facial nerve paralysis. In: Lee KJ, et al, eds: *Essential Otolaryngology Head and Neck Surgery*, 8th ed, 2003, Appleton and Lange, pp. 169–191.

Chang CY, Cass SP: Management of facial nerve injury due to temporal bone trauma, *Am J Otol* 20:96–114, 1999.

Danner CJ: Facial nerve paralysis, *Otolaryngol Clin North Am* 41:619–632, 2008.

Fattah AY, Gurusinghe AD, Gavilan J, et al: Facial nerve grading instruments: systematic review of the literature and suggestion for uniformity, *Plast Reconstr Surg* 135(2):569–579, 2015.

Gidley PW, Gantz BJ, Rubinstein JT: Facial nerve grafts: from cerebellopontine angle and beyond, *Am J Otol* 20:781–788, 1999.

O TM: Medical management of acute facial paralysis, *Otolaryngol Clin North Am* 51(6):1051–1075, 2018.

Ramsey MJ, DerSimonian R, Holtel MR, et al: Corticosteroid treatment for idiopathic facial nerve paralysis: a meta-analysis, *Laryngoscope* 110(3 Pt 1):335–341, 2000.

Ruckenstein MJ: Evaluating facial paralysis, expensive diagnostic tests are often unnecessary, *Postgrad Med* 103:187–188, 191–192, 199.

Rudman KL, Rhee JS: Habilitation of facial nerve dysfunction, *Otolaryngol Clin North Am* 45:513–530, 2012.

CHAPTER 45

SURGERY FOR VERTIGO

Scott E. Mann, MD and Stephen P. Cass, MD

KEY POINTS

1. Most forms of vertigo are not managed surgically. Most patients with vertigo can attain significant improvement with conservative nonsurgical measures.
2. Ménière's disease is a clinical diagnosis based on these features:
   - Two or more definitive episodes of vertigo lasting 20 minutes to 12 hour
   - Hearing loss involving the low to mid-frequencies on at least one occasion before, during, or after an episode of vertigo
   - Fluctuating aural symptoms (hearing, tinnitus, or aural fullness)
3. Surgical treatment options for medical failure in Ménière's disease include:
   - Intratympanic steroid perfusion
   - Endolymphatic sac surgery
   - Intratympanic gentamicin ablation
   - Surgical labyrinthectomy
   - Vestibular nerve section
4. There is no surgical procedure that reliably improves hearing in Ménière's disease.
5. Benign paroxysmal positional vertigo (BPPV) arises from free-floating endolymph particles, most commonly in the posterior semicircle canal.
   - Most cases can be treated by particle repositioning (Epley maneuver)
   - Recurrent BPPV is common
6. Vertigo provoked by loud sound (Tullio's symptom) or pressure changes (Hennebert's symptom) are cardinal symptoms of superior semicircular canal dehiscence.

Pearls
1. Vestibular compensation is a central nervous system process that is critical for improvement of the vestibulo-ocular reflex and gait stability after loss of peripheral vestibular (labyrinthine) function. Supervised vestibular physical therapy helps to expedite this process.
2. BPPV commonly follows an episode of vestibular neuritis. In this situation, vestibular physical therapy (in addition to canalith repositioning) is often helpful to promote full recovery.
3. Superior semicircular canal dehiscence can mimic other otologic diseases because it can present with conductive hearing loss similar to otosclerosis, ear fullness, and autophony similar to a patulous eustachian tube and vertigo similar to Ménière's disease.
4. The key finding that distinguishes conductive hearing loss due to superior semicircular canal dehiscence (SSCD) from that caused by otosclerosis is an intact ipsilateral stapedial reflex.

QUESTIONS

1. **What is the role of surgery in the treatment of vertigo?**
   Most forms of vertigo are not managed surgically. Management of patients with vertigo and balance disorders demands diagnostic acumen, clinical judgment, and both medical and surgical skills. The most important step in treating vertigo is correctly identifying the cause. Only then can appropriate treatment recommendations be made. Though surgery is an option for some causes of vertigo, often it is not the first treatment offered. Many patients with a condition amenable to surgical treatment can attain significant improvement with conservative measures alone. However, surgical intervention can be highly successful when patients are carefully selected.

2. **What are the most common vertigo conditions with surgical options?**
   - Ménière's disease
   - BPPV
   - Superior semicircular canal dehiscence

3. **What are some alternatives to surgery in patients with vertigo?**
As stated, the most important step in treating vertigo is identifying the correct cause. The appropriate nonsurgical treatment is dictated by an accurate diagnosis. Some common forms of conservative management include:
   - Vestibular rehabilitation therapy
   - Pharmacologic therapy (diuretics, migraine medications, vestibular suppressants)
   - Dietary changes
   - Canalith repositioning maneuvers

4. **Which patients should be considered for surgical intervention?**
As a general rule, surgery should only be considered for the treatment of vertigo if a patient meets the following three criteria:
   - Vertigo caused by unilateral peripheral vestibular dysfunction, with absolute certainty of which side is affected
   - Vertigo must be disabling
   - No signs or symptoms of central vestibular system dysfunction that could impair postoperative vestibular compensation

5. **How does the American Academy of Otolaryngology-Head and Neck Surgery advise reporting of vertigo control in Ménière's disease?**
At 18 to 24 months following treatment, divide the number of episodes per 6 months by the number of episodes in the 6 months prior to treatment.
   - Grade A: complete control (0%)
   - Grade B: substantial control (1% to 40%)
   - Grade C: partial control (41% to 80%)
   - Grade D: no control (81% to 120%)
   - Grade E: worse (>120%)
   - Grade F: secondary treatment required due to disabling vertigo

6. **What are the surgical options for the treatment of Ménière's disease?**
Procedures to control vertigo in Ménière's disease can be divided into ablative and nonablative procedures. Ablative procedures include gentamicin middle ear perfusions, labyrinthectomy, and vestibular nerve section. These procedures permanently reduce or eliminate aberrant vestibular signaling from the affected side. The most common nonablative procedures are endolymphatic shunt surgery and intratympanic steroid perfusion. The ablative procedures have greater vertigo control rates than the nonablative procedures but require vestibular compensation to limit posttreatment disequilibrium

7. **What are the possible types of endolymphatic shunt surgery?**
   - Shunting: placement of synthetic shunt to drain endolymph
   - Drainage: incision of the sac to allow endolymph drainage
   - Decompression: to improve sac function of endolymph absorption

8. **Describe the sham surgery trial by Thomsen et al., 1981.**
   - Double-blinded, placebo-controlled study
   - Compared cortical mastoidectomy without decompression versus endolymphatic shunt
   - Study conclusion: "We are therefore of the opinion that the impact of surgery on the symptoms of Ménière's disease is completely nonspecific and unrelated to the actual shunt procedure."
   - Validity of the sham study has been questioned and endolymphatic surgery continues to be a popular surgical procedure in many centers

9. **What is a vestibular nerve section?**
A vestibular nerve section is a procedure in which the vestibular division of the eighth cranial nerve is selectively divided to remove vestibular function from the affected side (Fig. 45.1). The approaches that can be used to perform vestibular nerve section include:
   - Middle fossa
   - Retrolabyrinthine
   - Retrosigmoid
   - Translabyrinthine (see Chapter 44)

10. **What are the potential complications of vestibular nerve section?**
   - Facial paralysis
   - Hearing loss
   - Cerebrospinal fluid leak
   - Persistent disequilibrium

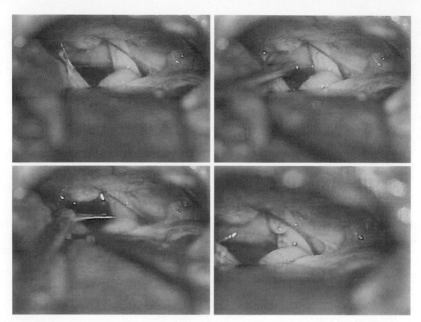

Fig. 45.1 Vestibular nerve sectioning (retrosigmoid approach).

11. **What is the most reliable treatment for vertigo due to Ménière's disease?**
Labyrinthectomy is the most reliable surgical treatment, although hearing is sacrificed. In this procedure, all of the vestibular neuroepithelium can be removed. This effectively ends all aberrant information produced by the diseased ear, and hearing function cannot be preserved.

Cochlear implantation has been successfully used to restore hearing ability after surgical labyrinthectomy.

12. **What is BPPV and when is the treatment surgical?**
BPPV is a condition in which free-floating otolith particles within semicircular canals activate the canal ampulla and cause vertigo during head movements. These particles can often be repositioned with maneuvers such as the Epley maneuver. Recurrence is common but maneuvers can be repeated as often as needed. However, if the symptoms are intractable or recurrences are frequent, surgery can be considered. The surgical options available include:
- Posterior semicircular canal occlusion: this procedure plugs the posterior semicircular canal, preventing free-floating particles from activating the canal ampulla (Fig. 45.2).
- Vestibular neurectomy: this procedure eliminates all vestibular function from the affected ear and is very rarely used for BPPV alone.
- Singular neurectomy: this procedure removes the innervation to the posterior canal ampulla. It was the first surgical procedure for BPPV but is technically difficult and carries a significant risk of hearing loss.

13. **What is Tullio's phenomenon?**
- Sound-induced dizziness, vertigo, or nystagmus
- First described by Tullio in 1928 who demonstrated that fenestration of the bony labyrinth renders it sound sensitive
- Tullio's phenomenon can be a present in patients with otologic conditions causing abnormal thinning or dehiscence of the bony labyrinth

14. **What is semicircular canal dehiscence?**
Semicircular canal dehiscence is loss of otic capsule bone overlying the superior semicircular canal that creates a "dehiscence" or "inner ear fistula" (Fig. 45.3).

15. **What are the characteristic clinical symptoms of SSCD?**
- Sound-, pressure-, or vibration-induced vertigo
- Hearing loss: usually with a low-frequency air-bone gap loss with better than 0-dB bone conduction threshold (bone conduction hyperacusis)
- Autophony (voice seems unusually loud), pulsatile tinnitus, and a "blocked ear" feeling

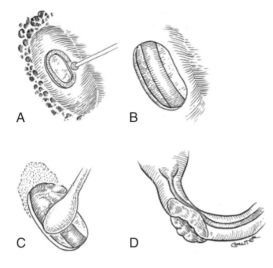

A   B

C   D

Fig. 45.2 A–D, Technique for plugging semicircular canal. (From Myers E: *Operative Otolaryngology Head and Neck Surgery* (Vol 2), Philadelphia, 1997, Saunders, figure 117–144.)

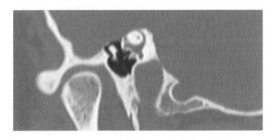

Fig. 45.3 CT scan showing superior semicircular canal dehiscence (oblique sagittal view).

16. **What testing is used to confirm a diagnosis of superior semicircular canal dehiscence?**
    - Vestibular evoked myogenic potentials demonstrate abnormally low thresholds.
    - High-resolution computed tomography scan of the temporal bone reveals dehiscence of the bony covering that separates the superior canal from the dura mater (see Fig. 45.2).
    - Stapedial reflex testing can be used to distinguish whether conductive hearing loss is due to SSCD or otosclerosis. In otosclerosis, the ipsilateral stapedial reflex will be lost once the patient has significant conductive hearing loss. In patients with SSCD, the ipsilateral stapedial reflex will continue to be intact on testing despite conductive hearing loss.

17. **What causes SSCD?**
    The cause is not understood and may be multifactorial. In the developmental hypothesis, the cause is thought to be due to incomplete ossification of the semicircular canals. SSCD is also noted when chronic increased intracranial pressure is present and can be found in association with temporal-mastoid encephalocele.

18. **What are the treatment options for SSCD?**
    - Educate the patient on the condition and offer reassurance
    - PE tubes can be helpful to reduce pressure-induced vertigo
    - Earplugs can be helpful to reduce exposure to loud sounds
    - Surgery to plug or resurface the affected semicircular canal when the patient fails other measures or has intractable symptoms

19. **What surgical techniques are used in SSCD?**
    - Middle fossa craniotomy to expose the superior semicircular canal is the traditional approach. The dehiscence is then plugged or resurfaced.
    - Transmastoid approaches can also be used to plug the semicircular canal and have been shown to be as effective as the middle cranial fossa approach.

20. **Intratympanic (IT) steroids or gentamicin: which is better when treating Ménière's disease?**
    IT steroids are a nonablative option and are thought to be effective for vertigo in approximately 70% of patients with no risk for increased hearing or vestibular function loss.

    IT gentamicin is an ablative option with efficacy in 90% of patients but with an increased rate of hearing loss compared to IT steroids.

BIBLIOGRAPHY

Banakis Hartl RM, Cass SP: Effectiveness of transmastoid plugging for semicircular canal dehiscence syndrome, *Otolaryngol Head Neck Surg.* 158(3):534–540, 2018.

Bhattacharyya N, Gubbels S, Swartz S, et al: Clinical practice guideline: benign paroxysmal vertigo (update), *Otolaryngol Head Neck Surg.* 156:S1–S47, 2017.

Cass SP: Surgery for vertigo. In: Myers E, editor: *Operative Otolaryngology Head and Neck Surgery* (Vol 2), Philadelphia, PA, 1997, Elsevier, pp. 1396–1432.

Kemink JL, Telian SA, Graham MD, et al: Transmastoid labyrinthectomy: reliable surgical management of vertigo, *Otolaryngol Head Neck Surg* 101:5–10, 1989.

Lopez-Escamez JA, Carey J, Chung WH, et al: Diagnostic criteria for Ménière's disease, *J Vestib Res* 25:1–7, 2015.

Minor LB: Superior canal dehiscence syndrome, *Am J Otol* 21:9–19, 2000.

Schwartz SR, Almosnino G, Noonan KY, et al: Comparison of transmastoid and middle fossa approaches for superior canal dehiscence repair: a multi-institutional study, *Otolaryngol Head Neck Surg* 161(1):130–136, 2019.

Thomsen J, Bretlau P, Tos M, Johnsen NJ: Placebo effect in surgery for Ménière's disease, *Arch Otolaryngol* 107:271–277, 1981.

Zhou G, Gopen Q, Poe DS: Clinical and diagnostic characterization of canal dehiscence syndrome: a great otologic mimicker, *Otol Neurotol* 28:920–926, 2007.

CHAPTER 46

NEUROTOLOGY

Nathan D. Cass, MD and Samuel P. Gubbels, MD, FACS

KEY POINTS

1. Neurotology involves the treatment of patients with lateral skull base disorders, encompassing surgery of the entire temporal bone and associated approaches to the middle fossa, posterior fossa, and brainstem.
2. The cerebellopontine angle (CPA) is the junction of the cerebellum and pons, in which a variety of pathologies may arise, of which vestibular schwannomas comprise the vast majority (70%–90%). A cistern of cerebrospinal fluid (CSF) is found at the CPA, which is known as the pontocerebellar cistern. Many critical neurovascular structures traverse this cisternal region: CNs VI, VII, and VIII and the anterior inferior cerebellar artery (AICA) and its branches, including the internal auditory artery.
3. Treatment options for vestibular schwannomas include observation, radiation, and surgery. The choice depends on the tumor size, location, and hearing status.
4. The translabyrinthine approach will destroy any residual hearing.

Pearls

1. In jugulotympanic paragangliomas, otoscopic examination may reveal a vascular middle ear mass pulsating against the tympanic membrane, which blanches upon pneumatic otoscopy. This is known as *Brown's sign* and is observed in approximately 50% of cases.
2. The jugular foramen contains the internal jugular vein (IJV) and CNs IX, X, and XI. The smaller *pars nervosa* comprises the anteromedial portion and contains CN IX; the larger *pars vascularis* is located posterolaterally and contains the vasculature as well as CNs X and XI. The inferior petrosal sinus traverses the *pars nervosa* to empty into the medial aspect of the jugular bulb in the *pars vascularis*.

QUESTIONS

1. **What is neurotology?**
   Neurotology, also known as neuro-otology, involves the treatment of patients with lateral skull base disorders. In contrast to otology (dealing with middle ear and mastoid disease), neurotology encompasses surgery of the entire temporal bone and associated approaches to the middle fossa, posterior fossa, and brainstem. However, most neurotologists practice both otology and neurotology.

2. **When were the beginnings of neurotology as a field?**
   In the 1960s, using the nascent technology of the operating microscope and the dental drill, Dr. William House of the House Ear Institute pioneered the middle cranial fossa (MCF) and translabyrinthine (TL) approaches to the internal auditory canal (IAC) and cerebello-pontine angle (CPA), in collaboration with Dr. William Hitselberger (neurosurgeon). Prior to this work, CPA tumors were resected only via the RS approach, which had a number of limitations. For this, Dr. William House is known as the "father of neurotology." Many other pioneers followed, expanding and elaborating on these approaches to treat skull base disorders.

3. **What are the key anatomic regions involved in neurotologic surgery?**
   Neurotologists operate on the temporal bone and the spaces within or adjacent to it—IAC, CPA, and jugular foramen—and occasionally on the brainstem, clivus, and paraclival region, including the petrous apex. The temporal bone consists of multiple embryologically distinct portions: tympanic, petromastoid, squamous (including the zygomatic process), and styloid processes. The superior face of the temporal bone forms the floor of the middle fossa, and the posterior face forms the anterior limit of the posterior fossa. The petrous portion is roughly pyramidal, with its apex pointing medially toward the midline. Fig. 46.1 shows the temporal bone and its landmarks.

4. **What is the IAC and what structures does it contain?**
   The IAC is the path by which cranial nerves (CNs) VII and VIII travel from their origin at the brainstem, known as the root entry zone, to the inner ear (also known as the otic capsule) (CN VIII), and through the temporal bone (CN VII). This bony canal runs approximately 1 centimeter in an antero-superolateral direction through the petrous

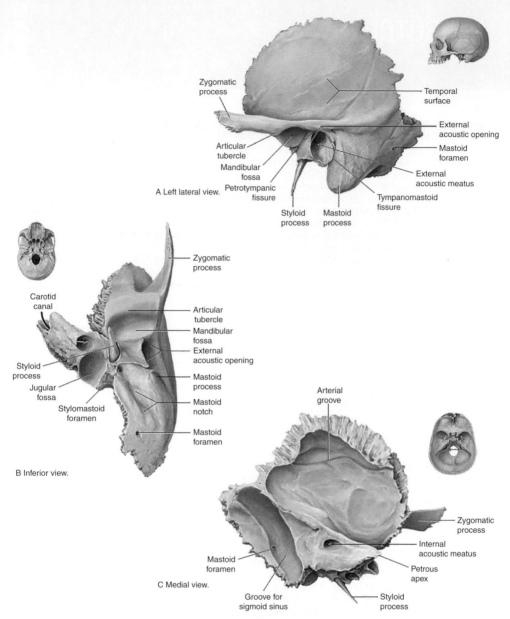

Zygomatic process

Temporal surface

External acoustic opening

Articular tubercle

Mastoid foramen

Mandibular fossa

A Left lateral view.

Petrotympanic fissure

External acoustic meatus

Tympanomastoid fissure

Styloid process

Mastoid process

Carotid canal

Zygomatic process

Articular tubercle

Mandibular fossa

External acoustic opening

Styloid process

Mastoid process

Jugular fossa

Stylomastoid foramen

Mastoid notch

Mastoid foramen

Arterial groove

B Inferior view.

Zygomatic process

Internal acoustic meatus

Mastoid foramen

Petrous apex

C Medial view.

Groove for sigmoid sinus

Styloid process

Fig. 46.1 The temporal bone. Source: https://doctorlib.info/medical/anatomy/37.html

temporal bone. The medial opening is known as the porus acusticus or the internal auditory meatus. At the lateral end or fundus, bony partitions separate the nerves into their respective canals. The facial nerve runs anterosuperiorly, the cochlear nerve anteroinferiorly, the superior vestibular nerve posterosuperiorly, and the inferior vestibular nerve posteroinferiorly (Fig. 46.2). The transverse or falciform crest divides the superior and inferior portions from one another, and the vertical "Bill's bar" (named for Dr. William House) divides the facial nerve from the superior vestibular nerve. Additional contents of the IAC include the nervus intermedius (the portion of the facial nerve supplying the sensory and parasympathetic fibers), as well as the internal auditory artery (a terminal branch of the AICA that supplies the otic capsule).

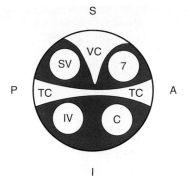

Fig. 46.2 Nerve divisions at the fundus of the internal auditory canal. S, superior; I, inferior; P, posterior; A, anterior; TC, transverse crest; VC, vertical crest (Bill's bar); 7, facial nerve; C, cochlear nerve; SV, superior vestibular nerve; IV, inferior vestibular nerve
Source: http://med.stanford.edu/sm/ohns-skull-base-surgery-atlas/01.1_surgical-anatomy.html

5. **What is the CPA and what does it have to do with neurotology?**
   The brainstem is divided into three sections, from superior to inferior: the midbrain, pons, and medulla. The CPA is the junction of the cerebellum and pons, in which a variety of pathologies may arise. A cistern of cerebrospinal fluid (CSF) is found at the CPA, which is known as the pontocerebellar cistern. Many critical neurovascular structures traverse this cisternal region: CNs VI, VII, and VIII and the anterior inferior cerebellar artery (AICA) and its branches, including the internal auditory artery. Neurotologists are specifically trained to provide safe and reliable access to this difficult-to-reach area for tumor removal.

6. **Which tumors are found in the CPA?**
   Vestibular schwannomas comprise the majority of CPA tumors (70%–90%). These tumors arise from Schwann cells of the vestibular portion of the vestibulocochlear nerve, at the transition area between the central and peripheral nervous systems, known as the Obersteiner-Redlich zone. Vestibular schwannomas were originally (and erroneously) termed acoustic neuromas and are sometimes still referred to by that name. The incidence of vestibular schwannomas is 3 to 7 per 100,000 individuals. Meningiomas are also common (5%–15%), followed by epidermoids (6%). The following are rare tumor types that can also be found in the CPA: lipoma, hemangioma, hemangioblastoma, other cranial nerve schwannomas, endolymphatic sac tumors, arachnoid cysts, and lymphomas.

7. **What symptoms are associated with CPA or IAC pathology?**
   Compromise of structures that traverse the CPA and IAC leads to loss of function. CN VIII dysfunction leads to hearing loss, tinnitus, vertigo, and/or imbalance. CN VII involvement leads to facial weakness and paralysis. Ischemia from AICA damage leads to cranial neuropathies, cerebellar stroke, and ischemic damage to the inner ear. In very large tumors, brainstem compression can occur, with subsequent hydrocephalus or altered mental status. Tumors extending cranially can affect the CN V, and those extending caudally can affect the lower cranial nerves (CNs IX–XII). A study of more than 500 patients with vestibular schwannoma showed that the most common presenting symptom was unilateral hearing loss (86%), followed by unsteadiness (61%) and tinnitus (57%); the less common symptoms were headache (36%), facial paresthesia (29%), aural pressure sensation (28%), and blurry vision or diplopia (22%).

8. **How is a vestibular schwannoma diagnosed?**
   Magnetic resonance imaging (MRI) is the gold standard for diagnosing vestibular schwannoma, while computed tomography (CT) imaging has poor ability to identify CPA/IAC pathology. MRI readily distinguishes between many types of masses of the CPA and IAC, although a definitive diagnosis cannot be made without histologic analysis. Vestibular schwannomas enhance on postcontrast T1 MRI imaging and may be hypo- or hyperintense on T2. Meningiomas possess similar imaging features but with a characteristic "dural tail" morphology. Epidermoids are nonenhancing, exhibit T2 hyperintensity, and restrict diffusion on diffusion-weighted imaging (DWI) sequences. Arachnoid cysts are isointense in the CSF and nonenhancing on postcontrast T1. Jugulotympanic (JT) paragangliomas (PGLs) are hyperintense on T2, are enhanced with contrast on T1, and exhibit characteristic "salt-and-pepper" flow voids.

9. **What risk factors exist for vestibular schwannoma?**
   Ninety-five percent of vestibular schwannomas are sporadic, with the remainder related to neurofibromatosis type 2 (NF2), a genetic disorder. Patients with NF2 possess a mutant copy of the *neurofibroma 2* (*NF2*) tumor suppressor gene on chromosome 22, which transcribes the protein merlin. Merlin is involved in cytoskeleton-membrane linking, contact inhibition, cell adhesion, motility, signaling, and proliferation. Patients with NF2 typically develop bilateral vestibular schwannomas, as well as other schwannomas, intracranial meningiomas, and ependymomas.

Table 46.1 Koos Grading System for Vestibular Schwannoma

GRADE	DEFINITION
I	Tumor lies entirely within the IAC
II	Tumor extends into the pontocerebellar cistern
III	Tumor contacts, but does not compress, the brainstem
IV	Tumor compresses the brainstem

10. **How are vestibular schwannomas staged?**
    There are a variety of staging systems; the Koos classification is simple and commonly used (Table 46.1).

11. **What are the treatment options for patients with vestibular schwannoma?**
    Three options exist: observation, radiation, and surgery. Unless the tumor is very large or causing compressive symptoms, many patients are initially observed. Between 40% and 70% of tumors demonstrate stability or even regress in size over time when measured linearly. Observation has the advantage of avoiding the risks of treatment but results in predictable loss of hearing over time; if the tumor continues to grow, other complications may also ensue. Radiation treatment is aimed at preventing tumor growth and usually results in excellent short-term results with minimal morbidity. However, long-term hearing outcomes are poor and mirror that of observation. Radiation also introduces a small potential for radiation-induced tumor growth or malignant transformation. Surgery is performed in a variety of clinical conditions, including young patients, large tumors, presence of mass-related complications, attempts at hearing preservation, and patient preference. Subtotal resection with or without postoperative radiation may be performed when the tumor is adherent to the facial nerve or cochlear nerve (if preoperative hearing exists) and may be utilized to prevent loss of the functions served by these nerves.
    Drugs targeting the merlin signaling pathway are being investigated as a medical alternative to radiation and surgery for patients with NF2, given the risks associated with treating multiple tumors with these modalities.

12. **What type of radiation is administered for vestibular schwannoma?**
    Precise targeting of the tumor is achieved with a delivery method known as "stereotactic radiosurgery" (SRS): radiation delivered from numerous angles with the beams converging at one point to deliver focused radiation with much smaller doses to the surrounding tissues.

13. **How is the retrosigmoid approach performed?**
    In the RS approach the tumor is approached posteriorly, permitting visualization of the posterior fossa and CPA. Cerebellar retraction is required. This approach does not provide good visualization of the IAC but with drillout this may improve, albeit at some risk of violation of the otic capsule and resultant hearing loss (if hearing still exists). In addition, drilling is performed intradurally, and the approach requires more detachment of the posterior neck musculature, both of which may contribute to the long-term headaches that often occur postoperatively. This approach is often used for intracisternal tumors of all sizes and can be performed with or without the aim of hearing preservation.

14. **How is the middle cranial fossa approach performed, and what are its other uses?**
    In MCF the tumor is approached superiorly, requiring a technically demanding drillout of the IAC without violation of the labyrinth. In some cases, the facial nerve may be between the tumor and the dissection, potentially putting it at higher risk. Drilling is performed extradurally, but temporal lobe retraction is required, which occasionally leads to (usually temporary) aphasia, word-finding difficulties, or seizures, especially in older adults. This approach is favored for intracanalicular tumors in younger patients with preserved hearing. The MCF approach is also used to repair middle fossa encephaloceles and/or CSF leaks and to repair superior semicircular canal dehiscence.

15. **How is the translabyrinthine approach performed?**
    In TL the tumor is approached laterally, traversing the temporal bone and bony labyrinth to gain access to the IAC and CPA. Drilling is entirely extradural, no brain retraction is required, and the approach can be used for tumors of any size. Unfortunately, complete and permanent hearing loss is expected. This approach is favored in any tumor in which hearing has already been lost or is not expected to be salvageable with resection or in large tumors in which TL offers the least risk to other neurovascular structures.

16. **How likely is hearing preservation during resection of vestibular schwannoma?**
    The likelihood of preserving existing hearing is proportional to the preoperative hearing level and inversely proportional to the size of the tumor. The TL approach is not compatible with the preservation of hearing.

17. What complications can occur with the resection of vestibular schwannoma?

In addition to the loss of hearing described above, other cranial neuropathies may occur. Facial nerve deficits can result from nerve stretching due to tumor dissection or disruption of the vasculature. Trigeminal neuropathy, seen with some large tumors, predisposes patients to exposure keratopathy in the setting of facial paralysis, as they are unable to sense impending dryness. Historically, the rate of CSF leak was approximately 10% in all approaches, although recent series have expounded rates as low as 1% to 3%. Leaks may be managed conservatively with bed rest, placement of a lumbar drain, or return to the operating room if persistent or of large volume. Meningitis or intracranial hemorrhage may also occur following skull base surgery, although they are infrequently encountered.

18. What is the jugular foramen and how is it approached?

The internal jugular vein (IJV) and CNs IX, X, and XI exit the skull via the jugular foramen. The smaller *pars nervosa* comprises the anteromedial portion and contains CN IX; the larger *pars vascularis* is located posterolaterally and contains the vasculature and CNs X and XI. The inferior petrosal sinus traverses the *pars nervosa* to empty into the medial aspect of the jugular bulb in the *pars vascularis*, forming the IJV. Dr. Ugo Fisch of Switzerland pioneered infratemporal fossa and transtemporal approaches to the jugular foramen for surgical resection of such tumors, which often involves transposition of the facial nerve to improve access.

19. What are jugulotympanic paragangliomas (PGLs), and how are they diagnosed?

Jugulotympanic (JT) PGLs, also known as glomus tumors (a historical misnomer), constitute the most common type of tumor involving the jugular foramen, although schwannomas, meningiomas, and other tumors may also occur. PGLs are neuroendocrine tumors derived from neural crest cells that arise in extraadrenal autonomic paraganglia, both sympathetic and parasympathetic. JT PGLs arise from the jugular bulb (glomus jugulare), or Arnold's or Jacobson's nerves within the middle ear (glomus tympanicum); the most common presentation involves pulsatile tinnitus, hearing loss, aural fullness, or lower cranial neuropathies. Examination may display a vascular middle ear mass pulsating against the tympanic membrane, which blanches upon pneumatic otoscopy, known as *Brown's sign*, and is seen in approximately 50% of cases.

20. How are jugulotympanic paragangliomas staged?

Two classification systems for JT PGLs are in use: Fisch and Glasscock-Jackson (Tables 46.2 and 46.3).

21. What is the proper workup of jugulotympanic paraganglioma?

CT imaging is essential to assess the involvement of the jugular bulb, evidenced by erosion of the adjacent bone; MRI/MRA/MRV may also be obtained if jugular bulb extension is confirmed. Over the last 15 years, research on the genetics of these tumors has led to radical changes in the recommended workup and surveillance. All patients

Table 46.2 Fisch Classification System for Jugulotympanic Paragangliomas

TYPE	
A	Tumor limited to middle ear cleft (i.e., glomus tympanicum)
B	Tumor limited to tympanomastoid complex
C	Tumor involves infralabyrinthine temporal bone or extends to carotid canal
C1	Limited involvement of the vertical portion of carotid canal
C2	Invades the vertical portion of carotid canal
C3	Invades the horizontal portion of carotid canal
D	Tumor extends intracranially
D1	<2-centimeter intracranial extension
D2	>2-centimeter intracranial extension

Table 46.3 Glasscock-Jackson Classification System For Glomus Jugulare

TYPE	
I	Small tumor involving the jugular bulb, middle ear, and mastoid
II	Tumor extending under the IAC; may have intracranial extension
III	Tumor extending into the petrous apex; may have intracranial extension
IV	Tumor extending beyond the petrous apex into the clivus or infratemporal fossa; may have intracranial extension

Table 46.4 Pittsburgh Staging System for Temporal Bone Carcinoma

T STAGE	
T1	Tumor limited to the EAC without bony erosion or soft tissue extension
T2	Tumor with limited EAC erosion or limited (<0.5 centimeters) soft tissue involvement
T3	Tumor eroding the full thickness osseous EAC with limited (<0.5 centimeters) soft tissue involvement, tumor involving the middle ear and/or mastoid, or patients presenting with facial paralysis
T4	Tumor eroding the cochlea, petrous apex, medial wall of the middle ear, carotid canal, jugular foramen, or dura or with extensive (>0.5 centimeters) soft tissue involvement

with known JT PGL should undergo genetic testing. Biochemical screening (urine metanephrines and catechol-amines) should be performed to ascertain whether the JT PGL is a secreting tumor and to rule out additional pheochromocytoma/PGL. If the biochemical or genetic screening is positive, whole-body MRI is recommended to screen for additional tumors, and lifelong follow-up with an endocrinologist or geneticist is recommended.

22. **What is the proper management of jugulotympanic paragangliomas?**
    Management options are similar to CPA tumors, such as observation, radiation, or surgical resection. Historically, surgery has produced significant morbidity with regard to cranial neuropathies. SRS is commonly used to treat such tumors. Surgery is indicated for tumors limited to the middle ear cleft (glomus tympanicum) or in debulk-ing the middle ear component to control bothersome pulsatile tinnitus. Surgery may also be performed for large tumors; to avoid morbidity, partial resection with postoperative SRS is performed when feasible. Of course, if ad-ditional PGLs are discovered due to a genetic disorder, a multi disciplinary discussion should be undertaken with an endocrinologist before treatment is pursued.

23. **Which lesions involve the clivus and how are they accessed?**
    Other than meningiomas, bony tumors are most commonly encountered in the clivus, including chordomas, chondrosarcomas, and osteosarcoma. Other possibilities include epidermoid, cholesterol granuloma, heman-giopericytoma, plasmacytoma, nasopharyngeal carcinoma, craniopharyngioma, pituitary tumors, or metastases. Endoscopic transsphenoidal surgery may be performed in some cases or combined with other approaches. Lateral skull base approaches include the RS, retrolabyrinthine/posterior petrous approach, the Kawase approach, and to-tal petrosectomy. The RS approach may be utilized for paraclival access but risky brainstem retraction is required to access the central clivus. The retrolabyrinthine approach is helpful for small tumors if the hearing is intact. This involves the MCF approach combined with mastoidectomy, skeletonizing, preserving the sigmoid sinus and bony labyrinth, and removing the posterior and middle fossa dural plates. The surgeon then looks anteriorly past the labyrinth to access the prepontine cistern and clivus. The Kawase approach involves MCF with a drillout of the anterior petrous apex (Kawase triangle) and sacrifice of the superior petrosal sinus. Total petrosectomy is the removal of the entire temporal bone to better access the clivus. Other approaches designed to allow for drainage of cystic lesions of the petrous apex (primarily cholesterol granulomas) include the infracochlear and infralabyrin-thine approaches.

24. **Do neurotologists only treat benign tumors?**
    Although most of the tumors discussed in this chapter are benign, neurotologists also treat cancers of the temporal bone and base of the skull. Chondrosarcoma and osteosarcoma have also been reported. Squamous cell carcinoma (SCC) of the external auditory canal (EAC) and temporal bone is staged using the Pittsburgh criteria (Table 46.4). SCC of the cheek, auricle, and parotid may grow to involve the mastoid bone and/or the vertical seg-ment of the facial nerve. Other tumors that may involve the temporal bone include basal cell carcinoma, adenoid cystic carcinoma, and acinic cell carcinoma.

25. **What are the surgical options for cancers of the temporal bone?**
    Sleeve resection involves removing the skin of the EAC and the TM; used only for very small T1 tumors, some surgeons consider the procedure to be oncologically unsound. For most T1 and T2 tumors, lateral temporal bone (LTB) resection, parotidectomy, and neck dissection are performed. LTB resection involves performing a mastoidectomy, skeletonizing the facial nerve tympanic and mastoid segments down to the stylomastoid foramen, extending the drillout circumferentially around the EAC, and finally excising the tympanic segment of the temporal bone in continuity with the skin of the EAC. A T3 tumor requires subtotal temporal bone resection, and a T4 tumor requires total temporal bone resection.

Bibliography

Arriaga M, Curtin H, Takahashi H, Hirsch BE, Kamerer DB: Staging proposal for external auditory meatus carcinoma based on preoperative clinical examination and computed tomography findings, *Ann Otol Rhinol Laryngol* 99:714–721, 1990.

Cass SP, Sekhar LN, Pomeranz S, Hirsch BE, Snyderman CH: Excision of petroclival tumors by a total petrosectomy approach, *Am J Otol* 15:474–484, 1994.

Coughlin AR, Willman TJ, Gubbels SP: Systematic review of hearing preservation after radiotherapy for vestibular schwannoma, *Otol Neurotol* 39:273–283, 2018.

Evans DGR. Neurofibromatosis type 2, Handb Clin Neurol 132:87–96, 2015.

Fayad JN, Schwartz MS, Slattery WH, Brackmann DE: Prevention and treatment of cerebrospinal fluid leak after translabyrinthine acoustic tumor removal, *Otol Neurotol* 28:387–390, 2007.

Fischer G, Fischer C, Remond J: Hearing preservation in acoustic neurinoma surgery, *J Neurosurg* 76:910–917, 1992.

Fishbein L, Merrill S, Fraker DL, Cohen DL, Nathanson KL: Inherited mutations in pheochromocytoma and paraganglioma: why all patients should be offered genetic testing, *Ann Surg Oncol* 20:1444–1450, 2013.

Friedmann DR, Grobelny B, Golfinos JG, Roland JT Jr: Nonschwannoma tumors of the cerebellopontine angle, *Otolaryngol Clin North Am* 48:461–475, 2015.

Hunter JB, Francis DO, O'Connell DP, et al. Single institutional experience with observing 564 vestibular schwannomas: factors associated with tumor growth, *Otol Neurotol* 37:1630–1636, 2016.

Jackson CG, Glasscock ME III, Harris PF: Glomus tumors. Diagnosis, classification, and management of large lesions, *Arch Otolaryngol* 108:401–410, 1982.

Lees KA, Tombers NM, Link MJ, et al: Natural history of sporadic vestibular schwannoma: a volumetric study of tumor growth, *Otolaryngol Head Neck Surg* 159:535–542, 2018.

Merkus P, Taibah A, Sequino G, Sanna M: Less than 1% cerebrospinal fluid leakage in 1803 translabyrinthine vestibular schwannoma surgery cases, *Otol Neurotol* 31:276–283, 2010.

Oldring D, Fisch U: Glomus tumors of the temporal region: surgical therapy, *Am J Otol* 1:7–18, 1979.

Rosenberg SI: Natural history of acoustic neuromas, *Laryngoscope* 110:497–508, 2000.

Sughrue ME, Yeung AH, Rutkowski MJ, Cheung SW, Parsa AT: Molecular biology of familial and sporadic vestibular schwannomas: implications for novel therapeutics, *J Neurosurg* 114:359–366, 2011.

Sun CX, Robb VA, Gutmann DH: Protein 4.1 tumor suppressors: getting a FERM grip on growth regulation, *J Cell Sci* 115:3991–4000.

Tschudi DC, Linder TE, Fisch U: Conservative management of unilateral acoustic neuromas, *Am J Otol* 21:722–728, 2000.

Volsky PG, Hillman TA, Stromberg KJ, et al: Hydroxyapatite cement cranioplasty following translabyrinthine approach: long-term study of 369 cases, *Laryngoscope* 127:2120–2125, 2017.

Wiegand DA, Fickel V: Acoustic neuroma—the patient's perspective: subjective assessment of symptoms, diagnosis, therapy, and outcome in 541 patients, *Laryngoscope* 99:179–187, 1989.

CHAPTER 47

TEMPORAL BONE TRAUMA

Vincent Eusterman, MD, DDS

KEY POINTS

1. The temporal bone is made up of five components (squamous, tympanic, petrous, mastoid, styloid), and fractures generally follow natural lines of weakness at the sutures, canals, and foramina in the bone.
2. The petrous bone is extremely solid and protects the auditory and vestibular organs within the otic capsule in temporal bone trauma.
3. CT scan classification of temporal bone fractures often does not correlate with the signs and symptoms of the fracture; physical examination still offers the most clinical relevance.
4. The classification of temporal bone fractures has shifted from the anatomic axis of the petrous ridge to the otic capsule, sparing or disrupting, to focus on the functional sequelae and complications of these fractures.
5. Persistent CSF drainage after conservative therapy requires surgical intervention to prevent meningitis.

Pearls

1. Clinical diagnosis of temporal bone fracture can be made based on three physical findings: hemotympanum, postauricular ecchymosis (Battle's sign), and periorbital ecchymosis (Raccoon sign).
2. CSF fistulae occur in 17% of temporal bone fractures and most leaks stop within 7 to 10 days using conservative therapy.
3. CSF leaks beyond 10 days have a 33% to 88% risk of meningitis and require surgical intervention.
4. The most common site of injury to the facial nerve is in the perigeniculate region in 80% to 93% of patients.
5. The most common hearing loss associated with temporal bone trauma is conductive hearing loss.

QUESTIONS

1. **What are the common causes of temporal bone trauma?**
   Temporal bone trauma can be classified as blunt or penetrating. Blunt trauma is most commonly the result of motor vehicle accidents (31%), followed by assaults, falls, and motorcycle accidents. Penetrating trauma is almost exclusively due to gunshot wounds. Temporal bone trauma is most common in the second through fourth decades of life and in males. Of fractures, 90% are associated with intracranial injuries and 9% are associated with cervical spine injuries. Sixty percent are open fractures, draining bloody otorrhea or CSF fluid, and 8% to 29% occur bilaterally.

2. **What important structures in and coursing through the temporal bone are subject to injury during temporal bone trauma?**
   The temporal bone is extremely complex; it houses ossicles, cochlear and vestibular organs, the vestibulocochlear nerve (IIX), the facial nerve (VII), the carotid artery, and the jugular vein. Other nerves passing near or through the temporal bone are the abducens nerve (VI), glossopharyngeal nerve (IX), vagus nerve (X), and spinal accessory nerve (XI), which can also be injured during temporal bone trauma. The multiple sutures, foramina, and canals in the skull base weaken the bone and are responsible for the fracture patterns seen in temporal bone trauma.

3. **The temporal bone is made up of five portions; what are they?**
   The *squamous portion* is a flat plate that is the lateral wall of the middle cranial fossa housing the middle meningeal artery; it includes the zygomatic arch and glenoid fossa. The *tympanic portion* is a horseshoe-shaped, incomplete ring of bone that makes up most of the external auditory canal. Medially, it forms the tympanic sulcus, which holds the tympanic membrane annular ligament. The *styloid process* projects inferiorly from the vaginal process of the temporal bone. It lies anterior to CN VII and lateral to the carotid artery. The *petrous portion* is the pyramid-shaped medial portion of the temporal bone that separates the middle and posterior cranial fossae. It is extremely solid and protects the auditory and vestibular organs within the otic capsule. The internal auditory canal is located medially on the posterior surface. The inferior surface contains the carotid canal and jugular foramen. The posterior part of the petrous bone contains the *mastoid*, which is filled with air cells and lined with a mucous membrane.

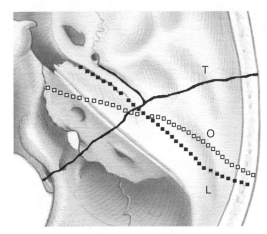

Fig. 47.1 Temporal bone fractures, longitudinal (L), transverse (T), and oblique (O).

4. **How are temporal bone fractures classified?**
   Temporal bone fractures are traditionally described as either longitudinal or transverse; however, most fractures are in an *oblique* or *mixed pattern* (Fig. 47.1). Current literature supports the nomenclature of "*otic capsule-sparing* or *disrupting*" to emphasize the functional sequelae and complications of the fracture. *Longitudinal fractures* account for 80% of cases, and most are otic capsule sparing. They are caused by temporoparietal blunt trauma and extend from the squamous portion, down the EAC, and through the middle ear (often disrupting the ossicular chain), parallel to the long axis of the petrous pyramid to the foramen lacerum. Facial nerve injury occurs in 20% of cases, and conductive hearing loss (CHL) is common but sensorineural loss (SNHL) is not. Tympanic membrane rupture and ear canal lacerations are common and can be associated with cerebrospinal fluid (CSF) otorrhea. *Transverse fractures* are less common and account for 20% of temporal bone fractures. Injury usually results from severe blunt trauma to the occiput or frontal regions. Fractures often begin at the foramen magnum and cross the long axis of the petrous pyramid at right angles and can have a higher incidence of otic capsule disruption. They have a 50% facial nerve injury rate, including severe SNHL or mixed (CHL + SNHL) hearing loss, with intense vertigo. The tympanic membrane is usually intact and CSF leaking into the middle ear presents as rhinorrhea via the eustachian tube.

5. **What physical signs should you look for when evaluating someone with suspected temporal bone fracture?**
   - *Facial nerve weakness* may be sudden or delayed in onset; documentation is important because sudden loss of function may require urgent intervention.
   - *Hearing loss* may be conductive, sensorineural, or both; hearing can be tested in the awake patient with a 512-Hz tuning fork and deferred in the unconscious patient.
   - *Nystagmus* results from vestibular injury or perilymphatic fistula. Sudden severe vertigo with SNHL is associated with disruption of the otic capsule.
   - *Tympanic membrane and external auditory canal lacerations* are often observed in longitudinal fractures.
   - *Hemotympanum* is blood within the middle ear space.
   - *CSF otorrhea* occurs most often through a lacerated eardrum with longitudinal fractures.
   - *CSF rhinorrhea* occurs through the eustachian tube with an intact TM, which is commonly observed in transverse fractures.
   - *Battle's sign* is postauricular ecchymosis arising from bleeding from the mastoid emissary vein.
   - *Raccoon eyes* is periorbital ecchymosis arising from middle and anterior cranial fossa fractures from meningeal tears that cause venous sinus bleeding into the orbit.

6. **What complications are associated with temporal bone fracture?**
   - *Facial nerve injury* is common and may be temporary or permanent.
   - *CSF leak* is common and generally improves within 7 days.
   - *Hearing loss* is common and may be conductive, sensorineural, or both.
   - *Vertigo* is common and may be mild to very severe and constant or positional.
   - *Vascular injuries* are uncommon, except in severe blunt or penetrating trauma where angiography for carotid, vertebral, and middle meningeal artery injuries may be required.
   - *Facial hypesthesia or hypoesthesia* is uncommon and caused by injury to the trigeminal nerve on the surface of the petrous bone in Meckel's cave.

- *Diplopia* is uncommon and due to abducens nerve injury as it courses through Dorello's canal.
- *Cholesteatoma* may be a late finding from displaced canal skin or tympanic membrane skin into the middle ear or mastoid spaces.

7. Which are the best imaging studies for temporal bone trauma?

Patients with severe head trauma often have a computed tomography (CT) scan of the head to assess for intracranial hemorrhage. Additional imaging of the temporal bone with axial and coronal thin-section high-resolution CT scanning with bone algorithms is indicated in the presence of facial paralysis, CSF leakage, EAC fracture and canal disruption, vascular injury, and conductive hearing loss. Carotid angiography, MRA, or CTA may be indicated for patients with transient or persistent neurologic deficits. Conventional radiographs no longer play a role in the evaluation of patients with suspected temporal bone fracture.

8. What are ways to detect a CSF fistula from a temporal bone fracture?

Noninvasive techniques for identifying CSF fistula include protein electrophoresis for beta-2-transferrin, which is specific for CSF. HRCT can demonstrate potential sites of a CSF fistula in approximately 70% of patients. CT cisternography with intrathecal contrast can be useful when not initially detected on HRCT. Intrathecal fluorescein used correctly in a diluted dose (0.5 mL 5% solution in 10 mL CSF reinjected) can identify otorrhea or rhinorrhea when collected on pledgets and examined under a Wood's lamp for green florescence.

9. What are the most likely sites of facial nerve injury in temporal bone fractures?

The most common site of facial nerve injury is in the *perigeniculate region* in 80% to 93% of patients, possibly due to tethering by the GSPN. Damage can also occur in the "horizontal" or tympanic segment and in the labyrinthine segment by direct injury or nerve edema (Fig. 47.2).

10. How is an injured facial nerve evaluated in an obtunded or unconscious patient?

Facial nerve evaluation begins after the stabilization of serious and life-threatening injuries. Facial nerve examination by gross facial function in the unconscious patient can be elicited as a grimace in response to painful stimuli. Patients with immediate onset of paralysis can be tested using the *Hilger nerve stimulator*, using minimal nerve excitability testing (NET) and maximum stimulation test (MST) between days 3 and 7 postinjury. If no loss of stimulability occurs, the patient is observed. If the nerve loses stimulability within 1 week of injury, facial nerve exploration is considered. *Electroneuronography* (ENoG) uses bipolar stimulating and recording electrodes. If ENoG demonstrates more than 90% degeneration of the compound muscle action potentials at 6 days and more than 95% in 14 days, recovery is unlikely and surgical exploration may be indicated. Traditional *electromyography* (EMG) performed by monopolar intramuscular recording electrodes shows voluntary activity (innervated muscle) and fibrillation potentials (denervated muscle). EMG is the most useful 2 to 3 weeks after paralysis and offers little additional information in the acute setting regarding the decision to operate.

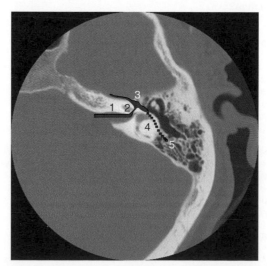

Fig. 47.2 CT image of the facial nerve through the left temporal bone, including the following segments from proximal to distal: (1) meatal segment, (2) labyrinthine segment, (3) perigeniculate area, (4) "horizontal" or tympanic segment and descending to the stylohyoid foramen as the (5) "vertical" or mastoid segment.

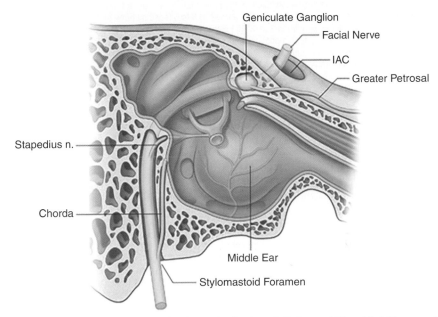

Fig. 47.3 Temporal bone drawing with the removal of the incus and malleus bones for the transmastoid/supralabyrinthine approach to the geniculate ganglion. (From • **geniculate_ganglion** in https://www.operativeneurosurgery.com.)

14. **What causes CSF otorrhea and rhinorrhea and what are the dangers?**
    CSF leaks occur in 17% of temporal bone fractures and represent a serious risk of meningitis. Fractures in the floor of the middle cranial fossa drain into the middle ear (epitympanum and antrum) and mastoid air cells. *CSF otorrhea* results when the tympanic membrane is perforated and *CSF rhinorrhea* results when the tympanic membrane is intact and CSF exits through the eustachian tube. CSF fistulas of 7 days or less have a 5% to 10% incidence of meningitis. From 57% to 85% of fistulas treated conservatively will close in 1 week. This includes head of bed elevation, bed rest, and stool softeners to keep the CSF pressure gradient below the tensile strength of the healing barrier. For fistulas lasting more than 7 to 10 days the risk of meningitis can be as high as 88%, and they should be closed surgically. To date, no studies have shown a statistically significant effect of antibiotic prophylaxis in patients with posttraumatic CSF fistula.

15. **How is persistent CSF fistula treated?**
    If spontaneous resolution does not occur with conservative treatment, lumbar drainage is attempted for 72 hours, and surgical exploration can be considered. Otic capsule-disrupting fractures with profound sensorineural hearing loss are treated with mastoidectomy and middle ear obliteration. Otic capsule–sparing fracture treatment depends on the location of the fracture and accessibility, but most are closed through a mastoidectomy and facial recess approach.

16. **What are the types of vertigo that occur following temporal bone trauma?**
    There are five types of posttraumatic vertigo. The most common form of posttraumatic vertigo is a *concussive injury* to the membranous labyrinth. These patients have positional vertigo with a normal VNG, requiring only symptomatic treatment. Otic capsules that disrupt temporal bone fractures produce a *severe ablative vertigo* with intensity that will decrease after 7 to 10 days and then decrease steadily over the following 1 to 2 months, leaving an unsteady feeling that lasts 3 to 6 months until compensation occurs. Intense nystagmus (third degree) is present initially, with the fast component beating away from the fracture site. This nystagmus progressively diminishes in intensity and then disappears over time. *Posttraumatic benign positional vertigo* is usually delayed on onset and is treated using the Epley maneuver. *Posttraumatic vertigo* and *fluctuating SNHL* may indicate a perilymphatic fistula that is initially treated with conservative measures and can require surgical closure. Last, *posttraumatic endolymphatic hydrops* may develop much later and presents as fluctuating hearing loss, tinnitus, and aural fullness with vertigo.

17. **What kinds of hearing loss are seen with temporal bone trauma? How are they treated?**
    Conductive hearing loss (CHL) is the most common type of hearing loss associated with temporal bone trauma. It is usually temporary and caused by blood in the middle ear, edema, or tympanic membrane perforation. It

may be persistent if the injury results in failure of the perforation to heal or an ossicular discontinuity. Surgical exploration of the middle ear with CHL is usually performed 3 to 6 months after injury, as 75% of these patients return to normal. *Sensorineural hearing loss* (SNHL) is less common and results from an otic capsule disruption injury. It may also occur from a perilymphatic fistula, noise injury, concussion injury, or direct injury to the central auditory system. Longitudinal fractures commonly produce a CHL with high-tone SNHL from inner ear concussion. Transverse fractures commonly produce severe SNHL or mixed (SNHL and CHL) loss.

CONTROVERSIES

18. **Should a paralyzed facial nerve be explored after temporal bone fracture?**
    Recommendations for surgery are based on three poor prognostic factors for spontaneous improvement: (1) immediate onset of paralysis, (2) worsening on ENoG testing, and (3) evidence of nerve transection or bony impingement on CT scan.

    Pros: Patients with immediate onset of complete facial paralysis following temporal bone trauma have a relatively poor prognosis. This is often due to transection of the facial nerve and the time of injury. Extensive data from nonrandomized studies in the treatment of Bell's palsy support the use of ENoG in the prognosis of an intact facial nerve that meets the criteria for degeneration. Data on its use to guide treatment of traumatic facial paralysis are only emerging and confined to case series, which suggest a favorable prognosis in patients with degeneration to less than 90% of normal within 6 days or less than 95% of normal within 14 days after injury (Fig. 47.4).

    Cons: Approximately 50% of patients with immediate-onset, complete paralysis recover normal or near-normal facial function. Surgical indications for posttraumatic intertemporal facial paralysis are poorly defined and randomized controlled studies of surgical versus nonsurgical treatments do not exist. Most recommendations for exploration of the facial nerve are based on opinion and data from case series to identify poor prognostic factors and the population most likely to benefit from surgery. The use of ENoG criteria for temporal bone trauma surgery is limited, as it has been studied more in Bell's palsy. More than 90% of individuals without poor prognostic factors listed above are likely to recover near-normal facial function (House-Brackmann grade 1 or 2) with conservative treatment.

19. **Should patients with CSF fistula due to temporal bone fracture receive antibiotics to reduce the risk of meningitis?**
    Ratilal et al. showed in a meta-analysis that the incidence of meningitis in temporal bone fractures *without* CSF fistula is low and antibiotic prophylaxis has no role in these cases. The incidence of meningitis in patients *with*

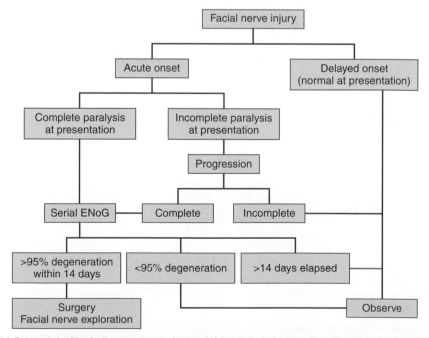

Fig. 47.4 Proposed algorithm for the management of traumatic injury to the facial nerve. (From Massa N: Intratemporal bone trauma. Available at http://emedicine.medscape.com/article/846226-overview.)

CSF fistula ranges from 2% to 88%, with the most significant factor being the duration of leakage. According to Brodie, the use of antibiotic prophylaxis in temporal bone fractures with CSF leak remains controversial due to the inadequate number of patients for meta-analysis. In contrast, his study of 320 patients showed a reduced incidence of meningitis in patients who received prophylactic antibiotics.

BIBLIOGRAPHY

Alvi A, Bereliani A: Acute intracranial complications of temporal bone trauma, *Otolaryngol Head Neck Surg* 119:609–613, 1998.

Brodie HA: Prophylactic antibiotics for posttraumatic cerebrospinal fluid fistulae. A meta-analysis, *Arch Otolaryngol Head Neck Surg* 123:749–752, 1997.

Brodie HA: Management of temporal bone trauma. In: Flint W, Haughey BH, Haughy K, et al, eds: *Cumming's Otolaryngology: Head and Neck Surgery*, 6th ed, Philadelphia, 2014, Mosby Elsevier, pp 2220–2233.

Brodie HA, Thompson TC: Management of complications from 820 temporal bone fractures, *Am J Otol* 18:188–197, 1997.

Chang CY, Cass SP: Management of facial nerve injury due to temporal bone trauma, *Am J Otol* 20:96–114, 1999.

Dahiya R, Keller JD, Litofsky NS, et al: Temporal bone fractures: otic capsule sparing versus otic capsule violating clinical and radiographic considerations, *J Trauma* 47:1079–1083, 1999.

DiBiase P, Arriaga MA: Post-traumatic hydrops, *Otolaryngol Clin North Am* 30:1117–1122, 1997.

Fisch U: Surgery for Bell's palsy, *Arch Otolaryngol* 107:1–11, 1981.

Gantz B, Rubinstein JT, Gidley P, et al: Surgical management of Bell's palsy, *Laryngoscope* 109:1177–1188, 1999.

Ghorayeb BY, Yeakley JW: Temporal bone fractures: longitudinal or oblique? The case for oblique temporal bone fractures, *Laryngoscope* 102:129–134, 1992.

Johnson F, Semaan MT, Megerian CA: Temporal bone fracture: evaluation and management in the modern era, *Otolaryngol Clin North Am* 41:597–618, 2008.

Kang HM, Kim MG, Boo SH, et al: Comparison of the clinical relevance of traditional and new classification systems of temporal bone fracture, *Eur Arch Otorhinolaryngol* 269:1893–1899, 2012.

Leech PI, Paterson A: Conservative and operative management of cerebrospinal fluid leakage after closed head injury, *Lancet* 1:1013–1111, 1973.

MacGee EE, Cauthen JC, Brackett CE: Meningitis following acute traumatic cerebrospinal fluid fistula, *J Neurosurg* 33:312–316, 1970.

Massa N: Intratemporal bone trauma. Available at http://emedicine.medscape.com/article/846226-overview.

Morgan WE, Coker NJ, Jenkins HA: Histopathology of temporal bone fractures: implications for cochlear implantation, *Laryngoscope* 104:426–432, 1994.

Patel A, Groppo E: Management of temporal bone trauma, *Craniomaxillofac Trauma Reconstr* 3:105–113, 2010.

Rafferty MA, McConn-Walsh R, Walsh M: A comparison of temporal bone fractures classification systems, *Clin Otolaryngol* 31:287–291, 2006.

Ratilal BO, Costa J, Sampaio C: Antibiotic prophylaxis for preventing meningitis in patients with basilar skull fractures, *Cochrane Database Syst Rev* 1, 2006, CD004884.

Resnick DK, Subach BR, Marion DW: The significance of carotid canal involvement in basilar cranial fracture, *Neurosurgery* 40:1177–1181, 1997.

Ulrich K: Verletzungen des gehorlorgans bel schadelbasisfrakturen (ein histologisch und klinissche studie), *Acta Otolaryngol Suppl* 6:1–150, 1926.

CHAPTER 48

PEDIATRIC ENT ANATOMY AND EMBRYOLOGY WITH RADIOLOGY CORRELATES

Stephen S. Newton, MD and David M. Mirsky, MD

QUESTIONS

1. **How does the size and shape of the external auditory canal differ between children and adults?**
   In adults, the EAC has a near-sigmoid shape with the cartilaginous portion angling posteriorly and superiorly and the bony portion angling anterior inferiorly. Pulling the helix posterosuperiorly straightens the EAC and allows for better visualization of the tympanic membrane. In the infant the EAC is nearly straight. It then elongates and changes shape until approximately 9 years of age when it is nearly adult size.

2. **What is a dimeric tympanic membrane?**
   The tympanic membrane is made up of three layers: an inner membranous layer, a middle fibrous layer that gives rigidity to the membrane, and an outer squamous layer. If a tympanic membrane perforation does not heal with the fibrous layer incorporated, then that newly healed portion has only two layers (dimeric) and results in a thin, floppy segment. This thinner segment is more easily retracted into the middle ear and can affect the conduction of sound to the ossicles.

3. **Why are the tympanic membrane and ossicles required for normal hearing?**
   Sound, as it is presented to us, travels through air while our hearing organs within the inner ear are bathed in fluid. If we attempt to transmit sound from air to fluid there is a 99.9% loss in energy, which is known as an impedance mismatch. The impedance mismatch is overcome by a series of mechanical advantages including a tympanic membrane that is 21 times the size of the stapes footplate and ossicles that create a lever force of 1.3×. Together these overcome the mismatch in impedance and allow for near full transmission of all sound energy into the inner ear.

4. **What are the innervations of the tensor tympani and stapedius muscles?**
   The tensor tympani is derived from the first pharyngeal arch and thus is innervated by a branch of the fifth cranial nerve. The stapedius muscle is derived from the second arch and thus is innervated by a branch from the seventh cranial nerve. The dampening effects of these two muscles can result in a reduced sound transmission of 15 dB.

5. **Why is the stapes shaped like a stirrup?**
   The stapedial artery is transiently present in fetal development, connecting the future external carotid arterial system with the internal carotid system. This vessel goes through the middle ear and the primordial stapes, creating the structure of the stapes known as the obturator foramen. A persistent stapedial artery (Fig. 48.1) is very rare and may be associated with pulsatile tinnitus, conductive hearing loss, and an absent ipsilateral foramen spinosum.

6. **What are the two most common congenital abnormalities of the ossicles?**
   The two most common ossicular abnormalities are a congenitally fixed stapes and incudostapedial discontinuity. Isolated abnormalities of the stapes are more likely to be unilateral, whereas congenital abnormalities of the other ossicles are more likely to be bilateral.

7. **Which nerves run through the middle ear?**
   Jacobson's nerve is a branch of CN IX and runs across the tympanic promontory innervating the middle ear mucosa and eustachian tube, providing parasympathetic innervation to the parotid gland. Arnold's nerve is a branch of the vagus nerve that gives sensory innervation to the external auditory canal. This nerve is sometimes stimulated when cleaning the ear and can make a patient cough. The chorda tympani nerve branches from the descending portion of the facial nerve (Fig. 48.2) and runs medial to the malleus before exiting the middle ear through the petrotympanic fissure. Finally, the facial nerve may be dehiscent superior to the oval window or may be positioned within the middle ear in congenitally malformed ears.

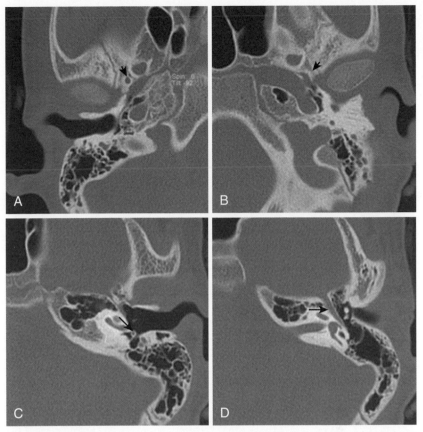

Fig. 48.1 Persistent stapedial artery. Axial CT images reveal **(A)** a normal foramen spinosum on the right (*arrowhead*) and **(B)** an absent foramen spinosum on the left (*arrowhead*). Images acquired more cephalad through the left ear illustrate the course of the persistent stapedial artery **(C)** ascending in a small canal on the surface of the posterior cochlear promontory (*arrow*), **(D)** resulting in an enlarged anterior tympanic segment of the facial nerve canal (*arrow*).

8. **What are the named segments of the facial nerve that run through the temporal bone and which is the narrowest?**
   The *internal auditory canal segment* of the facial nerve is 7 to 8 millimeters in length and runs superior to the cochlear nerve (think of the mnemonic "7-Up/Coke down"). The *labyrinthine segment* extends from the internal auditory canal to the geniculate ganglia; this is the narrowest segment and most prone to damage secondary to trauma and/or swelling. The *tympanic segment* runs from the geniculate ganglion to the second genu, running in the medial wall of the tympanic cavity over the round window and below the bulge of the lateral semicircular canal. The final segment is the *mastoid* or *vertical segment* (Fig. 48.2).

9. **What is the cochleariform process and what is its relationship to the facial nerve?**
   The cochleariform process is a curved ridge of bone that houses the tendon of the tensor tympani muscle. This ridge of bone is also a good landmark denoting the anterior position of the tympanic portion of the facial nerve.

10. **What are the boundaries of the sinus tympani?**
    The borders of the sinus tympani are formed by the ponticulus superiorly and subiculum inferiorly. This space is difficult to visualize during surgery without the use of a mirror or angled endoscope. Clinically, this area is important during surgery for cholesteatoma, as the cholesteatoma may have grown into the sinus and can be difficult to extract.

11. **What is the promontory of the middle ear?**
    This bulge on the medial surface of the middle ear represents the prominence of the basal turn of the cochlea.

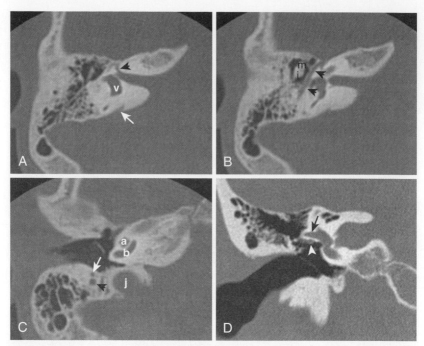

Fig. 48.2 Facial nerve. Axial CT images demonstrate the course of the facial nerve (*black arrowheads*), including **(A)** the labyrinthine segment, **(B)** the tympanic segment, and **(C)** the mastoid segment. Coronal reformat CT image **(D)** illustrates the course of the tympanic segment (*white arrowhead*) passing under the lateral semicircular canal (*arrow*). Relevant anatomy includes **(A)** the vestibule (v) and vestibular aqueduct (*white arrow*), **(B)** the interrelationship between the head of the malleus (m) and body of incus (i) in the epitympanum, and **(C)** the apical and basal turns of the cochlea (a and b), the jugular bulb (j), and the chorda tympani (*white arrow*).

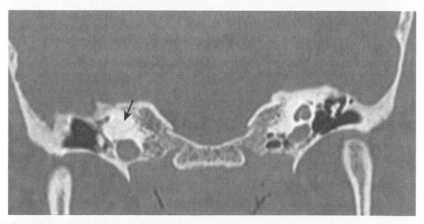

Fig. 48.3 Complete labyrinthine aplasia. Coronal reformat CT image shows complete absence of all inner ear structures on the right (*arrow*) representing arrested otic placode development prior to the third week of gestation.

12. **What are some commonly described developmental abnormalities of the cochlea and when does developmental arrest occur?**
    - Cochleovestibular aplasia, formerly known as a Michel deformity (arrest third week): complete absence of cochlear and vestibular structures (Fig. 48.3)
    - Cochlear aplasia (arrest late third week): absent cochlea; normal, dilated or hypoplastic vestibule; and semicircular canals
    - Common cavity (arrest fourth week): cochlea and vestibule form a common space (Fig. 48.4)

- Incomplete partition Type I (arrest fifth week): cystically enlarged cochlea without internal architecture; dilated vestibule; mostly enlarged internal auditory canal
- Cochlear hypoplasia (arrest sixth week): distinctly recognizable separation of cochlear and vestibular structures; small cochlear bud
- Incomplete partition Type II, formerly known as a Mondini deformity (arrest seventh week): cochlea with 1½ turns, cystically dilated middle and apical turn (cystic apex), slightly dilated vestibule (Fig. 48.5)

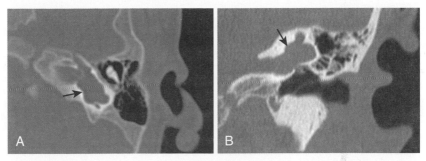

Fig. 48.4 Common cavity malformation. (A) Axial and **(B)** coronal reformat CT images demonstrate a featureless common cavity representing a rudimentary cochlea, vestibule, and semicircular canals (*arrows*). In this anomaly, otic placode development is arrested in the fourth gestational week, following differentiation into the otocyst.

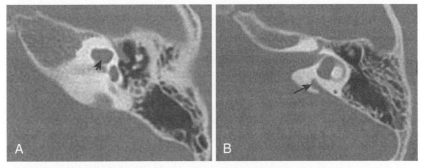

Fig. 48.5 Cochlear incomplete partition type II. (A) Axial CT image reveals deficiency of the interscalar septum between the middle and apical turns (*arrowhead*) in this patient with a **(B)** large vestibular aqueduct (*arrow*).

13. **Of the above developmental deformities, which are the most common?**
    Incomplete partition type II followed by a common cavity.

14. **What is the most common finding on a computed tomography (CT) scan of a profoundly deaf child?**
    The most common finding is a radiographically normal inner ear. It is presumed that the malformation is limited to the membranous labyrinth, which cannot be seen by imaging modalities and represents 90% of children with profound hearing loss.

15. **Why are children more prone to nasoseptal hematomas?**
    The cartilage of children is more pliable and less likely to fracture. The bending or buckling of cartilage can create a shearing force that results in separation of the perichondrium and the cartilage and bleeding within this space.

16. **What supplies blood to the nasal septum?**
    The anterior ethmoidal artery, posterior ethmoidal artery, sphenopalatine artery, and greater palatine artery and a branch of the superior labial artery.

17. **What is Kiesselbach's plexus?**
    Kiesselbach's plexus is an area of the anterior cartilaginous septum where four different arteries form a vascular network (anterior ethmoidal, sphenopalatine, greater palatine, and the septal branch of the superior labial artery). This is a common area for epistaxis because of the rich vascular network, tendency for the mucosa to dry out, and

digital manipulation, especially in children. It is estimated that 90% of all nasal bleeds come from this region of the septum. Pressing the nasal ala inward, toward the septum, applies pressure on this area.

18. **What structure drains under the inferior turbinate?**
The nasolacrimal duct carries tears from the lacrimal sac and opens into the nasal cavity just under the inferior turbinate. The nasolacrimal canal is formed by the lacrimal bone and maxilla. A congenial nasolacrimal duct cyst is caused when the membrane fails to cannulate and may present as a nasal mass extending from under the inferior turbinate and epiphora.

19. **What paranasal sinuses are present at birth? Describe the development of the paranasal sinuses.**
    - **Ethmoid:** the anterior and posterior ethmoid sinuses are the most developed sinuses and are present at birth.
    - **Maxillary:** the maxillary sinuses are present at birth but are only millimeters in size. The maxillary sinuses then undergo a biphasic growth pattern with rapid development in the first 3 years and then again between the ages of 7 to 12 years.
    - **Frontal:** the frontal sinuses are generally not present at birth and develop as extensions of ethmoid air cells anteriorly and superiorly into the frontal bone. At 2 years of age this development starts in the vertical phase of growth with near adult size achieved by the early teen years. Approximately 5% of people do not develop a unilateral frontal sinus and another 5% never develop any frontal sinuses.
    - **Sphenoid:** pneumatization of the sphenoid bone does not start to occur until 3 to 4 years of age and reaches adult size by 12 to 15 years of age.

20. **What are the developmental spaces of the nasal frontal region that are possible paths for dermoid, encephalocele, and nasal gliomas?**
During development, dural projections extend through the anterior neuropore (primitive frontonasal region) and approximate with the subcutaneous region. This includes the *fonticulus frontalis* (a transient fontanelle between the inferior frontal bone and nasal bone), the *foramen cecum*, and the prenasal space. When these spaces close, failure of involution can result in nasal dermoids, encephaloceles, and nasal gliomas.

21. **How does ossification and normal development of the nasofrontal region affect imaging characteristics and choice of imaging for congenital nasal frontal masses?**
In the first 6 to 8 months of life, the nasal frontal process, nasal bones, and ethmoid bones are unossified with CT attenuation similar to brain and nasal cartilage. The normal nasal secretions can give the false impression of a bony dehiscence in this region with possible connection to the frontal nasal mass. In addition, the frontal process, nasal bones, and crista galli lack fat in the first 8 months of life, resulting in similar intensity to brain on T1-weighted images. Because of this variability, magnetic resonance imaging (MRI) is the modality of choice for assessing the nasofrontal region in young children.

22. **Which muscles form the paratubal support for the eustachian tube?**
The tensor veli palatini, tensor tympani, levator veli palatini, and salpingopharyngeus. The tensor veli palatini is the primary dilator of the eustachian tube, which allows for equalization of pressure between the nasopharynx and the middle ear space with contraction.

23. **How does the eustachian tube vary between infants and adults?**
Besides being significantly smaller, the infant eustachian tube is either in a horizontal direction or 10 degrees from horizontal, whereas the adult eustachian tube is at a 45-degree angle. It is believed that this angle in infants affects the function of the tensor veli palatini.

24. **What are the divisions of the pharynx and their boundaries?**
The pharynx is divided into the nasopharynx, oropharynx, and hypopharynx.
    - Nasopharynx: superior to the soft palate, posterior to the choanae, with the skull base as the superior extent
    - Oropharynx: superior border is the soft palate, inferior boundary is the base of tongue (level of the hyoid), and the anterior borders are the palatoglossal arch and circumvallate papillae
    - Hypopharynx: level of the epiglottis down to the level of the inferior border of the cricoid cartilage

25. **Why are neonates considered obligate nasal breathers?**
In neonates the larynx is elevated with the epiglottis in apposition to the soft palate. This allows the infant to drink and breathe simultaneously, but this also means that infants have difficulty breathing through their mouths (Fig. 48.6).

26. **What is the anatomy of the tonsillar fossae?**
The palatine tonsils are surrounded by the tonsillar fossa, which is made up of the palatoglossus muscle (anterior tonsillar pillar) anteriorly and the palatopharyngeus muscle (posterior tonsillar pillar) posteriorly.

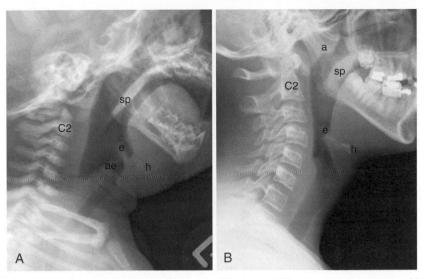

Fig. 48.6 Normal airway. Lateral radiographs in **(A)** a 13-day-old and **(B)** a 14-year-old illustrate normal airway anatomy. a, Adenoids; sp, soft palate; e, epiglottis; ae, aryepiglottic folds; h, hyoid; C2, odontoid process.

27. **What supplies blood to the palatine tonsils?**
    Five arteries primarily provide the blood supply: dorsal lingual artery, ascending palatine artery (facial artery), tonsillar branch of the facial artery, ascending pharyngeal artery (external carotid), and the lesser palatine artery (descending palatine artery). The venous drainage is via the peritonsillar plexus into the lingual and pharyngeal veins and then to the internal jugular vein. While not supplying the palatine tonsils, the internal carotid artery is approximately 2.5 centimeters posterolateral to the tonsils.

28. **What is Waldeyer's ring?**
    Heinrich von Waldeyer was an anatomist who described the lymphoid tissue in the posterior nasopharynx and oropharynx. The ring named in his honor is composed of the lingual tonsils, pharyngeal tonsils (adenoids), and palatine tonsils. This ring of the immune system samples pathogens that enter the upper aerodigestive pathway and is involved in the synthesis of humoral immunoglobulins and production of lymphocytes.

29. **What is a bifid uvula and what is its potential significance?**
    A bifid uvula is an abnormality in closure of the most posterior aspect of the soft palate resulting in a uvula with a forked tip. This may signify a possible submucosal cleft, where the mucosa of the secondary palate is normal but the underlying muscular sling may be incomplete with irregular attachments. This may result in abnormal motion of the palate and poor closure of the velopharynx, leading to speech and swallowing difficulties secondary to velopharyngeal insufficiency.

30. **Which pharyngeal arches develop into the larynx and how does this affect its innervation?**
    The larynx develops from the fourth and sixth pharyngeal arches. The fourth arch is associated with the superior laryngeal nerve and the sixth arch is associated with the recurrent laryngeal nerve.

31. **What is the narrowest part of the larynx in children and adults?**
    The narrowest part of the infant larynx is the cricoid cartilage. This is in contrast to the narrowest part of the adult larynx, which is the rima glottis or glottic opening. Because the narrowest part of the airway in young children is a rigid cartilaginous ring, an endotracheal tube that is too large may cause ischemic injury to the surrounding mucosa and result in scarring and eventual subglottic stenosis.

32. **Why does the recurrent laryngeal nerve wrap around the aortic arch on the left and subclavian artery on the right?**
    The sixth arch, which is important in laryngeal development, is also important in the development of the aortic arch and subclavian artery. Portions of the sixth arch descend to form these great vessels and carry the recurrent

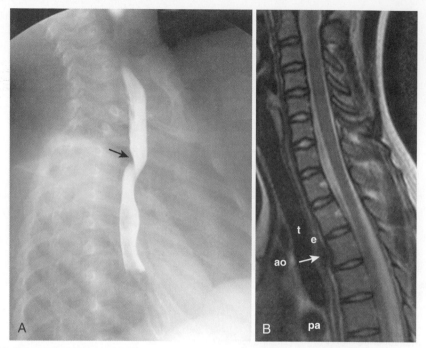

Fig. 48.7 Aberrant subclavian artery. (A) Oblique image from an esophagram shows an extrinsic posterior indentation on the esophagus (*black arrow*). **(B)** Sagittal T2-weighted image of the cervical spine in a different patient reveals an aberrant right subclavian artery (*white arrow*) coursing posterior to the trachea (t) and esophagus (e). pa, Pulmonary artery, ao, aorta.

laryngeal nerve with them. A nonrecurrent laryngeal nerve on the right is a rare entity associated with an aberrant right subclavian artery (abnormal development of the sixth arch) (Fig. 48.7).

33. **How do congenital airway and esophageal obstruction affect amniotic fluid levels during pregnancy?**
Abnormalities or compression of the upper airway or esophagus can decrease or prevent the infant's ability to swallow amniotic fluid, resulting in polyhydramnios.

34. **What is CHAOS?**
CHAOS stands for "congenital high airway obstruction syndrome." It is a failure of the airway to recannulate during embryologic development of the larynx (laryngeal atresia) (Fig. 48.8) or upper trachea. If this is not identified prenatally the survival rate is very low because the patient is unable to be ventilated, unless there is a corresponding tracheoesophageal fistula.

35. **Describe the normal shape of tracheal rings and how they are different from the cricoid cartilage.**
The cricoid cartilage is a complete cartilaginous ring, whereas the tracheal rings are incomplete with a membranous wall that is shared with the esophagus. This C-shaped tracheal ring allows for the needed rigidity to maintain the airway throughout respiration but also allows for larger boluses of food to pass through the esophagus.

36. **What supplies blood to the trachea?**
The lateral pedicles that run the length of the trachea and esophagus supply blood to the trachea. These pedicles obtain their blood supply from the inferior thyroid, subclavian, supreme intercostal, internal thoracic, innominate, and superior and middle bronchial arteries.

37. **What is Killian's triangle?**
Also known as Killian's dehiscence, this is a weakened area of the pharyngeal wall located between the inferior constrictor and the cricopharyngeus muscle. Excessive pressure within the lower pharynx and impaired relaxation/spasm of the cricopharyngeus during swallowing can lead to a diverticulum of this region called a Zenker's diverticulum.

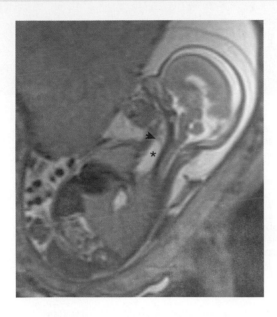

Fig. 48.8 Laryngeal atresia. Sagittal HASTE image from a fetal MRI reveals a high airway obstruction at the level of the larynx (*arrowhead*), with distension of the distal trachea (*asterisk*) secondary to failure of the airway to recannulate during embryogenesis.

BIBLIOGRAPHY

Ahmad SM, Soliman A: Congenital anomalies of the larynx, *Otolaryngol Clin North Am* 40:177, 2007.
Hedulund G: Congenital frontonasal masses: developmental anatomy, malformations, and MR imaging, *Pediatr Radiol* 36:647–662, 2006.
Jackler RK: Congenital malformations of the inner ear. In: Cummings CS, et al, eds: *Otolaryngology – Head and Neck Surgery*, 2nd ed, 1993, Mosby-Yearbook, pp. 152–159.
Lacout A, Marscot-Dupuch K, Smoker WR, et al: Foramen tympanicum, or foramen of Huschke: pathologic cases and anatomic CT study, *Am J Neuroradiol* 26(6):1317–1323, 2005.
Park HY, Han DH, Lee JB, et al: Congenital stapes anomalies with normal eardrum, *Clin Exp Otolaryngol* 2(1):33–38, 2009.
Poje CP, Rechtweg JS: Structure and function of the temporal bone. In: Wetmore RF, Munts HR, McGill TJ, eds: *Pediatric Otolaryngology Principles and Practice Pathways*, 2nd ed, 2012, Thieme.
Salassa JR, Pearson BW, Payne WS: Gross and microscopical blood supply of the trachea, *Ann Thorac Surg* 24(2):100–107, 1977.
Sennaroglu L, Saatci I: A new classification for cochleovestibular malformations, *Laryngoscope* 112:2230–2241, 2002.
Sibergleit R, Quint DJ, Mehta BA, et al: The persistent stapedial artery, *Am J Neuroradiol* 21(3):572–577, 2000.
Spaeth J, Krugelstein U, Schlondorff G: The paranasal sinuses in CT-imaging: development from birth to age 25, *Int J Pediatr Otorhinolaryngol* 39(1):25–40, 1997.

CHAPTER 49

THE ACUTE PEDIATRIC AIRWAY

Erin Hamersley*, DO, LCDR, MC, USN and Tendy Chiang, MD

KEY POINTS

1. The assessment of the acute pediatric airway patient includes general appearance (degree of distress), vital signs, skin color, and level of consciousness.
2. Stridor is not a diagnosis but rather a symptom or physical sign of turbulent airflow. Localization of the site of turbulence can be guided by the phase(s) of respiration in which stridor is present.
3. In general, a rapid onset of airway compromise requires immediate attention, whereas chronic mild stridor without distress can be managed in an outpatient setting.
4. Croup is a common viral infection in children. Most cases can be managed conservatively on an outpatient basis; atypical, severe, or recurrent episodes requiring prolonged medical management require further evaluation.
6. Always ask about the possibility of foreign body aspiration when evaluating a pediatric patient with acute airway obstruction.

Pearls
1. The pediatric airway is significantly smaller than the adult airway; inflammation and narrowing of the airway can be far more clinically significant in an infant than a similar degree of edema in an adult.
2. Multilevel airway obstruction should be considered in children with syndromes.
3. Bilateral choanal atresia classically presents with respiratory distress and cyanosis at birth that is relieved with crying.
4. Respiratory distress with inspiratory or biphasic stridor in the setting of a strong cry raises suspicion for bilateral true vocal cord paralysis.
5. Epiglottitis can frequently be managed nonoperatively with medical management. Younger patients are more likely to require operative intervention.
6. Urgent intervention is necessary if there is suspicion of button battery ingestion.

QUESTIONS

1. **How does an infant's airway differ anatomically from an adult's?**
   An infant's larynx is one-third the size of an adult larynx. The subglottis is the narrowest segment of the pediatric airway compared with the glottis in an adult. The average diameter of a term infant's subglottis is about 3.5 millimeters compared with 10 to 14 millimeters for an adult.
   The neonatal larynx is initially located at vertebral level C2–3, allowing for the supraglottic structures to interdigitate with the soft palate. This protects and optimizes the airway for infant feeding (suck-swallow-breathe pattern). The larynx descends throughout development to level C7 by adulthood.

2. **What unique physiologic and mechanical properties of the pediatric airway increase the risk of respiratory compromise in infants versus adults?**
   The narrow nature of the infant airway makes it much more susceptible to respiratory compromise compared with adults. Poiseuille's law states that resistance is inversely proportional to the radius to the fourth power. As such, minimal swelling produces significant narrowing of the airway in infants and children. For instance, 1 millimeters of obstruction in the infant subglottis (4 millimeters) leads to a 16-fold increase in resistance and a 75% decrease in airway cross-sectional area. In an adult the same 1 millimeter of obstruction causes only 30% decrease in cross-sectional area and a 2-fold increase in resistance (Fig. 49.1). Additionally, greater chest wall compliance allowing for easier collapse and higher oxygen consumption at baseline, and a smaller lung capacity leads to faster oxygen desaturation in children.

3. **What is stridor? What is stertor?**
   Stridor is a harsh, high-pitched noise produced by turbulent airflow in the airway. It can resemble a squeak or whistle. Stridor is not a diagnosis or disease in itself but rather a symptom that indicates narrowing or obstruction of the upper airway. *Stertor* resembles snoring and indicates nasal or pharyngeal obstruction.

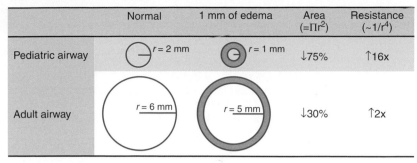

	Normal	1 mm of edema	Area ($=\Pi r^2$)	Resistance ($\sim 1/r^4$)
Pediatric airway	$r = 2$ mm	$r = 1$ mm	↓75%	↑16x
Adult airway	$r = 6$ mm	$r = 5$ mm	↓30%	↑2x

Fig. 49.1 Impact of minimal swelling on the pediatric versus adult airway. According to Poiseuille's law, resistance is inversely proportional to the radius to the fourth power. A minimal amount of edema in the pediatric airway will have a more significant impact on airway diameter and resistance compared with the same amount of edema in an adult. (Adapted from Albert D, Boardman S, Soma M: Evaluation and management of the stridulous child. In: Flint PW, Haughey BH, Lund VJ, et al., eds, *Cummings Otolaryngology: Head & Neck Surgery*, 5th ed, Philadelphia, 2010, Mosby, pp. 2896–2911.)

4. **Identify the three types of stridor.**
   Inspiratory stridor reflects airflow impairment above or at the level of the vocal cords. It is generally high pitched when occurring at the vocal cords and may be low pitched (stertor) when obstruction is above the vocal cords (pharynx or supraglottic larynx).
   Expiratory stridor is classically caused by obstruction in the distal trachea or bronchi. It gives rise to a more prolonged, sonorous sound and a prolongation of the expiratory phase of respiration.
   Biphasic stridor has both an inspiratory and expiratory component and is suggestive of a fixed lesion. This typically suggests a narrowing of the subglottic region, although fixed narrowing in other locations can also result in this sound.

5. **What are the signs of impending respiratory failure?**
   - Biphasic stridor or quiet breathing after prolonged stridor and increased work of breathing
   - Suprasternal and/or subcostal retractions
   - Abdominal breathing/accessory muscle use
   - Nasal flaring
   - Diaphoresis
   - Mental status changes
   - Neck hyperextension or a "tripod" position (sitting leaning forward with chin up, mouth open, and bracing hands on the bed)
   - Tachypnea, tachycardia
   - Given compensatory mechanisms (tachypnea, tachycardia), oxygen desaturation is a late and ominous sign that frequently indicates impending decompensation
   - Pallor and cyanosis can accompany hypoxia

6. **What is the differential diagnosis of respiratory distress that presents immediately at birth?**
   Airway obstruction that is present at birth is characteristic of a fixed anatomical narrowing of the airway. This can be due to obstruction at the level of the nose, oral cavity/oropharynx, hypopharynx, larynx, or trachea (Table 49.1).

7. **What are the possible causes of neonatal nasal obstruction?**
   The differential diagnosis includes rhinitis, piriform aperture stenosis, nasolacrimal duct cysts, midline nasal masses, and choanal atresia. Because neonates are obligate nasal breathers until 4 to 6 months of age, the classic presentation of respiratory distress from neonatal nasal obstruction results in difficulty breathing/cyanosis that is relieved with crying.

8. **What is choanal atresia?**
   Choanal atresia is a failure of the posterior nasal cavity to communicate with the nasopharynx, postulated to represent the failure of the nasobuccal membrane to rupture. Two thirds of cases are unilateral and usually present later in life with chronic rhinorrhea and congestion. Bilateral atresia usually presents in the neonatal period with cyanotic events during feeding that are relieved with crying. Fifty percent to 75% of patients will have an associated congenital anomaly.
   Suspicion for the diagnosis often arises with respiratory distress at birth and/or with failure to pass catheters through the nose. Diagnosis is made with flexible nasal endoscopy and computed tomography, which is also used for operative planning. Treatment is surgical resection of the atretic plate to create patent choanae.

Table 49.1 Differential Diagnosis of Neonatal Airway Obstruction by Anatomic Site

SITE OF OBSTRUCTION	DIFFERENTIAL
Nose	Rhinitis, piriform aperture stenosis, nasolacrimal duct cyst, nasal mass, choanal atresia, encephalocele or meningocele, midface hypoplasia (Crouzon's, Down syndrome, etc.)
Oral cavity/oropharynx	Micrognathia (Pierre Robin, Treacher Collins, etc.), macroglossia (Down syndrome), lingual thyroid, masses, cysts
Larynx	Laryngomalacia, vocal fold paralysis, subglottic stenosis, laryngeal web, laryngeal atresia, cysts or masses
Trachea	Tracheomalacia/bronchomalacia, tracheal stenosis or atresia, extrinsic/vascular compression (vascular ring, double aortic arch, pulmonary artery sling, etc.), complete tracheal rings

Albert D, Boardman S, Soma M: Evaluation and management of the stridulous child. In: Flint PW, Haughey BH, Lund VJ, et al, eds, *Cummings Otolaryngology: Head & Neck Surgery*, 5th ed, Philadelphia, 2010, Mosby, table 205-1.

9. **Name a common genetic syndrome with which choanal atresia is associated.**
   Choanal atresia is a component of the CHARGE syndrome:
   - C = Coloboma
   - H = Heart anomalies
   - A = Atresia of the choanae
   - R = Retardation of growth and development
   - G = Genitourinary disorders (hypoplasia for males)
   - E = Ear anomalies and/or hearing loss

10. **What is Robin sequence? What are other causes of obstruction at the same level?**
    Robin sequence (RS) describes a triad of micrognathia, glossoptosis, and airway obstruction. Micrognathia leads to glossoptosis, ultimately causing airway obstruction at the level of the base of tongue and oropharynx. Glossoptosis can prevent fusion of palatal shelves at the midline, resulting in a U-shaped cleft palate.
    RS can occur in isolation or with a syndrome (Treacher Collins, Stickler, Nager syndrome, and many others). Presence of a syndrome with mandibular hypoplasia should raise suspicion for multilevel obstruction.

11. **Discuss the evaluation and management of children with Robin sequence.**
    In addition to a complete history and physical, flexible fiberoptic/rigid laryngoscopy, bronchoscopy, sleep endoscopy, and polysomnogram are commonly used to characterize the degree of obstruction.
    Many cases of RS can be managed with supplemental oxygen, prone positioning, placement of a nasopharyngeal airway, and/or continuous positive airway pressure (CPAP). Failure to thrive, obstructive sleep apnea, and respiratory failure require escalation of management.
    Definitive surgical management options include tongue-lip adhesion, mandibular distraction, and tracheostomy.

12. **Name four congenital laryngeal anomalies that cause respiratory distress. What is the most common congenital laryngeal anomaly?**
    - Laryngomalacia (most common)
    - Collapse of the supraglottic larynx resulting in inspiratory stridor
    - May result from aryepiglottic fold shortening, redundant supraglottic tissue, and/or hypotonia
    - Vocal fold paralysis
    - Congenital subglottic stenosis
    - Congenital laryngeal web

13. **What is the cause of bilateral vocal fold paralysis?**
    Bilateral vocal cord paralysis (BVCP) is most commonly idiopathic (46%). Other causes include Chiari malformation, cerebral palsy, hydrocephalus, spina bifida, birth trauma, and hypoxia. Workup consists of an MRI of the brain to evaluate for intracranial abnormalities, genetic consultation to evaluate for chromosomal abnormalities, and laryngoscopy with palpation of the cricoarytenoid joint to delineate BVCP from joint fixation.

14. **How does bilateral vocal fold paralysis present and how is it managed?**
    Patients typically present at birth with respiratory distress and inspiratory or biphasic stridor. Awake flexible fiberoptic laryngoscopy should be performed to evaluate supraglottic architecture and cord mobility. Recording the endoscopy can be helpful for diagnosis given the rapid respiratory rate in infants. The mainstay of treatment is tracheotomy; however, some children are able to proceed with observation. Those without tracheostomy require

Table 49.2 Clinical Characteristics of Airway Infections by Location

	SUPRAGLOTTITIS	LARYNGITIS	CROUP	TRACHEITIS
Age	2–7 years	Any	6 months–3 years	6 months–8 years
Onset	Rapid*	Slow	Slow	Rapid
Prodrome	None or mild URI*	URI	URI	URI*
Fever	High*	No	None or low grade*	High*
Hoarseness	No but voice muffled and speech limited due to severe pain*	Yes*	Yes	Yes
Stridor	Usually none. Inspiratory stridor is a late finding indicating severe infection/obstruction	Absent	Inspiratory initially, may progress to biphasic in severe cases	Biphasic
Cough	None	Variable	Barky*	Barky
Odynophagia/ drooling	Yes*	No	No	No
Toxic appearance	Yes	No	No	Yes*
Pathogen	*Haemophilus influenza,* type B Group A beta-hemolytic streptococci	Multiple viruses	Parainfluenza virus Respiratory syncytial virus (RSV)	*Staphylococcus aureus* *Moraxella catarrhalis*

*Indicates classic feature.
Adapted from Duncan NO: Infections of the airway in children. In: Flint PW, Haughey BH, Lund VJ, et al, eds, *Cummings Otolaryngology: Head & Neck Surgery*, 5th ed, Philadelphia, 2010, Mosby, table 197-1.

careful follow up to ensure appropriate growth as their respiratory requirements change with increasing activity. Most cases of idiopathic BVCP demonstrate recovery of function in time, and decannulation is often possible.

15. **How do infections of the different divisions of the larynx differ in presentation? Which pathogens are most commonly associated with each?**
    See Table 49.2.

16. **What radiographic findings are classically found in supraglottitis, croup, and bacterial tracheitis?**
    (Fig. 49.2).
    - Supraglottitis: "Thumb sign" on lateral neck x-ray. Thickening and rounding of the epiglottis with loss of the normal air space of the vallecula.

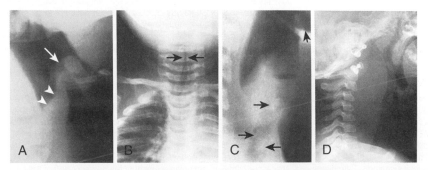

Fig. 49.2 Imaging characteristics of pediatric airway infections. **A,** Supraglottitis. Rounded epiglottis (*white arrow*), thickened aryepiglottic folds (*white arrowheads*), and distension of the hypopharyngeal space. **B,** Croup. Narrowed subglottis (*black arrows*), showing a "steeple sign." **C,** Bacterial tracheitis. Tracheal lumen obscured by sloughed mucosa (*black arrows*). Note normal epiglottis (*black arrowhead*). **D,** Retropharyngeal abscess. Widened retropharyngeal soft tissues compared with the vertebral bodies. (Adapted from Duncan NO: Infections of the airway in children. In: Flint PW, Haughey BH, Lund VJ, et al., eds, *Cummings Otolaryngology: Head & Neck Surgery*, 5th ed, Philadelphia, 2010, Mosby, pp. 2803–2811, figures 197-8, 197-3, 197-10, and 197-13.)

- Croup: "Steeple sign" on AP neck x-ray. Narrowing at the level of the subglottis.
- Bacterial tracheitis: "Pseudomembranes" on lateral neck x-ray. Irregular tracheal borders indicative of thick, purulent secretions or sloughing mucosa.

17. What is another name for supraglottitis? Describe the change in incidence in the last several decades.

Epiglottitis is another name for supraglottitis but this is somewhat inaccurate because this clinical entity typically involves the entire supraglottis. Most cases of supraglottitis were due to hemophilus influenza type b (HIB), the incidence of which dropped dramatically following implementation of the HIB vaccine in 1988.

18. Discuss the presentation and management of supraglottitis.

Patients with supraglottitis most commonly present with high fever, odynophagia (pain with swallowing), dysphagia (difficulty swallowing), voice change (muffled voice, hoarseness), and difficulty tolerating secretions. Stridor and respiratory distress are less common presenting signs but suggest impending airway obstruction, which is a surgical emergency. These patients will often assume the "tripod" position and appear anxious. A lateral neck radiograph may demonstrate the "thumb sign". Patients in acute distress should not undergo exams or procedures that may precipitate complete airway obstruction. Stable patients who are not in distress may be evaluated with flexible laryngoscopy to confirm the diagnosis.

The mainstay of management is to obtain and maintain a patent airway. In stable patients, admission with close airway surveillance is recommended. Children in acute distress or those felt to progress to respiratory failure should be taken directly to the operating room to secure the airway. Parents are counseled that intervention spans a wide spectrum from direct laryngoscopy or fiber-optic endotracheal intubation to tracheotomy; however, in most cases, this is not necessary. Airway intervention is more common in younger patients, with a mean of 4 years of age (almost two thirds are 2 years old or younger). Anxiety-provoking maneuvers should be avoided when handling a patient with a tenuous airway; all instrumentation and interventions should be performed in the operative suite.

If operative intervention is necessary, direct laryngoscopy should be performed after the airway is secured to obtain swab cultures from the epiglottis and evaluate for an abscess at the lingual surface of the epiglottis. Intravenous antibiotics should be started and a 10- to 14-day course should be completed. Extubation can generally be accomplished within 48 hours when supraglottic edema improves and an air leak is present around the endotracheal tube.

19. How is croup managed?

Croup is very common; 3% to 5% of all children have one episode in their lifetime. Most cases can be managed conservatively with supportive care only. For more significant symptoms, corticosteroids have been shown to decrease hospitalization rates and severity of disease. Generally one dose of dexamethasone is sufficient and nebulized racemic epinephrine can also be used to decrease airway edema. Between 85% and 99% of patients can be managed as outpatients. Hospitalized patients should be treated with repeated doses of intravenous dexamethasone and racemic epinephrine until symptoms resolve. Only 1% to 5% of patients require intubation for severe airway obstruction.

Direct laryngoscopy should be considered in very young children or those with recurrent or severe croup to rule out underlying airway pathology (i.e., subglottic stenosis, hemangioma, subglottic cyst, etc.).

20. How is bacterial tracheitis managed?

Though severity of symptoms is usually not as dramatic as in acute epiglottitis, airway obstruction is not infrequent with bacterial tracheitis and management includes rigid bronchoscopy with debridement of secretions and sloughed mucosa. Seventy-five five to ninety percent require intubation and repeated endoscopies for recurrent plugging and crusting. Extubation can be achieved after fever resolves, secretions diminish, and an air leak is present around the endotracheal tube. Intravenous antibiotics are directed toward *Staphylococcus aureus*, and then adjusted based on culture and sensitivity results for a 10- to 14-day course.

21. Describe how pharyngeal infections can lead to airway obstruction.

Peritonsillar, parapharyngeal, and retropharyngeal abscesses can all present with airway obstruction and require surgical drainage for management. All three infections tend to present with fevers, sore throat, and dysphagia. Peritonsillar abscesses present with a "hot potato" voice and possible stertor, because the level of obstruction is at the oropharynx. The obstruction is a result of anterior, medial, and often inferior displacement of the tonsil and palatal fullness. Airway symptoms are usually milder than with parapharyngeal and retropharyngeal abscesses. Parapharyngeal and retropharyngeal abscesses tend to present with decreased neck mobility in addition to the above symptoms. Retropharyngeal abscesses cause anterior displacement of the posterior wall of the pharynx into the airway lumen, whereas parapharyngeal cause a lateral and posterior encroachment on the airway. Airway obstruction is more likely and severe with retropharyngeal abscesses. Management of the airway should be carefully planned in patients with large abscesses. Care should be taken with sedation because endotracheal intubation can be challenging or even impossible and the airway can be lost. Tracheostomy may have to be considered. See Fig. 49.2, panel D.

22. **When evaluating a pediatric patient with acute airway obstruction, what should always be included in the history of present illness?**
    Always ask whether there is concern for or possibility of foreign body (FB) aspiration. About half of aspiration events are not witnessed. If the foreign body does not immediately cause airway obstruction, symptoms can be more subtle and mimic other airway infections, asthma, or pneumonia. A high index of suspicion should be maintained for FB aspiration and history regarding possible aspiration events should always be included when working up children with airway symptoms.

23. **What are risk factors for foreign body aspiration?**
    FB aspiration is most common in toddlers between 1 and 3 years of age. This is because they are more likely to explore their environment with their mouths, they have poor coordination of swallowing, they lack posterior dentition necessary for chewing food properly, they lack an appreciation of what is edible, and they are likely to be playing while eating. Other risk factors include male gender, developmental delay, and neurologic impairment.

24. **Which items have the highest risk for aspiration?**
    Vegetable matter, typically in the form of incompletely chewed food, is the most common item aspirated. Nuts, seeds, and beans are the most common types of food. Other common objects include small plastic or metal toys or pieces. Coins are the most common esophageal foreign bodies.

25. **What are the symptoms of foreign body aspiration?**
    Symptoms vary depending on the location of the foreign body and how long it has been present.
    * Larynx: FB in the larynx can cause an airway emergency requiring emergent intervention. Patients can present with obstruction, cough, hoarseness, and stridor. Delay in diagnosis can allow edema to progress and cause a partial obstruction to become a complete obstruction.
    * Trachea: Symptoms include stridor, wheezing, dyspnea, and coughing. Hoarseness is absent in comparison to laryngeal FB.
    * Bronchi: This is the most common location for airway FBs to lodge (80% to 90%). The classic triad of cough, wheeze, and decreased unilateral breath sounds may not always be present but nearly all patients will have at least one of these symptoms.
    * Esophagus: Dysphagia, odynophagia, drooling, and vomiting are common symptoms of esophageal foreign bodies. Esophageal FBs are more common than airway FBs. Common sites of esophageal FB are at the cricopharyngeus and at the level where the esophagus crosses the aortic arch.

26. **What is the x-ray of choice in diagnosis for airway foreign bodies?**
    Inspiratory and expiratory chest radiographs. The lodged FB allows air to enter but not escape, thus air trapping or hyperinflation can be appreciated on x-ray and exaggerated by the expiratory phase. These views can be difficult to obtain in children, thus lateral decubitus radiographs can be helpful to allow the patient's body weight to assist expiratory excursion. Other changes seen on plain films include atelectasis and pneumonia. Radiopaque objects and those in the bronchi are more likely to be detected on x-ray. A negative film should not rule out FB aspiration, as between 25% and 50% of patients can have completely normal radiographs.

27. **What is the management of foreign body aspiration? Which situations require urgent intervention?**
    Management includes direct laryngoscopy and bronchoscopy for evaluation and endoscopic removal of the foreign body. Intubation and treatment with steroids are considered for those patients with severe obstruction, mucosal damage, or significant airway edema. Bronchial foreign bodies can result in post-obstructive pneumonia distal to the point of obstruction. Always consider evaluation of the esophagus when a child presents with airway obstruction or a positive history and has a normal bronchoscopy because esophageal foreign bodies can cause effacement of the airway. Coins in the esophagus have a high rate of passage through the GI tract and watchful waiting can be considered in older children and those in the distal esophagus when there are no signs of airway compromise.
    Urgent intervention is necessary for acute or potential airway obstruction, concern for esophageal injury, or suspicion of disc battery ingestion.

28. **Discuss button battery ingestion and describe the differences in management compared with ingested coins.**
    A button battery can be mistaken for a coin on imaging. The most reliable way to differentiate the two is by observing the characteristic "double halo" or "double ring" sign on AP view. On lateral view a step-off may be present, however in slimmer button batteries this may be absent.
    The incidence of button battery ingestion has remained relatively stable (about 10 to 12 per million per year) but there has been a dramatic rise in complications and fatalities over the past 10 years as more household objects utilize batteries and battery size has increased. Though hearing aid batteries are the most commonly ingested battery, they are smaller, pass more easily, and pose less of a risk of serious injury to the aerodigestive tract.

Button batteries can lead to significant mucosal injuries within 2 hours of ingestion, thus urgent intervention is required. Patients should be taken to the operating room emergently, regardless of NPO (nothing by mouth) status, for removal. Direct laryngoscopy and bronchoscopy should be considered to assess for tracheal involvement, particularly when the negative pole is anterior. Prior to removal in early stage ingestions (less than 12 hours from time of ingestion) if there is no clinical concern for esophageal perforation, mediastinitis, or sepsis, honey or sucralfate can be administered to decrease the rate of initial injury. Following removal, if there is no visible evidence of an esophageal perforation, irrigation with 0.25% sterile acetic acid is recommended to decrease the progression of liquefactive tissue necrosis. Twelve percent of young children who ingest batteries greater than 20 millimeters in diameter will experience a major complication, such as perforation, tracheoesophageal fistula, major vessel injury, esophageal stricture, vocal cord paralysis, or cervical spine injury. Evaluation with an esophagram prior to resuming a diet should be performed to rule out perforation. Contrasted imaging of the chest should be considered in patients with severe injuries in close proximity to major vascular structures.

Disclosure: The views expressed in this article reflect the results of research conducted by the author and do not necessarily reflect the official policy or position of the Department of the Navy, Department of Defense, nor the United States Government.

BIBLIOGRAPHY

Acevedo JL, Lander L, Choi S, et al: Airway management in pediatric epiglottitis: a national perspective, *Otolaryngol Head Neck Surg* 140:548–551, 2009.

Albert D, Boardman S, Soma M: Evaluation and management of the stridulous child. In: Flint PW, Haughey BH, Lund VJ, et al: eds: *Cummings Otolaryngology: Head & Neck Surgery*, 5th ed., 2010, Mosby, pp. 2896–2911.

Daniel SJ: The upper airway: congenital malformations, *Paediatr Respir Rev.* S260–S263, 2006, S.

DeRowe A, Massick D, Beste DJ: Clinical characteristics of aero-digestive foreign bodies in neurologically impaired children, *Int J Pediatr Otorhinolaryngol* 62(3):243–248, 2002.

Duncan NO: Infections of the airway in children. In: Flint PW, Haughey BH, Lund VJ, et al: eds: *Cummings Otolaryngology: Head & Neck Surgery*, 5th ed., 2010, Mosby, pp. 2803–2811.

Holinger LD, Poznanovic SA: Foreign bodies of the airway and esophagus. In: Flint PW, Haughey BH, Lund VJ, et al: eds: *Cummings Otolaryngology: Head & Neck Surgery*, 5th ed., 2010, Mosby, pp. 2935–2943.

Jatana KR, Chao S, Jacobs IN, Litovitz T: Button battery safety: industry and academic partnerships to drive change, *Otolaryngol Clin North Am* 52(1):149–161, 2019.

Jatana KR, Litovitz T, Reilly JS, et al: Pediatric button battery injuries: 2013 task force update, *Int J Pediatr Otorhinolaryngol* 77:1392–1399, 2013.

Kuo M, Rothera M: Emergency management of the paediatric airway. In: Graham JM, Scadding GK, Bull PD, eds: *Pediatric ENT.* 2007, Springer, pp. 183–188.

Messner AH: Congenital disorders of the larynx. In: Flint PW, Haughey BH, Lund VJ, et al: eds: *Cummings Otolaryngology: Head & Neck Surgery*, 5th ed., 2010, Mosby, pp. 2866–2875.

Nisa L, Holtz F, Sandu K: Paralyzed neonatal larynx in adduction. Case series, systematic review, and analysis, *Int J Pediatr Otorhinolaryngol* 77:13–183, 2013.

Pasagolu I, Dogan R, Demircin A, et al: Bronchoscopic removal of foreign bodies in children: retrospective analysis of 822 cases, *Thorac Cardiovasc Surg* 39:95–98, 1991.

Sidell DR, Kim IA, Coker TR, et al: Food choking hazards in children, *Int J Pediatr Otorhinolaryngol* 77:1940–1946, 2013.

Stroud RH, Friedman NR: An update on inflammatory disorders of the pediatric airway: epiglottitis, croup, and tracheitis, *Am J Otolaryngol* 22:268–275, 2001.

CHAPTER 50

CHRONIC PEDIATRIC AIRWAY DISEASES

Ryota Kashiwazaki, MD and Jeremy D. Prager, MD, MBA

KEY POINTS

1. In the evaluation of pediatric airway disorders, flexible fiber-optic laryngoscopy is the best initial examination modality in the stabilized patient. Additional exams, such as direct laryngoscopy and bronchoscopy, may be indicated.
2. Laryngomalacia and unilateral vocal cord paralysis are the first and second most common causes of stridor in the infant.
3. Choose the smallest endotracheal tube that provides adequate ventilation and limit the total duration of time the patient is intubated to minimize the risk of subglottic stenosis.
4. Current management of RRP is based on repeat endoscopic excision of airway lesions emphasizing removal of disease while preserving function.
5. Pediatric aspiration is most commonly evaluated using modified barium swallow studies and/or fiber-optic endoscopic evaluation of swallowing. Both can be used to facilitate selection of a safe diet.

> **Pearls**
> 1. Laryngomalacia is the most common cause of stridor in the infant. In most cases, it resolves by the age of 2 years without surgical intervention.
> 2. The most common cause of subglottic stenosis is iatrogenic scarring related to endotracheal intubation.
> 3. In the setting of chronic aspiration, pediatric otolaryngologists must maintain a high index of suspicion for laryngeal cleft.
> 4. Infantile hemangiomas are the most common tumors of infancy. Oral propranolol is considered first-line therapy.

QUESTIONS

1. **List the three most common congenital disorders of the larynx.**
   In order of most to least common: laryngomalacia, vocal cord paralysis, and subglottic stenosis.

2. **What is stridor?**
   Stridor is an audible breath sound due to turbulent airflow from airway narrowing.

3. **What is the most common cause of stridor in the neonate and infant?**
   Laryngomalacia.

4. **Describe the characteristics of laryngomalacia.**
   There are several theories regarding the etiology of laryngomalacia, including short aryepiglottic folds (folds of tissue between epiglottis and arytenoid cartilages), poor neuromuscular control of the supraglottis, and inflammatory insults to the larynx. Inspiratory stridor occurs with collapse of supraglottic tissue on inspiration. Affected infants typically present with intermittent inspiratory stridor within the first 2 weeks of life. Stridor is usually worse with feeding, while supine, or while agitated. The child may need to take breaks while feeding to breathe. Most cases are self-limited, with resolution of symptoms by age 18 months. However, approximately 10% of patients experience significant upper airway obstruction resulting in feeding difficulties, failure to thrive, pectus excavatum, apneic episodes, cyanosis, and hypoxia. These patients warrant consideration for surgical intervention.
   Patients may have associated gastroesophageal reflux disease. This condition may contribute to airway edema, further compromising the airway. Acid suppression may improve mild cases of laryngomalacia and is often instituted empirically, though there are growing concerns about the long-term use of these medications.
   Diagnosis is made with awake flexible fiber-optic laryngoscopy.

5. **What is the typical size of the pediatric airway?**
   Airway size is determined based on the narrowest portion of the airway. In the pediatric population, this is the subglottis at the level of the cricoid cartilage. In a term infant, the subglottic lumen measures 4.5 to 5.5 millimeters.

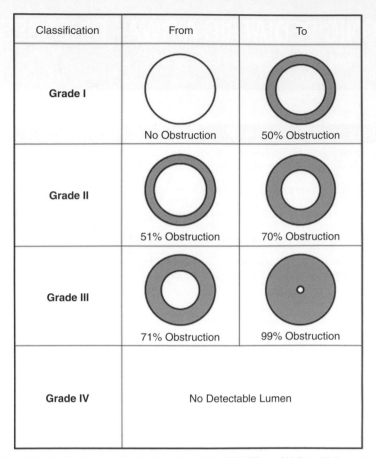

Classification	From	To
Grade I	No Obstruction	50% Obstruction
Grade II	51% Obstruction	70% Obstruction
Grade III	71% Obstruction	99% Obstruction
Grade IV	No Detectable Lumen	

Fig. 50.1 The Myer-Cotton classification system. (Used with permission. Myer CM III, O'Connor DM, Cotton RT: Proposed grading system for subglottic stenosis based on endotracheal tube size, *Ann Otol Rhinol Laryngol* 103:319, 1994.)

6. **How is an endotracheal tube size chosen?**
   Endotracheal and tracheostomy tube sizes are based on the inner diameter of the tube. For example, a 4.0 endotracheal or tracheostomy tube correlates to an inner diameter of 4 millimeters. The smallest tube that provides adequate ventilation should be chosen. Several size-predictive formulas exist and are based on parameters such as age, height, weight, and/or finger width. One commonly used formula is based on the age of the patient: inner diameter = 4 + age/4. This formula is more accurate for older children.

7. **Describe the characteristics of subglottic stenosis.**
   Subglottic stenosis (SGS) is narrowing of the subglottis and can be either congenital or acquired. Congenital SGS occurs in the absence of a history of endotracheal intubation or other causes of acquired stenosis. Causes of congenital SGS include an elliptical cricoid, congenital narrowing (as in Down syndrome), and trapped first tracheal ring.
   Acquired stenosis is more common than congenital SGS and endotracheal intubation is the most common cause. Duration of intubation and endotracheal tube size are the two most important factors in the development of stenosis. Stenosis occurs as a result of pressure necrosis and subsequent scar formation. Prevention of subglottic stenosis via selection of the proper endotracheal tube, a short duration of intubation, and appropriate cuff pressure is ideal. Other causes include neck trauma, laryngeal procedures, caustic ingestions, radiotherapy, and tracheal infection. Diagnosis is made at the time of direct laryngoscopy and bronchoscopy.

8. **Describe the most commonly used grading system for subglottic stenosis.**
   The Myer-Cotton classification system is the most widely used system for grading the degree and severity of subglottic stenosis (Fig. 50.1).

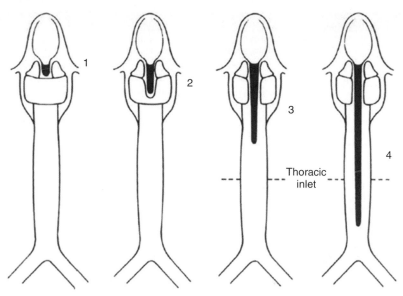

Fig. 50.2 Benjamin-Inglis classification system. Type 1: The cleft is isolated to the supraglottic interarytenoid region located above or at the level of the vocal cords. Type 2: The cleft extends into the upper portion of the cricoid but not through the inferior border. Type 3: The cleft extends through the inferior border of the cricoid cartilage and can variably extend into the cervical trachea. Type 4: The cleft extends into the thoracic trachea and may extend to the carina. (From Chien W, Ashland J, Haver K, et al: Type 1 laryngeal cleft: establishing a functional diagnostic and management algorithm, *Int J Pediatr Otorhinolaryngol* 70(12):2073–2079, 2006.)

9. **How is subglottic stenosis treated?**
   Surgical methods of managing subglottic stenosis include endoscopic and open transcervical techniques. Choice of method depends on many patient factors, including degree of stenosis, comorbid conditions, and age of the lesion. Thin web-like lesions that are identified early, when the scar is immature, may be amenable to endoscopic procedures including scar lysis by balloon dilation. More mature, thicker lesions with greater superior-inferior dimension may require augmentation or resection procedures. Augmentation procedures involve placing cartilage grafts into the airway to make the lumen bigger. Resection procedures involve removing the affected segment and anastomosing the airway.

10. **What is the underlying embryologic defect that leads to the development of a laryngeal cleft?**
    The tracheoesophageal septum forms from two opposing ridges in the midline of the primordial aerodigestive tract into what will eventually become the larynx/trachea and the esophagus. The septum forms in a caudal to cranial direction. Laryngeal clefts are a result of incomplete development and fusion of the tracheoesophageal septum, resulting in abnormal communication between the airway and the hypopharynx/esophagus.

11. **Describe the most commonly used classification system for laryngeal clefts.**
    The Benjamin-Inglis system is the most commonly used classification system (Fig. 50.2).

12. **Discuss the typical presentation of laryngeal clefts.**
    The presentation of this anomaly depends on the severity of the defect. For type I and some type II laryngeal clefts, symptoms may be subtle and include hoarse voice, mild stridor, chronic cough, lingering upper respiratory infections, and recurrent pneumonia. Because the presentation may be subtle, a high index of suspicion is needed to make the diagnosis. More severe types of laryngeal clefts present at birth with respiratory distress and aspiration with oral intake.

13. **Which syndromes are associated with laryngeal cleft?**
    See Table 50.1.

14. **What is the most common cause of unilateral vocal cord paralysis?**
    Iatrogenic complications are the leading cause of unilateral vocal fold paralysis, with patent ductus arteriosus ligation resulting in left vocal cord paralysis being the most frequent cause. Other surgical procedures that can lead

Table 50.1 Syndromes Associated With Laryngeal Cleft	
Opitz-Frias	Characterized by craniofacial anomalies such as cleft lip and palate, genitourinary abnormalities, and midline airway malformations such as laryngeal cleft
Pallister Hall syndrome	Congenital hypothalamic hamartoblastoma, hypopituitarism, polydactyly, imperforate anus, cardiac abnormalities, and renal malformations
VACTERL association	**V**ertebral anomalies, **A**nal atresia, **C**ardiac anomalies, **T**racheoesophageal fistula, **E**ar malformation, **R**enal anomalies, **L**imb anomalies
CHARGE syndrome	**C**oloboma, **H**eart disease, choanal **A**tresia, growth and mental **R**etardation, **G**enital anomalies, **E**ar anomalies

to unilateral vocal fold paralysis include repair of tracheoesophageal fistulas and esophageal atresia repair. Birth trauma may also result in vocal cord paralysis.

Unilateral vocal cord paralysis also may be congenital in origin. Arnold-Chiari malformations can lead to vocal cord paralysis but are classically thought to cause bilateral rather than unilateral paralysis. Other less commonly encountered causes of unilateral paralysis include neoplasms of the central nervous system, neck, or mediastinum causing recurrent laryngeal nerve dysfunction.

15. Describe the clinical course of unilateral vocal cord paralysis.

Unilateral vocal cord paralysis presents with stridor, a weak cry, and feeding difficulty with possible aspiration. This condition is the second most common cause of stridor in the infant. The diagnosis is made with an awake, flexible fiber-optic laryngoscopy. Further workup may be needed in patients in whom an underlying cause is not apparent (idiopathic). Imaging the course of the recurrent laryngeal nerve from skull base to mediastinum may be performed to identify potential etiologies. Patients with difficulty feeding may benefit from evaluation for aspiration via modified barium swallow or fiber-optic endoscopic evaluation of swallowing.

Seventy percent of idiopathic causes of unilateral vocal cord paralysis are expected to resolve spontaneously, most within 6 months of age. Cases of iatrogenic paralysis are less likely to resolve, with 35% of patients noted to recover function at 16-month follow-up. For those patients who are severely symptomatic, vocal cord medialization (injection laryngoplasty, thyroplasty, and ansa cervicalis to recurrent laryngeal nerve reinnervation procedures) may improve speech and swallow function at the cost of increasing airway narrowing at the glottis.

16. What is an infantile hemangioma?

Infantile hemangiomas are benign vascular neoplasms that develop during infancy as a result of disordered angiogenesis. These lesions may occur throughout the body but are most commonly found within the head and neck, including the airway. Symptoms and signs are dependent on the location and natural history of the hemangioma. These are the most common benign tumors of infancy.

17. What signs and symptoms could indicate the presence of an airway hemangioma?

Infantile hemangiomas of the airway present in early infancy during the rapid proliferative phase with symptoms of progressive airway compromise. Patients may present with biphasic stridor or a chronic cough, which may be misdiagnosed as croup. Failure to respond to standard treatment should lead to consultation with ENT. A particularly high degree of suspicion is warranted in the stridulous child with cutaneous hemangiomas of the lower face (beard distribution). Up to 50% have a synchronous airway lesion. Diagnosis of an airway hemangioma is made on fiber-optic laryngoscopy and/or direct laryngoscopy in the operating room. Plain films of the neck may also reveal an asymmetric narrowing of the subglottis.

18. What is the standard treatment of a subglottic infantile hemangioma?

While many infantile hemangiomas do not require treatment, those in the airway warrant intervention to prevent airway compromise. Oral propranolol is considered first-line therapy. Systemic corticosteroid therapy may be considered if there are contraindications or inadequate response to propranolol therapy. The treating physician should monitor for rebound growth following cessation of medical therapy. In many centers, a multidisciplinary team of providers will likely be involved in the treatment of vascular malformations.

Surgical therapy is an option for those patients who are not adequately treated with medical therapy alone. Endoscopic treatment includes laser treatment and steroid injection into the lesion. In addition, the lesion may be excised via an open transcervical approach. Finally, tracheostomy may be needed in some patients in order to bypass the site of obstruction in the subglottis until spontaneous involution occurs.

19. What is tracheomalacia?

Tracheomalacia is collapsibility of the trachea. It is diagnosed during rigid or flexible bronchoscopy when there is a greater than 50% loss of airway diameter during coughing. Lateral chest x-rays during inspiratory and expiratory phases may also demonstrate collapsibility of the tracheal airway. Tracheomalacia presents as expiratory stridor (sometimes biphasic), barky cough, and prolonged or recurrent pulmonary infections. This condition may be classified as extrinsic or intrinsic.

Intrinsic tracheomalacia occurs if the tracheal cartilage is weak, malformed, or absent. Many children with intrinsic tracheomalacia outgrow the condition during the first few years of life. Management for these children includes the potential need for early intervention for pulmonary illnesses, inhaled steroids for airway edema, and the understanding that the barky cough is not necessarily croup. A condition commonly associated with intrinsic tracheomalacia is tracheoesophageal fistula with or without esophageal atresia.

Extrinsic tracheomalacia implies that a structure outside of the airway is compressing the tracheal cartilage. This is most commonly related to cardiac and vascular anomalies. A barium esophagram may suggest a vascular ring encircling the airway. Rigid bronchoscopy and computed tomography or magnetic resonance imaging are also diagnostic of vascular ring.

20. **What is recurrent respiratory papillomatosis?**
RRP is a neoplasm of the airway that is caused by human papilloma virus (HPV). It is the most common benign neoplasm of the pediatric larynx, leading to symptoms of dysphonia and stridor. This disease does occur in adults and tends to be less aggressive.

21. **What are the most common types of HPV that lead to RRP?**
HPV types 6 and 11 are the most common types that lead to RRP.

22. **How is RRP transmitted?**
Vertical transmission via contact through an infected birth canal is the proposed method of disease transmission from mother to child. However, the overall risk of contracting RRP from a mother with active genital condylomata at the time of birth is generally low (1 in 231–400). Cesarean section is of limited use to prevent vertical transmission. The American Academy of Pediatrics and the American College of Obstetricians and Gynecologists do not currently recommend cesarean section solely to protect the neonate from HPV infection.

23. **List the risks factors for the development of RRP.**
   • First-born child
   • Teenage mother
   • Vaginal delivery (it should be noted that several cases exhibit in utero transmission)

24. **How is RRP treated?**
There is no single treatment modality that has been shown to eradicate RRP once and for all. The current mainstay of therapy is surgical reduction of disease burden (to debulk as much disease as possible while maintaining normal morphology and anatomy). Methods include cold steel excision with or without powered instrumentation (e.g., microdebrider) or laser excision (carbon dioxide, potassium titanium phosphate).

Adjuvant medical treatments also exist, although none have demonstrated efficacy in double-blind randomized controlled trials. The most well-known adjuvant therapy is topical injection of the antiviral medication cidofovir. It is important to keep in mind that cidofovir is a potential carcinogen. The use of this medication requires thorough counseling with families and is reserved for difficult to treat lesions and patients requiring at least four procedures within 12 months. Refer to RRP Task Force consensus statements for more information.

Although robust studies are lacking, there appears to be a great interest in transitioning away from cidofovir toward bevacizumab, a recombinant monoclonal antibody therapy. Local intralesional injections have met with some success, but a recent case series reported on the dramatic successes of systemic therapy. Additional therapies on the horizon include DNA vaccines and programmed death-1 pathway inhibitors.

25. **How is RRP prevented?**
HPV vaccination is likely the most important mode of prevention, as evidenced by a recent study performed in Australia. The authors reported a reduction of annual RRP incidence from 0.16 to 0.02 per 100,000 children. Currently, a 9-valent HPV vaccine is available in the United States.

26. **Define aspiration. How does it differ from penetration?**
Aspiration occurs when a material passes from the upper airway below the true vocal cords. Alternatively, penetration occurs when a material enters the larynx but not past the true vocal cords. Penetration deep into the larynx is a risk factor for aspiration.

27. **List the four phases of swallowing.**
See Table 50.2.

28. **How do abnormalities of the phases of swallowing contribute to aspiration?**
Any abnormality, whether anatomic or functional, of any phase of swallowing can contribute to swallowing dysfunction and ultimately result in aspiration. Dysfunction can be broken down into the affected phase of

Table 50.2 Four Phases of Swallowing

Oral preparatory phase	Bolus formation
Oral propulsive phase	Transport of bolus to the pharynx
Pharyngeal phase	Transport of the food bolus from the pharynx into the esophagus. During this phase, the nasopharynx is closed, breathing stops, the vocal cords adduct, the larynx rises, and the base of the tongue and pharyngeal muscles propel the bolus to the esophagus
Esophageal phase	Peristaltic contraction of the esophagus moves the bolus from the upper esophageal sphincter into the body of the esophagus, through the lower esophageal sphincter, and into the stomach

swallowing. For example, vocal cord paralysis can result in abnormal glottic closure during the pharyngeal phase of swallowing and possible aspiration. Neurologic disorders, on the other hand, can result in muscular weakness and dysfunction of any phase of swallowing.

29. **Which anatomic abnormalities may predispose a pediatric patient to aspiration?**
    Cleft palate, tracheoesophageal fistula, laryngeal cleft, macroglossia, and micrognathia are all examples of anatomic abnormalities of the head and neck that can lead to dysfunctional swallow and aspiration.

    It is important to note that neurologic conditions, hypotonia, and some syndromes (e.g., Down syndrome) are highly associated with aspiration during oral intake. Providers should keep this in mind when caring for these select patient populations.

30. **Discuss the workup of suspected pediatric aspiration.**
    Evaluation for aspiration includes obtaining a history consistent with aspiration (coughing and choking with feeds, recurrent pneumonia, wheezing, respiratory distress, etc.) as well as supportive radiographic or endoscopic testing. Modified barium swallow studies (MBS) are used to evaluate the oral cavity, pharynx, and upper esophagus during swallowing. During MBS, different consistencies of barium preparations are given to the patient during fluoroscopy of the upper aerodigestive tract. Penetration and aspiration with different consistencies may be noted and recommendations regarding safe oral intake can be made.

    Flexible or fiber-optic endoscopic evaluation of swallowing (FEES) is an additional method of evaluating the airway during oral intake. FEES relies on the direct visualization of swallow via a nasopharyngeal fiber-optic examination. During the examination, the patient is asked to swallow foods of varying consistencies. MBS and FEES each have their strengths and weaknesses as tools for the evaluation of aspiration. Patients may undergo both exams in order to gain the greatest amount of information regarding their disease process.

BIBLIOGRAPHY

Benjamin B, Inglis A: Minor congenital laryngeal clefts: diagnosis and classification, *Ann Otol Rhinol Laryngol* 98:417–420. 1989.
Bouhabel S, Hartnick CJ: Current trends in practices in the treatment of pediatric unilateral vocal fold immobility: a survey on injections, thyroplasty and nerve reinnervation, *Int J Pediatr Otorhinolaryngol* 109:115–118, 2018.
Cole F: Pediatric formulas for the anesthesiologist, *Am J Dis Child* 94:672–673, 1957.
De Bruyne P, Ito S: Toxicity of long-term use of proton pump inhibitors in children, *Arch Dis Child* 103(1):78–82, 2018.
Derkay CS, Bluher AE: Update on recurrent respiratory papillomatosis, *Otolaryngol Clin North Am* 52(4):669–679, 2019.
Derkay CS, Volsky PG, Rosen CA, et al: Current use of intralesional cidofovir for recurrent respiratory papillomatosis, *Laryngoscope* 123(3):705–712, 2013.
Derkay CS, Wiatrak B: Recurrent respiratory papillomatosis: a review, *Laryngoscope* 118:1236–1247, 2008.
Fraga JC, Jennings RW, Kim PC: Pediatric tracheomalacia, *Semin Pediatr Surg* 25(3):156–164, 2016.
Ida JB, Thompson DM: Pediatric stridor, *Otolaryngol Clin North Am* 47(5):795–819, 2014.
Jacobs IN, Finkel RS: Laryngeal electromyography in the management of vocal cord mobility problems in children, *Laryngoscope* 112:1243–1248, 2002.
King BR, Baker MD, Braitman LE, et al: Endotracheal tube selection in children: a comparison of four methods, *Ann Emerg Med* 22:530–534. 1993.
King EF, Blumin JH: Vocal cord paralysis in children, *Curr Opin Otolaryngol Head Neck Surg* 17:483–487, 2009.
Krowchuk DP, Frieden IJ, Mancini AJ, et al: Subcommittee on the management of infantile hemangiomas clinical practice guideline for the management of infantile hemangiomas, *Pediatrics* 143(1): e20183475. 2019.
Myer CM III, O'Connor DM, Cotton RT: Proposed grading system for subglottic stenosis based on endotracheal tube sizes, *Ann Otol Rhinol Laryngol* 103:319–323, 1994.
Olney DR, Greinwald JH Jr, Smith RJ, et al: Laryngomalacia and its treatment, *Laryngoscope* 1109:1770–1775. 1999.
Prager JD: Empirical proton pump inhibitor therapy in children, *Otolaryngol Head Neck Surg* 144(12):1124–1125, 2018.
Schwartz T, Faria J, Pawar S, Siegel D, Chun RH: Efficacy and rebound rates in propranolol-treated subglottic hemangioma: a literature review, *Laryngoscope* 127(11):2665–2672, 2017.
Truong MT, Messner AH, Kerschner JE, et al: Pediatric vocal fold paralysis after cardiac surgery: rate of recovery and sequelae, *Otolaryngol Head Neck Surg* 137:780–784, 2007.
Wertz A, Ha JF, Driver LE, Zopf DA: Pediatric laryngeal cleft repair and dysphagia, *Int J Pediatr Otorhinolaryngol* 104:216–219, 2018.

PEDIATRIC ADENOTONSILLAR DISEASE AND OBSTRUCTIVE SLEEP-DISORDERED BREATHING

Norman R. Friedman, MD

CHAPTER 51

KEY POINTS

1. There are no studies to date that demonstrate significant alterations in the immune system following an adenotonsillectomy.
2. Penicillin is the initial drug of choice for culture-positive streptococcal infections. Resistance to penicillin or first-generation cephalosporins has not been reported.
3. Obstructive sleep apnea (OSA) requires a polysomnogram (PSG) to make the diagnosis. Obstructive sleep-disordered breathing (oSDB) is a clinical diagnosis.
4. Ibuprofen is no longer contraindicated as a pain option following an adenotonsillectomy.
5. Post-tonsillectomy bleeding can be a life-threatening complication and should be evaluated by an otolaryngologist.

Pearls
1. The classic rash associated with scarlet fever appears on the neck and face and then spreads and looks like sunburn with tiny bumps. The rash will blanch when one presses on it.
2. If mononucleosis is suspected, amoxicillin should be avoided because it may cause a salmon-colored rash.
3. A submucous cleft palate is associated with a higher incidence of postadenoidectomy velopharyngeal insufficiency.

QUESTIONS

1. **How is tonsillar hypertrophy graded?**
   Tonsil size is graded as 1 to 4 according to the percentage projection from the anterior tonsillar pillar toward the midline. A 1+ tonsil projects 0% to 25% from the anterior tonsillar pillar toward the midline, 2+ projects 25% to 50%, 3+ projects 50% to 75%, and 4+ projects 75% to 100%. Tonsils graded 4 are sometimes referred to as "kissing" tonsils because they touch in the midline.

2. **What is the function of the tonsils and adenoid?**
   The tonsils and adenoid are predominantly B-cell lymphoid structures that probably play a role in secretory immunity. They are appropriately positioned for exposure to inhaled and ingested antigens, which can induce immunoglobulin and lymphokine production. Hyperplasia is thought to result from B-cell proliferation during exposure to high doses of antigen. Tonsils and adenoids are immunologically most active between the ages of 4 and 10 years, and tend to involute after puberty. There are no studies to date that demonstrate significant alterations in the immune system following an adenotonsillectomy.

3. **What are tonsilloliths?**
   Tonsillar concretions, or tonsilloliths, are whitish, cheesy, malodorous, foul-tasting lumps that can form in the tonsillar crypts. They arise from bacterial growth and retained debris, and although they are often asymptomatic, tonsilloliths can cause problems with halitosis, foreign body sensation, and otalgia. Conservative management includes gargling and expression and removal of tonsilloliths by the patient using cotton swabs or a dental water jet device.

4. **How does bacterial tonsillitis present?**
   Sudden onset of throat pain, odynophagia, enlarged erythematous tonsils with exudate, halitosis, fever, malaise, and tender cervical nodes are classic symptoms and signs of acute tonsillitis. The classic rash associated with scarlet fever appears on the neck and face and then spreads and looks like sunburn with tiny bumps. The rash

will blanch when one presses on it. Viral pharyngitis tends to be milder in presentation and usually without exudates. There may be an associated cold, cough, conjunctivitis, diarrhea, and rash. Epstein-Barr virus (EBV) is a notable exception.

5. **Name the most common infectious etiologic agents involved in adenotonsillar disease.**
   Group A β-hemolytic streptococcus (GABHS) is the most common cause of acute tonsillitis and can be associated with such serious sequelae as rheumatic fever and poststreptococcal glomerulonephritis. Numerous other organisms, however, are commonly associated with adenotonsillar disease, including non-GABHS bacteria and beta-lactamase-producing organisms such as *Bacteroides* species, nontypeable *Haemophilus* species, *Staphylococcus aureus*, and *Moraxella catarrhalis*. Common viral pathogens include adenovirus, coxsackievirus, parainfluenza, enteroviruses, EBV, herpes simplex virus, and respiratory syncytial virus.

6. **Describe the otolaryngologic manifestations of mononucleosis.**
   Mononucleosis is caused by EBV and often produces an exudative tonsillitis that may appear indistinguishable from bacterial infections. Signs and symptoms of mononucleosis include high fever, malaise, generalized lymphadenopathy, enlarged tonsils with yellow-gray exudates, odynophagia, dysphagia, palatal petechiae, and hepatosplenomegaly. Useful lab results include lymphocytosis and the presence of atypical lymphocytes, as well as a positive Monospot and heterophil antibody titers. If mononucleosis is suspected, amoxicillin should be avoided because it may cause a salmon-colored rash.

7. **How should adenotonsillar infection be treated?**
   It can be difficult to distinguish viral from bacterial tonsillitis/pharyngitis. Most viral infections are self-limited and require only supportive care. If a bacterial infection is suspected, a rapid streptococcus detection test should be performed. If the test results are negative, a throat culture should be performed. Penicillin is the initial drug of choice for culture-positive streptococcal infections. Resistance to penicillin or first-generation cephalosporins has not been reported. Tetracyclines, sulfonamides, and quinolones should not be used for treating GABHS infections. If a child is a suspected strep carrier, the most effective treatment is clindamycin for 10 days.

8. **What is a peritonsillar abscess? How does it present?**
   A peritonsillar abscess is a collection of pus in the potential space that surrounds the tonsil, between the tonsillar capsule and the superior constrictor muscle of the lateral pharyngeal wall. This process develops when infection penetrates the tonsillar capsule and enters the peritonsillar space. Over half of patients who present with peritonsillar abscess have a history of prior tonsillitis. Symptoms include throat pain, fever, dysphagia, a "hot potato" or muffled voice, trismus, and drooling. Examination reveals infected, swollen tonsils. The peritonsillar area is inflamed and swollen, usually unilaterally, with a bulge in the soft palate superior to the tonsil and displacement of the uvula toward the contralateral side.

9. **How is a peritonsillar abscess managed?**
   Needle aspiration or incision and drainage with recovery of pus can be diagnostic and therapeutic and has been shown to be effective more than 90% of the time. This procedure can usually be performed in the office or emergency department. After drainage, an antibiotic with gram-positive and anaerobic coverage, such as amoxicillin or clindamycin, is recommended. Tonsillectomy is recommended if a patient has had more than one peritonsillar abscess. It is performed after complete resolution of the infection. In selected cases, a quinsy tonsillectomy (tonsillectomy in the presence of abscess) is indicated, such as when drainage fails to adequately treat the abscess, or sometimes in children, who often require a general anesthetic for drainage anyway.

10. **How is obstructive sleep apnea (OSA) different from obstructive sleep disordered breathing?**
    OSA is a diagnosis that requires an abnormal polysomnogram. oSDB is a clinical diagnosis with the following features: snoring with associated gasping, labored breathing, and daytime symptoms that may include hyperactivity, inattention, poor concentration, and excessive sleepiness (Box 51.1).

11. **What are the indications for requesting a polysomnogram?**
    According to the American Academy of Otolaryngology/ Head and Neck Surgery (AAO/HNS) clinical practice guideline, one should obtain a preoperative polysomnogram prior to an adenotonsillectomy in the following circumstances: obesity, Down syndrome, craniofacial abnormalities, neuromuscular disorders, sickle cell disease, mucopolysaccharidoses, <2 years of age, or if history and physical examination are discordant.

12. **What does one assess during a sleep study?**
    The information contained in a sleep study allows one to evaluate sleep quality, degree of obstruction, and gas exchange (Box 51.2).

13. **What are the criteria to diagnose pediatric OSA?**
    Most clinicians agree and recent research suggests that an obstructive apnea/hypopnea index greater than five events per hour is clinically relevant.

Box 51.1 Clinical Features of oSDB

I Nighttime symptoms:
  1 Habitual snoring
  2 Gasping, pauses, labored breathing
  3 Other symptoms that may be related to SDB include night terrors, sleep walking, and secondary enuresis
II Daytime symptoms:
  1 Feeling unrefreshed after sleep
  2 Attention deficit
  3 Hyperactivity
  4 Emotional lability
  5 Temperamental behavior
  6 Poor weight gain
  7 Daytime fatigue
  8 Other symptoms that are suggestive of disruptive breathing patterns include daytime mouth breathing or dysphagia

---

Box 51.2 Standard Components of a PSG Report

Sleep efficiency: Total sleep time divided by total recording time. This indicates how well the child slept.

Sleep architecture: Another indication of how well the child slept. An elevated amount of Stage 1 sleep suggests a disrupted sleep pattern. The amount of REM sleep is important because REM sleep is associated with muscle atonia. In the absence of REM sleep, one may underestimate the severity of obstruction.

Oxygen distribution and nadir: The oxygen distribution gives an indication of the gas exchange. The nadir is important because it helps determine if a child should be admitted for observation following a tonsillectomy.

End-tidal CO_2 distribution: Some children may not have may obstructive events but rather prolonged periods of partial obstructive hypoventilation that can only be detected by an elevated end-tidal CO_2.

Obstructive index: Total number of obstructive respiratory events (obstructive apneas, obstructive hypopneas, and mixed apneas).

Central index: Total number of central apneas and central hypopneas.

Other Elements

Video: Comments on the appearance of the child during sleep. Some children may not have an elevated obstructive index but may look pitiful, with retractions, loud snoring, and paradoxical respirations (where the chest and abdomen, instead of rising up and down together, looks like a see-saw).

Morning-after questionnaire: To ensure the parent feels that the sleep patterns were typical during the study.

---

14. **Does nasal patency matter?**

Yes. A more patent nasal passage allows one to move air more easily into the upper airway. With a more patent nasal airway, the higher volume of air entering the pharynx will distend the upper airway and make it less likely to collapse.

15. **Does an adenotonsillectomy cure OSA?**

Adenotonsillectomy is not universally curative for OSA. Studies often have differing criteria for success of resolution of OSA after surgery. A large, multicenter retrospective review of treatment outcomes for OSA after adenotonsillectomy in 2010 showed the following factors were associated with less improvement: age >7 years, obesity, presence of asthma, and more severe OSA preoperatively (apnea/hypopnea index (AHI) >10 events/hour). In the first randomized controlled trial of pediatric OSA, the success of tonsillectomy compared to watchful waiting was 79% vs. 46%.

16. **What are nonsurgical treatment options for residual OSA?**

- One study in children with mild residual OSA (AHI >1 but <5 events/hour) who were treated with antiinflammatory therapy consisting of oral montelukast and intranasal nasal steroid for 12 weeks had normalization of their AHI.
- Positive airway pressure is a nonsurgical treatment for OSA. Positive pressure is applied via a nasal mask to splint open the upper airway. Effectiveness is determined by how compliant the child is.
- For children who have malocclusion and a contracted maxilla, rapid maxillary expansion has resulted in a dramatic improvement.

17. **What diagnostic tests are available to help identify the anatomic site of obstruction of a child with OSA?**

A cine MRI or drug-induced sleep endoscopy (DISE) will facilitate identification of sites of anatomic obstruction. Currently, there is a lack of consensus on the role of DISE prior to tonsil surgery. In 2021, the AAO/HNS published a DISE consensus statement on its role. Most surgeons agree that DISE is a very good tool to use for children with moderate to severe OSA who have had a previous tonsillectomy. More surgeons are using DISE prior to tonsillectomy if the child has an increased risk of persistent OSA.

18. **Besides a tonsillectomy, what other surgical options are there to treat OSA?**
Additional surgical interventions after adenotonsillectomy include an inferior turbinate reduction, palate procedures, lingual tonsillectomy, posterior tongue base reduction, and supraglottoplasty. Upper airway stimulation has not been approved for pediatric patients; however, a research study is in progress for children with Down syndrome.

19. **What are the indications for performing an adenotonsillectomy?**
The most common indication is oSDB, followed by recurrent tonsillitis. Other less common indications include dysphagia due to large tonsils and suspected malignancy. AAO-HNS guidelines recommend surgical intervention for recurrent tonsillitis under the following circumstances: seven infections in a 12-month period, five infections per year for 2 consecutive years, or three infections per year for 3 consecutive years.

20. **What are the clinical criteria for a throat infection to be counted as an acute tonsillitis to meet the AAO/HNS criteria for an adenotonsillectomy?**
See Box 51.3.

21. **What are the modifying factors for children with recurrent tonsil infections that one should consider when making a decision to recommend surgery?**
Modifying factors include multiple antibiotic allergies/intolerance; periodic fever, aphthous stomatitis, pharyngitis, and adenitis (PFAPA); or history of more than one peritonsillar abscess.

22. **List the contraindications for tonsillectomy and adenoidectomy.**
    1. Bleeding disorders
    2. Anemia
    3. Poor anesthetic risk due to uncontrolled medical illness
    4. Acute infection

23. **How are tonsils removed?**
The tonsil is dissected along the plane between the tonsillar capsule and the superior constrictor muscle. Tonsillectomy can be performed using either a "cold" or "hot" technique, and the merits of one over the other are much debated. In "cold" dissection, a superior mucosal incision is created with a knife and then blunt dissection separates the tonsil from the tonsillar bed. The tonsil is then amputated at its inferior aspect, often using a snare. The "hot" technique employs electrocautery to cut and coagulate simultaneously. Some studies suggest that "cold" dissection may lead to less postoperative pain; however, there may be less intraoperative blood loss with electrocautery. Other devices have also been introduced for tonsillectomy, including lasers and ultrasonic and radiofrequency devices. Proponents cite advantages such as less postoperative pain; however, these advantages remain to be proven.

24. **Tonsillotomy vs. tonsillectomy: which is better?**
Partial intracapsular tonsillectomy (PIT), also known as tonsillotomy, is a procedure that has been gaining popularity, especially in Europe. As opposed to a tonsillectomy, PIT is a subtotal removal of the tonsils.

25. **Are any special precautions required in performing tonsillectomy and adenoidectomy on children with Down syndrome?**
Approximately 12% of patients with Down syndrome have atlantoaxial instability. Cervical spine manipulations should be undertaken with the greatest of care when positioning these patients for surgery because neck extension may cause spinal cord compression. One also should be aware that these children have smaller airways and so should initially be intubated with a tube that is smaller than their age-appropriate size.

Box 51.3 Clinical Criteria for an Acute Tonsil Infection

Presence of a sore throat and at least one of the following:
1 Cervical lymphadenopathy (2-centimeters or tender lymph nodes)
2 Tonsillar exudates
3 Positive group A β-hemolytic streptococcus culture
4 Fever greater than 38.3°C

Table 51.1 Complications of Tonsillectomy and Adenoidectomy	
I. Acute	Airway obstruction due to edema
	Postobstructive pulmonary edema
II. Subacute	Postoperative hemorrhage
	Dehydration and weight loss
III. Delayed	Velopharyngeal insufficiency
	Nasopharyngeal stenosis

26. **In patients with long-standing adenotonsillar obstruction, what pulmonary problem can occur after adenotonsillectomy?**
    Pulmonary edema. The long-term obstruction by adenotonsillar tissue produces a state of increased positive end-expiratory pressure (PEEP). With removal of the obstructing tissue, the excess PEEP is suddenly relieved and fluid moves into the interstitial and alveolar spaces, resulting in pulmonary edema with decreased blood oxygen saturation. This can occur intraoperatively or a few hours later. Treatment involves diuresis for mild cases or intubation with reestablishment of increased PEEP in severe cases.

27. **List possible complications of tonsillectomy and adenoidectomy.**
    See Table 51.1.

28. **What are the criteria to admit a child postoperatively after T&A for overnight monitoring?**
    - Younger than 3 years of age with a diagnosis of SDB.
    - Abnormal polysomnogram with either an obstructive apnea/hypopnea index of ≥10 events per hour or an oxygen saturation nadir <80%.
    - A child who has complications following the surgery, which may include hypoxemia, obstruction, or poor oral intake. Social factors may also play a role, especially if there is not a reliable mode of transportation to return to the hospital or the family lives far from the hospital.
    - Although the AAO/HNS clinical practice guideline advocates for preoperative polysomnogram for children with certain comorbidities, if a sleep study was not performed one should strongly consider hospital observation since one would not know the severity of the obstruction. It is also reasonable to have a low threshold to observe a child with complex heart disease.

29. **Should one administer perioperative antibiotics?**
    The AAO-HNS guidelines strongly recommend against the routine administration of antibiotics postoperatively. There is no evidence that antibiotics aid recovery and there is the risk of adverse reactions, including rash, upset stomach, allergy, and inducing bacterial resistance.

30. **What should be given for post-tonsillectomy pain?**
    Tylenol with codeine is contraindicated due to an black box warning. Both codeine and hydrocodone are metabolized to a more active compound. For hydrocodone, the analgesic activity is attributed to hydromorphone, not hydrocodone. Since the conversion to hydromorphone occurs via the CYP2D6 pathway (the same pathway codeine uses when converting to morphine) the concern for variability in response between ultrarapid and poor metabolizers exists – oversedation in ultrarapid metabolizers and minimal pain relief in poor metabolizers.
    Nonsteroidal antiinflammatory drugs (NSAID) use has been controversial but has become more acceptable since 2011. A Cochrane review demonstrated NSAID safety with the exception of ketorolac. Particularly in the immediate postoperative period, NSAIDs may theoretically induce some platelet dysfunction. It may be prudent to wait for at least a few hours prior to ibuprofen administration after an adenotonsillectomy to allow for clot maturation.

31. **What does the postoperative management of adenotonsillectomy involve?**
    Expect significant pain and fatigue for approximately 1 week, and often longer in teenagers and adults. Children should plan to take 7 to 10 days off from school, and strenuous activity should be avoided for 2 weeks. Pain control is important to promote oral intake of liquids and to prevent dehydration. Diet may be advanced as tolerated; many recommend a soft diet.
    Throat and/or ear pain (referred pain), halitosis, and low-grade fevers are normal after surgery. No further bleeding should occur. If fresh blood is seen, it should be brought to the attention of the otolaryngologist immediately. There may be some blood-tinged saliva around postoperative days 5 to 7, when the "scab" falls off the surgical site. If this does not stop within several minutes, or if it should worsen, medical attention should be sought.

32. **What is the incidence of postoperative tonsillectomy bleeding?**
    The rate of primary hemorrhage (occurring within 24 hours of surgery) ranges from 0.2% to 2.2%. The rate of secondary hemorrhage (occurring more than 24 hours after surgery) has been cited as anywhere from 0.1% to 3%.

33. **How is postoperative bleeding managed?**
    A patient presenting to the emergency department with a post-tonsillectomy bleed should be examined by an otolaryngologist. The tonsillar fossae should be carefully examined, looking for active bleeding sites or evidence of a clot. If active bleeding is encountered, it should be controlled with cautery and/or suture ligation. If no abnormality is seen and only minimal bleeding is reported, then observation is reasonable. If a clot is present without active bleeding, the patient should be admitted for overnight observation, ready for surgery in case bleeding should reoccur. Depending on the history, a hematocrit and coagulation profile may be drawn. The threshold for admission and intervention should be lower in smaller children, who have a lower blood volume to begin with.

34. **What problems are caused by the adenoid?**
    The adenoid can become acutely and chronically infected. Symptoms may be difficult to differentiate from bacterial or viral upper respiratory infections and are often mislabeled as "sinusitis." Adenoiditis commonly presents as fever, purulent rhinorrhea, nasal obstruction, and otalgia. Postnasal drip, congestion, chronic cough, and halitosis can occur during chronic infections.

    Adenoid hypertrophy can cause nasal obstruction, contribute to obstructive sleep apnea, and result in hyponasal speech. Chronic hypertrophy and mouth breathing can also cause alterations in craniofacial growth. "Adenoid facies" is characterized by an open mouth, facial elongation, a high arched palate, an open anterior bite with protrusion of the upper incisors, and flattened midface. It is also believed that adenoid play a role in patients with recurrent otitis media or effusions by mechanically obstructing the eustachian tubes and by providing a bacterial nidus for infection.

35. **How is the adenoid evaluated?**
    In patients with suspected adenoid hypertrophy, breathing and speech should be assessed. Words that emphasize nasal emission such as "mommy" can be useful in demonstrating hyponasality. The nose should be examined for other causes of obstruction such as enlarged turbinates. The adenoid cannot be seen by looking in the mouth or the anterior nose, but it is generally assumed that children with significant obstructive symptoms who require tonsillectomy will also have enlarged adenoids. The adenoid is visualized at the time of surgery and removed accordingly. Lateral neck radiography and fiber-optic endoscopy can be used to assess the adenoid if there is diagnostic uncertainty.

36. **What nonsurgical therapies are available for adenoiditis or adenoid hypertrophy?**
    1. Antibiotics are used to treat infectious adenoiditis.
    2. Nasal steroid sprays can improve adenoidal hypertrophy.

37. **List the indications for adenoidectomy.**
    1. Recurrent acute or chronic adenoiditis
    2. Nasal obstruction with chronic mouth breathing
    3. Hyponasal speech
    4. Craniofacial growth abnormalities
    5. Obstructive sleep apnea
    6. Recurrent otitis media or persistent effusion in patients who have undergone prior tympanostomy tube placement (adenoidectomy usually performed in conjunction with a subsequent tube placement procedure)

38. **How is the adenoid removed?**
    Adenoidectomy is performed transorally, and the nasopharynx is visualized using a laryngeal mirror. Tissue can be removed by the following methods:
    1. Curetting is the traditional method for adenoidectomy. The curette is positioned high in the nasopharynx against the septal vomer and then swept inferiorly, thereby cutting out the adenoid tissue. Hemostasis is achieved by packing followed by suction cautery.
    2. Suction cautery can be used to fulgurate the adenoid tissue. This method is associated with less intraoperative blood loss and is ideal for smaller adenoids, although it can also be used routinely.
    3. The microdebrider can be used to shave away adenoid tissue. Care must be taken to avoid injury to surrounding structures when using powered instrumentation.

39. **Why can velopharyngeal insufficiency (VPI) occur after adenoidectomy?**
    VPI occurs when there is incomplete closure of the soft palate against the posterior pharyngeal wall during speech and swallowing. VPI results in hypernasal speech and nasopharyngeal regurgitation. In children, adenoid tissue significantly adds to the bulk of the posterior pharyngeal wall. An adenoidectomy reduces this bulk and can lead to incomplete closure. Most cases are temporary, but persistent or severe cases may require speech therapy and/ or surgical treatment.

    The incidence of VPI after adenoidectomy ranges from 1/1500 to 1/10,000 in healthy patients. The incidence is much higher in patients with palatal disorders.

40. **Why should one always inspect and palpate the palate prior to adenoidectomy?**
A submucous cleft palate is associated with a higher incidence of postadenoidectomy VPI. Signs of a submucous cleft include a bifid uvula, zona pellucida, and notching of the posterior hard palate. In the presence of these findings, a superior pole adenoidectomy is recommended. This procedure removes obstructing tissue from the choanal area but preserves bulk in the posterior pharyngeal wall.

BIBLIOGRAPHY

Baugh RF, Archer SM, Mitchell RB, et al: American Academy of Otolaryngology–Head and Neck Surgery Foundation: clinical practice guideline: tonsillectomy in children, *Otolaryngol Head Neck Surg* 144(Suppl 1):S1–S30, 2011.

Bhattacharjee R, Kheirandish-Gozal L, Spruyt K, et al: Adenotonsillectomy outcomes in treatment of obstructive sleep apnea in children: a multicenter retrospective study, *Am J Respir Crit Care Med* 182(5):676–683, 2010.

Casselbrant ML: What is wrong in chronic adenoiditis/tonsillitis anatomical considerations, *Int J Pediatr Otorhinolaryngol* 49:S133–S135, 1999.

Francis DO, Chinnadurai S, Sathe N, et al: *Tonsillectomy for Obstructive Sleep-Disordered Breathing or Recurrent Throat Infection in Children.* Rockville, MD: Agency for Healthcare Research and Quality; 2017. AHRQ comparative effectiveness review 16(17)-EHC042-EF.

Goldsmith AJ, Rosenfeld RM: Tonsillectomy, adenoidectomy, and UPPP. In: *Surgical Atlas of Pediatric Otolaryngology*, 2002, BC Decker, pp 380–405.

Jones KL: Chromosomal abnormality syndromes: Down syndrome. In: *Smith's Recognizable Patterns of Human Malformation*, 5th ed, 1997, Saunders, pp 8–10.

Kheirandish L, Goldbart AD, Gozal D: Intranasal steroids and oral leukotriene modifier therapy in residual sleep-disordered breathing after tonsillectomy and adenoidectomy in children, *Pediatrics* 117(1):e61–e66, 2006.

Koltai PJ, Solares CA, Koempel JA, et al: Intracapsular tonsillar reduction (partial tonsillectomy): reviving a historical procedure for obstructive sleep disordered breathing in children, *Otolaryngol Head Neck Surg* 129:532–538, 2003.

Marcus CL, Brooks LJ, Draper KA, et al: American Academy of Pediatrics: diagnosis and management of childhood obstructive sleep apnea syndrome, *Pediatrics* 130(3):e714–e755, 2012.

Marcus CL, Brooks LJ, Draper KA, et al: American Academy of Pediatrics: diagnosis and management of childhood obstructive sleep apnea syndrome, *Pediatrics* 130(3):576–584, 2012.

Marcus CL, Moore RH, Rosen CL, et al: Childhood Adenotonsillectomy Trial (CHAT). A randomized trial of adenotonsillectomy for childhood sleep apnea, *N Engl J Med* 368(25):2366–2376, 2013.

Mitchell RB, Archer SM, Ishman SL, et al: Clinical practice guideline: tonsillectomy in children (update)—executive summary, *Otolaryngol Head Neck Surg* 160(2):187–205, 2019.

Mitchell RB, Archer SM, Ishman SL, et al: Clinical practice guideline: tonsillectomy in children (update)—executive summary, *Otolaryngol Head Neck Surg* 160(Suppl 1):S1–S42, 2019.

Odhagen E, Stalfors J, Sunnergren O: Morbidity after pediatric tonsillotomy versus tonsillectomy: a population-based cohort study, *Laryngoscope* 129(11):2619–2626, 2019.

Odhagen E, Sunnergren O, Hemlin C, et al: Risk of reoperation after tonsillotomy versus tonsillectomy: a population-based cohort study, *Eur Arch Otorhinolaryngol* 273(10):3263–3268, 2016.

Parikh SR, Archer S, Ishman SL, Mitchell RB: Why is there no statement regarding partial intracapsular tonsillectomy (tonsillotomy) in the new guidelines? *Otolaryngol Head Neck Surg* 160(2):213–214, 2019.

Tan HL, Gozal D, Kheirandish-Gozal L: Obstructive sleep apnea in children: a critical update, *Nat Sci Sleep* 5:109–123, 2013.

Wiatrak BJ, Woolley AL: Pharyngitis and adenotonsillar disease. In: Cummings CW, Fredrickson JM, Harker LA, et al, eds: *Otolaryngology Head & Neck Surgery, Vol 5*, 3rd ed, 1998, Mosby, pp 188–215.

CHAPTER 52

CONGENITAL MALFORMATIONS OF THE HEAD AND NECK

Owen A. Darr, MD and Christian R. Francom, MD

KEY POINTS

1. A Sistrunk procedure involves removal of a thyroglossal duct cyst along with the central portion of the hyoid bone, resulting in decreased recurrence rates of the congenital cyst.
2. Tracheoesophageal anomalies are usually evident at birth because of significant feeding issues and require urgent intervention.
3. Newborns are obligate nasal breathers for at least the first month of life, and the presence of bilateral choanal atresia is a life-threatening airway.
4. Hemangiomas are typically absent at birth, proliferate over the first year of life, and eventually involute.
5. Lymphatic malformations are not true tumors but grow proportionally with the patient and can rapidly expand with bleeding, infection, or trauma.

Pearls

1. Branchial cleft anomalies track deep to the structures of their own arch and superficial to the structures of the subsequent arch.
2. Always evaluate for a normal thyroid gland prior to removing a thyroglossal duct cyst.
3. The pseudotumor of infancy (SCM tumor) responds to conservative treatment by 1 year of age in 80% of cases.
4. A stridulous child with a concomitant hemangioma, particularly in the "beard distribution" of the face, should raise suspicion for a subglottic hemangioma.

QUESTIONS

1. **What is the differential diagnosis for a congenital or pediatric neck mass?**

    The differential diagnosis for a pediatric mass of the head and neck can be organized based on anatomic distribution or possible etiology. The mnemonic "KITTENS" (K: congenital anomalies; I: infectious/inflammatory; T: trauma; T: toxic; E: endocrine; N: neoplasms; S: systemic disease) is useful for guiding a comprehensive list. The lesion varies according to anatomic distribution, age at presentation, and growth history.

    Congenital lesions represent the most common neck mass in children and are most often cystic. Midline lesions may be dermoid cysts or thyroglossal duct cysts, while branchial cleft anomalies are observed in the lateral neck. Acquired masses, such as lymphadenitis or atypical mycobacterial infections, are most often infectious or inflammatory. Neoplasms are relatively rare in the pediatric population but must always be considered in the differential; Hodgkin and non-Hodgkin lymphomas, neuroblastoma or rhabdomyosarcoma may initially present as a neck. See Table 52.1 for a detailed list.

    All pediatric neck masses require a detailed history and physical examination. Laboratory analysis may be helpful in establishing a diagnosis or ruling out more aggressive lymphoproliferative processes. Ultrasound imaging is useful in differentiating solid or cystic lesions, while cross-sectional imaging by CT or MRI provides more details regarding anatomic considerations. While some masses may be diagnosed through noninvasive measures, many will require surgical biopsy for a definitive diagnosis.

2. **How does a thyroglossal duct cyst develop?**

    During development, the thyroid diverticulum forms at the midline base of the tongue (foramen cecum). The developing thyroid descends through the neck, anterior to or through the hyoid bone, and comes to rest in its final position in the lower neck, inferior to the cricoid cartilage. The tract that the thyroid follows from the base of the tongue to the anterior neck (thyroglossal duct) normally obliterates; however, if this process is incomplete, a thyroglossal duct cyst may persist anywhere from the foramen cecum to the pyramidal lobe of the thyroid gland. The most common location is anterior or superior to the hyoid in the midline or slightly paramedian. Thyroglossal duct cysts are the most common congenital neck masses found in pediatric patients and may account for up to one-third of pediatric neck masses.

Table 52.1 Differential Diagnosis of Congenital Neck Mass

LOCATION	DIAGNOSIS	FEATURES
MIDLINE		
	Thyroglossal duct cyst	Overlies hyoid or thyroid notch, elevates with swallowing or tongue protrusion
	Dermoid cyst	Moves with skin, typically submental
	Teratoma	Firm, CT showing calcification, rare in neck
	Plunging ranula	Midline or slightly lateral, cystic, extends to floor of mouth
LATERAL		
	Branchial cleft cyst	Along anterior border of SCM, fluctuant, periodic infections
	Lymphatic malformation	Soft, compressible, often extends posterior to SCM, transilluminate
	Pseudotumor of SCM	Firm, painless, discrete, fusiform mass in newborn
EXTENSIVE		
	Lymphatic malformation	Thin-walled, macrocystic vs. microcystic, variable anatomic involvement
	Vascular malformations	Red/bluish mass, pulsatile (AVM), strawberry (hemangioma), size may increase with crying

Adapted from Wetmore R, Potsic W: Differential diagnosis of neck masses. In: Cummings CW, Frederickson JM, Harker LA, et al, eds: *Otolaryngology Head and Neck Surgery*, 3rd ed, St. Louis, 1998, Mosby, pp 248–261.

3. **What needs to be seen on imaging before removing a thyroglossal duct cyst?**
It is important to identify the presence of a normal thyroid gland prior to the excision of a thyroglossal duct cyst. In rare instances the thyroid gland can arrest its descent during development, and what is perceived as a thyroglossal duct cyst may actually be the patient's only functional thyroid tissue. Surgery to excise this lesion could then leave the patient hypothyroid and require lifelong supplementation.

4. **What are the complications of an untreated thyroglossal duct cyst?**
An untreated thyroglossal duct cyst may become infected and require antibiotics, aspiration, or incision and drainage. Large cysts can result in dysphagia, dysphonia, and airway obstruction in severe cases. While uncommon (<1% of cases), thyroglossal duct cysts can harbor malignant thyroid cells, most commonly a well-differentiated thyroid cancer such as papillary thyroid carcinoma.

5. **How is a thyroglossal duct cyst managed surgically?**
The standard of care for thyroglossal duct cyst removal is a Sistrunk procedure in which the entire thyroglossal duct cyst, duct, central hyoid bone, and a cuff of the suprahyoid musculature from the base of the tongue are removed. Recurrence rates following this procedure are less than 5%.

6. **What is the differential diagnosis for a midline congenital neck mass?**
Thyroglossal duct cyst, dermoid, teratoma, plunging ranula, lymph node, thymic cyst, foregut duplication cyst, and laryngocele.

7. **What is the difference between a teratoma and a dermoid?**
Teratomas and dermoids may be differentiated histologically: a teratoma is made from all three germ cell layers (endoderm, ectoderm, and mesoderm) and dermoid cysts are only made from two germ cell layers (ectoderm and mesoderm). Teratomas are often larger and more symptomatic than dermoids and are frequently found on prenatal ultrasound. Dermoids are much more common than teratomas. Surgical excision is the preferred treatment for both, and incomplete excision may result in recurrence.

8. **How do branchial anomalies develop?**
An understanding of embryology is necessary for the treatment of branchial anomalies. By the fourth week of gestation, an embryo constructs a set of branchial precursors that will eventually develop into the structures of the face, neck, pharynx, and mediastinum. There are six branchial or pharyngeal arches; however, the fifth involutes, so they are numbered one through four and six. The arches are separated externally by clefts (or "grooves") and internally by pouches. Each branchial arch is lined externally by ectoderm and internally by endoderm with a core of mesenchyme constructed of mesoderm, somites, and neural crest cells. In normal development the clefts and

pouches are replaced by mesenchymal tissue and develop into their designated structures. Branchial anomalies develop if portions of the clefts or pouches persist.

9. **How are branchial anomalies classified?**
Branchial anomalies are classified by the arch/pouch/cleft of origin and are based on the presence or absence of an internal or external opening. Branchial cysts have no internal or external openings, sinuses have either an internal or external opening, while fistulae have both internal and external openings.

10. **Which structures are associated with each branchial arch?**
Each branchial or pharyngeal arch has an associated artery and cranial nerve, muscles innervated by the nerve, and cartilaginous/skeletal structures. See Table 52.2.

11. **What is the relationship between a branchial anomaly and its associated structures?**
Branchial anomalies run deep to their own structures and are superficial to the structures of the next branchial arch. This is important surgically.

12. **A newborn presents with a lump along the sternocleidomastoid muscle and torticollis away from the lesion. What is the diagnosis?**
Fibromatosis coli, or pseudotumor of the sternocleidomastoid (SCM) muscle, presents as a firm, round mass of the lateral neck in a newborn's first month of life. This process is associated with torticollis due to shortening of the affected SCM; the infant will have a head preference away from the mass. As the name suggests, pseudotumor of infancy is not a neoplastic process but rather the result of muscular inflammatory changes and fibrosis from birth trauma, ischemia of muscle, or intrauterine positioning. It is characterized histologically by dense fibrous tissue and the absence of striated muscle. Treatment includes physical therapy for the associated torticollis to lengthen the affected muscle. More than 80% of cases resolve by 1 year of age.

13. **What is in the differential for a nasofrontal/midline congenital nasal mass?**
Nasal dermoids are by far the most common congenital nasofrontal masses. They present as noncompressible lesions anywhere from the glabella to the columella and often have an associated pit with a hair tuft. Left untreated, they can lead to complications including local soft tissue infection, deeper meningitis or brain abscesses, and soft tissue/skeletal deformities. Surgical excision is the only treatment option. They may maintain an intracranial connection that must be investigated with imaging prior to surgery; thus skull base reconstruction can be planned if necessary.

Gliomas are sequestered glial tissues but do not have herniated dural tissue or cerebrospinal spinal fluid (CSF). They present as a red or bluish lump, are firm and noncompressible, and may maintain a fibrous stalk that connects to the central nervous system. Imaging is required prior to surgical resection.

Encephaloceles are herniations of brain tissue and meninges through a skull base defect. They are soft and compressible, may be pulsatile, and transilluminate with light due to the presence of CSF. They may enlarge with crying, Valsalva, or compression of the internal jugular vein (Furstenberg sign). There is a definite intracranial connection, and imaging is required for the evaluation. While MRI is the preferred imaging modality for all nasofrontal masses, CT may add complementary information, such as demonstration of a bifid crista galli at the anterior skull base.

14. **What is choanal atresia?**
The absence of communication between the nasal passage and nasopharynx is known as choanal atresia. This is most likely due to a failure of the nasobuccal membrane to canalize between the fifth and sixth weeks of fetal development but may also involve abnormal neural crest cell migration, as in Treacher-Collins syndrome. Choanal atresia is most often unilateral, most commonly on the right side. Up to one-half of unilateral cases and 75% of bilateral cases are associated with other congenital anomalies such as Treacher-Collins or CHARGE syndrome.

The diagnosis of choanal atresia can be clinically suggested by the inability to pass a 6F catheter from the nose to the pharynx. Nasal endoscopy will confirm the diagnosis of atresia or stenosis, and a CT scan is necessary to elucidate whether the atretic plate involves only soft tissue (membranous) or bone.

Bilateral choanal atresia is typically apparent in newborns due to respiratory distress or cyanosis with oral feeding, as newborns are obligate nasal breathers for the first 1 to 2 months of life. Surgical intervention is indicated within the first month of life upon discovery. Unilateral atresia may go undiagnosed for several years and present later in childhood due to unilateral rhinorrhea and nasal obstruction. Repair of the unilateral cases can be deferred until after 3 years of age unless there are significant obstructive symptoms affecting daytime activity or sleep.

15. **What are the most common congenital subglottic lesions?**
Congenital subglottic stenosis (SGS) is defined as a subglottis with a diameter of <3.5 millimeters and can only be diagnosed as congenital prior to any airway instrumentation, including intubation. Congenital SGS may be the result of an underlying elliptical cricoid, where the transverse diameter of the cricoid measures less than the anterior-posterior diameter. Patients with congenital SGS may present in the first few years of life with symptoms of airway obstruction, including recurrent or persistent episodes of croup. They may have inspiratory or biphasic stridor. Management depends on severity and may include observation, medical management, or surgery.

Table 52.2 Structures Associated with Branchial Arch

PHARYNGEAL ARCH	ARTERY	CRANIAL NERVE	SKELETAL ELEMENTS	MUSCLES
1	Maxillary	Trigeminal (V)	Head and neck of malleus, incus body, maxilla, mandible, Meckel's cartilage, upper portion of auricle, zygoma, squamous portion of temporal bone, sphenomandibular ligament, anterior malleolar ligament	Muscles of mastication (temporalis, masseter, and pterygoids), mylohyoid, anterior belly of digastric, tensor tympani, tensor veli palatini
2	Stapedial artery (embryologic) and caroticotympanic artery (adult)	Facial nerve (VII)	Manubrium of malleus, long process of incus, stapes suprastructure (the footplate comes from the otic capsule), lesser cornu and upper body of hyoid, styloid process, Reichert's cartilage Stylohyoid ligament, lower portion of auricle	Muscles of facial expression (orbicularis oculi, orbicularis oris, fronto-occipitalis, buccinator), posterior auricular, stapedius, posterior belly of digastric, stylohyoid
3	Common and internal carotid artery	Glossopharyngeal (IX)	Greater cornu and lower body of hyoid	Stylopharyngeus
4	Left: arch of aorta Right: subclavian artery	Superior laryngeal branch of vagus (X)	Laryngeal cartilages (derived from the fourth arch cartilage, originate from lateral plate mesoderm)	Constrictors of pharynx, cricothyroid, levator veli palatini
5	Does not develop	Does not develop	Does not develop	Does not develop
6	Ductus arteriosus on the left; pulmonary artery on right	Recurrent laryngeal branch of vagus (X)	Laryngeal cartilages (derived from the sixth arch cartilage; originates from lateral plate mesoderm)	Intrinsic muscles of larynx

Tracheostomy, endoscopic intervention, and open airway reconstruction are all surgical options, depending on the severity and other patient factors.

Patients with subglottic hemangiomas may present with a clinical picture similar to that of patients with congenital SGS. These patients generally develop respiratory symptoms between one and four months of life. Diagnosis is made using endoscopic evaluation and sometimes radiographic studies. Patients with a cutaneous hemangioma in the "beard distribution" will have a subglottic hemangioma approximately 50% of the time. Subglottic hemangiomas follow the typical growth patterns of other infantile hemangiomas, including rapid growth in the first 6 months of life, a plateau phase until around 1 year of age, and an involution phase during which most regression will take place by 4 to 7 years of age. In cases where the lesion is more severe, medical and surgical options are available. If caught early, beta blocker therapy is often effective in halting progression and prompting early involution. Systemic or intralesional steroids, laser therapy, open laryngeal surgical resection, and tracheostomy are also options.

16. What is a laryngotracheal cleft?

A posterior laryngeal or laryngotracheal cleft is a congenital anomaly caused by insufficient fusion of the posterior tracheoesophageal septum. This abnormality is relatively rare and presents with varying degrees of severity. Most commonly, children present with recurrent aspiration (liquids > solids), coughing, choking, hoarseness, and possibly a history of recurrent pneumonia.

They are classified into four types based on the length of the cleft:

Type 1: interarytenoid cleft with absence of the interarytenoid muscle (above the level of the true vocal folds).

Type 2: extends below the level of the true vocal folds into the upper cricoid.

Type 3: involves the entire cricoid with or without extension into the cervical trachea.

Type 4: cleft extends into the thoracic trachea.

Management of type 1 and 2 laryngeal clefts is often endoscopic, with laser treatment of the intercleft groove and endoscopic suture repair of the posterior defect. Some type 1 laryngeal clefts may also be treated more conservatively with injection of voice gel or filler, such as carboxymethylcellulose, into the interarytenoid groove. Type 3 and 4 laryngotracheal clefts require open surgical repair.

17. Name five types of tracheoesophageal anomalies and discuss their presentation and diagnosis.

- Esophageal atresia with distal tracheoesophageal fistula (≈85%)
- Isolated esophageal atresia without fistula (≈8%)
- Tracheoesophageal fistula without atresia, "H-type" (≈5%)
- Esophageal atresia with proximal tracheoesophageal fistula (≈1%)
- Esophageal atresia with proximal and distal tracheoesophageal fistula (≈0.5%–1%)

Many of these anomalies are detected on prenatal ultrasound and may be evaluated after delivery. When esophageal atresia is present, a neonate will present with copious oral secretions due to the inability to swallow saliva. There will likely be episodes of coughing and respiratory distress with feeds in the first few days of life. Symptoms depend on the severity of atresia and anatomy of the tracheal fistula. A nasogastric tube cannot be passed when atresia is present. However, the H-type fistula often presents later, due to maintained patency of the esophagus, as chronic feeding difficulties and recurrent respiratory distress or pneumonia become apparent. Diagnosis can be made using barium esophagram and/or endoscopy.

18. Discuss the two basic categories of tracheal anomalies and common etiologies.

Intrinsic tracheal anomalies are caused by improper tracheal development. Such malformations include tracheomalacia, tracheal stenosis (often with complete tracheal rings), or tracheal agenesis (not compatible with life).

The trachea may also have partial or complete obstruction caused by *extrinsic* compression by surrounding structures. Examples include vascular compression (e.g., innominate artery, double aortic arch, right aortic arch with persistent ductus or ligamentum arteriosum, pulmonary artery sling), masses in the neck (thyromegaly, congenital cysts, lymphatic malformations), or mediastinum (teratoma, lymphoma, thymic mass).

19. Which other types of cysts can involve the upper airway?

There are several other types of congenital or pediatric cysts that may be found in the upper airway, including the larynx, pharynx, and oral cavity. A **vallecular cyst** is a mucosalized cyst that may be discovered in the vallecula, the area between the epiglottis and the base of the tongue. Vallecular cysts are often congenital but may grow over time before a child presents with difficult breathing, noisy breathing, feeding difficulties, or cyanosis with feeding.

Subglottic cysts are a cause of infant or pediatric stridor. A subglottic cyst may present as progressive stridor in a child with a history of intubation or prior airway instrumentation. This may appear as an asymmetric fullness of the subglottis on flexible laryngoscopy. Recurrence risks are high after excision by marsupialization; therefore serial laryngoscopic procedures may be required.

Foregut duplication cysts are congenital mucosalized cysts that parallel the normal aerodigestive tract. They may involve the deep tongue or pharyngeal structures. Laryngeal cysts, such as saccular cysts or laryngoceles, are uncommon in children.

20. What are the most common anomalies of the external auricle?

Lop ear refers to overfolding of the superior helical fold and is the most frequent congenital auricular deformity. Stahl's ear is the result of an abnormal fold in the scapha, which flattens the superior helix. Protruding ear or prominauris is the third most common; the subunits of the pinna are generally well formed; however, the postauricular angle (between the mastoid and auricle) is greater than the ideal of 25 to 30 degrees. In general, correction of these and other auricular deformities can be achieved by taping the ears into the correct anatomic position and molding the appropriate helical folds with dental wax and surgical tape. This is very effective if performed in the first 14 days of life, which correlates with continued levels of maternal estrogens in the newborn and increased hyaluronic acid in the auricular cartilage, making it more pliable. Tape is applied over a molding of wax or soft tubing and maintained for at least 2 weeks. Commercial molds are also available. After the first month of life, molding is generally less successful and requires a much longer taping period. If this window of opportunity is missed or taping is unsuccessful, then surgical otoplasty can be performed after the age of 7 or 8 years at the earliest.

21. **What is microtia and how are the different deformities described?**
    Microtia is a form of hypoplasia of the external ear. It may or may not be associated with atresia of the external auditory canal (EAC). There is a 2:1 preponderance of males to females, as well as right side to left. It may present as an isolated deformity in an otherwise healthy child but can be associated with other anomalies (e.g., Treacher-Collins syndrome, Goldenhar, branchio-oto-renal syndrome).
    Type I microtia refers to mild auricular hypoplasia. The external ear is smaller but has all identifiable subunits; however, they may appear constricted or hypoplastic. Type II deformities are those in which some structures of the normal auricle are recognizable; however, some subunits are deficient; reconstruction may require additional skin or cartilage grafting. Type III are severe deformities without identifiable landmarks; there may be a bud of conchal cartilage or merely a lobule ("peanut ear"). Reconstruction is complex, requiring cartilage and skin grafting to build and elevate the entire cartilage framework. Type IV is complete absence of the external ear ("anotia"), and reconstruction would require similar considerations. Initial workup should always include audiologic evaluation, and a bone-anchored hearing device should be considered before 1 year of age in cases of unilateral or bilateral conductive hearing loss. Many otolaryngologists also recommend renal ultrasound to screen for associated kidney anomalies.

22. **What ear anomalies arise from defects in the first branchial cleft?**
    The first branchial cleft (or "groove") gives rise to the EAC. It is paired with the first branchial pouch, which forms the eustachian tube and tympanic recess. Anomalies are divided into aplasia, atresia, stenosis, and duplication of the EAC. Aplasia occurs when the first branchial cleft does not develop. Atresia anomalies occur when the EAC is present but the lumen fails to develop, leaving a core of bone, fibrous tissue, or both. Stenosis occurs when the lumen is formed but narrowed and occurs in varying degrees of severity. Duplication occurs when the EAC develops normally but an additional tract persists between the canal and skin of the neck.

23. **What are the two general classes of vascular anomalies?**
    Vascular anomalies can be divided into vascular tumors and vascular malformations. Hemangiomas are the most common type of vascular tumors and the most common neonatal neoplasm in general. Rarely present at birth, hemangiomas are typically noted in the first 2 months of life and subsequently proliferate until 6 to 9 months. Involution is expected over the first several years of life (50% by 5 years of age, 70% by 7 years of age). Less common are congenital hemangiomas, which are present at birth and classified as rapidly involuting or noninvoluting congenital hemangiomas (RICH or NICH). Diagnosis is typically made clinically; however, biopsy may be indicated if there is uncertainty; immunohistochemical staining for glucose transporter 1 (GLUT1) is diagnostic. Hemangiomas may be treated with a beta blocker (oral propranolol) during the proliferation phase if large, symptomatic, or affecting function (airway, orbit). With the advent of medical therapies, surgical management has become less common.
    Vascular malformations (VMs) result from abnormal morphogenesis of vascular or lymphatic channels, without cellular hyperplasia or neoplastic changes. These lesions are present at birth; however, they may not be clinically visible or apparent. Unlike hemangiomas, there is no classic pattern of proliferation or involution; however, VMs may grow larger with changes in flow or volume of cystic spaces, as with infection, trauma, or hormonal changes. Low-flow lesions include capillary malformations, venous malformations, lymphatic malformations, and combined types. High-flow lesions may be arterial or arteriovenous malformations. Please see Chapter 56 for a more comprehensive discussion.

BIBLIOGRAPHY

Acierno S, Waldhausen J: Congenital cervical cysts, sinuses and fistulae, *Otolaryngol Clin North Am* 40:161–176, 2007.
Ahmad S, Soliman A: Congenital anomalies of the larynx, *Otolaryngol Clin North Am* 40:177–191, 2007.
Chandra R, Gerber M, Holinger L: Histologic insight into the pathogenesis of severe laryngomalacia, *Int J Pediatr Otorhinolaryngol* 61:31–38, 2001.
Lesperance MM, Flint PW: *Cummings Pediatric Otolaryngology*, 2015.
Matsuo K, Hayashi R, Kiyono M, et al: Nonsurgical correction of congenital auricular deformities, *Clin Plast Surg* 17:383–395, 1990.
Muriaki C, Quatela V: Reconstruction surgery of the ear. In: Cummings CW, Frederickson JM, Harker LA, et al, eds: *Otolaryngology Head and Neck Surgery*, 3rd ed, St. Louis, 1998, Mosby, pp 439–460.
Radowski D, Arnold J, Healy GB, et al: Thyroglossal duct remnants: preoperative evaluation and management, *Arch Otolaryngol Head Neck Surg* 117:1378, 1991.
Sandu K, Monnier P: Congenital tracheal anomalies, *Otolaryngol Clin North Am* 40:193–217, 2007.
Toynton SC: Aryepiglottoplasty for laryngomalacia: 100 consecutive cases, *J Laryngol Otol* 115:35–38, 2001.

CHAPTER 53

CLEFT AND CRANIOFACIAL DISORDERS

Gregory C. Allen, MD, FACS, FAAP

KEY POINTS

1. The etiology of cleft lip and palate is multifactorial, including both syndromic and nonsyndromic causes.
2. Embryologically, clefts of the lip and primary palate are due to failure of fusion between the medial nasal prominence and the maxillary prominence, the lateral nasal prominence, or both.
3. Fisher anatomic subunit and Millard rotation-advancement are the most common technique for repair of the unilateral cleft lip.
4. Velopharyngeal insufficiency (VPI) is hypernasality during speech or reflux of saliva or food into the nasopharynx during swallowing. VPI occurs when the nasopharynx and oropharynx are not successfully separated by complete palatal closure during particular speech sounds or during swallowing.

Pearls

1. A higher frequency of cleft lip and palate occurs in Native Americans, those of Asian descent, and those of Latin American descent (1:400). The lowest frequency is reported in African Americans (1:1500 to 2000). Cleft palate alone is fairly consistent among ethnic groups at 1:2000. There is a male predominance in cleft lip and palate and a female predominance in cleft palate alone.
2. Cleft lip and palate most commonly occur together (50%). Cleft palate alone occurs in 35% and cleft lip alone in 15%. Left unilateral cleft lip and palate is the most common.
3. There is a high association between cleft and other congenital anomalies.

QUESTIONS

1. **Who cares for children with cleft lip and palate?**
   It is generally agreed that a multidisciplinary team best treats children with cleft lip and palate. This team is usually composed of a diverse group of clinicians including otolaryngologists, plastic surgeons, pediatric dentists, orthodontists, occupational therapists, pediatricians, speech therapists, audiologists, social workers, geneticists, psychologists, and feeding specialists/nutritionists. Each team member provides expertise in an area needed in the treatment of children who are born with a cleft.

2. **Are there guidelines regarding the care of children with cleft lip and/or palate?**
   A report about children with special needs issued in 1987 by the Surgeon General of the United States stressed that the care of children with clefts should be comprehensive, coordinated, culturally sensitive, specific to the needs of the individual, and readily accessible. The Maternal and Child Health Bureau recognized that children with clefts and/or other craniofacial anomalies have special needs and in 1991 provided funding to the American Cleft Palate–Craniofacial Association (ACPA) to develop standards for their health care. As part of these parameters of care, it has been recommended that treatment of cleft and craniofacial conditions occur in a team setting. In 1993, the ACPA released *Parameters for Evaluation and Treatment of Patients With Cleft Lip/Palate or Other Craniofacial Anomalies.* These parameters have been revised several times, most recently in 2018, and serve as a basis for cleft teams to achieve and maintain accreditation.

3. **Summarize the guidelines for the cleft palate team.**
   - The team should consist of an operating surgeon, orthodontist, speech-language pathologist, and at least one additional specialist from otolaryngology, audiology, pediatrics, genetics, social work, psychology, and general pediatric or prosthetic dentistry, who meet face-to-face at least six times per year to evaluate and develop treatment plans for the team's patients.
   - The team should evaluate at least 50 patients per year.
   - The team should have at least one surgeon who operates on at least 10 primary cleft lips and/or palates per year.
   - The team should coordinate treatment and ensure that a primary care physician evaluates each patient.
   - The team should ensure that its members attend periodic, continuing education programs about cleft lip and palate.
   - Fig. 53.1 demonstrates example times/ages when specific concerns are most often addressed.

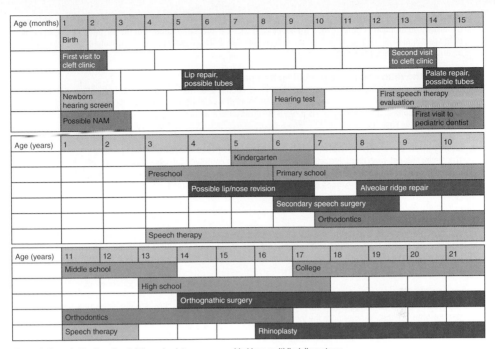

Fig. 53.1 Example timelines for cleft lip and palate care as provided by a multidisciplinary team.

4. **Describe the difference in frequency of clefting in regard to race and sex.**
   The overall reported frequency of children being born with a cleft lip and/or palate is approximately 1:700. A higher frequency of cleft lip and palate occurs in Native Americans, those of Asian descent, and those of Latin American descent (1:400). The lowest frequency is reported in African Americans (1:1500 to 2000). Cleft palate alone is fairly consistent among ethnic groups at 1:2000. There is a male predominance in cleft lip and palate and a female predominance in cleft palate alone.

5. **What are some of the causes of cleft lip/palate?**
   Clefts can be generally classified as syndromic or nonsyndromic. Single gene transmissions, chromosomal aberrations, teratogenic effects, or environmental exposures can cause syndromic clefting. Over 400 syndromes are associated with cleft lip/palate. Nonsyndromic clefts have a non-Mendelian inheritance pattern. There is not a clear understanding of the factors involved in the occurrence of cleft lip/palate. Concordance rates in monozygotic and dizygotic twins are 40% to 60% and 5%, respectively. These findings indicate a major genetic component, but environmental factors are also implicated. Recurrence rates for cleft lip/palate and isolated cleft palate range from 1% to 16% in cases of families with children born with nonsyndromic cleft lip and/or palate.

6. **Name some of the more common syndromes in which cleft lip/palate is a characteristic.**
   - Apert's syndrome
   - Stickler's syndrome
   - Treacher-Collins syndrome
   - 22q11 deletion syndrome (previously named velocardiofacial syndrome, Shprintzen syndrome, or DiGeorge complex syndrome)
   - Van der Woude syndrome
   - Goldenhar syndrome or hemifacial microsomia

7. **What is Pierre Robin or Robin (pr. Rō-băń) sequence?**
   Pierre Robin sequence was first described in the early 1800's but bears the name of Robin, a French stomatologist who wrote extensively on and drew attention to the constellation of findings beginning in 1923. It is usually described as micrognathia (small mandible), relative glossoptosis (tongue of normal size but relatively large compared to the small mandible), and airway obstruction. The constellation of findings is thought to occur from a single embryologic event that occurs between 6.5 and 10 weeks of embryologic development, resulting in a small

mandible. The relative macroglossia causes the tongue to sit high and posterior in the oropharynx, leading to upper airway obstruction at birth. A wide U-shaped cleft palate is present in most, but not all, patients due to inability of the palate to close normally because the tongue impedes it. Robin sequence is rarely isolated and can occur in a variety of craniofacial syndromes.

8. **What is the ratio of cleft lip to cleft lip and palate?**
   Cleft lip and palate is the most common occurrence, accounting for 50% of patients. Left unilateral cleft lip and palate is the most common, followed by right unilateral cleft lip and palate and then bilateral cleft lip and palate. Cleft palate alone occurs in 35% and is more often syndromic than cleft lip and palate or cleft lip alone. Cleft lip alone occurs in 15%.

9. **Distinguish between complete cleft lip and incomplete cleft lip.**
   The distinction between complete and incomplete cleft lip is controversial. Generally, a complete cleft lip is defined as a cleft with muscular diastasis of the orbicularis oris. This condition can usually be best determined by observing nostril symmetry or appearance with facial movement. A complete cleft may be present with a Simonart's band.

10. **What is a Simonart's band?**
    A Simonart's band is a thin remnant of tissue in the floor of the nasal vestibule bridging the medial and lateral lip elements across the cleft. The tissue may consist of skin and/or mucosa and subcutaneous tissue with or without a small amount of muscle fibers. The origin of the term is obscure, but many attribute it to Pierre Joseph Cécilien Simonart, a Belgian obstetrician (1817–1847).

11. **What is the primary palate and the secondary palate?**
    The primary and secondary palates are separated by the incisive foramen. The primary palate consists of the lip, alveolar arch, and palate anterior to the incisive foramen (the premaxilla). The secondary palate consists of the soft palate and the hard palate posterior to the incisive foramen (Fig. 53.2).

12. **How is the primary palate formed?**
    Primary palate formation occurs between weeks 4 and 7. The development of the primary palate is largely complete prior to formation of the secondary palate. During week 4 the frontonasal prominence forms, including nasal placodes. The nasal placode consists of ectodermal thickenings located on the lateral aspect of the prominence. By week 5 the frontonasal prominence elevates and forms medial and lateral nasal prominences around the nasal

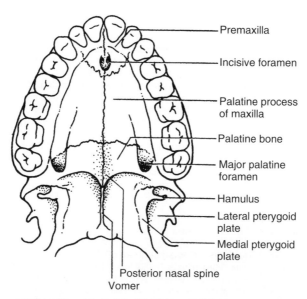

Fig. 53.2 Basic anatomy and divisions of the palate. (From Randall P, LaRossa D: Cleft palate. In: McCarthy JG, ed: *Plastic Surgery*, Philadelphia, 1990, Saunders.)

placode. Next, the placode invaginates and forms nasal pits. During weeks 6 and 7, the maxillary prominences enlarge and grow medially. This growth forces the medial nasal prominences toward the midline. With the fusion of both medial nasal prominences, the tip of the nose, central upper lip, and philtrum of the upper lip are formed. The lateral portion of the upper lip and maxilla is formed by fusion of the medial nasal prominence and maxillary prominence. Finally, the nasal alae are formed by fusion of the lateral nasal prominences with the maxillary prominence.

13. **How is the secondary palate formed?**
Formation of the secondary palate occurs between weeks 6 and 10 in three stages: growth, shelf elevation, and fusion. First, outgrowths from the maxillary processes extend vertically downward along the tongue. Next, the shelves quickly assume a horizontal position above the tongue. The palatal shelves then fuse, forming an intact secondary palate.

14. **Describe the embryologic failures in regard to the formation of a cleft lip and palate.**
A cleft lip is due to failure of fusion between the medial nasal prominence and the maxillary prominence, lateral nasal prominence, or both. Cleft palate formation is hypothesized to result from one of the following: defects in palatal shelf growth, delayed or failed shelf elevation, defective shelf fusion, failure of medial epithelial seam cell death, or failure of mesenchymal consolidation and differentiation.

15. **What is a submucous cleft? How is it diagnosed?**
A submucous cleft is a muscular diastasis in the palate with intact overlying mucosa. A submucous cleft is classically characterized by the triad of bifid uvula, a midline furrow along the length of the soft palate due to abnormal muscle insertion (zona pellucida), and a notch in the posterior margin of the hard palate. Submucous cleft palate can usually be seen on physical examination or nasopharyngoscopy. A midline furrow of the nasal surface of the posterior palate seen during phonation is a classic endoscopic finding.

16. **List some characteristics of the classic cleft nose deformity.**
   - Shortened columella with its base angled to the noncleft side
   - Nasal spine deviation to the noncleft side, with a similar deflection of the caudal septum toward the noncleft side and compensatory hypertrophy of the cleft side inferior turbinate
   - The lower lateral cartilage of the nose on the cleft side is rotated or displaced laterally in the nasal tip with the medial crura collapsed inferiorly and the lateral crura collapsed and buckled.
   - Deflection of the nasal tip toward the cleft side due to the above deficiencies
   - Relative stenosis or collapse of the nasal valve on the cleft side
   - Hypoplastic maxilla on the cleft side, causing lateralization of the alar base and widening of the nares
   - Broad nasal dorsum
   - Horizontal as opposed to vertical nostril orientation, as seen on basal view

17. **What specific role does the otolaryngologist play in the care of a child with cleft lip/palate?**
In some institutions, the otolaryngologist performs all surgical procedures involving cleft lip/palate repair, correction of velopharyngeal insufficiency (VPI), alveolar bone grafting, rhinoplasty, and orthognathic surgery. In other institutions, a plastic surgeon performs some or all of the previously listed procedures except for management of ear disease associated with cleft palate. Oral and maxillofacial surgeons may be involved in or perform alveolar bone grafting and orthognathic surgery procedures. A pediatric otolaryngologist should be involved with the complex feeding and airway issues that often occur in children born with cleft lip and/or palate.

18. **List the initial priorities for managing a newborn with cleft lip/palate.**
As in any newborn, airway management is of primary importance. Feeding and achieving adequate nutrition is the second priority for any newborn, including infants with cleft lip/palate (see Question 20).

19. **Discuss airway management in newborns with cleft lip/palate.**
For a child born with Pierre Robin sequence or more complex craniofacial anomalies, airway management is of much greater concern. Such children may have few signs of upper airway obstruction; however, severely affected children may require immediate attention. Intervention may be as simple as prone positioning, which is most effective in nonsyndromic cases. Surgical techniques for management are more often required in syndromic patients and may include glossopexy or tongue-lip adhesion (effectiveness is controversial), nasal airway placement, mandibular distraction osteogenesis, or tracheostomy tube placement.

20. **Describe the approach to feeding in infants with cleft lip/palate.**
Patients with cleft lip only may require little or no intervention, and many are able to breastfeed or use regular bottle nipples. Children with cleft palate or cleft lip/cleft palate are at a disadvantage, given the anatomic and functional deficits caused by a cleft. The inability to generate negative pressure within the oral cavity secondary to palatal insufficiency can lead to the expenditure of too much energy for feeding, long feeding times, and

subsequent poor weight gain or even dehydration. Strategies developed to assist these children include special feeding systems (e.g., Medela Special Needs Feeder, formerly called Haberman feeder, Mead Johnson squeeze bottle, Pigeon feeder, Dr. Brown's nipple/bottle) and the fabrication of a palatal obturator or prosthetic. The obturator not only acts to aid in feeding but can also be used to help reposition the protruded premaxilla, lengthen the columella, reposition lateral maxillary segments, and reshape the nostril (see Question 24).

21. **Discuss the underlying pathophysiology of middle ear disease in a child with cleft lip/palate.**
Studies since the 1960s have implicated eustachian tube dysfunction as the main cause of ear disease. Multiple investigations have supported the hypothesis that the eustachian tube in a child with cleft lip/palate is unable to open properly and ventilate the middle ear because the muscles of the palate are involved in eustachian tube physiology. When these muscles are abnormal, such as in a cleft palate, they cannot function normally to open and close the eustachian tube.

22. **What percentage of children with cleft palate have middle ear disease? How is it treated?**
Virtually all ($\geq$90%) children younger than 2 years of age with an unrepaired cleft have an effusion of the middle ear. Persistence of an effusion in young children leads to variable levels of hearing loss. Hearing loss during early childhood may lead to difficulties in speech and language development. The majority of centers treating children with clefts recommend tube placement during the first year of life or sooner if effusions become infected or hearing is markedly impaired. During either cleft lip or palate repair, the first set of tubes is often placed.

23. **When is the optimal time to perform a cleft lip repair?**
Commonly, the cleft lip is repaired between the ages of 2 and 6 months. After 10 weeks of age (corrected for prematurity if necessary), there is a decrease in respiratory complications following general anesthesia. The classic "rule of 10s" is often used at many centers. This rule requires children to be at least 10 weeks old, to weigh at least 10 lb, and to have a hemoglobin level of 10 mg/dL. Although these criteria are commonly used, they are largely of historical interest and are not based on scientific data. Efficient feeding, proven weight gain, and good general health are much more important for successful surgical repair. Obviously, other congenital anomalies, such as congenital heart disease, must take precedence over cleft repair.

24. **What is presurgical nasoalveolar molding (NAM)?**
Presurgical nasoalveolar molding (NAM or pNAM) is basically presurgical orthodontics (often termed presurgical orthopedics, since orthodontics implies that teeth are present). An anterior palatal obturator is fabricated. The obturator may help in feeding. The obturator is then progressively modified to move the lateral maxillary segments. A protuberant premaxilla can be moved posteriorly, and attachments can be added to lengthen the short columella. Nasoalveolar molding is most beneficial in wide complete bilateral clefts of the lip and palate, but increasing use is being seen in unilateral clefts.

25. **What is a cleft lip adhesion?**
In certain cases of wide unilateral or bilateral cleft lip, some surgeons perform a cleft lip adhesion. This procedure is a staged lip repair in which the first stage (adhesion) involves reapproximating medial and lateral lip elements and the orbicularis oris muscle. The first stage converts a complete cleft, either unilateral or bilateral, to a more easily repaired incomplete cleft. The second stage then uses one of the techniques in Question 26 as the formal lip repair.

26. **List the techniques used for formal repair of unilateral cleft lip.**
   - Fisher anatomic subunit repair: first published in 2004, the Fisher anatomic subunit repair of the lip has gained popularity since. It draws on portions of several previously published repairs, primarily those with triangular and quadrangular flaps.
   - Millard rotation-advancement repair: the medial lip element is rotated inferiorly and the lateral lip element is advanced into the resulting upper lip defect. The columellar flap is then used to lengthen the columella or create the nasal sill.
   - Tennison-Randell repair: the medial lip element is lengthened by introduction of a triangular flap from the inferior portion of the lateral lip element.
   - Hagedorn-LeMesurier repair: a quadrilateral flap developed from the lateral lip element is introduced to lengthen the medial lip element.

27. **List the techniques used for formal repair of bilateral cleft lip.**
   - Millard's repair involves complete elevation of the prolabium and reconstitution of the orbicularis across the premaxilla. In addition, Millard banked lateral segments of the prolabium as "forked flaps" that were meant to add columellar height at a later stage. The banking of forked flaps has recently fallen out of favor, with more emphasis now being placed on primary columellar lengthening and rhinoplasty.

- Veau repair: The Veau operation is a straight-line closure without elevation of the prolabial skin and correspondingly without any attempt to restore the continuity of the orbicularis oris, which is not favored because this results in incompetence of the oral sphincter.

28. **Describe recent developments in nasal and lip repair.**
First published in 2004, the Fisher anatomic subunit repair of the lip has rapidly gained popularity. It draws on portions of several previously published repairs, primarily those with triangular and quadrangular flaps. Small horizontal incisions are traded for better lip height, without compromise in length, as compared with Millard's technique. These horizontal incisions also seem to heal more predictably than the longer rotation incision of Millard.
　　Greyson and Cutting have introduced presurgical molding of the nasal tip and columella with acrylic outriggers, orthodontic elastics, and tapes attached to a palatal appliance (see Question 24).

29. **When should cleft palates be repaired?**
Timing of cleft palate repair is much more controversial than that of cleft lip repair. The goals of cleft palate repair include attaining normal long-term speech and avoiding deleterious effects on future facial growth. Patients with unrepaired clefts have the least amount of abnormal growth, but the speech impact of this approach is unacceptable. Recent research into speech development supports cleft palate repair before the age of 12 months, but for optimum outcomes some centers recommend closure at 8–10 months of age. Early repair avoids compensatory techniques that may impair speech and be difficult to unlearn. Studies have shown that children with clefts repaired before 12 months have improved speech outcomes compared with children who undergo repair closer to 24 months. Long-term follow-up has found no significant impact on growth in children with clefts repaired earlier.

30. **Name the more common methods of cleft palate repair.**
- Two-flap palatoplasty
- Wardill-Kilner V-Y advancement
- Von Langenbeck palatoplasty
- Furlow double-opposing Z-plasty

31. **List possible postoperative complications of cleft palate repair.**
- Bleeding
- Fistula or dehiscence
- Velopharyngeal insufficiency
- Postoperative upper airway obstruction

32. **What is velopharyngeal insufficiency (VPI)?**
VPI is hypernasality during speech or reflux of saliva or food into the nasopharynx during swallowing. VPI occurs when the nasopharynx and oropharynx are not successfully separated by complete palatal closure during particular speech sounds or during swallowing. Persistent VPI occurs in about 10% to 40% of children after cleft palate repair.

33. **How is VPI treated?**
An experienced speech and language pathologist should evaluate the presence, specific cause, and severity of VPI, often in conjunction with an imaging technique such as video nasopharyngoscopy or video fluoroscopy. Both medical and surgical methods for correction of VPI are available. Medical management includes speech therapy and oral appliances that aid in correcting the underlying problem. The majority of children undergo speech therapy before being referred for surgical management. Surgical management includes a variety of procedures aimed at attaining separation of the oropharynx from the nasopharynx during speech. Specific procedures include the pharyngeal flap, sphincter pharyngoplasty, Furlow palatoplasty, and posterior pharyngeal wall augmentation.

34. **What are the concerns as children reach older ages?**
As previously stated, the treatment of cleft lip and palate is best directed by a multidisciplinary team. Fig. 53.1 demonstrates example times/ages when specific concerns are addressed.
- As children reach elementary school age, dental and speech needs become more of a concern.
- In late elementary school and early middle school, orthodontic and alveolar cleft repair are usually addressed.
- In high school-age patients, orthodontics and secondary cosmetic surgical procedures are addressed.
- At skeletal maturity (16 to 18 years in females, 18 to 21 years in males), orthodontics and orthognathic surgical procedures are addressed.

35. **What are the adult concerns for patients with cleft lip and palate anomalies?**
It is the goal of team care that the majority of functional and cosmetic concerns will be addressed by the time a patient reaches adult age. In some instances, other circumstances prevent all concerns being addressed by this time. Functional and cosmetic concerns can be addressed at any age, even in adults. Many adults born with cleft and craniofacial disorders choose medical and/or surgical treatments to address these concerns.

CONTROVERSIES

36. **How is rhinoplasty approached in the child with cleft lip/palate?**
    The approach to correction of the cleft nose is controversial. Some experts recommend immediate or primary correction with cleft lip repair, whereas others who are concerned with potential disrupted growth recommend a much later repair when patients are in their late teens. Advocates of primary repair found that early repair creates better symmetry and hence symmetric growth. They also claim there is much less psychological stress with earlier repair. Advocates of later definitive repair claim that they avoid any potential disturbances in growth, produce less scarring, and avoid multiple surgeries due to unexpected changes caused by growth. Recently there has been increased support for limited primary rhinoplasty at the time of initial lip repair.

37. **What are advantages and disadvantages of earlier surgeries versus later or delayed surgeries?**
    For almost all of the required procedures in patients with cleft lip and/or palate, there are controversies, or advantages and disadvantages of early versus delayed intervention. Almost all of these controversies encompass improved function (early repair) versus lesser growth disturbance (delayed surgical intervention). The study of these effects is difficult without large, randomized trials.

BIBLIOGRAPHY

Byrd BH, Jhonny S: Primary correction of unilateral cleft nasal deformity, *Plast Reconstr Surg* 106:1276–1286, 2000.
Clark JM, Skoner JM, Wang TD: Repair of the unilateral cleft lip/nose deformity, *Facial Plast Surg* 19:29–39, 2003.
Fisher DM: Unilateral cleft lip repair: an anatomical subunit approximation technique, *Plast Reconstr Surg* 116(1):61–71, 2005.
Matthews MS, Cohen M, Viglione M, et al: Prenatal counseling for cleft lip and palate, *Plast Reconstr Surg* 101:1–5, 1998.
Murray JC: Gene/environment causes of cleft lip and/or palate, *Clin Genet* 61:248–256, 2002.
Randall P, Krogman WM, Jahins S: Pierre Robin and the syndrome that bears his name, *Cleft Palate J* 36:237–246, 1965.
Redford-Badwal DA, Mabry K, Frassinelli JD: Impact of cleft lip and/or palate on nutritional health and oral-motor development, *Dent Clin North Am* 47:305–317, 2003.
Rohrich RJ, Love EJ, Byrd S, et al: Optimal timing of cleft palate closure, *Plast Reconstr Surg* 106:413–421, 2000.
Seibert RW, Weit GJ, Bumsted RM: Cleft lip and palate. In: Cummings CW, et al, eds: *Otolaryngology-Head and Neck Surgery*. 3rd ed. Mosby, 1998, pp 133–173.
Shih CW, Sykes JM: Correction of the cleft-lip nasal deformity, *Facial Plast Surg* 18:253–262, 2002.
Thomas C, Mishra P: Open tip rhinoplasty along with the repair of cleft lip in cleft lip and palate cases, *Br J Plast Surg* 53:1–6, 2000.

CHAPTER 54

PEDIATRIC HEARING LOSS

Allison M. Dobbie, MD and Steven Leoniak, MD

KEY POINTS

1. Early identification of hearing loss, with intervention, is crucial to achieve optimal outcomes for speech and learning in children.
2. Suspect syndromic hearing loss in children with congenital hearing loss and other physical abnormalities.
3. Genetic evaluation of hearing loss requires detailed history and physical exam, family history/pedigree, audiometry and tympanometry, as well as molecular genetic testing. Genetic testing for hearing loss is rapidly evolving.

Pearls

1. In developed countries, the most common environmental, nongenetic cause of congenital hearing loss is cytomegalovirus infection.
2. Most nonsyndromic genetic hearing loss is caused by mutations in connexins 26 and 30, encoded by *GJB2* and *GJB6*.
3. Patients with an enlarged vestibular aqueduct or Mondini dysplasia should be tested for mutations in *SLC26A4*, which is associated with Pendred syndrome.
4. Alport syndrome is characterized by glomerulonephritis and progressive SNHL. It has a variable inheritance pattern but 85% of cases are X-linked and 15% are AR.
5. Usher syndrome should be considered in children with congenital severe-to-profound hearing loss in whom *GJB2* and *GJB6* are normal.

QUESTIONS

1. **How common is pediatric hearing loss?**
   Hearing loss is the most common birth defect and the most prevalent sensorineural disorder in developed countries. Each year in the USA, 4000 infants are born with bilateral profound hearing loss, and 8000 infants are born with unilateral or bilateral mild-to-moderate hearing loss. Congenital pediatric hearing loss can be categorized as genetic or acquired hearing loss.

2. **What is universal newborn hearing screening?**
   In 1993, the National Institutes of Health published a consensus statement endorsing screening of all newborns for hearing loss before hospital discharge. Prior to universal newborn hearing screening programs, testing was conducted only in high-risk infants, which resulted in identification of nearly 50% of congenital hearing loss after the critical period for speech and language development. All infants should have hearing screening before 1 month of age and 95% are now tested prior to discharge. Infants who do not pass newborn screening should have a follow-up medical and audiologic evaluation prior to 3 months of age.

3. **How are neonatal hearing screen tests performed?**
   There are two methods utilized for hearing screening at birth: otoacoustic emissions (OAE) and automated auditory brainstem response (AABR) testing. Both OAE and AABR tests are noninvasive and can be obtained during normal physiologic sleep in the setting of a newborn nursery or neonatal intensive care unit. Newborns who do not pass their hearing screens are referred to audiologists for further workup, typically with complete diagnostic auditory brainstem response testing.

4. **Why is early identification of hearing loss important?**
   Early identification and subsequent treatment of hearing loss has a substantial impact on the development of speech and language skills. Children with any degree of hearing loss who are treated by 6 months of age develop language skills comparable to their peers without hearing loss. Delayed diagnosis negatively impacts not only language skills but also academic performance, career opportunities, and psychosocial well-being.

5. **What is the most critical period for speech and hearing development?**

Hearing loss is most detrimental between birth and 3 years of age. It is during this critical period when children develop speech, auditory pathways, and emotional bonds to family members. Infants with profound hearing loss are unable to obtain auditory feedback, and without this feedback they cannot acquire the motor speech skills necessary for communication.

6. **Summarize the major milestones for development of speech and hearing.**

Infants younger than 3 months of age are startled by loud sounds and calmed by familiar voices. At 6 months of age, infants have the ability to localize sounds, and by 9 months of age they respond to their names and are able to mimic environmental sounds. By 18 months of age, infants react to sounds from any direction and are capable of following commands to perform simple tasks. Although most infants say "ma-ma" or "da-da" early on, the first obvious speech milestone occurs at about 1 year of age when infants learn their first meaningful words. By age 2 years, most normally hearing monolingual children have a vocabulary of 20 or more words.

7. **What are risk factors for early childhood hearing loss?**
- Family history of permanent childhood hearing loss
- Birth weight less than 1500 g
- Congenital craniofacial anomalies
- In utero infections (ToRCHeS)
- Maternal diabetes or alcohol/drug use
- Hyperbilirubinemia requiring exchange transfusion
- Apgar scores less than 5 at 1 minute and less than 7 at 5 minutes
- Neonatal exposure to ototoxic agents
- Mechanical ventilation for 5 days or longer
- Extracorporeal membrane oxygenation (ECMO)
- Postnatal infections associated with hearing loss
- Neurodegenerative disorders or sensorimotor neuropathies
- Head trauma
- Recurrent or persistent otitis media with effusion lasting for at least 3 months

8. **What are the causes of congenital hearing loss?**

Approximately 50% of all cases of congenital deafness are genetic, approximately 30% are from acquired/environmental causes, and 20% are cause unknown.

9. **How are genetic causes of hearing loss categorized?**

Genetic hearing loss is classified as syndromic (30%) or nonsyndromic (70%). Disorders that cause syndromic hearing loss are associated with congenital anomalies involving other organ systems. Nonsyndromic hearing loss is isolated to anomalies of the middle or inner ear and does not involve other organ systems or the external ear.

10. **What are the most common syndromes causing sensorineural hearing loss? Describe their features and modes of inheritance.**

Usher syndrome
- Autosomal recessive (AR) inheritance and the most common type of AR hearing loss
- The cause of up to 10% of congenital deafness but degree of hearing loss is variable
- Associated with variable vestibular dysfunction
- Associated with retinitis pigmentosa, which can cause progressive blindness
- Associated with mutations in genes *MYO7A*, *USH2A*, *CDH23*, and others

Pendred syndrome
- AR inheritance pattern
- Responsible for 5% to 10% of recessive hearing loss
- Associated with multinodular goiter, inner ear malformations including Mondini deformity, enlarged vestibular aqueduct, and abnormal perchlorate testing
- Mutations in the *SLC26A4* gene are common

Jervell and Lange-Nielsen syndrome
- Third most common cause of AR syndromic hearing loss
- Responsible for 1% of all cases of recessive hearing loss and commonly severe bilateral sensorineural hearing loss
- Associated with prolonged Q-T interval on ECG, which can cause sudden death
- Associated with mutations in the *KCNQ1* and *KCNE1* genes

Waardenburg syndrome
- Most common cause of autosomal dominant (AD) hearing loss
- Accounts for 2% of congenital hearing loss
- Severity of hearing loss is variable

- Associated physical findings include telecanthus, white forelock, hyperplastic high nasal root, hyperplastic medial eyebrows, and heterochromia irides
- Multiple genetic mutations exist, most commonly in the *PAX3* and *MITF* genes

Branchiootorenal syndrome
- AD inheritance pattern
- Children exhibit branchial cleft fistulas, renal abnormalities, and abnormal development of the inner, middle, or external ears including preauricular pits
- Associated with mutations in the *EYA1*, *SIX1*, and *SIX5* genes

Stickler syndrome
- AD inheritance
- Associated with cleft palate, osteoarthritis, myopia, and progressive sensorineural hearing loss
- Three types are recognized based on the molecular genetic defect: STL1 (*COL2A1*), STL2 (*COL11A1*), and STL3 (*COL11A2*)

11. **How is nonsyndromic hearing loss inherited? What are some nonsyndromic causes of genetic hearing loss?**

Most genetic hearing losses are caused by single gene Mendelian inheritance in the *absence* of a recognizable syndrome. Currently over 220 SNHL genes have been identified, and these numbers continue to grow. Eighty percent of nonsyndromic hearing loss is autosomal recessive, 15% is autosomal dominant, with the remainder X-linked or mitochondrial.

Mutation in the *GJB2* gene, which encodes the connexin-26 gap junction protein, causes 30% to 50% of all congenital profound hearing loss. *SLC26A4* mutations, present in Pendred syndrome and in children with enlarged vestibular aqueduct, are the second most common abnormality in congenital sensorineural hearing loss.

12. **Describe inner and middle ear anomalies that can cause hearing loss.**

Malformations of the inner ear are rare. They can be categorized into malformations of the bony and membranous labyrinth and those limited to the membranous labyrinth only. **Michel's aplasia** is complete failure of inner ear development (labyrinthine aplasia) and typically leads to complete deafness. **Mondini dysplasia** results in an incomplete partition in the cochlea; only the basal turn of the cochlea is developed, and the bony cochlea is restricted to 1.5 turns. This can present in early childhood or later in adult life, with hearing that ranges from complete loss to normal. Mondini dysplasia is inherited in an autosomal dominant pattern.

Membranous labyrinthine anomalies include **Siebenmann-Bing** (complete membranous labyrinthine) **dysplasia**, **Scheibe** (cochleosaccular) **dysplasia**, and **Alexander** (cochlear basal turn) **dysplasia**. Siebenmann-Bing dysplasia is extremely rare and has been reported in association with Jervell-Nielsen-Lange and Usher syndromes. Scheibe dysplasia is often noted in autosomal recessive congenital hearing losses. Alexander dysplasia may be related to familial high-frequency sensorineural hearing loss.

Enlarged vestibular aqueduct (EVA) is the most common inner ear anomaly seen on temporal bone imaging in patients with sensorineural hearing loss. It is described as a vestibular aqueduct that measures 1.5 millimeters or greater. Children can present with sensorineural or mixed hearing loss present at birth, progressive through childhood, or even fluctuating. Sudden or progressive hearing loss can occur spontaneously or with mild head trauma. Therefore children are urged to avoid situations that may result in head trauma such as contact sports.

Congenital middle ear ossicular anomalies can also occur and often result in varying degrees of conductive hearing loss. These can include malformed or entirely absent ossicles. Malleus head fixation is likely the most common ossicular abnormality and occurs secondary to incomplete pneumatization of the epitympanic space. Congenital absence of the incus's long process can occur, which leads to a maximal conductive hearing loss. Congenital stapes fixation may also be responsible for stable conductive hearing loss and require stapedectomy for hearing restoration.

13. **What are the most common causes of acquired pediatric hearing loss?**

Acute otitis media and chronic otitis media with effusion are the most common causes of conductive hearing loss in children. Fluid within the middle ear space inhibits vibration of the tympanic membrane, reducing sound conduction. Acquired hearing loss can also be caused by cholesteatoma when desquamated epithelium expands into the middle ear and mastoid spaces, which can erode middle ear ossicles, or even into the otic capsule.

14. **Which infections can lead to hearing loss in children?**

Toxoplasmosis, rubella, congenital cytomegalovirus (CMV), herpes, and syphilis (ToRCHeS) are infections that can be responsible for hearing loss if contracted in the perinatal period. Congenital CMV is the most common cause of nonhereditary sensorineural hearing loss in children. The prevalence of congenital CMV is 0.58%, and among those newborns infected, 12.8% experience hearing loss. Among patients with symptomatic CMV infections, the majority have bilateral hearing loss; in those with asymptomatic infection, unilateral loss is more common. The development of PCR testing for CMV has improved the accuracy and availability of CMV testing in recent years. CMV testing is not currently standardized or available universally in the United States; however, a number of pediatric advocacy initiatives are urging states to increase congenital CMV screening in patients who do not pass their newborn hearing screening.

Bacterial meningitis is thought to cause hearing loss in approximately 10% of infected children. This is usually caused by *Streptococcus pneumoniae*, group B streptococcus, *Neisseria meningitidis*, and, less commonly, by *Haemophilus influenzae* type b. The inflammatory process causes ossification of the cochlea resulting in hearing loss. Frequent audiometry is necessary and if there is hearing loss, a computed tomography (CT) scan of the temporal bones is obtained with attention to cochlear ossification. If ossification is realized, cochlear implantation may proceed urgently in order to preserve residual membranous cochlear architecture.

15. **What is the role of radiographic imaging in pediatric hearing loss?**
Temporal bone CT and brain/internal auditory canal magnetic resonance imaging (MRI) are the imaging modalities of choice to evaluate hearing loss. The risk of general anesthesia for MRI should be weighed with the risk of radiation for CT. Imaging has a higher diagnostic yield for bilateral hearing loss as opposed to unilateral hearing loss. Imaging is the only way to determine presence of an enlarged vestibular aqueduct, vestibular anomalies, or absent cochlear nerves. MRI is typically recommended prior to cochlear implantation, while CT is better at identifying enlarged vestibular aqueduct.

16. **What are some other adjunctive tests that may be helpful after hearing loss is diagnosed?**
In children with profound congenital deafness and absent vestibular function, an electrocardiogram (EKG) and/or cardiology consultation should be obtained to evaluate for the prolonged Q-T interval that is seen in Jervell-Nielsen-Lange syndrome. Urinalysis may be obtained to evaluate for microscopic hematuria in Alport syndrome. If hearing loss is present along with cleft palate, ophthalmologic consultation can be important in evaluating for Stickler syndrome. Furthermore, all children with nonsyndromic hearing loss are two- to three-fold more likely to have ophthalmologic problems.

17. **What are some medications used in the pediatric population that can cause ototoxicity?**
Aminoglycosides, erythromycin, cisplatin and other platinum-derived chemotherapeutics, and loop diuretics (e.g., furosemide) can all have ototoxic effects.

18. **What is auditory neuropathy spectrum disorder (ANSD)?**
In ANSD, children have a problem with neural processing causing decreased ability to understand speech despite an ability to respond to sound. Patients with ANSD may display robust OAEs (i.e., normal cochlear function) but have either an absent or a markedly dysmorphic AABR response in combination with varying degrees of hearing loss on pure tone and speech behavioral audiometry. This is sometimes called auditory nerve dyssynchrony. MRI is the imaging study of choice for children with ANSD.

19. **What role does genetic testing play in the diagnosis of congenital hearing loss?**
Comprehensive genetic testing is the diagnostic test of choice for children with bilateral sensorineural hearing loss. The diagnostic success rate of genetic testing is approximately 40% to 65% but negative genetic testing does not rule out a genetic cause of hearing loss. Genetic counselors are integral if genetic testing is pursed because the results can affect the whole family of the tested patient. If comprehensive genetic testing is unavailable, testing individual genes—for example, *GJB2* and *GJB6*—is possible. Unfortunately, genetic testing is rarely covered by insurance companies, so access to testing can be a barrier to diagnosis.

20. **What are the treatments for pediatric hearing loss?**
Hearing rehabilitation can be accomplished both surgically and nonsurgically. Behind-the-ear hearing aids are the most common nonsurgical treatment used in children, as they are more adaptable to a child's growing ear canal. Conductive hearing loss caused by otitis media and/or eustachian tube dysfunction may be improved with surgical tympanostomy tube placement. Other causes of conductive hearing loss (middle ear malformations) may benefit from middle ear exploration and ossicular reconstruction.

Bone-anchored hearing aids (BAHAs) are devices used to restore conductive hearing loss that cannot be treated with traditional hearing aids, such as in children with external auditory canal atresia or those with chronic otorrhea. Bone conduction hearing rehabilitation can be accomplished with a nonsurgical soft headband and attached device or a surgical osseointegrated implant. These devices bypass the conductive component of the hearing loss and stimulate the cochlea directly via vibration through the skull and otic capsule.

Cochlear implants are a surgical treatment for patients with profound hearing loss in whom hearing aids are not beneficial. A cochlear implant bypasses the nonfunctional cochlea and directly stimulates the cochlear nerve. In patients with bilateral profound hearing loss, excellent speech and language outcomes can be achieved with early implantation, often prior to 1 year of age.

BIBLIOGRAPHY

Cohen M, Phillips JA: Genetic approach to evaluation of hearing loss, *Otolaryngol Clin North Am* 45(1):25–39, 2012.

Force USPST. Universal screening for hearing loss in newborns: US Preventive Services Task Force recommendation statement, *Pediatrics* 122(1):143–148, 2008.

Goderis J, De Leenheer E, Smets K, et al: Hearing loss and congenital CMV infection: a systematic review, *Pediatrics* 134(5):972–982, 2014.

Kachniarz B, Chen JX, Gilani S, et al: Diagnostic yield of MRI for pediatric hearing loss: a systematic review, *Otolaryngol Head Neck Surg* 152(1):5–22, 2015.

Lasak JM, Allen P, McVay T, et al: Hearing loss: diagnosis and management, *Prim Care* 41(1):19–31, 2014.

Liming B, Carter J, Cheng A: International pediatric otolaryngology consensus recommendations: hearing loss in the pediatric patient, *Int J Pediatr Otorhinolaryngol* 90:251–258, 2016.

Parker M, Bitner-Glindzicz M: Genetic investigations in childhood deafness, *Arch Dis Child* 3:271–278, 2015.

Raveh E, Hu W, Papsin BC, et al: Congenital conductive hearing loss, *J Laryngol Otol* 116(2):92–96, 2002.

Rodriguez K, Shah RK, Kenna M: Anomalies of the middle and inner ear, *Otolaryngol Clin North Am* 40(1):81–96, 2007.

MICROTIA AND OTOPLASTY

Peggy E. Kelley, MD

QUESTIONS

1. **What is otoplasty?**
   Otoplasty is the manipulation of abnormally shaped cartilages to achieve a more natural-appearing shape of the external ear. This can be achieved by surgical and nonsurgical methods.

2. **What are the indications for otoplasty?**
   Otoplasty is not based on the ear shape but rather the patient's perception of the ear shape. If the ears are asymmetric or if their shape draws attention to the ears instead of the person's face, otoplasty may be indicated. If the patient sees only his or her ears in the mirror or is teased because of their size or shape, otoplasty can improve self-esteem.

3. **Which anatomic landmarks of the external ear are important in otoplasty? (Fig. 55.1)**
   The circumference of the external ear is described by the helix, lobule, and tragus. The inner folds of the ear consist of the antihelix and antitragus. The antihelix divides the external ear superiorly into the superior and inferior crus. Between the crura is the fossa triangularis. Between the helical rim and the antihelical fold is the scaphoid fossa. Between the antihelix and the tragus is the conchal bowl, which is divided by the root of the helix into the concha cymba above and the concha cavum below. The tragus overlies the ear canal opening.

4. **How are external ear malformations classified?**
   Various grading systems have been proposed for congenital malformations of the auricle. Most reliable for documentation or discussion between health care providers is an anatomic description of the abnormality, since no staging system is widely recognized. Description of the abnormality can help direct thought about reconstruction or correction. Commonly used terms are *protruding* or *prominent ears, lop ears, Stahl's ears, constricted ears, cryptotia, microtia,* and *anotia.*

5. **Describe the dimensions of a normal ear.**
   Ears are fully grown by 9 years of age. They do not change shape spontaneously beyond 12 months of age. Whereas no one size or shape is normal for all people, some approximate measurements can be helpful in assessing the degree of abnormality of an ear. Ear height is typically 55 to 65 millimeters, and width is from 30 to 45 millimeters. Width is usually 50% to 60% of the height. The ear is rotated so that the top is 15 to 30 degrees more posterior than the earlobe. At its midpoint, the ear protrudes from the scalp approximately 18 to 20 millimeters. The angle of protrusion of the ear from the head is usually <21 degrees in a female and <25 degrees in a male. The root of the helix is usually 75 to 95 millimeters posterior to the lateral canthus of the eye.

6. **What is a prominent or protruding ear deformity?**
   This common external malformation is diagnosed when the angle of the ear to the head is >35 degrees. It is most commonly a result of the lack of antihelical fold development. The ear then protrudes more than the 20 millimeters expected from the scalp and takes over the frontal profile. Instead of seeing a person's face, the eyes of the

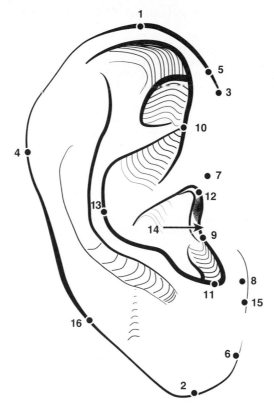

Fig. 55.1 Landmarks of the external ear: (1) superaurale, (2) subaurale, (3) preaurale, (4) postaurale, (5) otobasion superius, (6) otobasion inferius, (7) deepest point on the notch on upper margin of tragus, (8) lowest point on the lower border of tragus, (9) protragion, (10) concha superior (the intersection of the lower edge of the anterior end of the crus antihelicis inferius and the posterior border of crus helicus, (11) incisura intertragica inferior (the deepest point in the incisura intertragica), (12) incisura anterior auris posterior (the most posterior point on the edge of incisura anterior auris), (13) strongest antihelical curvature, (14) deepest lateral border of external auditory meatus, (15) lobule anterior (ear attachment line is drawn joining the otobasion superior and inferior – the point on this line just below the incisura intertragica where the cartilage ends is the landmark), and (16) lobule posterior (the most posterior point on the margin of lobule perpendicular to lobule anterior). (From Purkait R, Singh P: A test of individuality of human external ear pattern: its application in the field of personal identification. *Forensic Sci Int* 178(2–3):112–118, 2008.)

observer are drawn to the ears. A normal ear shape and angle of protrusion can be attained by gentle repositioning of the ear with finger pressure.

7. **What is a constricted or cup ear deformity?**
   This ear deformity is characterized by the inability of gentle finger pressure to attain a normal shape or position of the ear. A deficiency of skin, cartilage, or both restricts the opening up or "unfolding" of the ear into a normal shape with finger pressure.

8. **How is microtia or anotia characterized?**
   In the microtic ear, the cartilage shape is abnormal. The classic description is a cartilage remnant that looks like a rolled "peanut" positioned at the root of the helix. The lower portion of the microtic remnant is soft fatty tissue – the earlobe remnant. Superiorly, the remnant is composed of crumpled cartilage under the skin. An atypical microtia may have the beginnings of normal ear architecture but with obvious disruption in development. Anotia is absence of the external ear. A small earlobe remnant may be present and is often not in the expected location.

9. **Summarize the goals of otoplasty.**
   The primary goal of otoplasty is to make the patient (and often the parents) happy. The postoperative ear or ears should be symmetric. From the frontal view, you should have a small glimpse of both ears at the same time. On lateral view, the ear should have smooth contours with recognizable major anatomic features: helical rim,

antihelical fold with crus, scapha, conchal bowl, and lobule. The posterior view should exhibit appropriate scalp-to-ear distances (<20 millimeters).

10. **When should otoplasty be offered to a patient?**
The age at which otoplasty can be performed depends on the type of corrective surgery needed. The goal of timing is to avoid psychological insult to the child by completing the repair as soon as possible while balancing the maturity needed for participation and cooperation in surgical and postoperative care.

11. **What is the youngest patient age at which otoplasty can be performed?**
The first opportunity for the correction of abnormal ear shapes is within the first several days after birth. Reshaping with wax and tape within the first 96 hours of life can obviate the need for surgery in the future. The splint or molding technique requires 2 weeks of reshaping if applied during the neonatal period. Older infants may require longer periods of shape control. Recently, the use of a splint and double-sided tape for many months was reported in children up to 5 years of age as a means of avoiding surgical correction.

12. **What is the youngest patient age at which more complicated techniques can be performed?**
If the abnormality can be corrected by gentle finger pressure into a desired shape, then a permanent change in shape can be accomplished with the incisionless technique as early as age 2 years when cartilage is firm enough to hold sutures. If the abnormality cannot be corrected by gentle finger pressure, the child will need an open procedure and will need to be able to participate in the postoperative care and suture removal. An open otoplasty is typically performed as early as 5 to 6 years of age for very motivated children and parents but may be delayed until the child is ready. When microtia construction with autologous rib grafting is to be considered, the ribs must be large enough to carve. Some techniques can start as early as age 6 to 7 years but the newer 3D techniques require more rib and most children do not have enough rib stock until age 10 to 12 years.

13. **What are the options for protruding ear otoplasty?**
Open versus closed: Open techniques begin with skin excision and progress to weakening or thinning the cartilage, reshaping with mattress sutures, or dividing the cartilage and removal to reduce the conchal bowl. Closed options include tape and wax or splint application as well as the incisionless otoplasty described by Fritsch. Incisionless otoplasty employs permanent horizontal mattress sutures placed percutaneously.

   Cartilage sparing versus cartilage removal: Surgeons are highly opinionated as to whether cartilage can be reshaped with mattress sutures, scoring, or thinning by drilling or whether cartilage must be removed to attain a desirable ear shape. Either option can be used successfully, but often one option is adopted as preferred by an individual surgeon based on their own results.

14. **Describe the early complications of otoplasty for protruding ears.**
Hematoma is the major concern after open otoplasty. If a hematoma goes undiagnosed and untreated, perichondritis and loss of cartilage result. Persistent postoperative pain can be a sign of hematoma. Proper treatment consists of immediate evacuation of the clot and debridement of any necrotic tissue resulting from pressure of the hematoma, followed by reapplication of the compressive dressing. Other early complications include skin necrosis secondary to dressing pressure, skin hypersensitivity to pressure or temperature, and suture spitting. All of these, except suture extrusion, are avoided with the incisionless technique because no dressing is used postoperatively and no dead space for hematoma formation is raised during the procedure.

15. **What are the significant late complications of otoplasty for protruding ears?**
The most common late complication is unhappiness with the postoperative correction, usually because of undercorrection, asymmetry, or cartilage deformation over time. In an open procedure, scar hypertrophy or keloids may result.

16. **What is a "telephone ear" deformity?**
A telephone ear deformity describes the shape of an overcorrected midportion of the ear. The resultant shape is reminiscent of the original handpiece of a telephone with a separate receiver and a mouthpiece with a connecting narrower handle. The deformity is best appreciated on frontal view. Such overcorrection can be due to excessive removal of postauricular skin or mastoid soft tissue or by overtightening set-back sutures of the concha to the mastoid.

17. **What historical names should I know if I want to discuss otoplasty for protruding ears?**
Mustardé is known for the development of the horizontal mattress suture to reshape the antihelical fold (Fig. 55.2). This same horizontal mattress suture has been adapted to a percutaneous technique of incisionless otoplasty. Converse and Furness otoplasty techniques use cartilage repositioning and weakening in their otoplasties. Converse uses the cartilage weakening and repositioning to create the appearance of an antihelical fold. The Furness technique does not address the antihelical fold but focuses on the conchal bowl protrusion by suturing the bowl to

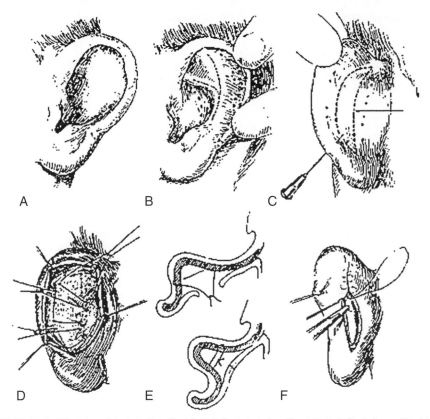

Fig. 55.2 The Mustardé technique of otoplasty. (From Wood-Smith D: Otoplasty. In: Rees TD, ed: *Aesthetic Plastic Surgery*, Philadelphia, 1980, Saunders, p. 851.)

the mastoid periosteum, rotating the ear posteriorly and thus decreasing protrusion. This technique is often used in conjunction with a technique for reshaping the antihelical fold.

18. **How is correcting a "cup" or constricted ear different from correcting a protruding ear?**
    A cup or constricted ear is missing enough skin, cartilage, or both so that a normal shape cannot be attained through the techniques used for protruding surgery. New skin or cartilage or advancement of tissue must be used to release the constricted part of the ear (Fig. 55.3).

    The deficiencies usually lie in the helical rim, scapha, and root of the helix. Techniques to unfurl and fan open have been described but may fail over time because the skin/soft tissue envelope collapses the new expanded cartilage shape. A preferred technique is to release the root of the helix as a V-Y advancement flap, incorporating the ridge of cartilage between the concha cavum and concha cymba. Several millimeters of length can be

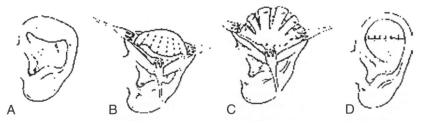

Fig. 55.3 Correction of severe cup ear deformity. (From Converse JH: Congenital deformities of the auricle. In: Converse JM, ed: *Reconstructive Plastic Surgery*, 2nd ed, Philadelphia, 1977, Saunders, p. 1708.)

borrowed and advanced into the height of the ear. Skin grafts are used if needed in the new fossa triangularis area, and the cartilage is reshaped with horizontal mattress sutures to add strength and stability over time.

19. **When does a lobule need to be corrected?**
The earlobe may angle forward, particularly in a cupped or protruding ear or with an abnormally long or flared caudal helical cartilage. The upper cartilage can be corrected, but the ear can still look abnormal if the earlobe is not repositioned. Resecting or repositioning this tail of cartilage will result in less anterior angulation of the lobule. Sometimes skin behind can be removed to assist in earlobe correction.

20. **Can a huge ear be reduced in size overall?**
Of course! Auricular reduction may be necessary to attain symmetry with a smaller opposite ear. Sometimes it is easier to reduce the larger ear than to expand the deficient one. All methods of reduction surgery involve geometric excision and closure. This approach decreases the chance of a notched scar along the sweeping helical rim.

21. **What can be done with a microtic ear?**
A person with microtia can be treated with a silicone prosthesis that is made to look like the opposite ear and attached with skin glues or, more recently, with bone-anchored screws and magnets.

Surgical correction can be attained with a buried silicone or Silastic ear mold, but the mold is prone to extrusion and malformation with the trauma of childhood play or sports. The long-term effects of a foreign body in children are also significant; thus this form of reconstruction should no longer be considered, particularly in children.

Synthetic biocompatible, porous, high-density polyethylene frameworks can be used with a temporalis fascia flap as a one- or two-stage operation. This procedure was popularized by Reinisch in the early 1990s. Concerns for long-term rejection or trauma have lessened with recent publications on long-term outcomes. This procedure can be done as early as 3 years of age, but an adult-sized ear is placed because the ear will not grow over time.

Brent described a four-stage autologous rib reconstruction. This form of reconstruction has been used for the past 40 years with good results. The first stage is the harvesting, carving, and placement of the autologous rib graft. Portions of three or four ribs (depending on the need for tragal reconstruction) are used to form the helical rim, antihelical fold, scapha, and fossa triangularis. The second stage rotates the microtic remnant earlobe onto the cartilage framework and attaches it there. The third stage is ear elevation away from the head with a skin graft. The fourth stage, if necessary, involves creation of a tragus and deepening of the conchal bowl. This type of reconstruction is typically begun after age 6 years, but it is usually recommended that boys wait until age 10 years for full cooperation. Usually 9 to 12 months are required to complete all four stages.

In the mid-1980s, another autologous rib reconstruction method was developed simultaneously by Nagata and Firmin. This two-stage operation is performed beginning at age 10 years and requires an evaluation for adequate costal cartilage volume. The first stage includes harvesting, fabrication of the three-dimensional costal cartilage framework, and grafting it into place. The second stage elevates the auricle to match projection. Results are more reliable with the topographic method of ear cartilage fabrication as carving is not as dependent on in situ rib width and depth. Magritz and others have developed variations on the work started by Firmin and Nagata to create an autologous rib-based framework.

22. **What does the future hold for microtia construction?**
Currently, the development of a bone-anchored hearing aid embedded in a silicone prosthetic ear is being trialed outside the USA. Ongoing research in tissue engineering with the goal of harvesting autologous chondrocytes continues to teach us more about cell growth and immunology, but there are no clinical applications currently available. 3D printing of the opposite ear as model to carve on the operative field is being performed in several centers. The future hope is for the 3D model to be able to be seeded with live cartilage that will reproduce and hold its shape over time so that the patient is not dependent on cartilage availability. The patient can therefore undergo construction sooner than waiting for rib stock to grow; they will not have a donor defect and will have an "implant" that will grow with them proportionally.

BIBLIOGRAPHY

Beahm EK, Walton RL: Auricular reconstruction for microtia part I: anatomy, embryology, and clinical evaluation, *Plast Reconstr Surg* 109(7):2473–2482, 2002.
Brent B: Microtia repair with rib cartilage grafts: a review of personal experience with 1000 cases, *Clin Plast Surg* 29:257–271, 2002.
Firmin F, Marchac A: A novel algorithm for autologous ear reconstruction, *Semin Plast Surg* 25(4):257–264, 2011.
Kamil SH, Vacanti MP, Vacanti CA, et al: Microtia chondrocytes as a donor source for tissue engineered cartilage, *Laryngoscope* 114(12):2187–2190, 2004.
Nagata S: A new method of total reconstruction of the auricle for microtia, *Plast Reconstr Surg* 92:187–201, 1993.
Romo T III, Reitzen SD: Aesthetic microtia reconstruction with Medpor, *Facial Plast Surg* 24:120–128, 2008.
Sorribes MM, Tos M: Nonsurgical treatment of prominent ears with the Auri method, *Arch Otolaryngol Head Neck Surg* 128:1369–1376, 2002.
Walton RL, Beahm EK: Auricular reconstruction for microtia: part II. Surgical techniques, *Plast Reconstr Surg* 110(1):234–249, 2002.
Yotsuyanagi T, Yokoi K, Sawada Y: Nonsurgical treatment of various auricular deformities, *Clin Plast Surg* 29:327–332, 2002.

CHAPTER 56

VASCULAR ANOMALIES

Pamela A. Mudd, MD, MBA and Nancy Bauman, MD

KEY POINTS

1. The head and neck is the most common site for vascular anomalies.
2. Infantile hemangioma is the most common tumor in infancy.
3. Vascular malformations are classified under the International Society for the Study of Vascular Anomalies (ISSVA) classification based on vessel involvement and flow characteristics (capillary, venous, arterial, lymphatic, combination).
4. Indications for treatment of vascular anomalies include impairment of organ or system function, ulceration, hemorrhage, or lesions that may lead to long-term functional or cosmetic problems.
5. Due to the increasingly recognized complexity of vascular anomalies, consultation by a multidisciplinary clinic is recommended to determine optimal workup and to optimize the discussion of prognosis, indications for treatment, and treatment options.

Pearls

1. GLUT-1 positivity distinguishes infantile hemangiomas (IHs) from vascular malformations and other vascular tumors.
2. Propranolol is the first-line treatment for infantile hemangioma (IH) unless contraindications for its use exist.
3. Infantile hemangiomas (IHs) affecting the beard distribution may be associated with subglottic hemangioma.
4. Lymphatic malformations (LMs) are low-flow vascular anomalies and further subclassified as microcystic, macrocystic, and mixed lesions, which affects the treatment of choice.
5. Pulsed- dye laser (PDL) is the treatment of choice for cutaneous capillary malformations such as port-wine stain.

QUESTIONS

1. **What are the four major classification schemes for vascular lesions, and what is the most useful and currently used nomenclature?**
   1. Descriptive
   2. Anatomic-physiologic (microscopic)
   3. Embryologic
   4. Biologic behavior

   Mulliken and Glowacki published a landmark paper in 1982 simplifying the nomenclature of vascular anomalies by classifying them based on cellular turnover and histology, which is most useful in the diagnosis, management, and prognosis of these lesions. The International Society for the Study of Vascular Anomalies (ISSVA) updated its consensus in 2018 to include causal genetic mutations.
   - **Vascular tumors** are characterized by rapidly enlarging endothelial proliferations and, in some cases, may spontaneously involute. These are further classified into benign, locally aggressive, and malignant tumors. This category includes infantile hemangioma (IH).
   - **Vascular malformations** are structural anomalies that are subcategorized based on channel type (simple: capillary, venous, arterial, lymphatic; or combined: combinations of vessel types) and flow characteristics (high vs. low), presence at birth, and growth characteristics. Unlike vascular tumors, there is no cellular proliferation but there may be progressive dilation of vascular channels.

2. **What is the most well-understood somatic genetic association for vascular malformations?**
   Virtually all venous malformations (VMs), lymphatic malformations (LMs), and arteriovenous malformations (AVMs) are now thought due to somatic PIK3CA genetic mutations.

3. **What is the most common tumor of infancy and what is the classic presentation?**
   Infantile hemangioma (IH) is the most common tumor of infancy, with an incidence of 1% to 2.6% at birth and ≈10% by 1 year of age. Eighty percent are noted within the first month of life, typically presenting at 2 to 4 weeks

of life. The female-to-male ratio is 3:1 and 60% occur in the head and neck. Superficial lesions are bright red or crimson, whereas deeper lesions may impart a bluish hue to the overlying skin. IH has a very characteristic cycle involving a proliferative phase (first 8 to 12 month of life), plateau phase, and a slow involution (beginning at about 12 months of age and involuting at variable rates, typically over 5 to 8 years). Most growth occurs during the early part of the proliferative phase and 80% of an infant's IH growth is reached by 5 months of age.

4. **What is the distinguishing cellular marker for hemangioma?**
GLUT-1 (glucose transporter isoform-1) shares common antigenicity to placental tissue and GLUT-1 positivity distinguishes IH from vascular malformations. Congenital hemangiomas, including rapid involuting congenital hemangioma (RICH) and noninvoluting congenital hemangioma (NICH), are GLUT-1 negative. These congenital hemangiomas do not show rapid growth during the first year of life, unlike IH.

5. **What are the indications for treatment for hemangiomas of the head and neck?**
Indications for treatment include functional compromise such as visual impairment, feeding difficulties, or airway compromise. Other indications for intervention include ulceration, bleeding, or infection and those suspected of inducing long-term deformity in cosmetically sensitive areas such as the nose. Psychosocial consequences are also taken into consideration if causing trauma to the patient or the family.

6. **What is the first-line treatment for infantile hemangiomas? What other treatments are available?**
If treatment is indicated, *propranolol* is currently the first-line treatment for infantile hemangiomas unless a contraindication exists. Propranolol is a nonselective betablocker, and although its mechanism of action is not fully understood, its use results in vasoconstriction, reduction of volume, softening, and involution of the lesion. Propranolol is efficacious in approximately 75% of lesions. It is unclear whether propranolol merely hastens involution or alters the natural outcome of the IH. Side effects include bronchospasm, hypoglycemia, GERD, hypotension, and somnolence. Beta blockers inhibit the process of hepatic gluconeogenesis and so should be held if a baby's oral intake is reduced due to gastrointestinal illness to lower the risk of hypoglycemic-induced seizures. Rebound growth of IH lesions is common if beta blocker therapy is stopped during the proliferative phase, so it is typically prescribed for a minimum of 4 months and often continued until the first birthday. All beta blockers do not have a similar efficacy and safety profile and only propranolol is FDA-approved for use in IH.

    Systemic or intralesional *steroids* were the mainstay of therapy prior to the use of propranolol. Systemic steroids afford similar efficacy, although serious adverse events, most commonly reversible growth retardation, are relatively common and make it less favorable than propranolol. Intralesional steroid injections have variable efficacy, often require multiple treatments at 6- to 8-week intervals, and carry a risk of hypopigmentation and atrophy. Periorbital lesions should be treated with caution as intralesional steroid injections around the orbit carry a risk of central retinal artery occlusion.

    Interferon α-2a is an angiostatic agent historically used for IH; however, due to its interference with myelination and the resultant risk of irreversible spastic diplegia when given to young infants in whom myelination is incomplete, it is not an ideal drug for IH.

    Photocoagulation of hemangiomas can be performed with pulsed dye (superficial), argon (ulcerated or active bleeding), and Nd:YAG (deep penetration into dermis) lasers.

    Surgical treatment is usually reserved for symptomatic lesions unresponsive to pharmacologic therapy. However, due to its rapid efficacy, surgical excision may be preferable to pharmacologic therapy in cases such as small eyelid lesions leading to amblyopia or astigmatism or lesions in which early intervention may prevent the development of serious cosmetic deformity. Surgical excision for cosmetic deformity is generally performed closer to 5 years of age when self-image adjusts, although it may be performed earlier if intervention will favorably affect the outcome of involution.

7. **How is beta blocker systemic and topical therapy dosed in infantile hemangiomas?**
The target dose of propranolol ranges from 1 to 3 mg/kg/d, with most practitioners advocating 2 mg/kg/d. Most practitioners start on an outpatient basis at 0.5 to 1.0 mg/kg/d after careful discussion with caretakers to hold propranolol therapy if oral intake is diminished for any reason due to risk of hypoglycemic induced seizures. Although criteria are controversial, in-house initiation may be indicated for babies who are premature; are under 6 weeks of age; have significant comorbidities; have a history of hypoglycemia, hypotension, or bradycardia; have PHACE syndrome; or are victims of poor social situations.

    Topical beta blocker therapy in the form of timolol 0.5% gel-forming solution may be effective in reducing superficial small infantile hemangiomas. Because timolol is systemically absorbed, dosing is generally limited to one drop twice daily for infants weighing ≥ 2 kg.

8. **What are the advantages and limitations of medical treatments for hemangiomas?**
See Table 56.1.

Table 56.1 Medical Treatment of Hemangioma

TREATMENT	MECHANISM OF ACTION	ADVANTAGE	MAJOR SIDE EFFECT(S)
Propranolol	Nonselective beta blocker Vasoconstriction vs. apoptosis effect vs. other	High response; oral medication	Hypotension, hypoglycemia, bronchospasm, sleep disturbance
Corticosteroid	Vasoconstriction vs. down regulation of angiogenic factors (VEGF) vs other	High response; oral medication	Growth retardation, adrenal crisis/Cushing's syndrome, gastric effects
Interferon α-2a	Antiviral angiostatic vs. other	Moderately effective but rarely used due to adverse events	Spastic diplegia (severe and nonreversible)
Vincristine	Chemotherapeutic agent Mitotic inhibition vs. other		Neurotoxic (also requires central access and 4 to 6 months of treatment), severe constipation

9. **What is Kasabach-Merritt syndrome?**
   Kasabach-Merritt syndrome is a complication of rapidly enlarging vascular lesions and is characterized by platelet trapping, hemolytic anemia, thrombocytopenia, and coagulopathy. This phenomenon is not a feature of IH and is most commonly associated with kaposiform hemangioendothelioma and tufted angioma. Many treatment modalities have been tried with varying success, including propranolol, corticosteroids, sirolimus, vincristine, cyclophosphamide, aminocaproic acid, radiation, embolization, and surgery.

10. **What is PHACE syndrome?**
    PHACE is an acronym for posterior fossa malformation, hemangiomas, arterial anomalies, cardiovascular anomalies (coarctation of the aorta), eye abnormalities (coloboma), and sternal abnormalities or ventral developmental defects.
    Any patient with a hemangioma greater than 5 centimeters in diameter should be worked up for PHACE syndrome, particularly for segmental lesions and those in the temporal area. Workup should include ophthalmology and cardiology consultation along with an MRI and MRA of the brain, neck, and aortic arch.
    Beta blocker (propranolol) therapy should be delayed until workup is complete and initiated with caution in patients with suspected PHACE syndrome, due to the low but present risk of ischemic stroke if intracranial arterial disease is present.
    The diagnostic criteria for PHACE syndrome continue to evolve based on major and minor criteria. Of note, approximately 30% of patients with face or scalp hemangioma >5 centimeters in diameter meet diagnostic criteria for PHACE syndrome.

11. **Hemangiomas in the beard distribution carry a risk of which related vascular anomaly? (Fig. 56.1)**
    Hemangiomas in the V3/beard distribution are associated with subglottic hemangioma in approximately 30% of cases. Conversely, approximately 13% of patients with subglottic hemangiomas have an IH in a beard distribution. Subglottic hemangiomas may be unilateral, bilateral, or circumferential. Imaging, typically MRI, is usually recommended to understand the extent of the lesion. Treatment modalities include systemic therapy with propranolol

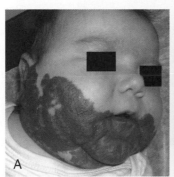 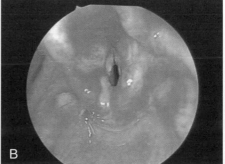

Fig. 56.1 A, Infant with beard distribution (V3) cervicofacial hemangioma. **B,** Segmental airway hemangioma as viewed under microlaryngoscopy in an infant with PHACE syndrome with beard distribution cervicofacial hemangioma. (Courtesy of David Low, MD.)

and/or steroids, local treatment with laser therapy, or surgical excision. A tracheotomy may be required to bypass obstruction in some cases until involution ensues. Observation without intervention of small subglottic hemangiomas in young infants is not advised as the lesions can grow to extreme size during the proliferative phase with minimal symptoms until nearly completely obstructive.

12. **What is a port-wine stain?**
A port-wine stain is a superficial isolated capillary vascular malformation typically present at birth and appearing as a sharply demarcated pink-red patch that darkens over time and grows proportionately with the child. For lesions warranting treatment, pulsed dye laser (PDL) is the gold standard treatment, with improved results if treated early in life. Nevus flammeus, also known as a "stork bite" or "salmon patch," is also a capillary malformation appearing over the nape of the neck or glabellar region that characteristically lightens during the first 2 years of life.

13. **Which syndrome is related to this vascular malformation? (Fig. 56.2)**
Sturge-Weber syndrome, also known as encephalotrigeminal angiomatosis, is characterized by a facial port-wine stain in the V1 (ophthalmic) distribution, glaucoma, bone and/or soft tissue overgrowth, seizures, mental retardation, and dural/leptomeningeal involvement.

14. **Sturge-Weber syndrome and port-wine stain share which genetic abnormality?**
Both Sturge-Weber syndrome and port-wine stains are due to an activating somatic mosaic mutation in the GNAQ gene.

15. **How are lymphatic malformations (LMs) classified? (Fig. 56.3)**
LMs are classified as macrocystic (formerly cystic hygroma), microcystic (formerly termed lymphangioma), or mixed. Macrocystic LM are composed of single or multiple cysts >1 cm³ in size. Microcystic LM are cysts <1 cm³. Mixed LMs contain both macrocystic and microcystic components.
    The de Serres staging system for LM is based on anatomic location and outcome of surgical treatment, with lesions involving bilateral supra- and infrahyoid spaces most difficult to manage. See Table 56.2.

16. **What are the mainstays of treatment for lymphatic malformations?**
Microcystic lesions are often more infiltrative and treatment is usually not curative. Treatment goals are to correct deformity and maintain function via surgery, coblation/radiofrequency, sclerotherapy, or laser excision/reduction. Macrocystic lesions are amenable to treatment with complete surgical excision or sclerosing agents such as doxycycline, bleomycin, ethanol, and OK-432 (picibanil). Acute enlargement of cysts may be secondary to bleeding within the lesion, response to other infectious conditions like viral upper respiratory infections, or acute infection of the cyst contents. Depending on the etiology and severity of associated symptoms, acutely enlarging lymphatic malformations may warrant observation, antibiotics, drainage, and/or systemic steroids. Most lesions return to their

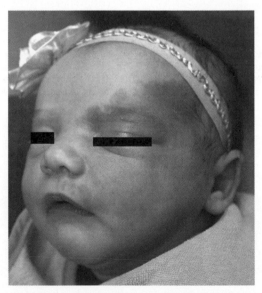

Fig. 56.2 Infant with port-wine stain (capillary vascular malformation) in V1/ophthalmic distribution associated with Sturge-Weber syndrome. (Courtesy of David Low, MD.)

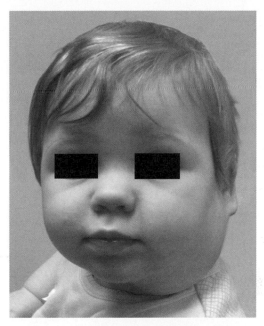

Fig. 56.3 Child with left-sided macrocytic lymphatic malformation. (Courtesy of David Low, MD.)

Table 56.2 de Serres Staging* of Head and Neck Lymphatic Malformations	
Stage 1	Unilateral infrahyoid
Stage 2	Unilateral suprahyoid
Stage 3	Unilateral infrahyoid and suprahyoid
Stage 4	Bilateral infrahyoid
Stage 5	Bilateral infrahyoid and suprahyoid

*From de Serres LM, Sie KC, Richardson MA. Lymphatic malformations of the head and neck. A proposal for staging. *Arch Otolaryngol Head Neck Surg* 121(5):577–582, 1995.

baseline size within 1 to 2 months of acute enlargement. In a Phase 2 trial, sirolimus, an mTOR (mammalian target of rapamycin) inhibitor, showed partial remission of disease in patients with massive lymphatic malformations, venolymphatic malformations, and a variety of other vascular anomalies while receiving ongoing treatment. Careful monitoring for toxicity, particularly of blood/bone marrow, is necessary but rarely requires cessation of treatment.

17. **What is the radiologic workup for lymphatic malformation? (Fig. 56.4)**
MRI with gadolinium and fat suppression, which shows marked high intensity of the homogenous lesion on T2 images, is very suggestive of LM. "Fluid-fluid" levels are commonly seen if there has been bleeding within a lesion. Ultrasound can be useful to assess change in the clinical setting.

18. **Which low-flow vascular malformation tends to involve muscle such as the tongue? (Fig. 56.5)**
Venous malformations tend to involve tongue muscles and may extend deep into the tissue. These lesions tend to swell with activity or in a dependent fashion. They can be painful, may clot, and may have palpable phleboliths (can be identified on US or CT scan). Lymphatic malformations are also seen in the tongue, though less frequently. Microcystic LMs often have a venous appearing exophytic verrucous component that can confuse the diagnosis. Imaging characteristics can help to differentiate venous from lymphatic malformations.

19. **Which high-flow vascular malformation can cause local soft tissue and bony destruction, often presenting in adulthood?**
Arteriovenous malformations (AVMs) are congenital lesions that often become apparent during childhood or early adulthood and grow rapidly during puberty or pregnancy. AVMs are characterized by the presence of a vascular

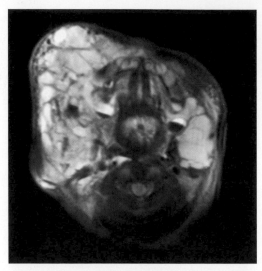

Fig. 56.4 T2-weighted MRI scan of a microcystic lymphatic malformation demonstrating fluid layering. (Courtesy of Children's Hospital of Philadelphia.)

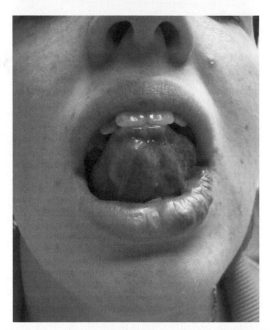

Fig. 56.5 Child with venous malformation affecting the tongue, floor of mouth, and lower lip. (Courtesy of David Low, MD.)

nidus representing a direct communication between arterial and venous systems, without an intervening capillary bed. Depending on the size and location, cure is elusive for many AVMs, as treatment requires complete destruction of the vascular nidus. The Schobinger clinical classification divides AVMs into four stages and aids in determining the appropriate time to pursue treatment. Stage I indicates quiescent vascular-appearing warm lesions that are asymptomatic; Stage II indicates expansion of the lesion with the development of a palpable thrill, audible bruit, and appearance of large, draining tense veins; Stage III is characterized by the onset of destructive local changes; and Stage IV is characterized by development of cardiac failure. More recently, radiologic staging systems have been proposed to better define the nidus characteristics and guide the best treatment or palliative options. Embolization of the nidus by interventional radiology combined, when possible, with surgical excision of the entire lesion is the current mainstay of treatment. The most common AVM embolic agents include ethanol, ethylene vinyl alcohol copolymer (Onyx), and cyanoacrylate.

BIBLIOGRAPHY

Adams DM, Trenor CC III, Hammill AM, et al: Efficacy and safety of sirolimus in the treatment of complicated vascular anomalies, *Pediatrics* 137(2);e20153257, 2016.

Dalakrlshnan K, Bauman N, Chun RH, et al: Standardized outcome and reporting measures in pediatric head and neck lymphatic malformations, *Otolaryngol Head Neck Surg* 152(5):948–953, 2015.

Bauman NM, McCarter RJ, Guzzetta PC, et al: Propranolol vs. prednisolone for symptomatic proliferating infantile hemangiomas: a randomized clinical trial, *JAMA Otolaryngol Head Neck Surg* 140(4):323–330, 2014.

Chang LC, Haggstrom AN, Drolet BA, Baselga E: Growth characteristics of infantile hemangiomas: implications for management, *Pediatrics* 122:360–367, 2008.

Dalla Costa R, Prindaville B, Wiss K: Doing the math: a simple approach to topical timolol dosing for infantile hemangiomas, *Pediatr Dermatol* 35(2):276–277, 2018.

Drolet BA, Frommlt PC, Chamlin SL, et al: Initiation and use of propranolol for infantile hemangioma: report of a consensus conference, *Pediatrics* 131:128–140, 2013.

Eivazi B, Werner JA: Management of vascular malformations and hemangiomas of the head and neck—an update, *Curr Opin Otolaryngol Head Neck Surg* 21(2):157, 2013.

Enjolras O, Wassef M, Mazoyer E, Frieden IJ, Rieu PN: Infants with Kasabach-Merritt syndrome do not have "true" hemangiomas, *J Pediatr* 130(4):631–640, 1997 J Pediatr. 1997 Apr;130(4):631–40.

Espinel AG, Bauman NM: Psychosocial impact of vascular anomalies on children and their families, *Otolaryngol Clin North Am* 51(1):99–110, 2018.

Garzon MC, Epstein LG, Heyer GL, et al: PHACE syndrome: consensus-derived diagnosis and care recommendations, *J Pediatr* 178:24–33, 2016.

Gilbert P, Dubois J, Giroux MF, Soulez G: New treatment approaches to arteriovenous malformations, *Semin Intervent Radiol* 34(3):258–271, 2017.

Glade RS, Richter GT, Jame CA, et al: Diagnosis and management of pediatric cervicofacial venous malformations: retrospective review from a vascular anomalies center, *Laryngoscope* 120(2):229, 2010.

Horbach SER, Rongen APM, O. TM, Waner M, van der Horst CMAM: Outcome measurement for vascular malformations of the head and neck, *Otolaryngol Clin North Am* 51(1):111–117, 2018.

ISSVA Classification of Vascular Anomalies. Available at issva.org/classification.

Kirkorian AY, Grossberg AL, Püttgen KB: Genetic basis for vascular anomalies, *Semin Cutan Med Surg* 35(3):128–136, 2016.

Mulliken JB, Glowacki J: Hemangiomas and vascular malformations in infants and children: a classification based on endothelial characteristics, *Plast Reconstr Surg* 69(3):412, 1982.

Padia R, Bly R, Bull C, Geddis AE, Perkins J: Medical management of vascular anomalies, *Curr Treat Options Pediatr* 4(2):221–236, 2018.

Sajan JA, Tibesar R, Jabbour N, et al: Assessment of pulsed-dye laser therapy for pediatric cutaneous vascular anomalies, *JAMA Facial Plast Surg* 15(6):434–438, 2013.

Tlougan BE, Lee MT, Drolet BA, et al: Medical management of tumors associated with Kasabach-Merritt phenomenon: an expert survey, *J Pediatr Hematol Oncol* 35(8):618–622, 2013.

CHAPTER 57

PEDIATRIC HEAD AND NECK TUMORS

Todd M. Wine, MD

KEY POINTS

1. The location of a neck mass is key to understanding the differential diagnosis.
2. Imaging studies are important in the evaluation of many masses of the head and neck.
3. A neck mass that presents with infectious symptoms may be due to an infected congenital lesion.
4. The choice of treatment of atypical mycobacterial infections of the neck must always consider the risks of the treatment versus the negative quality of life related to a prolonged neck mass and/or drainage.
5. Fine needle aspiration can often identify benign and malignant masses, but many masses will require a core or open biopsy for definitive diagnosis.

Pearls

1. The most common mass in the neck in children is a reactive lymph node. Lymphomas are the most common malignancy seen in the neck in children.
2. The key to a Sistrunk procedure is not just resecting the central portion of the hyoid bone but resecting tongue musculature between the hyoid bone and foramen cecum.

QUESTIONS

1. **What are the categories of neck masses in children that are important when creating a differential diagnosis?**
   - *Congenital neck masses* are those that are present at birth and secondary to defects occurring in embryology.
   - *Infectious neck masses* are those that present due to an infection and typically resolve with treatment of the infection. These are most commonly infected or reactive lymph nodes but can also occur in other tissues in the head and neck such as the salivary glands.
   - *Inflammatory masses* that do not have a known infectious cause such as those associated with Kawasaki's disease.
   - *Neoplastic lesions* of the neck including benign and malignant processes. These encompass malignant lymphadenopathy, benign and malignant salivary gland tumors, benign and malignant thyroid tumors, and tumors originating from neurologic, muscular, vascular, lymphatic, cartilaginous, or osseus tissues.
   - *Vascular malformations* (see Chapter 54).

2. **Which is the most common neck mass in children?**
   An enlarged lymph node is the most common reason that a child presents with a neck mass. The most common cause of enlarged lymphadenopathy is infection, either viral or bacterial. Viral causes of lymphadenopathy include adenovirus, rhinovirus, and enterovirus, which can all occur with a viral upper respiratory infection. Epstein-Barr virus causes mononucleosis, which consists of cervical lymphadenopathy, exudative tonsillitis, and hepatosplenomegaly.
   Bacterial causes of an enlarged lymph node most commonly include infections due to *Staphylococcus aureus* and *Streptococcus pyogenes*. Sometimes, the infected lymph node can suppurate and create a neck abscess. Other significant causes of bacterial lymphadenitis are atypical mycobacterium, *Bartonella henselae* (cat-scratch disease), and tuberculosis.

3. **Which presenting features suggest an acute infectious cause of a neck mass?**
   Fever, pain, acute swelling, erythema of the overlying skin, decreased neck range of motion, and odynophagia can indicate that a neck mass is secondary to an infectious cause. Concomitant upper respiratory tract symptoms, exposure to sick contacts, foreign travel, exposure to animals (cats, ticks), and the presence of immunodeficiency are all important historical features that can allow better understanding of the etiology of a neck mass.

4. **Which other type of neck lesions can present with an acute infection or inflammation?**
Congenital lesions including thyroglossal duct cysts, dermoid cysts, branchial cleft cysts, vascular malformations, and preauricular cysts can often present with acute swelling, erythema, pain, and fevers. The preferred treatment of these infectious exacerbations is antibiotic therapy. Incision and drainage should be performed only if necessary because they may complicate the definitive resection of the congenital mass. The resection of a congenital lesion is more easily accomplished after complete resolution of the infection.

5. **Which congenital neck masses occur in the midline neck?**
Thyroglossal duct cyst is the most common congenital neck mass. Thyroglossal duct cysts occur in the midline due to incomplete obliteration of the thyroglossal duct. The median thyroid anlage starts at the foramen cecum of the tongue and migrates caudally in the neck until it reaches its final anatomic position near the cricoid cartilage. The thyroglossal duct should obliterate, but occasionally this process is incomplete. A cyst can then form at that location with a tract that connects the cyst to the foramen cecum. Ectopic thyroid tissue can occur anywhere from the foramen cecum to the normal position of the thyroid gland.

   Dermoid cysts are benign cystic structures that can occur anywhere in the body. They frequently occur in the head and neck and can occur in the midline neck and mimic a thyroglossal duct cyst. Other common locations include the nose, oral cavity, orbit, and nasopharynx. Dermoid cysts arise due to entrapment of epithelial cells along lines of fusion. They usually contain other skin appendages including sebaceous glands, hair, or hair follicles. They can often be adherent to the overlying skin and may even have a small draining sinus.

   Teratomas are similar to dermoid cysts, with the exception that they contain cell types of ectodermal, mesodermal, and endodermal origin. They may present as a firm neck mass and can cause respiratory symptoms when they are very large. Treatment requires complete surgical excision.

   Laryngoceles occur as midline neck masses when they herniate through the thyrohyoid membrane (external laryngocele). If confined to the larynx, it is an internal laryngocele and will not likely present as a mass. Symptoms include hoarseness, dysphagia, and severe dyspnea, particularly when presenting in a neonate.

6. **What is the significance of the Sistrunk procedure used to resect a thyroglossal duct cyst?**
The earliest reports of thyroglossal duct cyst excision were plagued by a rate of recurrence as high as 50%. Resection of the hyoid bone along with cyst improved recurrence rates to 20%. Walter Sistrunk expanded that technique to include resection of the cyst, hyoid bone, and suprahyoid tongue musculature to ensure that the tract(s) connecting the cyst to the foramen cecum was adequately resected. This decreased the recurrence rate to near 5%. Removal of the cuff of lingual musculature is important because the tract may pass anterior or posterior to the hyoid and may be multiple.

7. **Which congenital neck masses occur in the lateral neck?**
Congenital lateral neck masses are most likely to be of branchial origin. Otherwise, congenital lateral neck masses can include vascular malformations and thymic cysts. Branchial anomalies presenting as a mass are most likely to be a cyst with or without a sinus, which may connect it to the skin or to an internal structure. Branchial anomalies are classified by their branchial origin. They can be first, second, third, or fourth branchial anomalies.

   The most common branchial anomaly is a second branchial cleft cyst. Second branchial cleft cysts occur in the upper neck and present as a cystic mass anterior to the sternocleidomastoid muscle. They can present as an acute, painful swelling of the neck that follows upper respiratory tract symptoms and often be confused with a suppurative lymph node. The differentiation between these two entities can be difficult, but imaging with contrast-enhanced computed tomography may be helpful. The infected cyst will have a circumferential thin wall compared to a thicker wall with more surrounding inflammation of an abscess.

   The second most common branchial anomaly is a first branchial cleft cyst. These occur in the infraauricular region and may occur anterior, inferior, or posterior to the lobule. These can be associated with the facial nerve and resection requires dissection of the facial nerve.

   Least common are branchial anomalies of the third and fourth arches, which typically present as left-sided infections in the lower neck. Thyroiditis may occur in the setting of a fourth branchial cleft cyst as the tract should extend through the thyroid gland. These cysts will often have a connection to the piriform sinus. Proper resection of a fourth arch anomaly requires hemithyroidectomy; otherwise, recurrence is more likely.

   Thymic cysts can occur in the lateral neck as thymic tissue originates from the third branchial arch and descends into the mediastinum via the thymopharyngeal duct. Thymic cysts usually occur in the left neck and can be unilocular or multilocular. The diagnosis is confirmed on pathology with the presence of Hassall corpuscles (concentric epithelioreticular cells and macrophages in the medulla).

   Vascular malformations are discussed in greater detail in Chapter 54. These include a range of pathologies that include venous malformation, lymphatic malformation, venolymphatic malformation, and arteriovenous malformation. These classically present in the posterior triangle of the neck.

8. **How does an atypical mycobacterial infection present?**
Atypical mycobacterium infections in the neck often present with a mass that is often firm, nontender, and located in the submandibular or preauricular regions. Classically, there is a violaceous discoloration to the overlying

skin. The skin may be thin with areas of fluctuance. Typically, there is no preceding illness, fever, weight loss, or night sweats. An intradermal tuberculin test will usually be negative or indeterminate. Computed tomography and magnetic resonance imaging may suggest an infectious cause by revealing fat stranding, a thick wall of the abscess cavity (if present), inflammation of the skin, and multiloculated appearance, although they are not diagnostic.

The clinical course may start as a discrete mass in the submandibular or periauricular regions. A course of antibiotics will have no significant effect. The mass may continue to enlarge, and it is not uncommon for violaceous skin changes to occur overlying a fluctuant component of the mass. The fluctuant area may progress to the point that the skin breaks down and a draining wound is created. The natural history is that this infection is self-limited and will heal without treatment. Unfortunately, the natural history is not typically expedient and may take many months to a couple of years for resolution.

9. **What are the treatment considerations for atypical mycobacterium?**
Treatment options consist of observation, medical management with antibiotics, surgical curettage, surgical excision, or any combination of these. The optimal treatment would be one that eradicates the disease quickly and does so with minimal short- and long-term risk to the patient. Prompt eradication is expected if complete surgical excision is performed. As such, many studies have supported complete excision as the optimal treatment for quicker time to resolution and better cosmetic outcomes. Unfortunately, the disease process often closely encounters the facial nerve or its branches. Complete excision can be associated with temporary nerve injury in approximately 20% to 30% and permanent nerve injury in 2% to 5% of cases. Other outcomes include higher incidence of poor scarring (21%), wound infection (14%), and recurrence (9%). While the risk of permanent injury is low, the risk is significant considering that the disease resolves, albeit more slowly, without surgery.

If complete surgical excision is deemed too risky, other treatment options consist of surgical incision and curettage of the purulent portion of the mass. This can help confirm the diagnosis and may help treat a draining or "about to drain" wound. Curettage may help decrease the duration of the draining wound.

Medical therapy with various antibiotics (clarithromycin, azithromycin, ethambutol, and rifabutin) may be helpful and antimicrobial therapy can be utilized alone or in combination with surgical treatment. The use of medical therapy is often debated, however, as there has been no research proving its efficacy over observation. Observation alone allows the disease to take its expectant course and most patients will have resolved the infection by 1 year.

10. **What is the differential for inflammatory but noninfectious lymphadenopathy?**
Kawasaki disease, also known as mucocutaneous lymph node syndrome, typically occurs in children aged less than 5 years. It is considered a vasculitis and presents with high fever for 5 days and four of the following signs: acute cervical adenopathy, nonexudative conjunctivitis, strawberry tongue, lip fissure, rash, erythema of palms and soles, edema of hands and feet, and desquamation. It may cause coronary artery aneurysm and cardiologic evaluation is necessary. Treatment consists of intravenous immunoglobulins and aspirin.

PFAPA (periodic fevers with aphthous stomatitis, pharyngitis, and cervical adenitis) causes recurrent high fever in children typically aged less than 5 years without signs of concomitant upper respiratory infections. Between episodes, they are likely asymptomatic. Diagnosis must rule out other causes of recurrent fevers and medical treatment can be helpful (steroids and/or cimetidine). Tonsillectomy is often curative.

Castleman disease is giant lymph node hyperplasia that causes concern due to the large size of lymph nodes. Fortunately, it is benign and excisional biopsy can be both diagnostic and curative.

Rosai-Dorfman disease consists of massive lymphadenopathy due to sinus histiocytosis occurring in patients aged less than 10 years. Diagnosis is made on biopsy of a lymph node. Treatment can be observational, but surgery, radiation, and chemotherapy may also play roles depending on severity of the disease.

Kikuchi-Fujimoto disease is a histiocytic necrotizing lymphadenitis typically occurring in 20- to 40-year-olds and may be unilateral or bilateral. Biopsy of the lymph node is required for diagnosis and resolution occurs in approximately 6 months.

11. **What are the reassuring sonographic findings of lymph nodes?**
   - Hypoechoic to muscle
   - Flat, oval-shaped, short axis:long axis <0.5, although submandibular and parotid nodes may be rounder
   - Echogenic hilum
   - Hilar vascularity seen in reactive or normal node
   - Surrounding edema
   - Sharp margins

12. **What are the sonographic features of malignant nodes?**
   - Markedly hypoechoic to muscle (except if papillary thyroid cancer)
   - Round shape
   - No echogenic hilus
   - Coagulation necrosis

- Eccentric cortical hypertrophy
- Cystic necrosis
- Ill-defined borders
- Peripheral or mixed vascularity
- Calcifications suggest metastatic thyroid cancer
- No surrounding inflammation

13. **Which is the most likely malignant pathology type found in the head and neck?**
Lymphomas (Hodgkin and non-Hodgkin) are the most common malignancy in the head and neck. Enlargement of lymph nodes is very common in children, and when it is not reactive lymphadenopathy, lymphoma is the primary pathology that must be considered. Ultrasound can be reassuring when a normal-appearing fatty hilum is identified. Otherwise, a persistently enlarged lymph node without resolution in time or antibiotic course may warrant biopsy to investigate further. Fine needle aspiration can often diagnose if a malignancy is present, but usually flow cytometry of a lymph node that has been completely excised is required to make the specific diagnosis that can help clarify the treatment of choice.

14. **Which is the most likely type of thyroid malignancy in a child?**
Papillary thyroid carcinoma is the most common thyroid malignancy in adults and children. Papillary thyroid carcinoma presents with a painless, firm thyroid nodule. Usually the nodule will be cystic and nonfunctioning. Fine needle aspiration is recommended to achieve the diagnosis. Suspicious lymph nodes in the central and lateral neck compartments should be biopsied at the same time. Nodal metastasis is quite common, but overall survival remains high (2.5% mortality). Treatment is most often total thyroidectomy with central and/or lateral neck dissections for biopsy for proven or highly suspicious lymph nodes, followed by radioactive iodine ablation.

15. **What are the common infectious or inflammatory lesions of salivary glands?**
Acute bacterial sialadenitis, viral sialadenitis, and juvenile recurrent parotitis. Acute bacterial sialadenitis occurs as unilateral, painful swelling with purulent drainage coming from the salivary duct. Treatment is with hydration, warm compress, massage, and sialogogues. Viral sialadenitis can occur due to coxsackievirus, cytomegalovirus, parainfluenza, or mumps.

16. **What pathologies are causes of benign salivary gland tumors?**
In children, the most common benign tumors are pleomorphic adenoma occurring in the parotid, submandibular, and minor salivary glands and hemangioma occurring in the parotid gland. Other benign pathologies exist and include Warthin's tumors (papillary cystadenoma lymphomatosum), basal cell adenoma, myoepithelioma, and lymphoepithelioma.
    Hemangioma of the parotid gland, and submandibular gland less commonly, presents at birth or shortly thereafter. Like hemangiomas occurring elsewhere, there is a rapid proliferative phase that occurs in the first few months of life followed by slow involution over a period of one to many years. Treatment of hemangioma classically is to allow involution over time and to medically treat with propranolol for more symptomatic lesions. Prior to propranolol, steroids and interferon were used. Surgical resection of hemangioma of the parotid gland is also an option but must be carefully considered due to an increased risk to the facial nerve.

17. **What pathologies are the most common causes of malignant salivary gland tumors?**
Mucoepidermoid carcinoma, acinic cell carcinoma, adenocarcinoma, adenoid cystic carcinomas, and carcinoma ex pleomorphic are possible salivary malignancies in childhood. Mucoepidermoid carcinoma is the most common malignant salivary mass in children, typically presenting in adolescence. Like benign tumors, treatment is with complete surgical excision with margins if possible. Neck dissection will be required in some malignancies, particularly if the lesion is of higher grade, lymph nodes are clinically suspicious, or there is evidence that the tumor has extraglandular extension or facial nerve invasion. Adjuvant radiotherapy is used if there is significant nodal involvement, extraglandular extension, perineural invasion, or incomplete excision. The risks and benefits of radiotherapy must be carefully considered in children due to the risk of second malignancy and other complications of radiation therapy.

18. **Which is the most common type of sarcoma occurring in the head and neck of children?**
Rhabdomyosarcoma (RMS) is the most common sarcoma occurring in the head and neck region of children. Approximately one third of RMS occurs in the head and neck, and within the head and neck the orbit is the most common site. The presenting symptoms will depend on the site of origin for the tumor. Tumors can be classified as parameningeal, which implies that they arise either along the anterior or lateral skull base, or nonparameningeal, occurring in oro/hypopharynx, parotid, external ear, or lateral neck. Ideally, complete surgical resection with wide margins results in the best long-term prognosis. Unfortunately, in the head and neck, wide margins are rarely possible without major functional impairment. Thus initial treatment involves obtaining tissue diagnosis. Although fine needle aspiration may identify a sarcoma, more detailed histologic typing by a pathologist experienced in sarcomas is required to allow proper treatment decisions. Therefore core or open biopsies are often required. Treatment

of head and neck sarcomas will often consist of chemotherapy (directed by the Intergroup Rhabdomyosarcoma Studies [IRS] protocols for rhabdomyosarcomas or Children's Oncology Group [COG] protocols for nonrhabdomyosarcomas), surgery, and radiation therapy.

19. **What are the other types of sarcoma?**
Fibrosarcoma, onrhabdomyosarcoma, hemangiopericytoma, osteosarcoma, chondrosarcoma, extraskeletal Ewing sarcoma, liposarcoma, and leiomyosarcoma.

20. **What are the types of neuroblastic neck masses?**
Neuroblastic masses include ganglioneuroma, ganglioneuroblastoma, and neuroblastoma. Neuroblastoma is the most common of these lesions and is the third most common malignancy in children. These three pathologies represent different stages of the same disease process, with neuroblastoma being the least differentiated, with the most malignant potential, and ganglioneuroma being the most differentiated, with likely no malignant potential. Typically, these are painless neck masses and symptoms are related to nerve (cranial nerves, sympathetic chain) or aerodigestive tract compression.

21. **What is the importance of creating a differential diagnosis as it pertains to investigating a neck mass?**
Creating an appropriate differential diagnosis for each patient presenting with a neck mass allows judicious consideration for the appropriate diagnostic tests to order, whether laboratory assessment or radiographic imaging. The history should dictate which imaging modality should be utilized, and this is particularly important when considering computed tomography scans. Through the cumulative effects of radiation exposure, two to three computed tomography scans of the head can increase the risk of brain cancer three-fold and 5 to 10 head CTs may increase risk of leukemia three-fold. As such, special consideration should be taken when considering each imaging study.

BIBLIOGRAPHY

Acierno SP, Waldhausen JH: Congenital cervical cysts, sinuses and fistulae, *Otolaryngol Clin North Am* 40(1):161–176, 2007.
Anne S, Teot LA, Mandell DL: Fine needle aspiration biopsy: role in diagnosis of pediatric head and neck masses, *Int J Pediatr Otorhinolaryngol* 72(10):1547–1553, 2008.
Fang QG, Shi S, Li ZN, et al: Epithelial salivary gland tumors in children: a twenty-five-year experience of 122 patients, *Int J Pediatr Otorhinolaryngol* 77(8):1252–1254, 2013.
Giacomini CP, Jeffrey RB, Shin LK: Ultrasonographic evaluation of malignant and normal cervical lymph nodes, *Semin Ultrasound CT MR* 34(3):236–247, 2013.
Huh WW, Fitzgerald N, Mahajan A, et al: Pediatric sarcomas and related tumors of the head and neck, *Cancer Treat Rev* 37(6):431–439, 2011.
Lee DH, Yoon TM, Lee JK, et al: Clinical utility of fine needle aspiration cytology in pediatric parotid tumors, *Int J Pediatr Otorhinolaryngol* 77(8):1272–1275, 2013.
Lindeboom JA, Kuijper EJ, Bruijnesteijn van Coppenraet ES, et al: Surgical excision versus antibiotic treatment for nontuberculous mycobacterial cervicofacial lymphadenitis in children: a multicenter, randomized, controlled trial, *Clin Infect Dis* 44(8):1057–1064, 2007.
Lindeboom JA, Lindeboom R, Bruijnesteijn van Coppenraet ES, et al: Esthetic outcome of surgical excision versus antibiotic therapy for nontuberculous mycobacterial cervicofacial lymphadenitis in children, *Pediatr Infect Dis J* 28(11):1028–1130, 2009.
Maddalozzo J, Alderfer J, Modi V: Posterior hyoid space as related to excision of the thyroglossal duct cyst, *Laryngoscope* 120(9): 1773–1778, 2010.
Moukheiber AK, Nicollas R, Roman S, et al: Primary pediatric neuroblastic tumors of the neck, *Int J Pediatr Otorhinolaryngol* 60(2): 155–161, 2001.
Owusu JA, Parker NP, Rimell FL: Postoperative facial nerve function in pediatric parotidectomy: a 12-year review, *Otolaryngol Head Neck Surg* 148(2):249–252, 2013.
Parker NP, Scott AR, Finkelstein M, et al: Predicting surgical outcomes in pediatric cervicofacial nontuberculous mycobacterial lymphadenitis, *Ann Otol Rhinol Laryngol* 121(7):478–484, 2012.
Pearce MS, Salotti JA, Little MP, et al: Radiation exposure from CT scans in childhood and subsequent risk of leukaemia and brain tumours: a retrospective cohort study, *Lancet* 380(9840):499–505, 2012.
Wei JL, Bond J, Sykes KJ, et al: Treatment outcomes for nontuberculous mycobacterial cervicofacial lymphadenitis in children based on the type of surgical intervention, *Otolaryngol Head Neck Surg* 138(5):566–571, 2008.
Whittemore KR Jr, Cunningham MJ: Malignant tumors of the head and neck. In: Bluestone C, Healy G, Simons J, eds: *Pediatric Otolaryngology,* 2014 Peoples Medical Publishing House, pp 1803.
Zeharia A, Eidlitz-Markus T, Haimi-Cohen Y, et al: Management of nontuberculous mycobacteria-induced cervical lymphadenitis with observation alone, *Pediatr Infect Dis J* 27(10):920–922, 2008.

FACIAL PLASTIC AND RECONSTRUCTIVE ANATOMY AND EMBRYOLOGY WITH RADIOLOGIC CORRELATES

CHAPTER 58

Fiyin Sokoya, MD and Adam M. Terella, MD

KEY POINTS

1. Formation of the head and neck structures is intimately related to the development of the pharyngeal arches, with each arch carrying an artery, nerve, cartilaginous bar, and muscle.
2. Palate formation requires midline fusion of the medial nasal prominences and palatal shelves. Incomplete fusion results in a spectrum of cleft palate deformities.
3. The superficial muscular aponeurotic system (SMAS) represents a discrete fascial layer that separates the subcutaneous fat from the underlying parotidomasseteric fascia and facial nerve.
4. When operating on the face, if dissection is kept superficial to the superficially situated musculature, the facial nerve should not be harmed.
5. When completing a facial fracture repair, it is often necessary to reestablish the vertical buttresses with rigid fixation.

Pearls
1. The forehead is composed of five anatomic layers, described by the mnemonic "SCALP." Identification of these layers is important for both cosmetic and reconstructive procedures in this region.
2. The galea aponeurosis can serve as a tension-bearing layer during scalp reconstruction.
3. The majority of facial mimetic muscles are superficially situated and receive facial nerve innervation from their deep surface.
4. With progressive age, descent of the suborbicularis orbital fat pad (SOOF) structures leads to deepening of the nasolabial crease.

QUESTIONS

APPLIED EMBRYOLOGY

1. **What are the pharyngeal arches? How are they significant to head and neck development?**
   Formation of the head and neck structures is intimately related to the development of the pharyngeal arches, with each arch carrying an artery, nerve, cartilaginous bar, and muscle. The formation of these arches begins at approximately 20 days of gestation, and by 28 days, five arches are visible. Each arch is lined by ectoderm and inside houses mesoderm and neural crest cells, which form an artery, nerve, cartilaginous bar, and muscle. Of note, the first arch cartilage develops into the maxillary process and mandible and carries the mandibular branch of the trigeminal nerve, the internal maxillary artery, and the muscles of mastication. The second arch carries CN 7 (facial nerve), the stapedial artery, and the muscles of facial expression.

2. **What primitive structures contribute to the formation of the face?**
   At the end of the fourth embryonic week, neural crest–derived facial prominences appear from the first pair of pharyngeal arches. Maxillary prominences are found laterally. The frontal nasal prominences develop into the forehead and frontal nasal process. On either side of the frontal nasal prominences are local thickenings that form nasal placodes. These placodes invaginate to form nasal pits and ultimately ridges of tissue that can be divided into lateral nasal prominence and medial nasal prominence (Table 58.1 and Fig. 58.1).

3. **How and when is the upper lip formed?**
   At approximately 6 weeks postconception, the paired maxillary prominences grow medially and contact the paired medial nasal prominences. As fusion of these structures occurs, the upper lip is formed. Ultimately, the maxillary prominences form the lateral lip and the medial nasal prominences form the philtrum, medial upper lip, columella, and nasal tip.

Table 58.1 Structures That Contribute to the Formation of the Face

PROMINENCE	STRUCTURES FORMED
Frontonasal	Forehead, bridge of the nose, medial and lateral nasal prominences
Maxillary	Cheeks, lateral portion of the upper lip
Medial nasal	Philtrum of the upper lip, crest, and tip of the nose
Lateral nasal	Alae of the nose
Mandibular	Lower lip

(From Wang TD and Milczuk HA: Cleft lip and palate. In: Lesperance MM, Flint PW, eds: *Cummings – Pediatric Otolaryngology*, Philadelphia, 2015, Saunders Elsevier.)

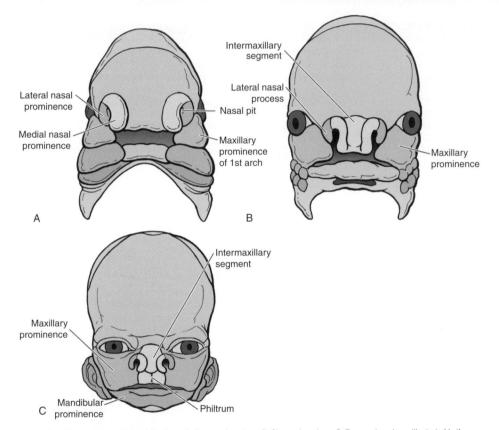

Fig. 58.1 Developmental anatomy of the face. A, Five-week embryo. **B,** Six-week embryo. **C,** Ten-week embryo. Illustrated is the relationship of the maxillary prominence and the nasal placodes, contributing to the lateral and medial nasal prominence. (From Chen EY, Sie KC: Developmental anatomy. In Lesperance MM, Flint PW, eds: *Cummings – Pediatric Otolaryngology*, Philadelphia, 2015, Saunders Elsevier.)

4. **Discuss the embryology of the nose.**
   In the 7-week embryo, five facial prominences contribute to the formation of the nose: the frontal nasal prominence, the paired medial nasal prominences, and the paired lateral nasal prominences. The frontal nasal prominence forms the nasal bridge, the medial nasal prominences fuse and form the nasal tip and columella, and the lateral nasal prominence forms the nasal alae.

5. **How is the primary palate (intermaxillary segment) formed?**
   Formation of the palate begins concurrently with the formation of the upper lip and nose at the end of the fifth week. In addition to contributing to the nose and upper lip, fusion of the two medial nasal prominences forms the intermaxillary segment. The *primary palate* includes the hard palate anterior to the incisive foramen.

6. **What is the secondary palate, and how is it formed?**
   The *secondary palate* refers to the portions of the palate posterior to the incisive foramen. It is formed by the medial migration and midline fusion of the two palatine shelves around the seventh week. These shelves are extensions of the maxillary prominences. Midline fusion proceeds from anterior to posterior, ending with creation of the uvula.

7. **Failed fusion of the intermaxillary segment to the maxillary prominences results in what deformity?**
   Failure of fusion of the intermaxillary segment and maxillary prominence results in cleft lip deformity. There is a wide spectrum of cleft lip deformities, including unilateral versus bilateral cleft lip and complete versus incomplete cleft lip.

8. **Failure of fusion of the palatal shelves will result in what deformity?**
   Failed fusion of the palatal shelves, and thus the secondary palate, results in a spectrum of palatal cleft abnormalities. The mildest form of the soft palate cleft is bifid uvula. A submucous cleft occurs when there is midline dehiscence of the palate musculature but the mucosa remains intact. The most extensive cleft is a bilateral complete cleft of the palate in which the vomer and premaxilla do not fuse with the palatal shelves.

9. **Discuss the embryologic development of the pinna**
   The pinna develops from the first (mandibular) and second (hyoid) branchial arches. Each arch contributes three *hillocks*. Traditionally it was thought that specific hillocks gave rise to specific ear anatomy, but there is now some debate on the subject. However, it is classically taught that the first hillock gives rise to the tragus. The second and third hillocks form the crus helicis. The fourth and fifth hillocks become the crura anthelicis and helix, respectively. The sixth hillock forms the antitragus.

10. **Developmental error in hillock formation and/or fusion results in what malformation?**
    Microtia is a malformation of the auricle. There can be a wide spectrum of presentation ranging from a small external ear with minimal structural abnormality to an ear with major external, middle, and inner ear structural aberrations including absence of the ear (anotia).

APPLIED ANATOMY

11. **What are the layers of the forehead and scalp?**
    The layers of the forehead are in continuity with layers in the scalp. An effective mnemonic, "SCALP," describes the five anatomic layers: (S) skin, (C) subcutaneous tissue, (A) galea aponeurosis, (L) loose areolar tissue, and (P) pericranium. The galea aponeurosis is a discrete fibrous layer that is important during both cosmetic and reconstructive procedures. This layer surrounds the entire skull and divides to envelope the frontalis and occipitalis muscles. It is continuous with the temporoparietal fascia (TPF) below the temporal line.

12. **Which four muscles are responsible for forehead and eyebrow movement?**
    The frontalis, procerus, paired corrugator supercilii, and paired orbicularis oculi muscles each independently contribute to brow positioning and forehead/glabellar rhytids. It is useful to classify these muscles as brow elevators or brow depressors. The frontalis muscle is the primary and sole elevator of the brow. The procerus, corrugator supercilii, and orbicularis oculi all act as brow depressors.

13. **What is the superficial muscular aponeurotic system (SMAS)?**
    The SMAS represents a discrete fascial layer that separates the subcutaneous fat from the underlying parotidomasseteric fascia and facial nerve. In the temporal region the SMAS is continuous with the temporal parietal fascia (TPF), and in the neck, it is continuous with the platysma. This layer is important in many facial plastic surgery procedures, such as face lifting (rhytidectomy) and soft tissue reconstruction, and represents an important surgical landmark.

14. **Describe the anatomic structures contributing to the malar prominence**
    The malar prominence is formed by the subcutaneous malar fat pad, which overlies the orbicularis oculi muscle. Deep to this muscle is the suborbicularis orbital fat pad (SOOF). With progressive age, the descent of these structures leads to deepening of the nasolabial crease.

15. **What is the relationship of the facial mimetic muscles to the facial nerve? Why is this anatomic relationship important?**
    The orbicularis oculi, platysma, and zygomaticus major and minor are considered superficially situated facial mimetic muscles and receive innervation from the facial nerve. These superficially situated muscles receive innervation from the deep surface.

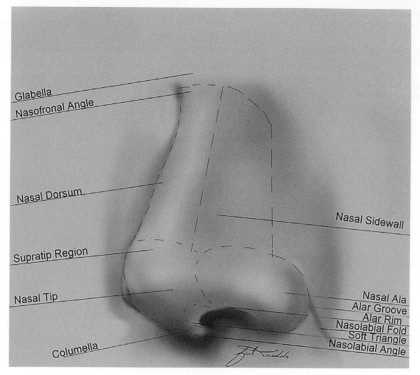

Fig. 58.2 Nasal aesthetic subunits and important external landmarks. (From Joseph AW, Truesdale C, Baker SR: Reconstruction of the nose, *Facial Plast Surg Clin North Am* 2019 Feb;27(1):43-54.)

16. **Which facial mimetic muscles receive innervation from the superficial surface?**
    Only the buccinators, levator anguli oris, and mentalis muscle lie in a plane deep to the facial nerve and thus receive innervation from the superficial surface.

17. **What is the primary blood supply to the face?**
    The primary arterial supply to the face consists of branches from the facial artery, which is a branch of the external carotid artery. The facial artery ascends over the body of the mandible anterior to the masseter muscle. It has a tortuous course, which is thought to help accommodate movement of the underlying mandible. As the facial artery passes across the face, branches of the facial nerve cross it superficially. The facial artery gives off several branches, including the superior and inferior labial arteries to the upper and lower lips and the angular artery to the lateral soft tissue envelope of the nose.

SURFACE ANATOMY

18. **What are the facial esthetic units?**
    The face can be divided into, and evaluated by, individual esthetic units. These esthetic units include the forehead and brow, periorbital region, cheeks, nose, perioral region, chin, and neck.

19. **What are the esthetic subunits of the nose?**
    There are nine esthetic units of the nose, including the nasal tip, dorsum, columella, paired sidewalls, paired alae, and paired soft tissue facets (Fig. 58.2). These esthetic subunits were proposed based on the observation that the nasal surface is made up of several concave and convex surfaces separated from one another by ridges and valleys.

20. **Describe the surface anatomy of the pinna.**
    The surface anatomy of the pinna can be organized into a series of fossae and prominences, or ridges, as illustrated in Fig. 58.3. The four fossae include the triangular fossa, concha cymba, concha cavum, and scaphoid fossa. The primary prominences include the helix, antihelix, crus, tragus, antitragus, and lobule.

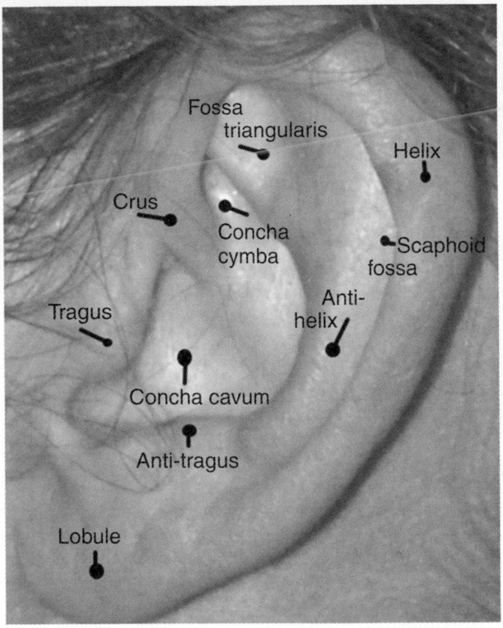

Fig. 58.3 The surface anatomy of the pinna is described as a series of prominences and depressions.

BIBLIOGRAPHY

Baker S: *Local Flaps in Facial Reconstruction*, 2nd ed, Philadelphia, 2007, Mosby.

Burget GC, Menick FJ: The subunit principle in nasal reconstruction, *Plast Reconstr Surg* 76(2):239–247, 1985.

Friedman O, Wang TD, Milczuk H: Cleft lip and palate. In: Flint PW, Haughey BH, Lund VJ, et al, eds: *Cummings Otolaryngology—Head & Neck Surgery*, 5th ed, Philadelphia, 2010, Mosby Elsevier.

Joseph AW, Truesdale C, Baker SR: Reconstruction of the nose, *Facial Plast Surg Clin North Am* 27(1):43–54, 2019.

Manson PN, Hoopes JE, Su CT: Structural pillars of the facial skeleton: an approach to the management of Le Fort fractures, *Plast Reconstr Surg* 66(1):54–62, 1980.

Ruder RO: Congenital malformation of the auricle. In: Papel ID, et al, eds: *Facial Plastic and Reconstructive Surgery*, 2nd ed, New York, 2002, Thieme.

Som PM, Naidich TP: Illustrated review of the embryology and development of the facial region, part 1: early face and lateral nasal cavities, *Am J Neuroradiol* 34(12):2233–2240, 2013.

Terella AM, Wang TD: Technical considerations in endoscopic brow lift. In: Azizzadeh B, Massry GG, eds: *Clinics in Plastic Surgery. Brow and Upper Eyelid Surgery: Multispecialty Approach*, Philadelphia, 2013, Elsevier.

Wang TD, Milczuk HA: Cleft Lip and palate. In: Lesperance MM, Flint PW, eds: *Cummings–Pediatric Otolaryngology*, Philadelphia, 2015, Saunders Elsevier.

CHAPTER 59

PRINCIPLES OF WOUND HEALING

Mofiyinfolu Sokoya, MD and Andrew A. Winkler, MD

KEY POINTS

1. The tenets of Halstead are highly important in good surgical wound healing.
2. Wound healing occurs in overlapping phases: inflammatory, proliferative, and remodeling phases.
3. A patient's metabolic issues should always be addressed to promote ideal wound healing. It is wise to prescribe a daily multivitamin.
4. Wounds heal best when kept continually moist (white petrolatum ointment), clean, and protected.
5. Keloid scars grow outside the border of the initial wound.

Pearls
1. Scar revision timing: most scars improve in appearance without revision 1 to 3 years after the inciting event. Patients should be counseled to wait at least 6 to 12 months before undergoing a scar revision surgery, unless there are obvious scar characteristics that are not expected to improve.
2. Dermabrasion is typically undertaken 8 to 12 weeks after the initial inflammatory phase, taking advantage of the end of the proliferative phase.

QUESTIONS

1. **What are the layers of skin?**
   The epidermis and dermis are the two main layers of skin. The epidermis is further separated into the stratum corneum, stratum lucidum, stratum granulosum, stratum spinosum, and stratum basale (from superficial to deep). The layers of the dermis include the papillary and reticular dermis.

2. **What is a scar?**
   A scar is an area of fibrosis that replaces normal skin after injury. A scar always forms after an injury, as it is the product of a normal wound healing process. Scars can be made less visible with various surgical and nonsurgical techniques.

3. **What is healing by primary intention?**
   Healing by primary intention healing occurs when the edges of the wound are brought together in direct contact, which may involve sutures, staples, or other closure methods. This is the most commonly used method of wound closure and results in a minimally visible surgical scar.

4. **What is healing by secondary intention? (Fig. 59.1)**
   Healing by secondary intention occurs when wound edges are not approximated, leaving an area of exposed subcutaneous tissue. This may result in greater wound contracture than seen in primary closure. This type of healing works best in concavities (e.g., temporal fossa, medial canthus, alar groove). It can be useful in scalp and forehead wounds. Advantages include low risk of infection, high rate of healing, acceptable cosmesis, and surveillance in cases where cancer may be incompletely excised.

5. **What is healing by tertiary intention?**
   Healing by tertiary intention is delayed primary closure. Wound edges are not closed immediately, but the defect is allowed to undergo the acute inflammatory phase in which phagocytosis of contaminated tissue occurs and the microbial count decreases. The wound edges are then brought together and closed.

6. **What are the three phases of surgical wound healing?**
   1. Inflammatory phase (injury to approximately 1 week)
   2. Proliferative phase (30 minutes to approximately 1 month)
   3. Remodeling phase (3 weeks to approximately 1 year)

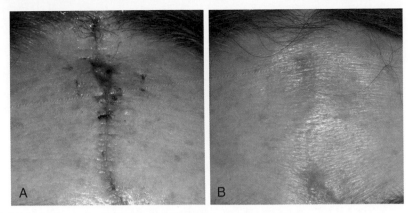

Fig. 59.1 A, B, Healing by secondary intention of a forehead wound.

7. **What occurs in a wound during the inflammatory phase?**

Local *vasoconstriction* occurs within the first 5 to 10 minutes and, then the coagulation cascade proceeds and a fibrin clot is formed. Activated platelets release several chemotactic factors that affect vascular tone. *Vasodilation* subsequently ensues secondary to histamine release. Next, the *cellular response* begins. Macrophage, neutrophil, and lymphocyte infiltration occurs, hallmarking the inflammatory phase. Importantly, only when inflammation subsides does collagen deposition begin. Therefore wounds with excess nonviable debris will experience a prolonged inflammatory phase.

8. **What is the proliferative phase?**

The proliferative phase begins with *reepithelialization* of the wound. This process begins at the time of the injury, and in primary closure it is completed in 24 hours. *Collagen synthesis* begins on day 2. Fibroblasts proliferate and produce type III collagen, elastin, and extracellular matrix. The final component of the proliferative phase is *wound contraction*, which is mediated by myofibroblasts. This contraction is centripetal and is maximal at 10 to 15 days. Contraction may be severe in inflamed wounds.

9. **What is the remodeling phase?**

Collagen remodeling and vascular maturation occur in the remodeling phase. Scars become pale, soft, and less protruding. Type III collagen initially deposited in the proliferative phase is converted into type I collagen. Collagen fibers become more organized into parallel bundles. Completion of remodeling may take 12 to 18 months, and even then, scars achieve only 70% to 80% of the tensile strength of normal skin.

10. **Which four local factors influence wound healing?**
    1. Oxygenation
    2. Infection
    3. Foreign bodies
    4. Venous sufficiency

11. **Which chemotactic and proliferative factors are released during wound healing?**
    - **Growth Hormone**: produced by the pituitary gland; promotes fibroblast proliferation
    - **Epidermal Growth Factor:** produced by platelets; promotes epithelial cell and fibroblast proliferation and migration; activates fibroblast and vascular formation
    - **Platelet Derived Growth Factor:** produced by platelets, macrophages, endothelial cells and keratinocytes; functions as a chemoattractant for neutrophils, macrophages, and fibroblasts. Also works as a mitogenic agent for fibroblasts, inducing production of collagen and hyaluronic acid.
    - **Fibroblast Growth Factor:** produced by macrophages, mast cells, lymphocytes, endothelial cells, and fibroblasts; promotes proliferation of vascular endothelial cells; is also mitogenic for keratinocytes and fibroblasts
    - **Transforming Growth Factor:** produced by platelets, fibroblasts, neutrophils, macrophages, and lymphocytes; promotes proliferation of epithelial cell and fibroblasts
    - **Insulin-Like Growth Factor:** produced by liver, plasma, and fibroblasts; promotes fibroblast proliferation and synthesis of extracellular matrix
    - **Tumor Necrosis Factor:** produced by macrophages, mast cells, and lymphocytes; promotes fibroblast proliferation

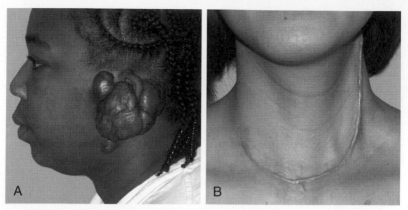

Fig. 59.2 A, A profound keloid scar stemming from ear piercings. **B,** A hypertrophic scar of a neck apron incision following thyroidectomy.

12. What are the tenets of Halstead?

These tenets address gentle handling of tissue, aseptic technique, sharp anatomic dissection, obliteration of dead space, careful hemostasis, and avoidance of wound tension. These principles are highly important to surgical wound healing.

13. How does wound desiccation affect healing?

A moist environment is essential for wound healing, particularly in reepithelialization. Dry, scabbed wounds heal more slowly than wounds with adequate humidity. Desiccation increases the energy expenditure of epithelial cells in wound closure, thereby lengthening wound healing time.

14. How are wound healing phases affected by oxygen?

Initial hypoxia by vasoconstriction and vascular disruption actuates the early phases of wound healing by activating platelets and endothelium. However, recovery of tissue oxygenation is required for adequate healing, and chronic hypoxia can disrupt all aspects of wound healing.

15. What are relaxed skin tension lines (RSTLs)?

These are lines of tension that are intrinsic to the skin and determined largely by the underlying collagen matrix. RSTLs typically lie parallel to wrinkles. Incisions made at 90-degree angles to RSTLs will gape open widely, while those lying parallel will close with minimal tension.

16. Describe the differences and similarities between hypertrophic scars and keloids (Fig. 59.2).

- Hypertrophic scars:
  - Remain within the boundaries of original tissue injury.
  - Tend to regress with time. Contain collagen fibers in a wavy, randomly organized pattern, parallel to the epithelial surface.
- Keloids:
  - Tend to overgrow the boundaries of the initial tissue injury.
  - May continue to enlarge with time.
  - Can be treated with intralesional corticosteroids, interferons, or radiation.
  - Contain thick collagen fibers, closely packed together, haphazardly oriented to the epithelial surface.

17. How do vitamin deficiencies affect wound healing?

Vitamin A is important in epithelialization, collagen synthesis, and cross-linking. Vitamin C is an important cofactor in lysine and proline hydroxylation in collagen synthesis. It is also important to neutrophil function and serves as a reductant in free radical formation ("antioxidant"). Vitamin E reduces collagen production, thereby decreasing wound tensile strength. Vitamin K is important to the production of clotting factors II, VII, IX, and X. Zinc is important to wound healing by promoting cell differentiation and fibroplasia.

18. Which lifestyle factors affect wound healing?

Smoking, through the effects of nicotine, leads to vascular compromise and causes wound tissue ischemia and delayed healing. Alcoholism is associated with global malnutrition, which is detrimental to the wound healing process.

19. **What is the ideal dressing for a surgical wound?**
An ideal dressing for a surgical wound would have the following characteristics: maintains a moist wound environment, absorbs exudate, and keeps the surgical site protected.

20. **What are the types of collagen?**
Type I collagen: Found in skin, bone, and tendons and supports connective tissue
Type II collagen: Found in cartilage, corneal stroma, and vitreous humor; promotes shock absorption and joint mobility
Type III collagen: Ubiquitous; promotes formation of fibrous elements
Type IV collagen: Found in basement membranes; forms a scaffold for filtration
Type V collagen: Ubiquitous; forms cytoskeleton around cells

21. **How does radiation affect wound healing?**
Radiation leads to diminished fibroblast, myofibroblast, and endothelial cell proliferation. There is also considerable ischemia of tissue due to hyalinization and sclerosis of blood vessels. This leads to overall delay and poor wound healing in radiated patients.

22. **What is the role of vacuum-assisted closure in otolaryngology?**
Vacuum-assisted closure may be used in skin grafts to remove fluid secretions that prevent revascularization and imbibition of the graft. They are also used to promote granulation in infected wounds that are healing by secondary intention. Vacuum-assisted devices must not be used in nasal, oral, tracheal, blood vessels, or neoplastic sites.

CONTROVERSIES

23. **What is the role of autologous platelet-rich plasma in wound healing?**
The theoretical principle of the use of platelet-rich plasma (PRP) in wound healing is that platelets are a potent source of growth factors and a concentrate of these growth factors potentially improves healing. Clinical reports studying the efficacy of PRP in reducing ecchymosis and edema have been mixed and its use remains controversial.

BIBLIOGRAPHY

English RS, Shenefelt PD: Keloids and hypertrophic scars, *Dermatol Surg* 25(8):631–638, 1999.
Fisher E, Frodel JL: Wound healing. In: Papel ID, Frodel J, eds: *Facial Plastic and Reconstructive Surgery,* Thieme, pp 15–25.
Gantwerker EA, Hom DB: Skin: histology and physiology of wound healing, *Facial Plast Surg Clin North Am* 19(3):441–453, 2011.
Guo S, Dipietro LA: Factors affecting wound healing, *J Dent Res* 89(3):219–229, 2010.
Hom DB, Sun GH, Elluru RG: A contemporary review of wound healing in otolaryngology: current state and future promise, *Laryngoscope* 119(11):2099–2110, 2009.
Terris DJ: Dynamics of wound healing. In: Bailey BJ, ed: *Otolaryngology: Head and Neck Surgery,* 1998, Lippincott-Raven.

CHAPTER 60

FACIAL ANALYSIS

Gabriela Heslop, MD and Geoffrey Ferril, MD

KEY POINTS

1. Symmetry and proportion are important to facial harmony. The individual subunits must balance each other to achieve an aesthetically pleasing result.
2. Ideal relationships have been established based on the relationship of soft tissue landmarks to each other. However, variations exist for different ethnicities.
3. When analyzing the nose, it is important to evaluate its relationship to the rest of the face in addition to its individual characteristics.
4. Photography and imaging software enhance physician-patient communication, surgical planning, and resident education.

Pearls
1. The Frankfort horizontal line allows for standardization in photographs and is the cornerstone for facial analysis.
2. Nasal rotation refers to movement of the tip along an arc from the Frankfort horizontal line.
3. Nasal projection refers to how far the tip projects from the face.

QUESTIONS

1. **What are the important soft tissue reference points of the face with regards to facial analysis?**
   Trichion: anterior hairline at the midline
   Glabella (G): most anterior point of the forehead on profile view
   Nasion (N): point of deepest depression at the root of the nose on profile view
   Nasal tip (T): most anterior point of nose on profile view
   Columellar point (Cm): most anterior point of the columella on profile view
   Subnasale (Sn): point where the nasal columella merges with the upper lip
   Labrale superioris (LS): vermillion border of the upper lip
   Labrale inferioris (LI): vermillion border of the lower lip
   Pogonion (Pg): most anterior point of the chin on profile view
   Menton (Me): lowest point of the chin
   Cervical point (C): innermost point between the submental area and the neck
   Fig. 60.1 illustrates these reference points.

2. **What is the Frankfort horizontal plane?**
   A line drawn from the superior aspect of the external auditory canal to the inferior aspect of the infraorbital rim on a lateral view (Fig. 60.2). In photographs, it is approximated by a line drawn from the superior tragus to the lower eyelid-cheek skin junction. This allows standardization for patient positioning in photographs, as well as for facial analysis.

3. **What is the facial plane?**
   A line drawn from the glabella to the pogonion. The facial plane should intersect the Frankfort horizontal plane at an angle of 80 to 95 degrees.

4. **What is the zero meridian of Gonzales-Ulloa?**
   A line perpendicular to the Frankfort horizontal line that goes through the nasion. The pogonion should be within 5 millimeters of this line.

5. **What are some important angles used for facial analysis?**
   Nasofrontal angle (Fig. 60.3A): intercept of G to N line with N to T line
   Nasofacial angle (Fig. 60.3B): intercept of G to Pg line with N to T line

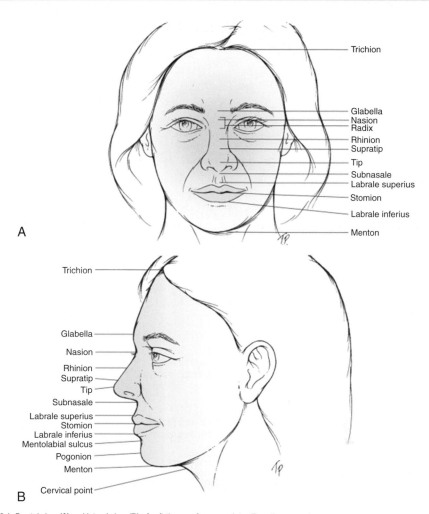

Fig. 60.1 Frontal view **(A)** and lateral view **(B)** of soft tissue reference points. (From Zimbler MS: *Cummings Otolaryngology Head & Neck Surgery*, pp 269–280. Copyright 2010, 2005, 1998, 1993, 1986 by Mosby, Inc. All Rights Reserved.)

Nasolabial angle (Fig. 60.3C): intercept of Cm to Sn line with Sn to LS line
Nasomental angle (Fig. 60.3D): intercept of N to T line with T to Pg line
Mentocervical angle (Fig. 60.3E): intercept of G to Pg line with Me to C line

6. **What is the aesthetic triangle of Powell and Humphreys?**
   This system incorporates the nasofrontal, nasofacial, nasomental, and mentocervical angles to relate all of the major components of the face in the evaluation of facial harmony (Fig. 60.4). The nasomental angle is considered the most important measurement because it is dependent upon nasal projection and chin position and shows the interdependence of individual facial features.

7. **What are ideal measurements of the angles mentioned above?**
   Nasofrontal angle: 115–130 degrees
   Nasofacial angle: 36–40 degrees
   Nasolabial angle: 90–95 degrees in males and 95–110 degrees in females
   Nasomental angle: 120–132 degrees
   Mentocervical angle: 80–95 degrees

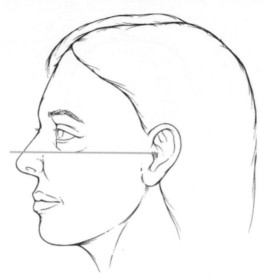

Fig. 60.2 Frankfort horizontal plane. (From Zimbler MS: *Cummings Otolaryngology Head & Neck Surgery*, pp 269–280. Copyright 2010, 2005, 1998, 1993, 1986 by Mosby, Inc. All Rights Reserved.)

8. **What is the rule of thirds?**
   The face can be divided into thirds of approximate equal vertical height on frontal view (Fig. 60.5A). The distance from the trichion to the glabella should equal the length from the glabella to the subnasale, which should equal the length from the subnasale to the menton.

9. **What is the rule of fifths?**
   The face can be divided into fifths of equal width on frontal view (Fig. 60.5B). The width of one eye should equal one fifth of the facial width. In other words, the intercanthal distance should approximate the width of the nose and the width from the lateral canthus to the ear.

10. **What are the subunits of the face?**
    Forehead, periorbital region, cheeks, nose, perioral region and chin, and neck

11. **What are the subunits of the nose?**
    The nose is divided into nine subunits. These are the paired sidewalls, ala, and soft tissue triangles and the unpaired dorsum, tip, and columellar subunits.

12. **What is the supratip break?**
    The transitional area from the dorsum to the tip where the lower and upper lateral cartilages overlap is called the supratip break. The nasal tip should ideally lead the dorsum by 1 to 2 millimeters, leading to a break in the line of the dorsum. This is an aesthetic that is more important in women than in men.

13. **What is the double break of the columella?**
    As the nasal tip transitions to the columella, it is seen making two breaks. The first break is the point at which the tip turns posteriorly and inferiorly onto the infratip lobule, while the second break occurs where the infratip lobule transitions to a flatter and more horizontal columella. The second break corresponds to the junction of the medial and intermediate crura.

14. **Where is the ideal location for the nasion?**
    The nasion ideally should lie at the level of the supratarsal crease on profile view. If it is too low, it may lead to overestimation of nasal projection.

15. **What are the characteristics of an ideal nasal base?**
    On base view, the nose should approximate an equilateral triangle. The columella should comprise two thirds of the height and the lobule comprises another third, leading to a columella:lobule ratio of 2:1.

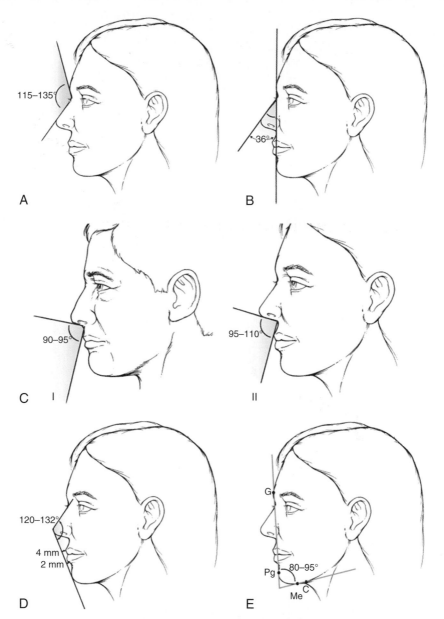

Fig. 60.3 A, Nasofrontal angle. **B,** Nasofacial angle. **C,** Nasolabial angle. Male (i) and female (ii). **D,** Nasomental angle. **E,** Mentocervical angle. (From Zimbler MS: *Cummings Otolaryngology Head & Neck Surgery*, pp 269–280. Copyright 2010, 2005, 1998, 1993, 1986 by Mosby, Inc. All Rights Reserved.)

The nostrils should be symmetric and appear pear shaped, with the widest portion at the nostril sill. The width of the lobule should be 75% of the width of the nasal base. On lateral view, the alar:lobule ratio should be 1:1 and there should be 2 to 4 millimeters of columellar show.

16. **What is nasal tip rotation?**
    Rotation refers to the movement of the nasal tip along an arc based at the external auditory canal. Increasing rotation refers to cephalic movement of the nasal tip along that arc, while caudal movement of the tip leads to derotation.

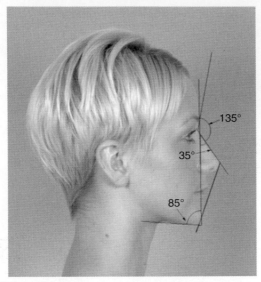

Fig. 60.4 Aesthetic triangle of Powell and Humphreys.

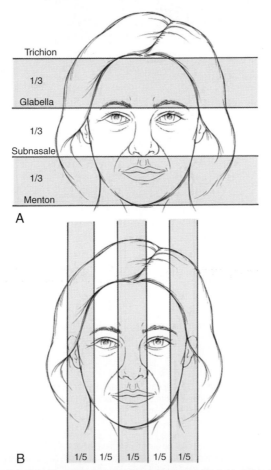

Fig. 60.5 A, Facial height. The facial height is divided into equal thirds. **B,** Facial width. The facial width is divided into equal fifths. (From Zimbler MS: *Cummings Otolaryngology Head & Neck Surgery*, pp 269–280. Copyright 2010, 2005, 1998, 1993, 1986 by Mosby, Inc. All Rights Reserved.)

17. **What is nasal tip projection?**
    Projection refers to the distance the nasal tip projects from the face.

18. **What are the methods used to assess nasal projection?**
    Joseph: described nasal projection in relation to the facial plane, defining the nasofacial angle, which is important in describing projection. The more acute the angle, the less the tip projection and vice versa.
    Simons: ratio of nasal projection to length of the upper lip should equal 1:1. The ratio of the length of the vermilion border (LS) to the Sn should equal the length of the nasal tip as measured from the Sn to the T.
    Goode: ratio of tip projection to nasal dorsum length should equal 0.55:1 to 0.6:1. A vertical line is drawn from the N to the alar facial groove. Tip projection is measured by the length of a horizontal line drawn from the T perpendicular to the vertical line. Nasal dorsum length is measured from N to T (Fig. 60.6).
    Crumley: ratio of tip projection to vertical height to nasal length should equal 3:4:5. Tip projection, vertical height, and nasal length are measured as described by Goode's method, and these sides should form a right triangle.
    Powell and Humphreys: ratio of nasal height to tip projection should equal 2.8:1. Height is measured by the length from N to Sn and projection is measured by a line drawn perpendicular to the line of nasal height through the T.

19. **What is a simple way to assess chin projection?**
    Draw a vertical line from the vermilion border of the LI. The Pg should approximate this line in males and should be 2 to 3 millimeters posterior to this line in females.

20. **How does chin projection affect nasal appearance?**
    An underprojected chin leads to a perceived increase in nasal size, while an overprojected chin leads to a perceived decrease in nasal size.

21. **How does forehead shape affect nasal appearance?**
    A prominent forehead leads to a perceived decrease in nasal size, while a retrusive forehead leads to a perceived increase in nasal size.

22. **What are two different ways to assess lip projection?**
    - A line is drawn from the Sn to the Pg. The upper lip should rest 3.5 millimeters anterior to this line and the lower lip should rest 2.2 millimeters anterior.
    - A line is drawn from the T to the Pg. This line is called the nasomental line. The upper lip ideally falls 2 millimeters posterior to this line and the lower lip 4 millimeters posterior.

23. **What accounts for an aesthetic eyebrow and what are the differences between the male and female brow?**
    The female brow ideally should start medially directly above the nasal ala, reach its highest point at the lateral limbus or lateral canthus, and end at an oblique line passing through from the nasal ala to the lateral canthus.

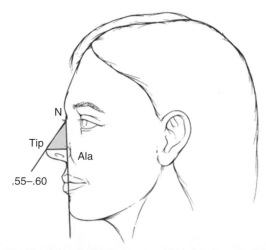

Fig. 60.6 Goode's method of tip projection. (From Zimbler MS: *Cummings Otolaryngology Head & Neck Surgery*, pp 269–280. Copyright 2010, 2005, 1998, 1993, 1986 by Mosby, Inc. All Rights Reserved.)

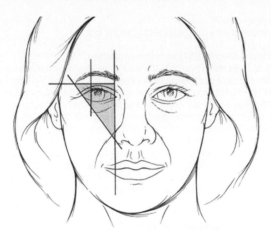

Fig. 60.7 Ideal eyebrow position. (From Zimbler MS: *Cummings Otolaryngology Head & Neck Surgery*, pp 269–280. Copyright 2010, 2005, 1998, 1993, 1986 by Mosby, Inc. All Rights Reserved.)

The medial and lateral aspects of the brow should be on the same horizontal plane. The medial aspect should be club-shaped and gradually taper laterally. Female brows tend to be thinner, more arched, and positioned above the supraorbital rim, while male brows tend to be thicker, straighter, and positioned at the supraorbital rim (Fig. 60.7).

24. **What is the value of computer imaging and digital photography in facial analysis?**
    It provides an opportunity for preoperative planning, patient education, establishing patient expectations, photo archiving, and resident teaching.

BIBLIOGRAPHY

Bernstein L: Esthetics in rhinoplasty, *Otolaryngol Clin North Am* 8:705–715, 1975.
Brennan GH: Correction of the ptotic brow, *Otolaryngol Clin North Am* 13:265–273, 1980.
Burstone CJ: Lip posture and its significance in treatment planning, *Am J Orthod* 53:262–284, 1967.
Crumley RL, Lanser M: Quantitative analysis of nasal tip projection, *Laryngoscope* 98:202–208, 1988.
Gonzalez-Ulloa M: Quantitative principles in cosmetic surgery of the face (profileplasty), *Plast Reconstr Surg Transplant Bull* 29:186–198, 1962.
Goode R: A method of tip projection measurement. In: Powell N, Humphreys B, eds: *Proportions of the Aesthetic Face,* 1984, Thieme-Stratton, pp 15–39.
Powell N, Humphreys B: *Proportions of the Aesthetic Face,* 1984, Thieme-Stratton.
Simons RL: Adjunctive measures in rhinoplasty, *Otolaryngol Clin North Am* 8:717–742, 1975.
Winkler A, Wudel JM: Preoperative evaluation and facial analysis in facial plastic surgery. In: Johnson JT, Rosen CA, eds: *Bailey's Head and Neck Surgery Otolaryngology,* 2014, Lippincott Williams & Wilkins, pp 2757–2771.
Zimbler MS: Aesthetic facial analysis. In: Flint PW, Haughey BH, Lund V, et al, eds: *Cummings Otolaryngology Head & Neck Surgery,* 2015, Saunders, pp 273–285.

CHAPTER 61

FUNCTIONAL AND COSMETIC RHINOPLASTY

Andrew A. Winkler, MD

KEY POINTS

1. A thorough understanding of the anatomy and physiology of the nose is paramount to performing successful rhinoplasty surgery.
2. Nasal tip support mechanisms must be respected, preserved, and/or addressed in rhinoplasty.
3. Preoperative goals, expected outcomes, and potential complications must be discussed at length between the surgeon and patient.

Pearls

1. Major nasal tip support mechanisms are (1) the size, strength, and resiliency of the lower lateral cartilages; (2) attachments of the lower lateral cartilages to the septum; and (3) the attachments of the lower lateral cartilages to the upper lateral cartilages.
2. The internal nasal valve comprises the upper lateral cartilage, nasal septum, and nasal floor. The Cottle maneuver helps to diagnose internal nasal valve collapse.
3. Endonasal (closed) rhinoplasty utilizes transcartilaginous or intercartilaginous incisions with hemitransfixion or transfixion incisions. External (open) rhinoplasty utilizes transcolumellar and marginal incisions.
4. A "pollybeak" deformity is a complication of rhinoplasty whereby supratip fullness results in the appearance of a parrot's beak; this can be the result of loss of tip support or supratip scar tissue.
5. A saddle nose deformity is a concavity of the midvault secondary to insufficient cartilage support of the middle third of the nose; this can be a result of rhinoplasty, septal hematoma, septal abscess, autoimmune disease, or cocaine use.

QUESTIONS

1. **What is rhinoplasty?**
   Rhinoplasty is a challenging surgical operation used to change the functional performance or aesthetic appearance of the nose through manipulation of bone, cartilage, and soft tissue.

2. **Who undergoes rhinoplasty?**
   An estimated 80% of rhinoplasty surgeries are performed on women, and it is the most common procedure performed in facial plastic surgery. Rhinoplasty is most common in the 22- to 34-year-old age group (44% of all), followed by the 35- to 60-year-old age group (31% of all).

3. **Why is rhinoplasty a challenging operation?**
   There are few surgical procedures in which the perception of success rests so substantially on the abilities of the surgeon. In cosmetic rhinoplasty, millimeter changes mean the difference between a satisfactory and a disappointing outcome. Rhinoplasty therefore requires a collaborative discussion of what the patient desires and how his or her expectations match surgical realities. The surgeon must have experience with numerous rhinoplasty techniques and have a thorough grasp of nasal anatomy (Figs. 61.1 and 61.2). The success or failure of rhinoplasty depends on the interplay of the patient's unique nasal anatomy and comorbidities, the surgeon's experience and ability, and the patient's preparation regarding realistic outcomes.

4. **How does one analyze the nose preoperatively for rhinoplasty?**
   While a comprehensive discussion of preoperative nasal analysis is beyond the scope of this chapter, there are several general points worth mentioning. Every initial rhinoplasty consultation includes six standard preoperative rhinoplasty photos, which provide a framework to analyze the nose. These views are the frontal, right/left oblique, right/left lateral, and basal views.

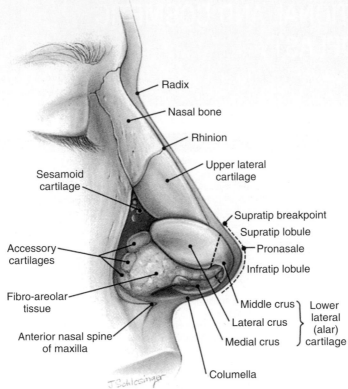

Fig. 61.1 Anatomy of the nose, frontal view. (From Winkler AA: *Open Septorhinoplasty: The Complete Operative Guide*, Cupertino, CA, 2013, Apple, Inc.)

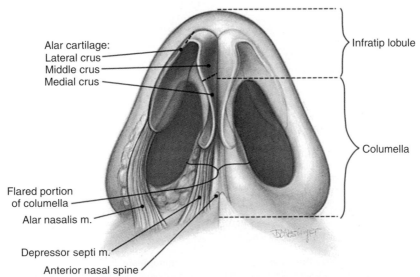

Fig. 61.2 Anatomy of the nose, basal view. (From Winkler AA: *Open Septorhinoplasty: The Complete Operative Guide*, Cupertino, CA, 2013, Apple, Inc.)

- **Frontal View:** on frontal view, the nose is divided horizontally into thirds. The upper third comprises the nasal bones, which should be symmetric and 75% of the intercanthal distance. The middle third, also called the "mid-vault," is formed by the upper lateral cartilages and the dorsal septal cartilage. A line connecting the glabella to the ipsilateral tip-defining point is called the brow-tip aesthetic line. It should be curvilinear, symmetric, and smooth. Deformities from trauma or prior surgery disrupt the brow-tip aesthetic line. A narrow middle third suggests the presence of nasal valve dysfunction (see Question 8). Nasal tip shape may be characterized as bulbous, narrow, bifid, boxy, or amorphous. The elegant tip forms a diamond shape with two tip-defining points, which are identified by the light reflex they produce. The tip defining points are ideally separated by less than 1 centimeter. Finally, the nostril rims should form a "gull-in-flight" relationship with the columella.

- **Lateral View:** the lateral view provides assessment of the profile of the nose and also the ala-tip complex. On lateral view, the length of the ala and tip should be roughly equal and there should be 2 to 4 millimeters of columella showing below the level of the nostril rim. The elegant nasal tip profile has a "double break" produced by (1) the tip-defining point and (2) a subtle angulation at the junction of the tip lobule with the columella. Additionally, a supratip break should be present between the nasal tip and the nasal dorsum.
- **Basal View:** the basal view is used to assess nasal base width and nasal tip symmetry. On basal view, the nose should form an equilateral triangle. The width of the columella compared to the width of the lobule should be 2:1. The tip should comprise one third of the total height, while the nostrils make up the remaining two-thirds on basal view.

5. **What is nasal tip rotation and nasal tip projection?**
   - **Tip Rotation:** rotational movement of the position of the tip along an arc formed from a fixed point at the superior tragus
   - **Tip Projection:** the anterior or posterior positioning of the nasal tip relative to the midface

6. **Define the nasofrontal, nasolabial, and nasofacial aesthetic angles (Fig. 61.3).**
   - **Nasofrontal Angle:** intersection of a line connecting the glabella and sellion and a line tangent to the nasal dorsum (ideally 115 to 130 degrees)
   - **Nasolabial Angle:** intersection of a line tangent to the columella and a line tangent to the upper lip, which forms a vertex at the subnasale (ideally 90 to 95 degrees in males and 95 to 110 degrees in females)
   - **Nasofacial Angle:** intersection of a line tangent to the nasal dorsum with a line from the glabella to the soft tissue pogonion (ideally 36 to 40 degrees)

7. **What is the internal nasal valve and why is it important?**
   The internal nasal valve is approximately 1 centimeter posterior to the nostril aperture and comprises the septum, caudal edge of the upper lateral cartilage, and nasal floor. The angle between the upper lateral cartilage and the septum is acute at this location and is susceptible to collapse. The anterior head of the inferior turbinate may crowd the internal nasal valve, though it is not strictly part of the nasal valve. This internal nasal valve behaves like a Starling resistor in that it shuts once a threshold flow rate is reached. If the triggering flow rate is relatively low, the patient perceives difficulty breathing through the nose.

8. **What is external nasal valve collapse?**
   The lower lateral cartilages form an incomplete ring around the nostril called the external nasal valve. They are designed to prevent the collapse of the soft tissue of the nose during nasal inspiration. External nasal valve collapse occurs when these cartilages are insufficient to support the soft tissue during inspiration.

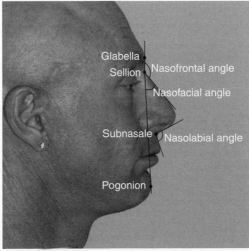

Fig. 61.3 Aesthetic angles of the nose from the lateral view.

9. **What is the Cottle maneuver?**
The Cottle maneuver is a dynamic nasal examination tool whereby the cheeks are distracted laterally, assessing for any subjective improvement in nasal airflow. This tool aids in diagnosing nasal valve incompetence.

10. **How are the incompetent internal and external valves corrected?**
Many suture and cartilage graft modalities have been described to correct nasal valve collapse. Cartilage spreader grafts are the most commonly used grafting technique to correct internal nasal valve incompetence. Spreader grafts are rectangular cartilage grafts that are sutured to either side of the dorsal septum to lateralize the upper lateral cartilages. External nasal valve collapse may be corrected by the butterfly graft, alar batten grafts, or flaring sutures, all of which provide greater stability to the ala.

11. **What are the major and minor support mechanisms for the nasal tip?**
Major (3)
- Size, strength, and resiliency of the lower lateral cartilages
- Attachments of the lower lateral cartilages to the septum at the medial crural footplate
- Attachments of the lateral crura of the lower lateral cartilages to the upper lateral cartilages, known as the scroll region

Minor (6)
- Interdomal ligament
- Cartilaginous dorsal septum (anterior septal angle)
- Sesamoid complex
- Attachment of the lower lateral cartilage to the overlying superficial musculoaponeurotic system
- Nasal spine
- Membranous septum

12. **Describe the incisions used in external (open) rhinoplasty.**
- **Transcolumellar:** a horizontal incision made at the narrowest, most convex portion of the columella. To prevent a straight-line scar, this incision is broken up with an "inverted V" at the midline.
- **Marginal:** a curvilinear incision that follows the caudal margin of the lower lateral cartilages. When combined with the transcolumellar incision, this allows the nasal tip to be degloved (Fig. 61.4).

13. **Describe the incisions used in endonasal (closed) rhinoplasty.**
- **Intercartilaginous:** Placed between the lower lateral and upper lateral cartilage to gain access to the nasal dorsum (Fig. 61.4). These incisions may be extended medially to the septum and continued as a hemitransfixion or full transfixion incision for access to the septum.

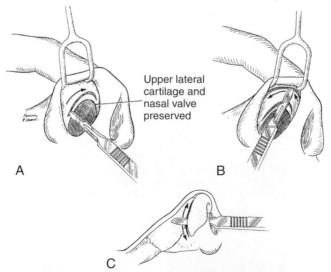

Fig. 61.4 The intercartilaginous incision **(A)** and marginal rim incision **(B)** are made on either side of the lateral crura of the alar cartilage. The intercartilaginous incision permits good access to the nasal dorsum **(C)**. (From Tardy ME Jr: Rhinoplasty. In: Cummings C, et al, eds, *Otolaryngology – Head and Neck Surgery*, 3rd ed, St. Louis, 1998, Mosby.)

- **Transcartilaginous:** a variant of the intercartilaginous incision. The transcartilaginous incision is made several millimeters caudal to the junction of the upper and lower lateral cartilages. The incision is carried through the lateral crural cartilage, which is removed, thereby performing a cephalic trim (see Question 17).

14. **What are the advantages and disadvantages of the two standard rhinoplasty approaches?**
Endonasal
   - Advantages: no external incisions, less operative time, significantly less tip edema
   - Disadvantages: compromised exposure, compromised tip support
   External/Open
   - Advantages: maximum exposure, accurate placement and suturing of grafts, greater accuracy in establishing relationships between the various parts of the nose, greater visualization helpful in surgeon training
   - Disadvantages: longer operative time, more postoperative edema, external scar

15. **What is the tripod concept of the nasal tip?**
The tripod concept is a simplified way to depict the structures that control the position of the domes of the nasal tip (see Figs. 61.1 and 61.2). The tripod consists of:
   - The paired medial crura of the lower lateral cartilages
   - The left lateral crus of the lower lateral cartilage
   - The right lateral crus of the lower lateral cartilage
      In this model, lengthening or shortening any of the members of the tripod will alter tip position.

16. **How is upward tip rotation achieved?**
Upward tip rotation can be achieved by repositioning the tip cartilages and securing them to the caudal septum. This is known as the "tongue-in-groove" technique. Cephalic rotation may also be accomplished by repositioning the lower lateral cartilages onto a graft that is attached to the caudal septum, known as a caudal septal extension graft. This nonanatomic cartilage graft is utilized if the caudal septum is positioned too far posteriorly. More subtle rotation is achieved by simply resecting cartilage from the cephalic portion of the lateral crus. Postoperative scar tissue forms in the resected void and scar contraction causes tip rotation in the cephalic direction. Another method to procure increased tip rotation is to transect, overlap, and suture the lateral crura. This shortens these two limbs of the "tripod" and causes the domes to rotate upward.

17. **What is done to correct the bulbous nasal tip?**
Bulbosity refers to convexity of the lateral crura that lies lateral to the nasal tip domes. This region of the lateral crura is flat in the aesthetic ideal, which allows the domes of the lower lateral cartilages to define and dominate the shape of the nasal tip. To correct bulbosity, many surgeons advocate for volume reduction of the cephalic border of the lateral crura, known commonly as a "cephalic trim." A cephalic strip of lateral crus cartilage is removed. The cartilage that remains behind is ideally kept entirely intact; that is, a "complete strip" is maintained. A weakened lateral crural strip puts the patient at high risk for scar contracture disfigurement and other anomalies. Most surgeons believe that a minimum of 5 to 8 millimeters of complete strip must be preserved to avoid a significant loss of support. Importantly, an adjunct to cephalic trim is the lateral crural strut graft, which is a 1-centimeter by 0.5-centimeter rectangular cartilage graft placed into a pocket beneath the lateral crus. This flattens the lateral crus, providing less bulbosity, and also strengthens the cartilage, which limits postoperative complications.

18. **What is a dorsal hump, how is it removed, and what is an "open-roof" deformity?**
The midvault cartilages and to a lesser extent the nasal bones contribute to dorsal humps. A variety of techniques and tools have been developed to treat unsightly dorsal humps. In the case of a small dorsal hump, rasps are used to reduce the hump with fine control. Larger humps are taken down using traditional osteotomes and/or piezoelectric tools. However, removing large portions of the dorsum may lead to an "open-roof" deformity. This deformity is analogous to cutting the peak off of an A-frame house. The nasal dorsum appears widened on frontal view and the cut edges of the nasal bones may be visible through the skin. To correct an open-roof deformity, osteotomies are made at the lateral aspect of the nasal bones. The mobile nasal bones are then pushed together medially, closing the open-roof defect.

19. **Which potential complications should be discussed with the patient prior to rhinoplasty surgery?**
Bleeding, infection, scarring, septal perforation, need for further procedures, failure to improve symptoms, and poor cosmetic result.

20. **What is a "pollybeak" deformity and how does it occur?**
The pollybeak deformity is a complication of rhinoplasty in which the postoperative appearance resembles the curved beak of a parrot because of supratip fullness. Pollybeaks are categorized by their cartilaginous or soft tissue etiologies. Cartilaginous pollybeak deformity results from loss of nasal tip support. This causes the nasal tip to descend, which allows the anterior septal angle to produce a convexity in the supratip region. Soft tissue

pollybeak occurs when scar tissue fills the supratip break. This may occur following over-resection of the nasal dorsum with resultant dead space, especially in a patient with thick or inelastic skin. The treatment of a pollybeak depends on the etiology. Intralesional steroids may improve soft tissue pollybeak, whereas tip support reconstruction may be necessary for cartilaginous pollybeak deformity.

21. **What is a saddle nose deformity?**
The saddle nose deformity is a concave depression of the midvault resulting from insufficient cartilage support in the middle third of the nose. This can be caused by an untreated septal infection, septal hematoma, cocaine abuse, inflammatory or autoimmune disease, and prior surgery.

22. **What is the inverted V deformity?**
An inverted V deformity occurs when the upper lateral cartilages lose their attachments to the nasal bones and/ or septum, which allows the nasal bones to be seen in relief through the skin. The inverted V deformity is typically a complication of rhinoplasty but may be seen with aging. Placement of spreader grafts resuspends the upper lateral cartilages to the septum and improves the inverted V.

23. **How long does it take to heal following rhinoplasty surgery?**
The majority of healing following primary rhinoplasty takes place during the first 8 weeks. However, a small amount of healing takes place for up to 18 months. Soft tissue swelling may take months to resolve completely, especially following open rhinoplasty. Patients must be made aware of this fact preoperatively so that they are not disappointed by their immediate postoperative results. Numbness or sensitivity of the nasal tip skin is commonplace following rhinoplasty due to neuropraxia of the nasopalatine nerve as it travels through the incisive canal. This typically resolves over 3 to 6 months. In addition, the nasal tip will feel very stiff after surgery due to scar tissue formation. However, as the scar tissue remodels over the first 3 to 6 months the nasal tip becomes more mobile. If revisions are necessary, it is wise to wait at least 6 months between operations.

CONTROVERSIES

24. **Which approach is superior: open or closed?**
Open rhinoplasty involves degloving the nasal tip and provides optimal exposure of the nasal skeleton. Although exposure is improved, it is at the expense of greater postoperative edema. Open rhinoplasty also produces a small external columellar scar, though this is typically very well tolerated. Closed rhinoplasty involves intranasal incisions to gain access to the nasal structures through the nostrils. Exposure is limited and tip work requires "delivery" of the lower lateral cartilages for direct visualization. Although closed rhinoplasty does not produce an external scar, it disrupts more of the nasal tip support mechanisms than the open approach.

The approach utilized depends on the goals of the surgery and expertise of the surgeon. Most experienced rhinoplastic surgeons prefer and advocate one approach over the other for general rhinoplasty, but few surgeons would argue against using the closed approach for addressing minimal defects and the open approach for correcting significant, severe nasal deformities.

25. **Do alloplastic implants have a role in rhinoplasty surgery?**
In many situations, the availability of cartilage for grafts is limited. Alloplastic implants, though not without inherent problems, can serve an important role. The most common implants used include polymeric silicone, expanded polytetrafluoroethylene (ePTFE; Gore-Tex, WL Gore and Associates Inc., Flagstaff, AZ, USA), porous high-density polyethylene (pHDPE; Mepor, Porex Technologies, Fairburn, GA, USA), polydioxanone plate (PDS Flexible Plate, Johnson & Johnson Company, Langhorne, PA, USA), and irradiated human rib cartilage. The surgeon must counsel patients on the increased incidence of infection and extrusion with their use when compared to autologous grafts in preoperative discussions.

BIBLIOGRAPHY

Byrd HS, Andochick S, Copit S, et al: Septal extension grafts: a method of controlling tip projection shape, *Plast Reconstr Surg* 100:999–1010, 1997.
Ferril GR, Wudel JM, Winkler AA: Management of complications from alloplastic implants in rhinoplasty, *Curr Opin Otolaryngol Head Neck Surg* 21:372–378, 2013.
Surgeons, A.S.o.P., 2012 Plastic Surgery Statistics Report. 2012.
Surgery, A.A.o.F.P.a.R., 2012 AAFPRS Membership Study. 2012.
Winkler AA, Soler ZM, Leong PL, et al: Complications associated with alloplastic implants in rhinoplasty, *Arch Facial Plast Surg* 14:437–441, 2012.
Winkler AA, Wudel JM: In Johnson JT, Rosen CA, editors: *Bailey's head and neck surgery—otolaryngology*, ed xx, Philadelphia, 2013, Wolters Kluwer Health/Lippincott Williams & Wilkins, pp xx–xx.
Winkler AA: *Open Septorhinoplasty: The Complete Operative Guide*, Cupertino, California, 2013, Apple, Inc., pp 67.
Winkler AA. Prerhinoplasty Facial Analysis. Medscape, 2014. [date of accession] https://emedicine.medscape.com/article/842545-overview.

CHAPTER 62

PERIORBITAL SURGERY

Alexandra Levitt, MD, MPH, Ryan Larochelle, MD and Sophie Liao, MD

KEY POINTS

1. Detailed knowledge of eyelid and orbital anatomy is crucial for any physician working in the periocular area.
2. There are a variety of surgical approaches to the orbit. The best choice depends on the size and location of the pathologic process.
3. Rejuvenation of the periocular area is best accomplished using a combination of neuromodulators, fillers, and surgical procedures.
4. The Asian eyelid differs from the Western eyelid. When performing blepharoplasty, careful surgical planning and clear patient expectations are necessary to achieve a satisfactory outcome.

Pearls

1. The seven bones that make up the orbit are the sphenoid, maxillary, ethmoid, lacrimal, zygoma, palatine, and frontal.
2. From anterior to posterior, the layers of the upper eyelid above the lid crease are as follows: skin, orbicularis oculi, orbital septum, preaponeurotic fat, levator aponeurosis, Müller's muscle, and conjunctiva.
3. Levator function is the most important variable in determining what type of ptosis surgery to perform.
4. When closing a full-thickness eyelid defect, either the anterior or posterior lamella must be vascularized to remain viable; therefore only one lamella may be repaired with a free graft.

QUESTIONS

1. **Name the seven bones of the orbit.**
   Sphenoid, maxillary, ethmoid, lacrimal, zygoma, palatine, and frontal.

2. **What are the distances of the anterior ethmoid foramen, posterior ethmoid foramen, and optic canal from the orbital rim?**
   This can be remembered by the mnemonic 24-12-6. The anterior ethmoid foramen is approximately 24 millimeters posterior to the orbital rim on the medial wall, the posterior ethmoid foramen is an additional 12 millimeters posterior, and the optic canal is a further 6 millimeters posterior.

3. **What are the eyelid lamellae?**
   The eyelid is often conceptualized as consisting of an anterior and a posterior lamella. The anterior lamella is composed of skin and the striated muscle fibers of the orbicularis muscle. The posterior lamella is composed of the tarsal plate and the palpebral conjunctiva. The anterior and posterior lamellae are separated by the orbital septum (the "middle" lamella).

4. **An object travels through the upper eyelid 12 millimeters superior to the lid margin. What structures does it travel through?**
   In the upper eyelid, the tarsus is typically not taller than 10 millimeters. Therefore at 12 millimeters the object will travel above the tarsus. The layers from anterior to posterior are the skin, orbicularis oculi, orbital septum, preaponeurotic fat, levator aponeurosis, Müller's muscle, and conjunctiva. Below 10 millimeters, the object would travel through the anterior and posterior lamellae, as defined above.

5. **What is the difference between dermatochalasis, blepharoptosis, and blepharochalasis?**
   Dermatochalasis refers to excess skin on the upper eyelid. When severe, it can hang down over the upper eyelid lashes and obstruct the superior visual field. Blepharoptosis refers to drooping of the eyelid, often due to levator dysfunction. Blepharochalasis is a rare syndrome in which episodic edema causes distortion and discoloration of the upper eyelid. Its etiology is poorly understood, but it is commonly considered to be a type of localized angioedema.

6. **How is dermatochalasis surgically addressed?**
Dermatochalasis repair is achieved via blepharoplasty. In this procedure, excess skin and occasionally orbicularis muscle are excised. If there is excessive preaponeurotic or orbital fat (herniation of the medial fat pad is commonly seen), it may be excised or sculpted to optimize lid contour by opening the orbital septum.

7. **How is blepharoptosis repaired?**
The two most common methods to repair blepharoptosis are external levator advancement (ELA) and internal levator advancement (ILA). ELA involves a skin incision at the lid crease, whereas ILA is a transconjunctival approach involving excision of variable amounts of conjunctiva, Muller's muscle, levator, and tarsus. When levator function is poor, such as in congenital ptosis, the upper eyelid can be tethered to the frontalis muscle to assist in eyelid elevation. This procedure is known as a frontalis sling.

8. **The contralateral eyelid occasionally falls after unilateral blepharoptosis repair. Why does this happen?**
Hering's law of equal innervation postulates that yoke muscles receive equal innervation. According to this law, innervation to the bilateral levator palpebrae superioris muscles is equal, and when one eyelid is ptotic the innervation increases in an attempt to clear the visual axis. The increased innervation to the contralateral eyelid can result in pseudoretraction. After repair of unilateral blepharoptosis, the drive to elevate the lids is decreased and descent of the contralateral eyelid may occur.

9. **What next steps are indicated in the treatment of biopsy-proven basal cell carcinoma of the lower eyelid?**
Lower lid basal cell carcinoma should undergo complete excision with frozen sections to confirm clear margins. Alternatively, patients can be referred to a Mohs surgeon for excision.

10. **What principles should be kept in mind when planning the reconstruction of an eyelid defect?**
Important principles include avoiding vertical tension and maintaining a good vascular supply. Minimizing vertical tension helps to avoid eyelid retraction. When a full-thickness defect is present, only one lamella can be repaired with a free graft. If both the anterior and posterior lamellae are replaced with free grafts, the rate of failure is high due to lack of blood supply.

11. **What is ectropion? What are the causes?**
Ectropion is outward turning of the eyelid margin. It may be secondary to a variety of etiologies of an involutional (senile), paralytic, mechanical, cicatricial, or congenital nature.

12. **What is entropion? What are the causes?**
Entropion is an inward turning of the eyelid. The different types of entropion include involutional, spastic, cicatricial, and congenital.

13. **How does the strategy for the repair of involutional ectropion and entropion differ?**
Both conditions typically require horizontal shortening of the eyelid. For ectropion, this is often sufficient. For successful entropion repair, reinsertion of dehiscent lower lid retractors on the tarsus may be required. Additionally, everting sutures may be placed to help correct entropion, while inverting sutures may be placed to help correct ectropion.

14. **If a patient with thyroid eye disease has proptosis, strabismus, and eyelid retraction, in what order should their correction be performed?**
As orbital decompression surgery can alter strabismus and strabismus surgery can alter eyelid position, decompression should be performed first, followed by strabismus surgery and then correction of eyelid retraction.

15. **Name five surgical incisions to approach the orbit.**
Transconjunctival, lateral canthotomy, upper lid skin crease, transcaruncular, and vertical lid split.

16. **During decompression of the orbital floor, what should be preserved to minimize dystopia and diplopia?**
The inferomedial orbital strut.

17. **What choices of orbital implant are available to fill an anophthalmic socket after enucleation or evisceration?**
Orbital implants can be autologous or alloplastic. A dermis fat graft is an example of an autologous implant. Alloplastic implants are used more commonly in the United States and can be divided into porous and nonporous implants. Porous materials allow fibrovascular ingrowth and include hydroxyapatite, porous polyethylene, and aluminum oxide. Nonporous materials include polymethylmethacrylate (PMMA) and silicone.

18. **What are the signs of an orbital compartment syndrome due to retrobulbar hemorrhage? What is the treatment?**
Signs include decreased vision, afferent pupillary defect, proptosis, and increased intraocular pressure. Diagnosis is clinical, not radiographic. Treatment involves lateral canthotomy and cantholysis to relieve orbital compartment pressure, which may be performed on both the upper and lower eyelids as necessary.

19. **When biopsy of the lacrimal gland is indicated, which lobe should be biopsied?**
The lacrimal gland has an orbital lobe and a palpebral lobe. Via a series of ducts, the orbital lobe drains into the palpebral lobe, which then drains onto the ocular surface. Biopsy of the palpebral lobe can cause injury to the tear outflow apparatus. Therefore, biopsies should be taken from the orbital lobe.

20. **What is a DCR? What approaches are available?**
DCR, or dacryocystorhinostomy, is a procedure to address nasolacrimal duct obstruction by creating a fistula between the lacrimal sac and the adjacent nasal cavity. It can be accomplished by an external approach through the skin overlying the sac or by an endoscopic approach through the nose.

21. **What are the most common reasons for DCR failure?**
Common canalicular obstruction and closure of the osteotomy secondary to fibrosis or scarring are the most common etiologies of treatment failure.

22. **What structure may be found within the fat pads of the lower eyelid? Why is it important to identify?**
The inferior oblique muscle runs between the medial and central fat pads of the lower eyelid and is thus particularly vulnerable to injury during lower lid blepharoplasty. Damage to this muscle may result in torsional diplopia.

23. **What age-related changes may be observed in the periorbital area?**
Involutional changes in the upper face include descent and laxity of soft tissues, fat atrophy, and decreased skin elasticity. On exam, these changes may result in findings such as more pronounced static and dynamic rhytids, brow and eyelid ptosis, upper eyelid dermatochalasis, and orbital fat prolapse secondary to weakening of the orbital septum.

24. **Name some nonsurgical treatments for periorbital aging.**
Botulinum toxin injections, dermal fillers, laser and light resurfacing, and chemical peels may be used independently or in combination to address the effects of periorbital aging.

25. **What is the lethal dose of botulinum toxin in an average-sized adult?**
Approximately 3000 units.

26. **What are some of the most commonly used dermal filler materials in the face?**
Hyaluronic acid: Juvederm (Allergan), Restylane (Galderma), Perlane (Medicis Aesthetics)
Poly-L-lactic acid: Sculptra (Valeant Aesthetics)
Calcium hydroxylapatite: Radiesse (Merz)
PMMA: Artefill/Bellafill (Suneva Medical)
Autologous fat

27. **List some of the complications of filler injection.**
The most serious reported complications of dermal filler injection are tissue necrosis and blindness, which result from intravascular injection. Infection has also been reported. Other complications or undesirable outcomes include migration of filler, erythema, bruising, pain, persistent tissue edema, Tyndall effect, and visible nodules due to injection technique or granulomatous inflammation.

28. **What is the advantage of using hyaluronic acid fillers?**
Hyaluronic acid fillers are reversible with the application of hyaluronidase, which is valuable both for cosmetic revision as well as for treatment of postprocedure vascular occlusion.

29. **List the major and minor complications of blepharoplasty.**
Major complications include retrobulbar hemorrhage, globe perforation, diplopia, and severe dry eye. Minor complications include eyelid malposition, eyelid hematoma, wound dehiscence, milia, and chemosis.

30. **Name the different techniques to lift the brow.**
Transblepharoplasty, direct, midforehead, temporal, pretrichial, coronal, and endoscopic brow lifts have all been described. These approaches vary with respect to incision site, dissection plane, and fixation method.

31. How is the Asian eyelid different from the Western eyelid?

The insertion point of the septum into the levator aponeurosis is lower in Asians. As a result, the fat behind the septum can move lower on the eyelid. This causes the eyelid crease to be lower or nonexistent and gives the appearance of a fuller lid. If a crease is present, it usually runs parallel to the lid margin, as opposed to the semilunar shape of the Western lid. Asian eyelids are also more likely to have an epicanthal fold.

BIBLIOGRAPHY

Baroody M, Holds JB, Vick VL: Advances in the diagnosis and treatment of ptosis, *Curr Opin Ophthalmol* 16(6):351–355, 2005.

Bray D, Hopkins C, Roberts DN: A review of dermal fillers in facial plastic surgery, *Curr Opin Otolaryngol Head Neck Surg* 18(4):295–302, 2010.

Chen WP, Park JD: Asian upper lid blepharoplasty: an update on indications and technique, *Facial Plast Surg* 29(1):26–31, 2013.

Custer PL, Kennedy RH, Woog JJ, et al: Orbital implants in enucleation surgery: a report by the American Academy of Ophthalmology, *Ophthalmology* 110(10):2054–2061, 2003.

Kahn DM, Shaw RB: Overview of current thoughts on facial volume and aging, *Facial Plast Surg* 26(5):350–355, 2010.

Knoll BI, Attkiss KJ, Persing JA, et al: The influence of forehead, brow, and periorbital aesthetics on perceived expression in the youthful face, *Plast Reconstr Surg* 121:1793–1802, 2008.

Koursh DM, Modjtahedi SP, Selva D, et al: The blepharochalasis syndrome, *Surv Ophthalmol* 54(2):235–244, 2009.

Levy LL, Emer JJ: Complications of minimally invasive cosmetic procedures: prevention and management, *J Cutan Aesthet Surg* 5(2):121–132, 2012.

Pedroza F, dos Anjos GC, Bedoya M, et al: Update on brow and forehead lifting, *Curr Opin Otolaryngol Head Neck Surg* 14(4):283–288, 2006.

Ramakrishnan VR, Hink EM, Durairaj VD, et al: Outcomes after endoscopic dacryocystorhinostomy without mucosal flap preservation. *Am J Rhinol* 21:753–757, 2007.

CHAPTER 63

LASERS, SKIN RESURFACING, AND HAIR RESTORATION

Andrew A. Winkler, MD

KEY POINTS

1. Skin resurfacing modalities and methods of action
   - Chemical peels: caustic injury
   - Dermabrasion: mechanical injury
   - Laser: thermal injury
2. Different types of chemical peels
   - Superficial chemical peels (epidermis): TCA 10% to 30%, Jessner's solution, glycolic acid 40% to 70%, and salicylic acid 5% to 15%
   - Medium chemical peels (superficial dermis): TCA 35% to 40%, combination of 35% TCA with other agents and phenol 88%
   - Deep chemical peels (deep dermis): TCA 50% and the Baker-Gordon phenol peel
3. Contraindications of skin resurfacing
   - Facelift surgery, medium or deep chemical peel, or laser resurfacing in the previous 6 months
   - For non-fractionated fully ablative lasers and dermabrasion: Isotretinoin use within 6 months
   - Active herpes simplex virus infection
   - Active skin disorders
4. Ablative lasers
   - CO_2 laser (10,600 nm) targets water
   - Erbium-YAG laser (2940 nanometers) targets water
5. Nonablative lasers
   - Vascular lasers: pulsed KTP (532 nanometers) and pulsed dye (585 nanometers) target hemoglobin
   - Infrared laser: Nd-YAG (1064 nanometers)
   - Intense pulsed light: IPL (550–1200 nanometers) laser targets melanin and hemoglobin

---

Pearls

1. The most important consideration prior to skin resurfacing is proper patient selection, especially with respect to the Fitzpatrick skin type (types I and II are the best candidates).
2. The Baker-Gordon formula's (phenol 88%, croton oil, septisol, and distilled water) depth of penetration is more dependent on the croton oil than on the concentration of phenol.
3. Pigmentary changes can result from any skin resurfacing modality (chemical peels, lasers, or dermabrasion). Hyperpigmentation tends to occur sooner and can be successfully treated with topical steroid therapy, while hypopigmentation tends to be a delayed phenomenon and is often permanent.
4. Ablative lasers cause vaporization of tissue and are comparable for resurfacing to medium and deep chemical peels and dermabrasion.
5. Phenol chemical peels are associated with cardiac toxicity and should be applied to individual facial subunits at 15-minute intervals to limit systemic absorption.
6. Follicular unit transplantation refers to the transfer of individual follicular units of hair (groups of one to four hairs). When evaluating the patient for hair restoration, the patient's age, medical history, family pattern of hair loss, and amount of donor area on the posterior scalp need to be determined.
7. Know the Norwood classification for androgenic alopecia.

QUESTIONS

SKIN RESURFACING

1. **Describe age-related changes of the skin.**
   The skin changes seen with aging include thinning of the dermis and epidermis, effacement of the epidermal-dermal junction (most consistent change), thinning of the subcutaneous fat, and loss of organization of elastic fibers and collagen. These changes contribute to increased skin laxity and wrinkling of the aged face.

Table 63.1 Fitzpatrick Skin Classification System

SKIN TYPE	SKIN COLOR	SUN REACTION
I	White or freckled	Always burns
II	White	Usually burns
III	White to olive	Sometimes burns
IV	Brown	Rarely burns
V	Dark brown	Very rarely burns
VI	Black	Never burns

2. **Describe the Fitzpatrick skin type classification system.**
The Fitzpatrick skin type classifies the degree of skin pigmentation and the ability to tan. Skin is graded from I to VI and predicts sun sensitivity, susceptibility to photodamage, and ability for melanogenesis (Table 63.1). It also provides important information related to risk factors for complications during skin resurfacing procedures. Types III through VI have a higher risk of pigmentary dyschromia (hypo- or hyperpigmentation) after skin resurfacing procedures.

3. **What are the different methods of skin resurfacing and how do they promote rejuvenation?**
The different methods are chemical peels, dermabrasion, and laser resurfacing. Superficial resurfacing (micro-dermabrasion and superficial chemical peels) exfoliates the epidermis only and stimulates regeneration and thickening of the epidermis. Medium and deep resurfacing (medium and deep chemical peels, dermabrasion, and lasers) penetrate into the superficial and deep dermis, inducing collagen production.

4. **What are the main indications for chemical peels and dermabrasion?**
Photodamage, fine wrinkles, pigmentary dyschromia, and acne scars.

5. **What are the agents used for superficial chemical peels?**
Superficial chemical peels (epidermis) can be prepared using 10% to 30% trichloroacetic acid (TCA), Jessner's solution (resorcinol, salicylic acid, lactic acid, and ethanol), glycolic acid 40% to 70% solution, and salicylic acid 5% to 15% solution.

6. **What are the agents used for medium-depth chemical peels?**
The medium-depth peel (papillary dermis) agents are trichloroacetic acid (TCA) 35% to 40% solution, a combination of 35% TCA with other agents (35% TCA + solid CO_2, 35% TCA + Jessner's solution, 35% TCA + 70% glycolic acid), and phenol 88% solution.

7. **What are the agents used for deep chemical peels?**
The deep chemical peel (reticular dermis) agents are trichloroacetic acid (TCA) 50% and the Baker-Gordon phenol peel (phenol 88%, croton oil, septisol, and distilled water). The addition of croton oil, an epidermolytic agent, increases the penetration of phenol into the dermis.

8. **What are the limitations associated with the use of phenol?**
Phenol is associated with cardiotoxicity (mostly premature ventricular contractions), hepatotoxicity, and nephrotoxicity. Phenol application requires intravenous hydration and cardiac monitoring for the development of arrhythmias. Facial subunits should be treated at 15-minute intervals to avoid toxicity.

9. **Describe the complications related to chemical peels.**
Complications associated with chemical peel resurfacing include milia formation (the most common complication of all resurfacing procedures), hyper- or hypopigmentation, scar formation, allergic or irritant dermatitis, bacterial or fungal (most commonly *Candida*) infection, and reactivation of herpes simplex virus (which could lead to scarring).

10. **What is dermabrasion?**
Dermabrasion is a method of mechanical skin resurfacing using a rotary burr, called a fraise. Fraises come in various shapes and coarseness grades. The goal depth of skin penetration in dermabrasion is the reticular dermis.

LASERS

11. **What is a laser?**
Laser stands for light amplification by stimulated emission of radiation. Laser light is collimated (parallel), coherent (with the same frequency and periodicity), and monochromatic (single wavelength) light.

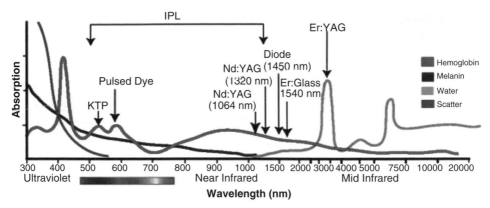

Fig. 63.1 Absorption spectrum of common tissue chromophores.

12. **What is IPL?**
    As opposed to laser light, IPL is a narrow band of wavelengths. Intense white light is passed through a filter, eliminating all wavelengths except for those desired to treat the target molecule.

13. **What is selective photothermolysis?**
    Selective photothermolysis is the property of maximal or preferential absorbance by the targeted tissue chromophore for a specific wavelength of light, thereby minimizing collateral damage to surrounding tissues (Fig. 63.1).

14. **What is ablative laser resurfacing?**
    Ablative laser resurfacing utilizes the principle of selective photothermolysis, wherein the target chromophore has a high absorbance peak, which allows for very rapid absorption of energy by the chromophore, causing steam formation and tissue vaporization. The most common ablative lasers are CO_2 and erbium-YAG.

15. **What is the difference between CO_2 and erbium-YAG lasers?**
    Erb-YAG energy is absorbed more efficiently in the skin (tenfold greater absorption) than the energy from the CO_2 laser. This leads to more precise tissue ablation with fewer adjacent thermal injuries. This, in turn, leads to a shorter recovery time, less erythema, and a lower risk of hypo- or hyperpigmentation. However, it produces less tissue tightening.

16. **What is nonablative and fractional laser resurfacing?**
    Nonablative resurfacing produces a thermal injury that does not lead to tissue vaporization. Rather, the energy is more slowly absorbed, leading to a more diffuse thermal injury. Fractional lasers utilize microbeams of light, rather than a single, larger column of light. This leads to islands of tissue within the treated area that are relatively unaffected by the laser. These unaffected areas promote much more rapid healing and decrease the risk of adverse reactions.

17. **How do lasers produce photorejuvenation?**
    They work by the induction of proliferation of fibroblasts with new collagen (types I and III) and elastin deposition in the papillary dermis. Infrared and visible light lasers are used with cooling mechanisms to protect the overlying epidermis.

18. **Is there a need for any preoperative treatment?**
    Yes. All patients undergoing laser resurfacing should receive antiviral prophylaxis and avoid sun exposure prior to resurfacing. The use of hydroquinone, isotretinoin, glycolic acid, and antibiotics is not well established.

19. **What are important considerations in patient selection for laser resurfacing?**
    One of the most important considerations is the skin type of the patient. The safest skin types are Fitzpatrick I and II. Types III–VI are more susceptible to pigmentary complications.

20. **What are the most common complications associated with laser skin resurfacing?**
    Milia, hypopigmentation, hyperpigmentation, scar formation, infection (viral, fungal, and bacterial), and contact dermatitis.

HAIR RESTORATION

21. **What are follicular units?**

    Hair follicles grow together in groups called follicular units (FUs). Each unit consists of one to four terminal hair follicles with its associated sebaceous gland, arrector pili muscle, blood supply, and neural plexus surrounded by a fine adventitial collagen sheath.

22. **Describe the hair cycle**

    Hair growth is a cyclical phenomenon with a period of growth (anagen), involution (catagen), and rest (telogen). In the normal scalp, 90% to 95% of the hairs are in the anagen phase, approximately 1% in the catagen phase, and 5% to 10% in the telogen phase. Each hair goes through this process 10 to 20 times during a lifetime. This cycle is regulated by a complex signaling system that is not yet fully understood.

23. **What is androgenic alopecia?**

    Androgenic alopecia (AGA) affects both men and women. Its onset is variable and seems to be determined by the presence of circulating androgens. The prevalence of AGA is also variable, affecting approximately 30% of males at 30 years of age and approximately 50% of 50-year-old males. This type of alopecia is nonscarring and has a characteristic pattern of variation in hair shaft diameter and the presence of miniaturized hairs, leading to their transformation into vellus-like follicles, which are then expelled. The exact mechanism by which androgens cause hair loss remains unclear. It is likely that, in susceptible follicles in the scalp, dihydrotestosterone (DHT) binds to the androgen receptor and the hormone receptor complex activates genes that gradually transform large terminal hairs into miniaturized hairs.

24. **How is androgenic alopecia is classified?**

    Androgenic hair loss in males, or male pattern baldness (MPB), often follows a characteristic pattern beginning with temporal recession followed by diffuse thinning of the crown area, eventually leading to complete hair loss in this region. Balding in this area enlarges and eventually meets the temporal recession. In the final stages of progression, the parietal and occipital fringes thin and recede. This stepwise progression was classified by Norwood, with a grading scale ranging from I to VII (Fig. 63.2).

25. **Describe female pattern baldness.**

    Because the role of androgens in alopecia in women remains uncertain, female pattern hair loss (FPHL) has become the preferred term for AGA in women. It affects approximately 20% of all women, with the onset being as early as the third decade, with a steady progression until acceleration during menopause. Diagnosis of FPHL is clinical, based on the characteristic appearance of the scalp. It normally does not require further workup, but patients should be asked about signs of hirsutism, acne, and menstrual and hormonal abnormalities. The most widely used classification system for FPHL was proposed by Ludwig (Fig. 63.3). The frontal hairline usually remains intact, and hair loss occurs on the top of the scalp and is arbitrarily divided into three degrees of severity.

25. **What are the nonsurgical treatment options for alopecia?**

    Without treatment, AGA advances at a rate of approximately 5% per year. Currently, two drugs are available for the treatment of AGA: minoxidil and finasteride. Minoxidil is a vasodilator, and its mechanism of action to promote hair growth is not well understood but seems to be independent of vasodilation. It causes an initial surge in hair growth, which quickly stops when the medication is stopped. Adverse effects include scalp irritation, dryness, itching, and redness. Finasteride is a competitive inhibitor of type 2 5α-reductase that inhibits the conversion of testosterone into DHT. It lowers the levels of DHT but has no affinity for other androgen receptors; therefore it does not interfere with the metabolic actions of testosterone. Adverse effects include decreased libido, erectile dysfunction, and ejaculatory dysfunction, which are reversible with discontinuation of the medication.

26. **How are follicular units (FUs) obtained?**

    FUs can be obtained through a single strip harvest or follicular unit extraction (FUE). The strip technique starts by determining and marking the donor area on the occipital scalp. The incision is made using a scalpel, beveling the knife along the axis of the follicles to avoid transection. The FUs are then dissected from the scalp strip and the donor area is closed. In the FUE technique, a sharp 1-millimeter punch is used to incise the midreticular dermis, stopping just above the subcutaneous tissue. This is done by observing the angle of the hair shaft in the scalp and using the punch on the same axis to avoid transection. Using forceps or a suction-assisted device, the top of the graft is then firmly grasped and pulled out. FUE minimizes the amount of scarring that occurs at the donor site.

27. **How are FUs transplanted?**

    This starts by dissecting the FUs and setting them apart into individual units of one, two, three, or four hairs. They are then transferred to the recipient site and inserted into small openings, which minimizes recipient site scarring and trauma to the local blood vessels but, more important, creates a snug fit for the FU. With an intentional design

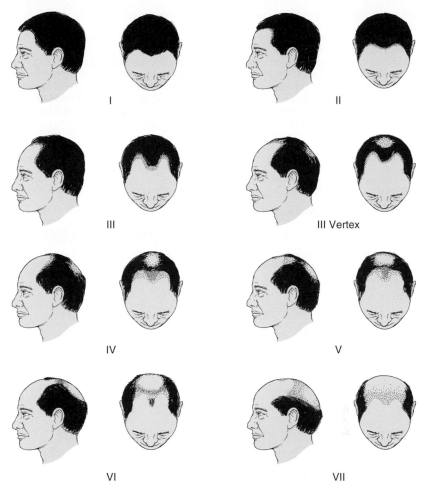

Fig. 63.2 Norwood classification of male pattern baldness. (Previously published in Flint PW, Haughey BH, Lund VJ, et al, eds: *Cummings Otolaryngology—Head and Neck Surgery*, 5th ed, Philadelphia, 2010, Mosby Elsevier, Figure 26-4, p 377.)

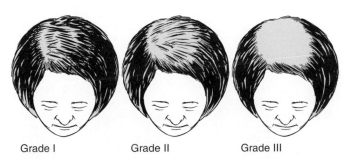

Fig. 63.3 Ludwig classification of female pattern baldness. (Previously published in Flint PW, Haughey BH, Lund VJ, et al, eds: *Cummings Otolaryngology—Head and Neck Surgery*, 5th ed, Philadelphia, 2010, Mosby Elsevier, Figure 26-5, p 377.)

based on data regarding the natural hairline, FU transplantation creates a natural-appearing treated hair-bearing scalp.

28. **What is postsurgical effluvium?**

    Postsurgical effluvium is the loss of preexisting hair in the FU following transplant and occurs to a small degree in some patients. This loss occurs at any point from the first 3 weeks to 3 months after surgery and is usually minor and unnoticed by the patient. Significant postsurgical effluvium occurs when a large number of transplanted grafts are placed in an area that contains a large proportion of miniaturized hairs. The degree of effluvium is unpredictable and can affect any patient, although it occurs more frequently in women. The patient needs to be reassured that hair will start growing again in the following 3 to 6 months.

BIBLIOGRAPHY

Alexiades-Armenakas MR, Dover JS, Arndt KA: The spectrum of laser skin resurfacing: nonablative, fractional, and ablative laser resurfacing, *J Am Acad Dermatol* 58(5):719–737, 2008.
Bernstein RM, Rassman WR: Follicular unit transplantation: 2005, *Dermatol Clin* 23(3):393–414, 2005.
Carniol PJ, Harmon CB: Laser facial resurfacing. In: Papel ID, ed: *Facial Plastic and Reconstructive Surgery*, New York, 2002, Thieme Medical, pp 241–246.
Fitzpatrick TB: The validity and practicality of sun-reactive skin types I through VI, *Arch Dermatol* 124(6):869–871, 1988.
Jackson A: Chemical peels, *Facial Plast Surg* 30(1):26–34, 2014.
Ludwig E: Classification of the types of androgenetic alopecia (common baldness) occurring in the female sex, *Br J Dermatol* 97(3):247–254, 1977.
Norwood OT: Male pattern baldness: classification and incidence, *South Med J* 68(11):1359–1365, 1975.
Smith JE: Dermabrasion, *Facial Plast Surg* 30(1):35–39, 2014.

CHAPTER 64

COSMETIC SURGERY FOR THE AGING NECK AND FACE

Andrew A. Winkler, MD

KEY POINTS

1. Facelift is a cosmetic procedure that involves elevating the tissues of the lower face and neck into a more youthful position.
2. There are several possible complications from facelift, including hematoma, nerve injury, skin necrosis, and contour irregularities.
3. Numerous facelift techniques have been described, each with their own risks and benefits.

Pearls
1. The most common complication from facelift surgery is hematoma. It occurs in up to 10% of cases and is more common in men.
2. The rate-limiting anatomy in facelift surgery is the position of the hyoid bone. A congenitally anterior hyoid bone relative to the chin forces the mentocervical angle (MCA) and lower face-throat angle (LFTA) to be more obtuse.
3. The most commonly injured nerve in facelift surgery is the great auricular nerve.
4. The most commonly injured motor nerve in facelift surgery is the marginal mandibular nerve.
5. The superficial musculoaponeurotic system (SMAS) contains the muscles of facial expression and is the tissue layer that is lifted in most facelift techniques.

QUESTIONS

1. **What is a facelift?**
   Facelift, or cervicofacial rhytidectomy, is a surgery that elevates the skin and soft tissues of the lower facial third and neck. The procedure involves elevating a skin flap around the ear, drawing the deeper tissues up superiorly, and fixating them to strong fascia. Facelift is generally considered a cosmetic procedure and is performed in the outpatient setting.

2. **What type of anesthesia is required?**
   Facelift can be performed under general anesthesia, IV sedation, or local anesthesia only.

3. **What aging stigmata are addressed with facelift?**
   When examining the aging face patient interested in facelift, it is useful to know what areas can be corrected with this procedure. The following aging issues can be addressed (Fig. 64.1):
   Sagging neck skin
   Platysmal bands
   Jowls
   Excess cervical fat
   A combination of facelift, liposuction, and platysmaplasty (see below) is used to correct these problems. Fine wrinkles are not treated by facelift.

4. **What is the SMAS?**
   The Superficial Musculoaponeurotic System (SMAS) is a continuous layer of the face that contains the muscles of facial expression. The SMAS layer is connected to the dermis, which allows these muscles to move the skin and convey emotion. These are the only muscles in the body that attach directly to skin, which highlights the importance of facial expression in social species such as our own.

5. **What is the most common complication of facelift and what are some risk factors?**
   Hematoma is the most common complication of facelift. This can range from major postoperative hematoma requiring emergent surgical evacuation to minor hematomas that are aspirated in clinic. The reported incidence

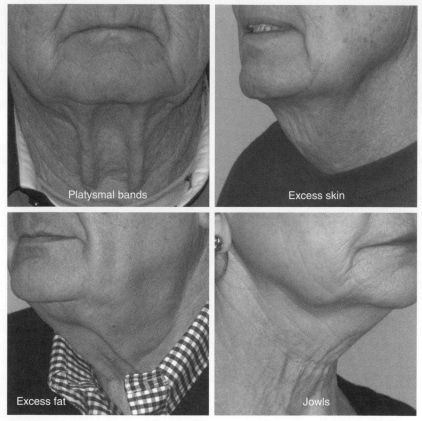

Fig. 64.1 Areas of the lower face and neck that can be improved with facelift surgery.

is 5% to 10%. Hematoma is more common in men due to differences in skin vascular perfusion around whiskers. Another significant risk factor is uncontrolled hypertension. When blood pressure is above 150/100 mmHg at admission, hematoma is 2.6 times more likely than in normotensive patients.

6. **Which is the most commonly injured nerve in facelift surgery?**
   The great auricular nerve – a sensory nerve originating from spinal levels C2 and C3. It innervates to the lower ear and periauricular skin and is found 6.5 centimeters below the external ear canal on the belly of the sternocleido-mastoid muscle. Injury to the great auricular nerve occurs in approximately 7% of cases.

7. **Which is the most commonly injured motor nerve in facelift surgery?**
   The marginal mandibular nerve – a motor nerve to the depressors of the oral commissure. Injury to the marginal mandibular nerve is thought to occur in less than 1% of cases and depends greatly on the facelift technique utilized.

8. **What are other complications of facelift surgery?**
   - Skin necrosis: most common in the area of preauricular skin followed by postauricular skin
   - Cobra-neck deformity: over-prominence of the platysmal bands due to overly aggressive removal of submental fat (Fig. 64.2).

9. **What are some popular facelift techniques?**
   Skin-only
   The skin-only facelift technique was the original procedure described. It is safe and reliable for the beginning surgeon. This technique employs subcutaneous dissection only. The skin is elevated off the underlying SMAS to a variable extent around the ear. Excess skin is trimmed and the incision is closed. The skin-only technique

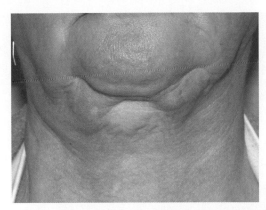

Fig. 64.2 Contour irregularities, such as the cobra-neck deformity pictured here, are possible complications of facelift surgery.

has the advantage of having minimal risk to the facial nerve. The main drawback of this technique is a lack of longevity, which is greatly improved with the SMAS techniques described below. Unfortunately, SMAS dissection procedures are poorly and inconsistently described in the literature. Generally accepted descriptions of the various techniques follow.

SMAS imbrication and plication (standard SMAS)

After elevation of a skin flap around the ear, the SMAS is incised on a line from the malar eminence to the angle of mandible (approximately 3 centimeters anterior to the tragus). Dissection then proceeds in a sub-SMAS level, which is an avascular and loosely adherent plane. Once freed, the SMAS is then repositioned in an anti-gravity direction and secured in position. Imbrication refers to overlapping the SMAS and securing it, whereas plication describes folding the SMAS over on itself near the ear and securing it with sutures. Often, in plication procedures a subcutaneous flap is elevated but no sub-SMAS dissection is performed.

Extended SMAS flap

Extended SMAS techniques simply imply that the amount of sub-SMAS dissection is increased relative to the standard SMAS procedure, especially in the area inferior to the border of the mandible. However, this can also imply a greater distance into the neck or anteriorly toward the oral commissure.

High SMAS flap

High SMAS is a variation of the SMAS imbrication wherein the SMAS is incised near the preauricular crease with an extension beneath the zygomatic arch. The SMAS is then carefully elevated off the parotid gland, where the facial nerve is protected. As the facial nerve branches exit at the anterior border of the parotid gland, they course directly beneath the SMAS within the masseteric fascia. The advantage of this technique is that the overlapping of SMAS along the zygomatic arch provides augmentation of this area, which is often a goal of treatment of the aging face.

Deep-plane

The deep-plane technique was originally described as a means to reposition the descended malar fat pad. Therefore it can be considered a midfacial adjunct to other SMAS techniques. The deep-plane lift begins with an extended SMAS procedure. Dissection proceeds until the zygomaticus major muscle is discovered. Here, the facial nerve branches will begin to ascend from the masseteric facia to innervate their muscles from below. Therefore dissection is transitioned from a sub-SMAS plane to a supra-SMAS plane (subcutaneous) to avoid injuring these facial nerve branches. In doing so, the zygomatico-cutaneous ligament (MacGregor's Patch) is encountered and released. This provides greater mobility of the SMAS flap.

Minimal access cranial suspension (MACS) lift

The MACS lift is a plication technique that utilizes only a preauricular incision and a limited skin flap dissection. Suspension sutures are used to superiorly reposition SMAS tissue vertically. These sutures pass down to the neck, jowls, and malar fat pad in a purse-string manner to achieve elevation. The main difficulty with this technique is contour irregularities from the bunching of the SMAS, though these typically flatten with time.

10. **What are some important reference angles and points with regards to facelift?**

Lower face-throat angle (90–105 degrees)

The LFTA describes the extent to which the submental tissues are tucked beneath the chin. It is the angle formed by connecting a line from the cervical point (posterior-most point in the submental area) to the menton (inferior-most point of the chin), with a line from the subnasale (junction of the columella and upper lip) to the pogonion (anterior-most point of the chin in the midline). The intersection of these lines is a virtual point called the gnathion (Fig. 64.3).

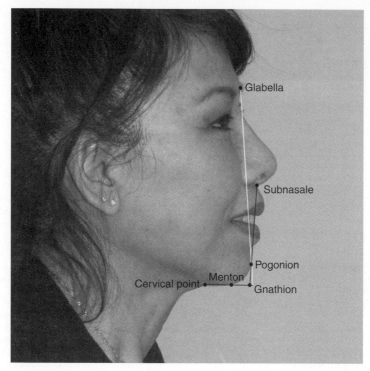

Fig. 64.3 The lower face-throat angle (black) and mentocervical angle (red) are useful to take note of in the pre- and postoperative period.

Mentocervical angle (80–90 degrees)

The MCA takes into account a broader area of the face and therefore better describes the relationship of the neck to the face. The MCA is formed by the intersection of a line from the cervical point to menton with a line from the glabella (anterior most point between the eyebrows) to the pogonion (Fig. 64.4).

11. **Which anatomic structures limit the improvement of the LFTA and the MCA?**
The values of the MCA and LFTA are reliant on the relationship of the hyoid bone to the mandible. The relative position of these anatomic entities to one another represents the limiting factor in any attempt to surgically manipulate the neckline.

12. **What can be done about platysmal bands?**
The corset platysmaplasty is the most popular technique to address platysma bands. The medial bands of the platysma are identified via a submental crease incision. They are then trimmed, incised at the hyoid bone, and imbricated together across the midline.

CONTROVERSIES

13. **SMAS vs. deep-plane facelifts**
The Deep Plane technique aimed at incorporating the malar fat pad within the SMAS flap. In doing so, the malar fat pad is repositioned in a superior direction during SMAS imbrication. In recent years, the pendulum has swung back toward less invasive facelift techniques. This is in part due to less risk of complications but perhaps more to a failure to realize the improved results touted by more extensive dissection techniques. Certainly, excellent results can be seen with any technique in the hands of an experienced surgeon.

14. **Drains and/or compression dressings**
The use of subcutaneous drains is controversial. Hematoma is the most common complication of this surgery and can even be life-threatening. Preventing this complication is foremost in the surgeon's mind. However, drains are uncomfortable and not necessary in the majority of patients. There is also controversy regarding their effectiveness to prevent life-threatening hematomas. Compression dressings wrapped around the head may reduce the risk of hematoma but may increase the risk of focal skin necrosis in susceptible patients.

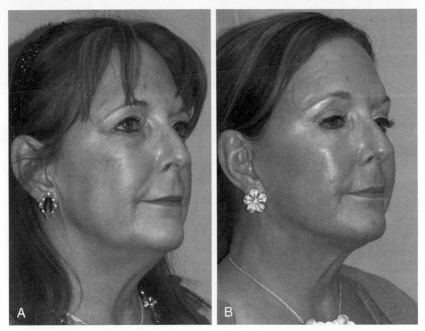

Fig. 64.4 (A) Before and (B) after images of a happy patient who underwent a modified MACS facelift (and other procedures).

BIBLIOGRAPHY

Daane SP, Owsley JQ: Incidence of cervical branch injury with "marginal mandibular nerve pseudo-paralysis" in patients undergoing face lift, *Plast Reconstr Surg* 111(7):2414–2418, 2003.

Feldman JJ: Corset platysmaplasty, *Plast Reconstr Surg* 85(3):333–343, 1990.

Griffin JE, Jo C: Complications after superficial plane cervicofacial rhytidectomy: a retrospective analysis of 178 consecutive facelifts and review of the literature, *J Oral Maxillofac Surg* 65(11):2227–2234, 2007.

Mayrovitz HN, Regan MB: Gender differences in facial skin blood perfusion during basal and heated conditions determined by laser Doppler flowmetry, *Microvasc Res* 45(2):211–218, 1993.

McCollough EG, Perkins S, Thomas JR: Facelift: panel discussion, controversies, and techniques, *Facial Plast Surg Clin North Am* 20(3):279–325, 2012.

McKinney P, Katrana DJ: Prevention of injury to the great auricular nerve during rhytidectomy, *Plast Reconstr Surg* 66(5):675–679, 1980.

Rees TD, Aston SJ: Complications of rhytidectomy, *Clin Plast Surg* 5(1):109–119, 1978.

Straith RE, Raju DR, Hipps CJ: The study of hematomas in 500 consecutive face lifts, *Plast Reconstr Surg* 59(5):694–698, 1977.

Tanna N, Lindsey WH: Review of 1000 consecutive short-scar rhytidectomies, *Dermatol Surg* 34(2):193–202, 2008.

Winkler AA, Wudel JM: Preoperative evaluation and facial analysis in facial plastic surgery. In: Johnson J, ed: *Bailey's Head and Neck Surgery Otolaryngology*, 5th ed, 2013, Lippincott Williams and Wilkins.

CHAPTER 65

BOTULINUM TOXIN AND FILLERS

Isabel Fairmont, MD, MS and Geoffrey Ferril, MD

KEY POINTS

1. Of the botulinum toxins available, Botox® has the longest record of safety and efficacy as well as the most FDA-approved indications. However, due to similar mechanism of action and widespread off-label use, Dysport®, Xeomin®, and Jeuveau® may also be used for cosmetic purposes.
2. Hyaluronic acid–based fillers are the most commonly used facial fillers.
3. Major adverse reactions to injection with facial fillers are rare and can largely be prevented through meticulous technique and injection into the correct plane.

Pearls

1. Botulinum toxin cleaves SNAP-25 at the presynaptic neuromuscular junction, inhibiting acetylcholine release. This leads to temporary muscle paralysis.
2. Upper eyelid ptosis secondary to botulinum toxin injection can be treated with alpha-2 adrenergic ophthalmic drops.
3. An understanding of a filler's rheologic and physicochemical properties, such as G′, helps the clinician select which products are the most suitable for a given clinical need.
4. Sculptra® acts by invoking a host tissue response that leads to the gradual ingrowth of type I collagen.

QUESTIONS

1. **What is botulinum toxin and what is its mechanism of action?**
   Clostridium botulinum produces botulinum exotoxin (BTX), of which there are seven serotypes (A-G). These potent neurotoxins cause flaccid paralysis by preventing the release of acetylcholine from presynaptic vesicles at the neuromuscular junction. This is accomplished by cleaving the SNARE complex of proteins (SNAP-25, synapto-brevin, and syntaxin) that allows the vesicles containing acetylcholine to fuse with the plasmalemma of the nerve terminal, leading to exocytosis. By preventing muscle contraction, BTX prevents the formation of facial rhytids from dynamic muscle movement.

2. **What are the formulations of botulinum toxin that are available in the United States?**
   There are currently four FDA-approved formulations of BTX-A:
   Botox and Botox Cosmetic (onabotulinumtoxinA, Allergan, Irvine, CA)
   Dysport (abobotulinumtoxinA, Valeant, Laval, Quebec)
   Xeomin (incobotulinumtoxinA, Merz, Frankfurt, Germany)
   Jeuveau® (prabotulinumtoxinA-xvfs, Evolus, Santa Barbara, CA)
   The only BTX-B formulation available is Myobloc (rimabotulinumtoxinB, Solstice Neurosciences, San Francisco, CA).

3. **What is botulinum toxin used for?**
   From a cosmetic standpoint, Botox Cosmetic, Dysport, Xeomin, and Jeuveau are all FDA approved for the tempo-rary improvement of glabellar lines. Botox Cosmetic also has an additional cosmetic indication for the temporary improvement of lateral canthal lines, otherwise known as crow's feet. Use of these products in other locations for aesthetic purposes is considered off-label.
   Other medical indications include the following:
   1. Botox®: overactive bladder, detrusor overactivity due to a neurologic condition, chronic migraine, upper and lower limb spasticity, cervical dystonia, axillary hyperhidrosis, blepharospasm, and strabismus
   2. Dysport®: cervical dystonia, upper and lower limb spasticity
   3. Xeomin®: chronic sialorrhea, upper limb spasticity, cervical dystonia, and blepharospasm
   4. Jeuveau®: no medical FDA-approved indications
   Other common off-label uses for botulinum toxin include facial tics, spasmodic dysphonia, myofascial pain syndrome, and sialorrhea.

4. **What is the onset and duration of botulinum toxin?**
   For cosmetic injections in the face, it takes 3 to 7 days for the effects of botulinum toxin to be seen, reaching maximal efficacy around 2 weeks after injection. This effect lasts for approximately 3 months. However, with repeated injection, the duration could extend to 4 to 6 months as the facial muscles atrophy. The return of normal muscle function occurs through axonal sprouting and production of new neuromuscular junctions.

5. **What is the lethal dose of Botox and what is a common dose for cosmetic purposes?**
   The LD_{50} (lethal to 50% of those injected) is 2500 to 3000 units in humans. For cosmetic purposes, use of 40 to 60 units per treatment is common.

6. **What are typical doses of Botox® for facial rhytids?**
   - Glabella: 20–40 units divided in 5 sites
   - Forehead: 10–30 units divided in 4–8 sites; inject at least 2 centimeters above the eyebrow
   - Crow's feet: 8–12 units on each side divided in 2–4 sites
   - Perioral area: 4–10 units divided in 2–6 sites
   - Chin: 2–8 units divided in 1–2 sites
   - Neck (platysmal banding): 10–40 units divided in 2–4 sites per band

7. **What are the depressors and elevators of the brow?**
   - Depressors: corrugator supercilii, procerus, depressor supercilii (part of the orbicularis muscle)
   - Elevator: frontalis
     These muscles are demonstrated in Fig. 65.1.

8. **What is the "Spock" look and how do you treat it?**
   The "Spock" look is caused by excessive elevation of the lateral brow while the medial brow remains relatively fixed. The look is due to overactivity of the lateral aspect of the frontalis and is easily treated by injecting botulinum toxin in that area to weaken its activity.

9. **What is a chemical brow lift?**
   Botox is injected in the superolateral orbicularis oculi muscle just below the eyebrow to weaken the orbicularis oculi's depressor function. This results in a 1- to 2-millimeter elevation of the brow.

10. **What are some common side effects of botulinum toxin?**
    Pain and bruising at the injection site are most common. Headache, dry mouth, tiredness, neck pain, and eye problems can also occur.

11. **What are some serious potential side effects of botulinum toxin?**
    Serious, potentially fatal, side effects include difficulty breathing, difficulty swallowing, dysphonia, dysarthria, loss of bladder control, and generalized weakness. This is most likely due to spread of the toxin from the injection site to other parts of the body. At usual cosmetic doses, these side effects are very unlikely.

12. **How does upper eyelid ptosis occur after botulinum toxin injection and how do you treat it?**
    Ptosis of the upper eyelid, or blepharoptosis, occurs by diffusion of the botulinum toxin to the levator palpebrae superioris or levator aponeurosis, usually by injection of botulinum toxin too close to the upper eyelid. It can best be prevented by injecting at least 1 centimeter above the orbital rim. Apraclonidine (Iopidine) and phenylephrine (Mydfrin) eye drops will selectively target alpha-2 and alpha-1 adrenergic receptors, respectively, leading to contraction of Müller muscle, which will decrease the ptosis.

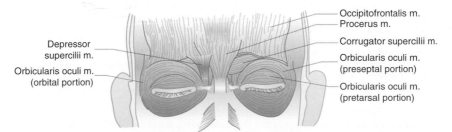

Fig. 65.1 Depressors and elevators of the brow. (From Biesman B: *Atlas of Cosmetic Surgery*. Philadelphia, 2009, Saunders, pp 483–503.)

13. **Can a patient be resistant to botulinum toxin?**
Yes. While rare, there are reports of patients developing resistance to botulinum toxin. This is felt to be due to the formation of antibodies to either the neurotoxin or the complexing proteins that accompany it. To avoid this possibility, it is recommended to use the smallest possible doses to achieve the desired effect and to wait at least 3 months between treatments.

14. **What precautions should patients take after botulinum toxin injection?**
The patient should avoid massaging or rubbing the injected areas as well as any skin treatments on the day of the procedure. Additionally, the patient should avoid any vibrational therapy such as the whirlpool or hydrotherapy. The patient ideally should avoid vigorous sports for a week after injection.

15. **What are some different types of fillers available for facial aesthetics?**
Broadly, fillers can be classified as absorbable or nonabsorbable. The only nonabsorbable filler available is Artefill (Suneva Medical, San Diego, CA), composed of polymethylmethacrylate microspheres. Its use has largely fallen out of favor due to the widespread success of absorbable fillers.
  Absorbable fillers can be divided into synthetic or natural products. Synthetic fillers include Radiesse (Merz, Frankfurt, Germany), composed of calcium hydroxylapatite, and Sculptra (Valeant, Laval, Quebec), composed of poly-L-lactic acid.
  Natural absorbable fillers account for the most commonly used facial fillers, with hyaluronic acid (HA) products comprising the bulk of this category. Other options include autologous fat and collagen, but collagen products are no longer used due to superiority of the HA products and fat.

16. **What is hyaluronic acid?**
Hyaluronic acid is the most common glycosaminoglycan in the skin. It is potently hydrophilic and binds to water, leading to volumization and hydration of the skin. Interestingly, hyaluronic acid is identical across all species, making it extremely unlikely to lead to allergic reaction. As such, no skin testing is needed prior to injection. Hyaluronic acid products are by far the most commonly used type of facial filler.
  Hyaluronic acid fillers available include Restylane (Valeant, Laval, Quebec), Juvéderm (Allergan, Irvine, CA), Revanesse (Prollenium Medical Technologies Inc., Ontario, Canada), Prevelle Silk (Mentor, Santa Barbara, CA), Belotero (Merz, Frankfurt, Germany), and Eleveess (Anika Therapeutics, Bedford, MA). The main differences between products are due to particle size and concentration of hyaluronic acid, which determine how soft and pliable the product is. Several products now also contain lidocaine for a more comfortable injection.

17. **How long do hyaluronic acid fillers last?**
Anywhere from 6 to 18 months.

18. **What are different methods of injection of facial fillers?**
• Serial puncture: injecting a series of small boluses
• Threading: tunneling the needle beneath the area of concern and injecting as the needle is withdrawn
• Fanning: injection of multiple threads radially by changing direction without withdrawing the needle
• Crosshatching: injection of multiple threads perpendicular to one another in a grid
    These techniques are demonstrated in Fig. 65.2.
    Threading is useful for lip and nasolabial fold augmentation. Fanning and crosshatching are particularly useful for filling in larger defects.

19. **What is the mechanism of action of Sculptra?**
Sculptra works through the process of neocollagenesis wherein the body gradually builds collagen over time in the areas where the product is injected. This leads to a gradual increase in volume over time as opposed to an immediate effect. Effects of Sculptra have been reported up to 3 years after treatment.

20. **What are complications that can result from injection of facial fillers?**
Common complications include ecchymosis, erythema, and edema at the site of injection. Asymmetry from over- or undercorrection can also be seen. Nodules and granulomas can form as a result of the inflammatory response to the filler but are usually rare. Nodules specifically have been reported for Sculptra but can be avoided by the depth and technique of injection. Finally, serious complications have been reported, including skin necrosis, blindness, and even death. These are due to accidental intravascular injection leading to occlusion of blood flow.

21. **What is the Tyndall effect?**
A complication of injecting hyaluronic acid too superficially, leading to a visible bump under the skin with a bluish discoloration. This can be prevented by deeper injection as well as beveling the needle away from the skin.

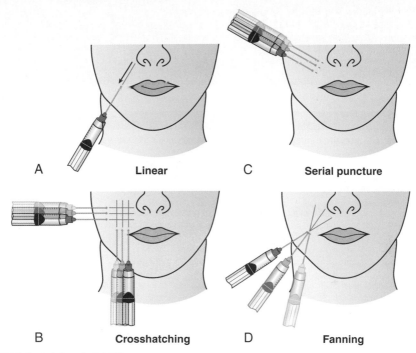

Fig. 65.2 Injection techniques for facial fillers.

22. **What is hyaluronidase and how is it used?**
    Hyaluronidase causes hydrolysis and breakdown of hyaluronic acid, allowing areas of overcorrection to be dissolved away. Its effect is usually seen within 24 hours.

CONTROVERSIES

23. **Should blunt-tip cannulas or needles be used for the injection of facial fillers?**
    Because of the risk of puncture of blood vessels due to needles, which can lead to bruising or other intravascular complications associated with the injection of fillers, some practitioners prefer using blunt-tip cannulas to minimize this risk. However, others feel it is still possible to puncture vessels with blunt-tip cannulas due to their small caliber.

BIBLIOGRAPHY

Carruthers A, Kane MA, Flynn TC, et al: The convergence of medicine and neurotoxins: a focus on botulinum toxin type A and its application in aesthetic medicine—a global, evidence-based botulinum toxin consensus education initiative: part I: botulinum toxin in clinical and cosmetic practice, *Dermatol Surg* 39:493–509, 2013.
Carruthers J, Fagien S, Matarasso SL, et al: Consensus recommendations on the use of botulinum toxin type a in facial aesthetics, *Plast Reconstr Surg* 114(Suppl 6):1S–22S, 2004.
Cohen JL: Understanding, avoiding, and managing dermal filler complications, *Dermatol Surg* 34(Suppl 1):S92–S99, 2008.
FDA-Approved Dermal Fillers. Available at https://www.fda.gov/medical-devices/cosmetic-devices/dermal-fillers-approved-center-devices-and-radiological-health.
Gilman GS: Cosmetic uses of neurotoxins and injectable fillers. In: Johnson JT, Rosen CA, eds: *Bailey's Head and Neck Surgery Otolaryngology*, 2014, Lippincott Williams and Wilkins, pp 3239–3251.
Kim JE, Sykes JM: Hyaluronic acid fillers: history and overview, *Facial Plast Surg* 27:523–528, 2011.
Kontis TC: Contemporary review of injectable facial fillers, *JAMA Facial Plast Surg* 15:58–64, 2013.
Vleggaar D: Facial volumetric correction with injectable poly-L-lactic acid, *Dermatol Surg* 31:1511–1517, 2005.
Walker TJ, Dayan SH: Comparison and overview of currently available neurotoxins, *J Clin Aesthet Dermatol* 7:31–39, 2014.

CHAPTER 66

FACIAL REANIMATION

Scott Hirsch, MD, Geoffrey Ferril, MD and Adam M. Terella, MD

KEY POINTS

1. The patient with facial nerve paralysis necessitates a thorough workup to delineate timing, mechanism, location, and extent of the injury.
2. Ophthalmologic care, whether medical and/or surgical, is crucial in the management of lagophthalmos due to facial nerve paralysis and should be instituted as early as possible.
3. Facial reanimation procedures are classified as static or dynamic, depending on whether facial movement may be achieved.
4. The elapsed time since nerve injury affects the viability of distal nerve fibers and, in turn, influences the appropriate type of reanimation procedure (neural reinnervation versus muscle transposition or static).

Pearls
1. In the setting of denervation, nerve and motor endplate fibrosis leads to muscle atrophy. Thus reinnervation procedures must be completed 12 to 18 months post injury before atrophic changes become permanent.
2. Electromyographic testing (EMG) is an invaluable tool to help determine whether spontaneous recovery is occurring.
3. After complete transection of the facial nerve and repair by tension-free reapproximation or an interposition graft, House-Brackman Grade 3 paralysis is the maximum amount of recovery achievable.

QUESTIONS

1. **Briefly describe the course of the facial nerve.**
   The facial nerve exits the brainstem, courses through the cerebellopontine angle, and then enters the temporal bone. After a complex course through the temporal bone, it exits the stylomastoid foramen and branches within the parotid gland into two main branches, the temporofacial and cervicofacial, at the pes anserinus. Traditionally, five terminal branches are present, including the temporal, zygomatic, buccal, marginal mandibular, and cervical branches.

2. **What is the most commonly used classification of facial nerve injury?**
   The House-Brackmann Grading Scale is the most commonly used in the literature. House and Brackmann staged injury from grades 1 to 6 (Table 66.1). Increasing grade corresponds to a decreasing likelihood of spontaneous recovery.

Table 66.1 Facial Nerve Grading Scale

GRADE	DESCRIPTION	CHARACTERISTICS
I	Normal	Normal facial function
II	Mild dysfunction	Slight weakness or synkinesis; normal symmetry at rest; complete eye closure with minimal effort
III	Moderate dysfunction	Noticeable weakness or synkinesis; normal symmetry at rest; complete eye closure with maximal effort
IV	Moderately severe dysfunction	Obvious weakness; normal symmetry at rest; incomplete eye closure
V	Severe dysfunction	Only perceptible movement; asymmetric at rest; incomplete eye closure
VI	Total paralysis	No movement

Adapted from House JW, Brackmann DE: Facial nerve grading system, *Otolaryngol Head Neck Surg* 93(2):146–147, 1985.

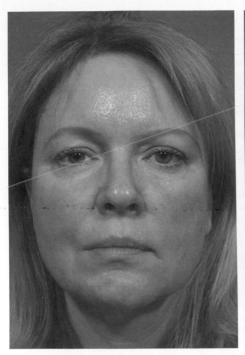 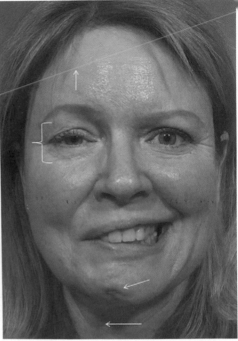

Fig. 66.1 Photographs of a patient with synkinesis after Bell palsy. The left photograph shows the patient in repose, and on the right, the patient is attempting to smile. The yellow arrow on the forehead shows the ipsilateral frontalis activation with smiling. The yellow bracket shows the palpebral narrowing. The arrows on the lower face show mentalis and platysmal activation with smiling. (From Pepper JP, Kim JC: Selective chemodenervation with botulinum toxin in facial nerve disorders, *Oper Tech Otolaryngol Head Neck Surg* 23(4):297–305, 2012.)

3. **What is synkinesis and what is the first-line treatment for this disorder?**
   Synkinesis is a hyperkinetic and uncoordinated mass facial movement seen with aberrant nerve fiber regeneration after facial nerve injury (Fig. 66.1). This involuntary synkinesia often occurs between the orbicularis oculi and orbicularis oris muscles or presents as increased lacrimation of the affected eye. Botulinum toxin, which blocks the presynaptic release of acetylcholine, is the first-line therapy. Results from Botox injections are improved when performed after facial rehabilitation.

4. **What key elements of the history and physical exam must be taken into account when approaching the patient with facial nerve paralysis?**
   It is important to consider the patient's medical history, mechanism of injury, presumed site of injury, timing of injury, presence and state of facial nerve, vestibulocochlear function, eye closure, facial symmetry, functional impairment, and individual expectations. Evaluating the ability of the patient to elevate their eyebrows, close their eyes, frown, smile, pucker their lips, puff the cheeks, and tense the neck allows for assessment of the terminal branches of the facial nerve.

5. **What exam findings differentiate between central and peripheral facial nerve lesions?**
   Paralysis limited to the lower facial muscles with intact forehead animation is usually a sign of a central lesion (because of bilateral innervation of the forehead muscles). Forehead-sparing paralysis can also result from a peripheral lesion that involves only the lower division of the facial nerve. A further distinguishing finding is the preservation of emotional facial motion with central facial paralysis, whereas peripheral facial paralysis impairs both voluntary and emotional facial animation.

6. **What is the role of electrodiagnostic testing following facial paralysis?**
   The goal of electrodiagnostic testing is to evaluate the degree of facial nerve injury and functionality of the facial musculature. It is useful in determining the prognosis for facial nerve recovery and stratifying patients into continued observation versus surgical intervention groups. Commonly utilized electrical tests are the maximum stimulation test (MST), nerve excitability test (NET), electroneuronography (ENoG), and electromyography (EMG).

7. **Discuss electromyography (EMG) testing and how it is useful in the setting of facial reanimation.**
   EMG is the study of depolarization potentials in a muscle fiber. With facial paralysis, EMG provides important information that can help determine the appropriate treatment options. Typically, resting muscles exhibit no spontaneous electrical activity. In the setting of denervation from facial nerve injury, electrical activity may be increased and *spontaneous fibrillation potentials* develop. Fibrillation potentials provide strong evidence that denervation has occurred. Conversely, *polyphasic action potentials* indicate the occurrence of reinnervation. Electrical silence is observed in completely denervated muscles with a nonfunctional motor end plate. If reinnervation is evident, observation is appropriate to determine the amount of recovery the patient may have.

8. **Is there a role for physical therapy in facial reanimation?**
   Yes. Physical therapy is often underutilized in the setting of facial nerve paralysis. Facial neuromuscular reeducation using surface EMG and biofeedback techniques has demonstrated improvements in facial movement and reduction in synkinesis in randomized trials.

9. **What is a potential sequela of paralysis of the orbicularis oculi?**
   Paralysis of the orbicularis oculi muscle may result in incomplete eye closure or *lagophthalmos*. Left untreated, paralytic lagophthalmos can lead to exposure keratitis, corneal ulceration, and blindness.

10. **Describe broadly the types of surgical rehabilitation utilized for facial paralysis.**
    Surgical techniques for the management of facial paralysis can be classified as either *static* or *dynamic*. Static procedures serve to restore symmetry and limit functional sequelae but do not restore facial movement. Dynamic procedures aim to restore movement and can be subdivided into *neural procedures* (cable grafting, cross-facial nerve grafting, XII to VII, V to VII), *microvascular free flaps* (gracilis flap), and other dynamic procedures (transposition of the temporalis or masseter and temporalis tendon transfer).

11. **Discuss treatment of the lower eyelid in the setting of facial paralysis.**
    The decision to treat the lower eyelid largely depends on lower lid laxity, which can be assessed by the snap test. Medial lower lid laxity can cause the inferior punctum to evert from the globe, resulting in epiphora. Correction is attained via medial canthoplasty. For excess lateral lower lid laxity contributing to scleral show or ectropion, a horizontal lid shortening procedure is indicated.

12. **What is ectropion?**
    Ectropion is the abnormal eversion of the lower eyelid in relation to the globe and can be associated with lower eyelid paralysis.

13. **Discuss treatment of the paralyzed upper eyelid.**
    Nonsurgical treatment includes topical lubricating drops and ointment, as well as taping the eyelid closed at night. Gold weight implantation at the level of the tarsal plate is the most common surgical procedure for managing upper eyelid paralytic lagophthalmos. Gold or platinum is often used because of their low reactivity and high density. The procedure can often be performed under local anesthesia and is reversible.

14. **In situations where the facial nerve is transected or resected, what is the technique of choice for repair?**
    In the acute setting, primary nerve anastomosis is the technique of choice for the repair of a completely disrupted facial nerve. Repair should occur as early as possible, ideally prior to Wallerian degeneration (within 72 hours). Success is largely dependent on the ability to reapproximate the disrupted segments *without tension*. Obtaining a tensionless repair may require mobilization or rerouting of the adjacent facial nerve segments.

15. **What are some alternative options to repair a transected facial nerve when a tension-free reapproximation is not possible?**
    For situations in which a tension-free reapproximation is not possible, an interposition nerve graft can be utilized. The two most popular nerves utilized for this purpose are the great auricular and sural nerves.

16. **When counseling patients in terms of House-Brackmann score after a primary neurorrhaphy or interposition graft facial nerve repair, what is the best possible outcome?**
    House-Brackmann Grade III (see Table 66.1).

17. **What is cross-facial nerve grafting?**
    Cross-facial nerve grafting is a two-stage procedure in which the functioning facial nerve and its branches are used to innervate contralateral paralyzed nerve branches by way of an interposition graft. The first stage involves identifying distal facial nerve branches (buccal and zygomatic) on the normally functioning side and coapting a

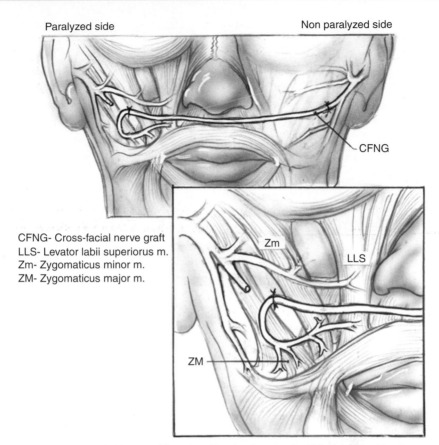

Paralyzed side

Non paralyzed side

CFNG

CFNG- Cross-facial nerve graft
LLS- Levator labii superiorus m.
Zm- Zygomaticus minor m.
ZM- Zygomaticus major m.

Zm

LLS

ZM

Fig. 66.2 Illustration of the cross-facial nerve graft from a buccal branch on the nonparalyzed left side to a buccal branch on the paralyzed side. (From Collar RM, Byrne PJ, Boahene KD: Cross-facial nerve grafting, *Oper Tech Otolaryngol Head Neck Surg* 23(4):258–261, 2012.)

sural nerve graft to these. The second stage, undertaken 9 to 12 months later, comprises secondary neurorrhaphies between selected paralyzed facial nerve branches and the cross-face nerve graft. This procedure relies on a contralateral, normal-functioning nerve and functional motor end plates on the paralyzed side. For this reason, the period of degeneration should ideally be less than 6 months (Fig. 66.2).

18. **What is meant by the term "nerve transposition"? What is the most common nerve transposition procedure?**
   A nerve transposition procedure involves coapting to the facial nerve trunk or distal branches to another cranial nerve. This technique is utilized when a proximal facial nerve stump is not available or viable but the distal nerve and motor end plates on the paralyzed side are viable. Several cranial nerves have been utilized for nerve transpositions, but the hypoglossal nerve (CN XII) and masseteric branch of the trigeminal nerve (CN V) remain the most commonly utilized due to relatively low donor site morbidity and close anatomic proximity to the facial nerve.

19. **What is the role of muscle transposition in the setting of facial paralysis?**
   Muscle transposition is usually used when nerve grafting is not possible because of the degradation of the distal nerve fibers and motor end plates. In this setting, transposition of the temporalis or masseter muscle can provide tone and dynamic reanimation to the lower face (Fig. 66.3).

20. **What are the advantages of temporalis tendon transfer versus temporalis muscle transposition?**
   The original temporalis muscle transfer described the transfer of the temporalis muscle belly over the zygomatic arch. This technique resulted in a significant cosmetic deformity in the temporal and zygomatic regions. The orthodromic temporalis tendon transfer technique prevents this deformity by avoiding the transfer of the muscle

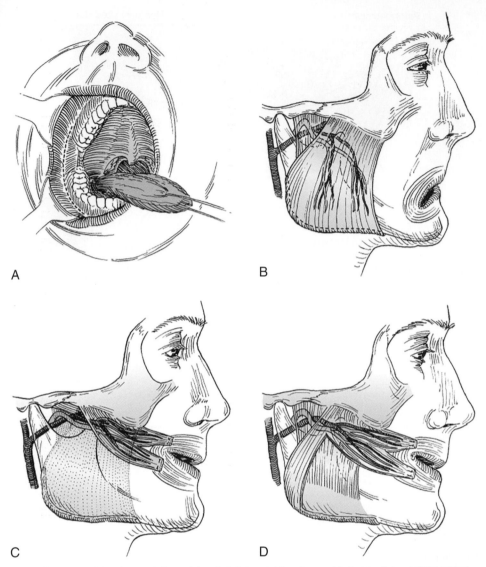

A

B

C

D

Fig. 66.3 Schematic depiction of a masseteric muscle transfer technique. **A**, Intraoral approach to the masseteric muscle; an external approach is sometimes preferred. **B**, Release of masseter muscle. **C** and **D**, The masseter is transposed so that the masseteric nerve supply is transferred intact with the muscle belly. (From Ridgway JM, Bhama PK, Kim JH: Rehabilitation of facial paralysis. In: Flint PW, Haughey BH, Lund VJ, et al, eds: *Cummings Otolaryngology: Head and Neck Surgery*, 6th ed, Philadelphia, 2015, Saunders Elsevier.)

over the arch. Instead, the temporalis tendon is disinserted from its attachment to the coronoid and transferred to the lateral commissure or melolabial fold.

21. **Discuss the role of microneurovascular free flaps in facial reanimation.**
    Microneurovascular free flaps utilize free tissue transfer, including soft tissue and the corresponding nerve and vascular supply, to rehabilitate a paralyzed face. They have the potential to offer emotional animation, in addition to good tone. They typically involve a two-stage procedure in which a cross-facial nerve graft is performed approximately 9 to 12 months prior to the flap. The microneurovascular flap is then anastomosed to the cross-facial graft and facial artery and vein.

22. **What is the most commonly utilized microneurovascular flap in facial reanimation?**
The most commonly utilized microneurovascular free flap is the gracilis flap. This muscle is found in the medial thigh and innervated by the anterior branch of the obturator nerve. The vascular supply is by way of the adductor branch of the profunda femoris artery and accompanying paired venae comitantes.

23. **What is the role of static procedures in the facial paralysis patient?**
Static procedures are used to address asymmetry in the facial paralysis patient. They do not provide restoration of facial movement and are thus used when dynamic procedures are not an option. Such procedures are commonly applied to the brow and midface to re-create resting symmetry, a melolabial fold, and improve nasal obstruction due to valve collapse.

BIBLIOGRAPHY

Bergeron CM, Moe KS: The evaluation and treatment of lower eyelid paralysis, *Facial Plast Surg* 24:231–241, 2008.
Catalano PJ, Bergstein MJ, Biller HF: Comprehensive management of the eye in facial paralysis, *Arch Otolaryngol Head Neck Surg* 121(1):81–86, 1995.
Clark JM, Shockley WW: Management and reanimation of the paralyzed face. In: Papel ID, Frodel J, Holt GR, et al, eds: *Facial Plastic and Reconstructive Surgery*, 2nd ed, 2002, Thieme Medical Publishers.
Diaz RC, Poti SM, Dobie RA: Tests of facial nerve function. In: Flint PW, Haughey BH, Lund VJ, et al, eds: *Cummings Otolaryngology: Head and Neck Surgery*, 6th ed, Philadelphia, 2015, Saunders Elsevier.
House JW, Brackmann DE: Facial nerve grading system, *Otolaryngol Head Neck Surg* 93(2):146–147, 1985.
Jowett N, Hadlock TA: Free gracilis transfer and static facial suspension for midfacial reanimation in long-standing flaccid facial palsy, *Otolaryngol Clin North Am* 51(6):1129–1139, 2018. doi: 10.1016/j.otc.2018.07.009.
Meltzer NE, Alam DS: Facial paralysis rehabilitation: state of the art, *Curr Opin Otolaryngol Head Neck Surg* 18(4):232–237, 2010.
Owusu JA, Stewart CM, Boahene K: Facial nerve paralysis, *Med Clin North Am* 102(6):1135–1143, 2011. doi: 10.1016/j.mcna.2018.06.011.
Pepper JP, Kim JC: Selective chemodenervation with botulinum toxin in facial nerve disorders, *Oper Tech Otolaryngol Head Neck Surg* 23(4):297–305, 2012.
Ridgway JM, Bhama PK, Kim JH: Rehabilitation of facial paralysis. In: Flint PW, Haughey BH, Lund VJ, et al, eds: *Cummings Otolaryngology: Head and Neck Surgery*, 6th ed, Philadelphia, 2015, Saunders Elsevier.

CHAPTER 67

SKIN GRAFTS AND LOCAL FLAPS

Adam M. Terella, MD and Emily S. Misch, MD, MPH

KEY POINTS

1. Apply the concept of the "reconstructive ladder" when assessing the complexity of the required reconstructive method. The more problematic the wound, the more complex the reconstruction.
2. Cutaneous flaps are classified according to their blood supply, configuration, location, or method of transfer.
3. Orienting a skin excision, wound closure, or local flap parallel to relaxed skin tension lines (RSTLs) will camouflage the resulting scar, limit closure tension, and result in an optimal esthetic outcome.
4. When utilizing a skin graft, the reconstructive surgeon must consider the vascularity of the recipient site and optimize contact between the graft and recipient bed.

Pearls
1. Utilization of a full-thickness skin graft, when possible, limits graft contraction and usually results in an improved texture and color match.
2. Avoiding injury to the dermal and subdermal plexus is critical for preserving the blood supply to random flaps.
3. Orient local flaps such that the final scar orientation and tension vector are away from distortable structures, such as the lower eyelids.
4. In designing a rotational flap, the arc of rotation (flap length) should be approximately four times the diameter of the defect.

QUESTIONS

SKIN GRAFTING

1. **Describe the concept of the "reconstructive ladder."**
   The goal of surgical management of a wound is to achieve rapid wound closure using the simplest method, while creating the best functional and cosmetic outcomes. The "reconstructive ladder" concept helps the reconstructive surgeon assess the complexity of the treatment required, beginning with the simplest modality and progressing in difficulty from there (Fig. 67.1).

2. **What are the three histologic layers of the skin?**
   The skin is composed of the epidermis, dermis, and subcutaneous connective tissue. The epidermis is composed of keratinizing stratified squamous epithelium and is separated from the dermis by a basement membrane. The dermis is subdivided into a thin papillary dermis overlying a thicker reticular dermis.

3. **What is a skin graft?**
   A skin graft is an island of epidermis with varying thicknesses of dermis that has been surgically removed from a donor site and transferred to a recipient site. The blood supply to the skin graft is dependent on the vascularity of the recipient site.

4. **When should a skin graft be utilized?**
   Skin grafts are best utilized to address superficial wounds that cannot be reasonably reconstructed with primary closure or a local flap. Wound size, location, and risk of distortion may often prohibit primary closure or the use of local flaps. To obtain the best cosmetic outcome the graft should be harvested from a site closely matching the color and texture of the skin surrounding the wound.

5. **Which two techniques can be used for harvesting skin grafts?**
   Skin grafts are harvested as full thickness or split thickness. Full-thickness skin grafts (FTSGs) consist of epidermis and the full thickness of the dermis. They are usually harvested deep into the dermis and within the superficial subcutaneous plane. Manual removal of excess subcutaneous tissue is performed prior to use. Split-thickness skin grafts (STSGs) consist of the epidermis and a variable portion of the underlying dermis. They are usually harvested utilizing a dermatome at a thickness of 0.012 to 0.025 in.

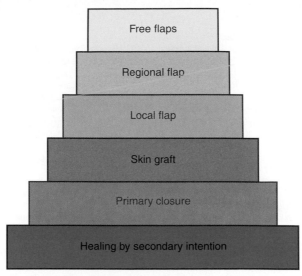

Fig. 67.1 The reconstructive ladder. (From Flint PW, Haughey BH, Lund V, et al: *Cummings Otolaryngology*, 3rd ed, Philadelphia, 2015, Saunders.)

6. **What factors will most affect skin graft viability?**

   Several factors directly influence skin graft viability. These include the vascularity of the recipient site, contact between graft and recipient site, and certain systemic illnesses such as diabetes or chronic hypoxemia. Irradiated tissue; exposed bone, cartilage, or tendon; infected tissue; or bleeding wounds tend to be unfavorable conditions for skin graft viability.

7. **What are the phases of skin graft survival?**

   Skin grafts initially survive by the diffusion of nutrition from serum at the recipient site through a process termed *plasma imbibition*. Between days 3 and 7, there is reestablishment of blood flow between preexisting graft capillaries and recipient end capillaries in a phase termed *inosculation. Revascularization* begins at approximately day 4 and is characterized by the ingrowth of new vessels into the graft.

8. **What are the advantages and disadvantages of a full-thickness skin graft?**

   Full-thickness grafts provide a better color match and better texture match and undergo less contraction than split-thickness grafts. Their increased thickness also makes them more appropriate for deeper defects. Disadvantages include reduced survival rate and longer healing time.

9. **What are the advantages and disadvantages of a split-thickness skin graft?**

   A split-thickness skin graft will have increased viability due to greater capillary exposure on the undersurface of the graft. This permits greater absorption of nutrients from the wound bed. In addition, because STSGs contain less tissue, revascularization occurs more quickly. The main disadvantage is that STSGs often result in poor texture and color matching. They are also more prone to contraction.

10. **What are the important points for postoperative care of skin grafts?**

    Skin graft dressings should aim to immobilize the graft on the recipient bed and minimize any shearing forces that will disrupt the developing blood supply. Often, this immobilization is accomplished with bolsters made of Xeroform™ or petroleum gauze. The dressing should remain in place for 5 to 7 days to enable adequate graft adherence to take place and help prevent desiccation.

11. **How should a skin graft donor site be managed?**

    Full-thickness donor sites are primarily closed when possible. Split-thickness skin graft donor sites are best treated with an occlusive dressing. Studies have shown that a moist, clean, healing environment allows wounds to heal more quickly.

12. **What are the four main mechanisms by which skin grafts fail?**

    The most common mechanisms of failure include (1) inadequate wound bed vascularity, (2) shearing forces that separate the graft from the bed and prevent revascularization, (3) hematoma or seroma formation that prevents contact of the graft to the bed, and (4) infection.

LOCAL FLAPS

13. **What is a local cutaneous flap?**
    A local cutaneous flap is an area of skin and subcutaneous tissue with direct vascular supply that is transferred to a site located adjacent to or near the flap. In contrast, a graft does not have its own blood supply.

14. **What are relaxed skin tension lines, and why are they important?**
    Relaxed skin tension lines (RSTLs) are lines intrinsic to aging skin. They manifest as creases and wrinkles oriented perpendicular to the underlying facial mimetic musculature (Fig. 67.2). In planning skin excisions, wound closures, or local flaps, it is desirable to orient the resulting closure or scar parallel to RSTLs. Wounds oriented parallel to RSTLs are well camouflaged and have minimal wound closure tension, thus resulting in a less apparent scar.

15. **What is the concept of facial aesthetic regions? Why is this concept important to the design of local flaps?**
    The face can be divided into specific "primary aesthetic regions," including the forehead, eyelids, cheeks, nose, lips, mentum, and auricles. Valleys, troughs, and creases represent the boundaries between facial esthetic regions. It is preferable to design flaps within the same esthetic region. Additionally, it is desirable to orient incisions, and thus scars, along the borders of esthetic units, because this will improve scar camouflage.

16. **How are cutaneous flaps classified?**
    Cutaneous flaps are commonly classified according to their blood supply, configuration, location, or method of transfer. When characterizing by blood supply, local flaps can be based on a random or axial pattern. Random flaps are based on the subdermal plexus and do not include blood vessels. An axial flap utilizes a dominant vessel

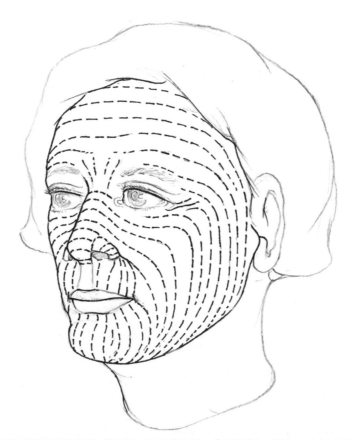

Fig. 67.2 Oblique view of the face illustrating relaxed skin tension lines. (From Patel KG, Sykes JM: Concepts in local flap design and classification, *Oper Tech Otolaryngol Head Neck Surg* 22(1):13–23, 2011.)

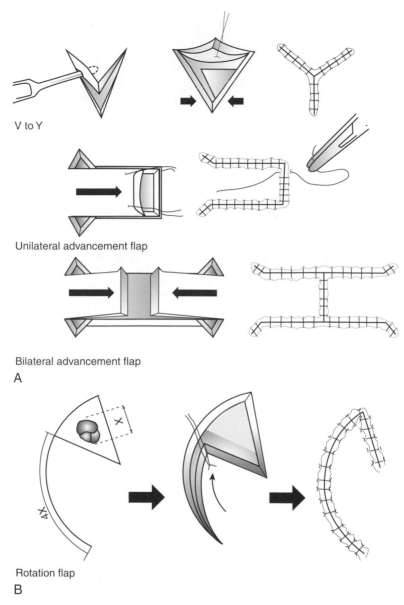

V to Y

Unilateral advancement flap

Bilateral advancement flap

A

Rotation flap

B

Fig. 67.3 A, B. Schematic representation of local flaps. The unilateral advancement, bilateral advancement, and rotational flaps are illustrated. The flap length should be approximately four times the diameter of the defect. (From Patel KG, Sykes JM: Concepts in local flap design and classification, *Oper Tech Otolaryngol Head Neck Surg* 22(1):13–23, 2011.)

for primary vascularity. The paramedian forehead flap, based on the supratrochlear artery, is a commonly used axial pattern flap.

17. **How are local flaps classified by method of transfer?**
    Pivotal and advancement flaps are commonly used local flaps. An advancement flap has a linear configuration and is advanced into a defect (Fig. 67.3A). They work best in areas of significant skin laxity because they involve stretching the skin of the flap. Advancement flaps have a length-to-width ratio of 1:1 or 2:1 and often create "dog-ear" or standing cone deformity. Pivotal flaps involve pivoting the tissue around a fixed point at the base of the pedicle (Fig. 67.3B). Examples of pivotal flaps include rotation, transposition, and interpolated-style flaps.

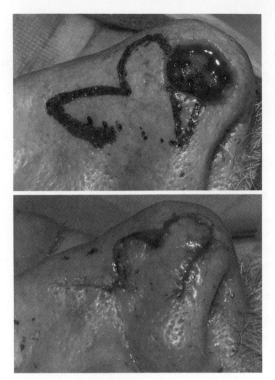

Fig. 67.4 Bilobed transposition flap used to close a nasal defect.

18. **How do rotational, transposition, and interpolated flaps differ?**

Rotational flaps pivot around the base of the flap and rotate toward the defect along an arc. Traditionally, rotation flaps travel along an arc of 30 degrees or less, with a radius two to three times the diameter of the defect and an arc length four to five times the width of the defect. Most also encompass the features of advancement flaps and are commonly labeled rotation-advancement flaps. A transposition flap is rotated over a segment of the normal skin to be placed at an adjacent recipient site. The donor site must be closed during the design process. Two commonly utilized transposition flaps are the rhombic flap and bilobed flap (Fig. 67.4). In contrast, the base of an interpolated flap is not contiguous with the defect. This arrangement creates a pedicle that crosses the intervening intact tissue. A second-stage procedure is required for the division and inset of the pedicle. An example of an interpolated flap is the paramedian forehead flap.

19. **Describe the concept of a V-Y advancement flap.**

The V-Y flap achieves advancement of tissue into a defect. A V-shaped incision is made and the secondary triangular donor defect is closed primarily. This primary closure serves to push the tissue into the defect. In closing the donor site primarily, the wound closure suture line assumes a Y configuration (see Fig. 67.3A).

20. **What three changes will a Z-plasty create in a scar contracture?**

A Z-plasty (Fig. 67.5) is designed with three limbs of equal length that form two triangular flaps. The two triangular flaps represent transposition flaps. The triangles represent angular flaps that are transposed with each other. This technique is useful to (1) interrupt scar linearity, (2) lengthen a scar contracture, and (3) change the orientation of a scar/contracture.

21. **What is the theoretical increase in scar length created by a 30-30-degree Z-plasty? A 45-45-degree Z-plasty? A 60-60-degree Z-plasty?**

A 30-30-degree Z-plasty will lengthen a scar by 25%. A 45-45-degree Z-plasty will lengthen a scar by 50%. A 60-60-degree Z-plasty will lengthen a scar by 75%.

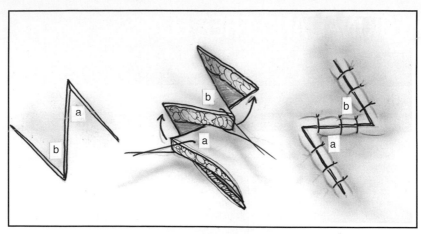

Fig. 67.5 A vertical scar is depicted on the left; 60-degree Z-plasty flaps are designed (a and b). After transposition, the central limb is lengthened and redirected, and the final scar is broken into three limbs (right). (From Frodel JL Jr: Creative uses of the Z-plasty technique, *Oper Tech Otolaryngol Head Neck Surg* 22(1):30–34, 2011.)

BIBLIOGRAPHY

Baker S: *Local Flaps in Facial Reconstruction*, 3rd ed, 2014, Saunders.
Borges AF: Pitfalls in flap design, *Ann Plast Surg* 9(3):201–210, 1982.
Brenner MJ, Moyer JS: Skin and composite grafting techniques in facial reconstruction for skin cancer, *Facial Plast Surg Clin North Am* 25(3):347–363, 2017.
Greer SE: *Handbook of Plastic Surgery*, 2006, Marcel Dekker.
Hudson DA: Some thoughts on choosing a Z-plasty: the Z made simple, *Plast Reconstr Surg* 106(3):665–671, 2000.
Kaplan B, Moy RL: Flaps and grafts for facial reconstruction, *Dermatol Surg* 21(5):431–440, 1995.
Papel ID: *Facial Plastic and Reconstructive Surgery*, 2nd ed, 2002, Thieme.
Patel KG, Sykes JM: Concepts in local flap design and classification, *Oper Tech Otolaryngol Head Neck Surg* 22(1):13–23, 2011.

CHAPTER 68

REGIONAL AND FREE FLAPS

Aurora G. Vincent, MD, FACS, Yadranko Ducic, MD, FACS and Fiyin Sokoya, MD

KEY POINTS

1. Every reconstructive plan should be tailored to the individual patient, taking into consideration not only the unique defect but also other perioperative and patient factors.
2. The ideal plan for one patient may not work for another.
3. Before surgery, always consider patient comorbidities (heart/lung disease, perioperative risk) and optimize patients for healing (diabetes control, thyroid-stimulating hormone [TSH], nutrition [albumin/pre-albumin], cessation of nicotine use, and psychosocial support).
4. When deciding on a reconstructive plan, always consider previous surgeries that the patient has had, donor site morbidity, and the patient's lifestyle and hobbies, in addition to general flap characteristics.
5. In general, both regional pedicled and free tissue flaps are very reliable and allow successful reconstruction of complex defects in the head and neck.
6. Remember that defect reconstruction does not have to occur at the time of injury; some cases may be better served with a delayed reconstruction, either all together or in part.
7. When choosing a flap, consider donor site morbidity, tissue type the flap provides and tissue type being reconstructed, bulk of the flap, and pedicle length.
8. When evaluating the defect, consider whether it should be altered or expanded for an improved cosmetic outcome and consider nearby features that are important not to distort or alter (e.g., facial subunits).
9. Not every large defect is best served with regional/free flap reconstruction, and not every small defect is best served with local tissue rearrangement.
10. Even if a defect could be closed with local tissue rearrangement, a regional or free flap may be preferable if it can:
    a. prevent distortion of facial features
    b. prevent undesirable tissue tethering or deformity
    c. allow easier healing by transferring well-vascularized, nonirradiated tissue into a wound.

Pearls
1. Free flaps
   Advantages
       Maximally versatile positioning, minimal bulk around the pedicle, osteocutaneous reconstruction, minimal distortion of surrounding features and tissues, reliable
   Disadvantages
       Operative time, time in hospital, microsurgical training, possible second surgical team
1. Regional pedicled flaps
   Advantages
       Shorter operating times, no microsurgical training necessary, can be used in vessel-depleted areas, reliable
   Disadvantages
       Limited position and reach given pedicled base, cosmetically undesirable bulk around the pedicle, few-to-no options for osteocutaneous reconstruction
3. Remember to evaluate if a patient needs a temporary tracheostomy or feeding tube.

QUESTIONS

1. **What is a regional or regional pedicled flap?**
   A regional flap is any group of tissue that is nourished by a named artery that can be surgically separated from its surrounding tissue and rotated, transposed, or interpolated into a new position. A regional flap remains pedicled at its base around the vessel(s) that provide(s) its nutrition.

2. **What are common regional flaps in head-and-neck reconstruction?**
   Pectoralis, deltopectoral, sternocleidomastoid (SCM), supraclavicular, trapezius, paramedian forehead, nasolabial, latissimusdorsi, submental, temporoparietofascial (TPF), abbe, temporalis (Table 68.1).

Table 68.1 Common Regional Flaps for Head and Neck Reconstruction

NAME AND TYPE	PEDICLE	CHARACTERISTICS AND USES
Pectoralis major (myocutaneous, myofascial)	Thoracoacromial artery	- Simple harvest with or without skin - Can easily reach the neck, occasionally reach the lower face - Can be very bulky - Shearing of skin paddle during harvest may lead to damage of perforating vessels and partial flap loss - Can disfigure the breast and be aesthetically undesirable, especially for women - Can be harvested with rib cartilage or bone for osteocutaneous reconstruction (but rib viability is often unreliable)
Deltopectoral (fasciocutaneous)	Internal mammary artery, perforating branches (2nd and 3rd)	- Simple harvest - Often used for cutaneous defects of the lower neck - May require a skin graft for donor site closure - Can be prone to distal-tip necrosis, especially when extended over the deltoid
Latissimus dorsi (myocutaneous, myofascial)	Thoracodorsal artery	- Used for large cutaneous defects of the face, neck, and scalp - Used for smile reanimation - Can be harvested with the patient in a supine or prone position - Can be very bulky if harvested with skin or thin and pliable if only muscle is harvested - Can be pedicled or free - Can have relatively small-caliber pedicle vessels
Trapezius (myocutaneous, myofascial)	Transverse cervical artery	- Used for cutaneous defects of the posterior and lateral neck or lower face - Can be harvested off the transverse or descending branches - May have a short arc of rotation and variable vascular anatomy - May need lateral decubitus positioning or intraoperative position changes for harvest and inset
Supraclavicular (fasciocutaneous)	Supraclavicular artery	- Used for cutaneous defects of the neck and lower face - In some cases can reach the oral tongue, buccal mucosa, and soft palate - Has excellent color match for facial defects - Can be prone to distal tip necrosis
Temporoparietal fascia (fascia only)	Superficial temporal artery	- Used in facial and skull base defects and microtia repair - Very thin, durable, and highly vascular - Harvest can risk damage to the frontal branch of the facial nerve and alopecia from hair follicle damage
Temporalis (myofascial)	Deep temporal artery	- Used for facial and skull base defects - Very robust, durable, reliable - Carries a risk of aesthetic deformity from temporal wasting
Abbe (myocutaneous)	Labial artery	- Full-thickness lip reconstruction
Nasolabial (fasciocutaneous)	Angular artery	- Used for cutaneous defects of the nose or cheek and oral cavity defects of the buccal mucosa and lips
Inferior turbinate (mucosal)	Angular artery (anteriorly), branches of the sphenopalatine artery (posteriorly)	- Used for intranasal and septal defects - Can be anteriorly or posteriorly based
Paramedian forehead (fasciocutaneous)	Supratrochlear artery	- Nasal reconstruction

(Continued)

Table 68.1 Common Regional Flaps for Head and Neck Reconstruction (*Cont.*)

NAME AND TYPE	PEDICLE	CHARACTERISTICS AND USES
Submental (myocutaneous)	Submental artery	- Oral cavity defects - Risk of failure to remove malignant cells when used for reconstruction of defects from oral cavity cancer resection
Sternocleidomastoid (myofascial, myocutaneous)	Occipital artery (superior third), superior thyroid artery (middle third), transverse cervical artery (inferior third) - 2 of 3 vessels need to be preserved	- Can be pedicled superiorly or inferiorly - Used for oral and pharyngeal defects and cutaneous defects of the neck and face - Can have poor viability of the skin flap due to variable vessel anatomy - Donor site contour abnormality
Latissimus dorsi (myofascial, myocutaneous)	Thoracodorsal artery and vein	- Used for neck and lower face defects - May require intraoperative position changes

3. What are the advantages of regional flap reconstruction?
   - Does not require microsurgical anastomosis or training for use
   - Can provide a large amount of tissue for reconstruction
   - Can provide an optimal match of skin tone and texture
   - Can be used in a vessel-depleted neck that lacks suitable local vessels required for free flap anastomosis
   - Often completed with shorter operating/anesthesia times than free flaps

4. What are disadvantages of regional flap reconstruction?
   - This can result in undesirable donor site morbidity and scarring. For example, a pectoralis myocutaneous or myofascial regional flap distorts the breast, which may be concerning, particularly for female patients.
   - Can have bulkiness at the pedicle with an undesirable cosmetic outcome
   - Are more at risk for distal tip necrosis from poor perfusion
   - Are limited in their positioning and reach, given that they are reliant on their pedicled base

5. What is a free flap, aka free tissue transfer?
   A free flap is any group of tissue that is nourished by a named artery and can be harvested, its artery and vein ligated, for transfer to a completely separate part of the body. The artery and vein(s) supplying a free flap are cut, thus making the tissue completely free from any attachments. The artery and vein require anastomosis to local vessels in the area of transfer to reestablish nutritional inflow and outflow and flap survival.

6. What are common free flaps used in head and neck reconstruction?
   Radial forearm, fibula, anterolateral thigh (ALT), rectus abdominis, latissimus dorsi, scapula/parascapular, lateral arm, jejunum, gracilis, sternohyoid/omohyoid (Table 68.2).

7. What are the advantages of free flap reconstruction?
   - Maximally versatile in terms of positioning, tissue bulk, tissue pliability/quality given the many donor options
   - Can achieve excellent cosmetic and functional results
   - Generally very reliable
   - Does not have a bulky pedicle
   - Variability of donor site and donor site morbidity

8. What are the disadvantages of free flap reconstruction?
   - Requires microsurgical vessel anastomosis
   - Often requires longer operating room/anesthesia times
   - May require a second surgical team
   - Often requires longer stays in the ICU and longer stays in the hospital after surgery

Table 68.2 Common Microvascular Free Flaps for Head and Neck Reconstruction

NAME AND TYPE	PEDICLE	CHARACTERISTICS AND USES
Radial forearm (fasciocutaneous, osteocutaneous)	Radial artery, venae comitantes ± cephalic vein	- Thin and pliable with a long pedicle - Versatile, with numerous uses including oral cavity, tongue, palate, face, pharynx, and larynx - Often good color match for head and neck defects - Need for donor site skin graft - Rare risk of hand ischemia
Anterolateral thigh (myocutaneous, septocutaneous)	Descending branch of lateral circumflex femoral artery, venae comitantes	- Pliable with a long pedicle - Large surface area - Versatile - Very bulky in some patients, thin in others - Variable pedicle course can make harvest challenging
Rectus abdominis (myocutaneous, myofascial)	Deep inferior epigastric artery and vein	- Often very bulky - Used when reconstruction requires tissue volume (such as total glossectomy and skull base defects) - Risk of abdominal hernia
Fibula (osteocutaneous – can be harvested with or without a skin paddle)	Peroneal artery and vein	- Most common flap used for osteocutaneous reconstruction (mandibular and maxillary repair) - Risk of ankle pain and instability - Risk of foot ischemia
Scapular/parascapular (fasciocutaneous, osteocutaneous)	Circumflex scapular artery and vein	- Harvest can include muscle, skin, and bone - Flexibility for 3D reconstruction - Used for closing large, complex midface and oromandibular defects or when fibular harvest is contraindicated - Lateral decubitus positioning during surgery (risk of brachial plexus injury) - Risk of shoulder weakness - Can be combined with latissimus dorsi harvest for a mega flap - Can be harvested as a chimeric flap with separate skin paddles
Lateral arm (fasciocutaneous)	Profunda brachii artery, venae comitantes	- Thickness depends on patient BMI - Used for oropharyngeal and cutaneous defects - Can have a small-caliber pedicle - Risk of radial nerve palsy
Latissimus dorsi (myofascial, myocutaneous)	Thoracodorsal artery and vein	- Used for skull base and scalp defects, facial reanimation - Useful for large, thin defects - May require intraoperative position changes
Jejunum (enteral)	Branches of the superior mesenteric artery and vein	- Used for circumferential pharyngoesophageal defects - Peristalsis affects swallowing - Production of succus entericus can cause dysgeusia and interfere with voice rehabilitation - Tolerates a shorter ischemia time (2 h)
Gracilis (myofascial)	Adductor artery and venae comitantes, obturator nerve	- Facial reanimation - Can add unnatural bulk to the face
Sternohyoid/omohyoid (myofascial)	Superior thyroid artery, middle thyroid vein, ansa cervicales	- Facial reanimation - Fast twitch, synchronous smile rehabilitation - Adds minimal bulk to the face

9. **What does it mean for a flap to be called fasciocutaneous, myocutaneous, myofascial, or osteocutaneous?**

   These terms refer to the different tissue types transferred. A fasciocutaneous flap includes transfer of skin and underlying fascia. A myocutaneous flap includes transfer of skin and muscle. Similarly, a myofascial flap includes transfer of muscle with its fascia but no cutaneous components. An osteocutaneous flap includes skin and bone. While different flaps can include multiple angiosomes, perforators, or branching vessels that supply subsections of the overall flap, all tissue transferred is based on a single, dominant arteriovenous pedicle.

10. **What is a perforator flap?**

    A perforator flap is one based on a perforating artery or an artery that travels through fascial planes to supply tissue. An ALT, for example, is a type of perforator flap, as the vessels supplying the skin perforate through the underlying muscle and fascia.

11. **Which patient factors are important to consider before reconstruction?**

    Previous surgery or trauma may compromise the integrity of a planned reconstruction if it is in the area of a flap's vascular pedicle. In addition, major comorbidities may affect a patient's suitability for surgery, including the ability to withstand long periods of anesthesia. Regardless of the reconstructive plan, continued tobacco, alcohol, and/or drug use can affect wound healing and the postoperative course. Poor nutrition, low thyroid hormone, and vitamin deficiencies can predispose patients to poor wound healing and fistula formation. Similarly, uncontrolled diabetes, poor hygiene, and preoperative infection can increase the risk for postoperative infection, poor wound healing, and flap compromise. Finally, patients with hypercoagulable disorders are at increased risk of vessel thrombosis and flap failure in both regional and free tissue transfer.

12. **What is an angiosome and why is it important in flap reconstruction?**

    An angiosome is an area of tissue supplied by a single dominant artery. Regional and free flaps are both supplied by a dominant artery and drained by a dominant vein or the venae comitantes that accompany the named artery. The network of arterioles and capillaries arising from the main artery define the limit of tissue that can be raised with the vascular pedicle, regardless of whether it will be transferred in a regional pedicled or free fashion. Tissue that does not receive adequate nutrition from the vascular pedicle will undergo necrosis if transferred during reconstruction.

13. **What are "choke" vessels, and what does it mean to "delay" a flap?**

    Choke vessels connect tissues of adjacent angiosomes. In the setting of delayed tissue transfer, a flap is initially incised and separated from its underlying tissue and then replaced in its native position, which encourages the choke vessels to dilate, thus improving nutritional blood flow to the flap, specifically its distal portion; later, when the flap is harvested during a second procedure, it is at a decreased risk of distal flap necrosis from poor blood supply.

14. **What considerations are unique to free flaps?**

    The pedicle caliber and length are important in assessing a patient for free tissue transfer. For example, a large scalp defect may be suitable for free flap reconstruction when it cannot be closed with local tissue rearrangement and when regional flaps cannot reach the defect. The free flap, however, will require a pedicle long enough to reach the superficial temporal vessels or vessels in the neck. If a flap has a short pedicle that does not reach local vessels for primary anastomosis, it may require vein grafts to increase its length. Vein grafts add sites of vessel anastomosis, however, and can increase the risk of vessel thrombosis and flap compromise.

15. **Can free flaps be innervated, and does that matter?**

    Some flaps can become sensate either spontaneously or after neurorrhaphy. In the setting of facial palsy, muscular flaps such as the gracilis, sternohyoid/omohyoid, or latissimus dorsi are transferred specifically to reanimate the smile; in addition to vessel anastomosis after inset, they undergo neurorrhaphy to allow restoration of voluntary muscular contraction.

16. **When should a single composite flap be used and when should multiple flaps be used in reconstruction?**

    Multiple free, regional, and local flaps can be used in concert to achieve an optimally functional and cosmetically desirable reconstruction. Sometimes, the best reconstruction includes a combination of methods from the "reconstructive ladder." For example, a composite defect of the unilateral mandible, buccal mucosa, and cheek could be repaired with a scapular free flap including two soft tissue components and one bony component. If this flap fails, however, then the entire reconstruction is lost. Alternatively, the same defect could be repaired with an osteocutaneous fibular free flap, restoring bone and oral cavity soft tissue, plus a second regional or free flap to restore the cheek skin. Similarly, the soft tissue defects could be repaired initially with one or more regional or free flaps, and an osteocutaneous free flap or autologous bone grafting could be performed later for mandibular rehabilitation.

17. **How does other therapy (radiation, chemotherapy) affect the reconstructive plan?**
   For optimal survival benefit, radiation and chemotherapy, if warranted in the treatment of cancer, should be started within 4 to 6 weeks of surgery. Thus delayed flaps should be avoided for surgical reconstruction before adjuvant cancer therapy. Similarly, flaps that require skin grafts in the area of planned radiation (such as an STSG over a muscle-only regional or free flap) should be avoided, as they require longer periods of healing and may delay the start of adjuvant therapy.

18. **What if the patient is a candidate for dental rehabilitation?**
   In the setting of mandibular and maxillary reconstruction, the surgeon should consider whether the patient will want and can afford dental implants, as this may affect the reconstruction plan. Adequate bone stock is required to support dental implants, and placement of a reconstructive plate supporting an osteocutaneous flap can affect the subsequent placement of dental implants.

19. **Will the patient be able to adequately breathe and eat after surgery?**
   Tissue transfer to the oral cavity and pharynx will add bulk and increase swelling that could compromise the airway; in such cases, a tracheostomy at or before the time of reconstruction should be considered. Similarly, after reconstruction of the aerodigestive tract in the head and neck, patients may have significant difficulty swallowing, or swallowing may not be advisable in the acute phases of healing. In such cases, a nasogastric tube, gastric tube, or other means of facilitating perioperative nutrition should be placed.

20. **What intraoperative considerations are important for successful free tissue transfer?**
   In general, fluid administration should be limited and vasopressors should be avoided. Further, shorter anesthetic times are beneficial compared to longer times. Intraoperative fluid administration of more than 7 total liters or more than 6 mL/kg/h has been associated with increased rates of flap failure. Hypovolemia, however, can lead to poor flap perfusion. Many studies suggest that vasopressor use does not increase flap-related complications, but many surgeons prefer crystalloid and colloid boluses to improve pressure before resorting to vasopressors. If vasopressors are necessary, dobutamine, dopamine, and norepinephrine are considered preferable to vasopressin for preserving flap flow and perfusion. Intraoperative times exceeding 18 hours have been associated with significantly more flap-related complications than shorter procedures.

21. **What is the Allen test, and why is it important before raising a radial forearm free flap?**
   Adequate perfusion of the hand is reliant on the ulnar artery after radial forearm harvest. If there is an incomplete superficial palmar arch and poor communication between the deep and superficial arches, hand ischemia could result after ligation of the radial artery. The Allen test assesses ulnar perfusion of the hand before radial artery ligation in radial forearm free flap harvest to prevent postoperative hand ischemia. To perform an Allen test, the patient first clenches his/her fist tight enough that the fingers and palm blanch, indicating blood has been drained. The surgeon then occludes both the radial and ulnar arteries in the wrist. The patient is asked to relax the hand; it should maintain a blanched appearance, indicating the surgeon is adequately blocking inflow from both radial and ulnar arteries. Next, the ulnar artery is released and the hand is observed. If perfusion and capillary refill of the thumb and index finger are restored, then adequate collateral flow exists for safe radial forearm harvest. If the results are equivocal, the test can be repeated intraoperatively with the aid of a Doppler probe. If there is inadequate collateral flow, a radial forearm flap should not be harvested from that arm.

22. **How is the forearm closed after radial free flap harvest?**
   The cutaneous defect of the forearm requires placement of a skin graft to cover the flexor tendons. This is usually accomplished using a split-thickness skin graft taken from the thigh. It is important to preserve the paratenon over the flexor tendons so that the skin graft will survive. The hand and forearm are immobilized postoperatively for 1 week to prevent shearing forces from tendon movement and graft failure.

23. **What is "three-vessel run-off," and why is this important for fibular free flap harvest?**
   The popliteal artery in the knee branches into the anterior tibial, posterior tibial, and peroneal arteries, which supply the leg and foot. Two vessels are often required to maintain adequate perfusion of the foot. A fibular free flap includes ligation of the peroneal artery, which can lead to foot ischemia if collateral flow through the anterior tibial and posterior tibial arteries is diminished by atherosclerotic disease or other factors. A lower-extremity angiogram, Doppler, magnetic resonance imaging, or ankle-brachial index should be performed to confirm perfusion of the foot before fibula harvest.

24. **How is the donor site closed after rectus abdominis harvest?**
   The rectus sheath requires primary repair after rectus abdominis harvest to prevent hernia formation. Superior to the arcuate line, closure of the posterior sheath alone is often adequate. However, inferior to the arcuate line, both anterior and posterior abdominal sheaths must be repaired, as the posterior sheath is composed of only transversalis fascia, which is inadequate to prevent hernia formation.

25. **How are microvascular free tissue flaps monitored?**
Free flaps are monitored by clinical exam, often every hour for the first 2 to 3 days after surgery, then with a gradually reduced frequency. Tissue color, temperature, turgor, and capillary refill are examined. A warm, pale flap that is soft to palpation with intact capillary refill is a healthy flap. Venous congestion can manifest with tissue mottling and increased firmness. Arterial compromise will result in an abnormally blanched flap that lacks capillary refill.

Further, flow through the pedicle is evaluated with Doppler, either internally or externally. In some cases, flap tissue can be pricked with a small needle to assess how quickly it bleeds. Quick return of dark, venous blood after pinprick suggests poor venous outflow and flap congestion, while a lack of any bleeding after pinprick suggests poor arterial flow. Normally, a flap should produce slow bleeding of bright red blood after pinprick.

26. **What are the signs of venous congestion?**
- Bluish discoloration
- Taut, firm on palpation
- Rapid bleeding of dark blood on pinprick

27. **What are signs of arterial compromise?**
- Pale discoloration
- Cool temperature
- Absent Doppler
- Absent bleeding on pinprick

28. **What are causes of microvascular free flap failure?**
Free flaps have an overall high success rate, estimated to be between 95% and 99%. Thrombosis is estimated to occur in 8% to 14% of cases, with failure rates of 1% to 9%. However, the success of a second flap attempt after initial flap failure is estimated to be approximately 73%. Venous thrombosis is the most common cause of free flap failure, and it is more likely to occur in the first 72 hours after flap inset. If recognized within 6 hours, flaps can be successfully salvaged in 50% to 85% of cases. Salvage rates are higher the sooner the flap compromise is noted. Arterial compromise is less common than venous thrombosis, but if it occurs it is most likely to occur within the first 24 hours after surgery.

29. **What is hirudotherapy, and when is it useful?**
Hirudotherapy is the application of leeches to a flap. Leeches secrete hirudin, which inhibits factor Xa and clot formation. They also extract venous blood from a flap. Hirudotherapy, or "leech therapy," is useful when there is partial venous congestion of a flap, as they can temporarily relieve congestion until inosculation and neoangiogenesis is sufficient to support a flap. Leeches can be applied to free or regional flaps. Patients on leech therapy often require close hemodynamic monitoring, frequent hemoglobin evaluations, and transfusions. Some patients may require sedation to tolerate leech therapy if, for example, the flap is in the oral cavity. Finally, leeches are known to be colonized with *Aeromonas hydrophilia*, so patients on leech therapy require prophylactic antibiotic treatment. Consider fluoroquinolones such as Levaquin for prophylactic treatment.

30. **How long can a flap survive ischemia?**
Musculocutaneous, myofascial, osteocutaneous, and fasciocutaneous flaps can often tolerate 4 hours of ischemia. However, enteric flaps can only tolerate 2 hours or less. Ischemia for longer periods than a flap can tolerate leads to a phenomenon known as reperfusion. In reperfusion, arteriovenous shunting occurs that prevents distal tissue perfusion. A reperfusion injury can result from the activation of neutrophils and the release of oxygen free radicals in flap tissues.

31. **Is anticoagulation therapy necessary after regional or free tissue transfer?**
No medications have ever been definitively shown to reduce the rate of thrombotic events after free tissue transfer. However, as thrombosis is the most common cause of flap failure, anticoagulation is common after surgery and heparin is the most commonly used agent, followed by aspirin and low-molecular-weight heparin (LMWH). Dextrans and prostaglandin E1 have also been used, and postoperative anticoagulation may decrease thrombotic events in the flap, but it is also useful to prevent venous thromboembolism elsewhere in the body. The benefits of anticoagulation should be weighed against the risk of excessive bleeding and hematoma formation.

32. **What is the cost of microvascular free flap reconstruction versus regional flap reconstruction?**
Longer operative times, increased length of hospital stay, increased time in the intensive care unit, and increased use of medications lead to a higher short-term cost of free flaps compared to pedicled flaps. However, these costs are often justified by the perceived benefits of improved long-term functional and esthetic outcomes achieved with free tissue transfer.

BIBLIOGRAPHY

Alam DS: The sternohyoid flap for facial reanimation, *Facial Plast Surg Clin North Am* 23(1):61–69, 2016.

Alam DS, Haffey T, Vakharia K, et al: Sternohyoid flap for facial reanimation: a comprehensive preclinical evaluation of a novel technique, *JAMA Facial Plast Surg* 15(4):305–313, 2013.

Brinkman JN, Derks LH, Klimek M, Mureau MA: Perioperative fluid management and use of vasoactive and antithrombotic agents in free flap surgery: a literature review and clinical recommendations, *J Reconstr Microsurg* 29(6):357–366, 2013.

Cannaday SB, Hatten K, Wax M: Postoperative controversies in the management of free flap surgery in the head and neck, *Facial Plast Surg Clin N Am* 24:309–314, 2016.

Carroll WR, Esclamado RM: Ischemia/reperfusion injury in microvascular surgery, *Head Neck* 22:700–713, 2000.

Chan D, Rabbani CC, Inman JC, Ducic Y: Cephalic vein transposition in the vessel-depleted neck, *Otolaryngol Head Neck Surg* 155(2):367–368, 2016.

Chepeha DB, Nussenbaum B, Bradford CR, et al: Leech therapy for patients with surgically unsalvageable venous obstruction after revascularized free tissue transfer, *Arch Otolaryngol Head Neck Surg* 128:960–965, 2002.

Chepeha DB, Teknos TN: Microvascular free flaps in head and neck reconstruction. In: Bailey BJ, Johnson JT, Newlands SD, eds: *Bailey's Head and Neck Surgery: Otolaryngology*, 4th ed, 2006, Lippincott Williams & Wilkins.

Chien W, Varvares MA, Hadlock T, et al: Effects of aspirin and low-dose heparin in head and neck reconstruction using microvascular free flaps, *Laryngoscope* 115:973–976, 2005.

Dort JC, Farwell DG, Findlay M, et al: Optimal perioperative care in major head and neck cancer surgery with free flap reconstruction: a consensus review and recommendations from the enhanced recovery after surgery society, *JAMA Otolaryngol Head Neck Surg* 143(3):292–303, 2017.

Hohman MH, Hadlock TA: Microneurovascular free gracilis transfer for smile reanimation, *Oper Tech Otolaryngol Head Neck Surg* 23:262–267, 2012.

Ishimaru M, Ono S, Suzuki S, Matsui H, Fushimi K, Yasunaga H: Risk factors for free flap failure in 2846 patients with head and neck cancer: a national database study in Japan, *J Oral Maxillofac Surg* 74:1265–1270, 2016.

Kruse ALD, Luebbers HT, Gratz KW, Obwegeser JA: Factors influencing survival of free-flap in reconstruction for cancer of the head and neck: a literature review, *Microsurgery* 30:242–248, 2010.

Lighthall JG, Cain R, Ghanem TA, et al: Effect of postoperative aspirin on microvascular free tissue transfer surgery, *Otolaryngol Head Neck Surg* 148(1):40–46, 2013.

Lo SL, Yen YH, Lee PJ, Liu CHC, Pu CM: Factors influencing postoperative complications in reconstructive microsurgery for head and neck cancer, *J Oral Maxillofac Surg* 75:867–873, 2017.

McCory AL, Magnuson JS: Free tissue transfer versus pedicled flap in head and neck reconstruction, *Laryngoscope* 112:2161–2165, 2002.

Motakef S, Mountziaris PM, Ismail IK, Agag RL, Patel A: Emerging paradigms in perioperative management for microsurgical free tissue transfer: review of the literature and evidence-based guidelines, *Plast Reconstr Surg* 135:290–299, 2015.

Pertruzzelli GJ, Brockenbrough JM, Vandevender D, et al: The influence of reconstructive modality on cost of care in head and neck oncology, *Arch Otolaryngol Head Neck Surg* 128(12):1377–1380, 2002.

Ross G, Yla-Kotola TM, Goldstein D, et al: Second free flaps in head and neck reconstruction, *J Plast Reconstr Aesthet Surg* 65:1165–1168, 2012.

Taylor GI, Palmer JH: The vascular territories (angiosomes) of the body: experimental study and clinical applications, *Br J Plast Surg* 40:113–141, 1987.

Urken M, Cheney M, Blackwell K: *Atlas of Regional and Free Flaps for Head and Neck Reconstruction: Flap Harvest and Insetting*, 2nd ed, 2011, Lippincott Williams & Wilkins.

Vincent AG, Bevans SE, Robitschek JM, Groom KL, Herr MW, Hohman MH. Sterno-omohyoid free flap for dual-vector dynamic facial reanimation. *Ann Otol Rhinol Laryngol*. 129(2):195–200.

CHAPTER 69

PRINCIPLES OF TRAUMA

Paul Montero, MD and Erik Peltz, DO

KEY POINTS

1. Manipulation of the traumatically injured airway during intubation attempts may lead to critical decompensation, which requires an immediate, emergent surgical airway.
2. Chest radiography in a trauma patient allows for rapid assessment of airway deviation, subcutaneous emphysema, pneumothorax, hemothorax, rib fractures, or mediastinal widening, which may be indicative of great vessel injury.
3. Any neck injury resulting from direct force that causes significant swelling, pain, or altered mental status should also be evaluated with CT angiography of the neck.

Pearls
1. A secured airway must always be verified by observation of equal chest rise/fall, bilateral breath sounds on auscultation, and CO_2 return. A chest radiograph can demonstrate the position of the endotracheal tube above the carina but does not necessarily rule out the possibility of esophageal intubation.
2. The burn patient should be rapidly assessed for associated inhalation injury with a low threshold for airway stabilization (intubation) if suspected.

QUESTIONS

INITIAL EVALUATION OF THE TRAUMA PATIENT

1. Describe the primary assessment of the trauma patient (ABCs).
   - **Airway:** Assess the patient's airway by observing and listening. Assess for bleeding, loose teeth, inhalation injury (in case of burn), and level of consciousness. A decreased level of consciousness (GCS ≤8) is an indication of the potential inability to protect the airway and need for elective intubation. Orotracheal intubation with in-line cervical stabilization is the method of choice; however, orofacial trauma or a difficult airway may require a surgical airway (see Chapter 77). In the setting of blunt or penetrating tracheal injury, intubation should ideally be performed in the OR. This is performed with adequate equipment for a surgical airway open and readily available and with the neck prepped and draped prior to intubation attempts. Manipulation of the traumatically injured airway during intubation attempts may lead to critical decompensation, which requires immediate emergency surgical airway.
   - **Breathing:** Assess by looking, listening, and feeling. Look for equal chest rise bilaterally. Auscultation can be difficult in the trauma bay but should be performed to evaluate for absence of breath sounds suggesting pneumothorax or hemothorax. Palpate for crepitus of the chest wall, suggesting rib fracture with potential underlying pneumothorax. Evaluate for "flail chest" – three or more ribs with fractures in two or more locations. Paradoxical respiration of this segment and impaired pulmonary mechanics can lead to both life-threatening hypoxia and hypercapnia. Additionally, this substantial injury mechanism is often associated with refractory, life-threatening hypoxia, even with mechanical ventilator support.
   - **Circulation:** Assess circulation with frequent vital sign assessments, pulse examination (all extremities), skin color/capillary refill, and mentation. Circulatory assessment may be challenging in the extremes of age, with concomitant heart disease, in athletes and pregnant women, and with medications, hypothermia, and pacemakers.
   - **Disability:** A brief neurologic exam and assessment based on the Glasgow Coma Scale is essential, particularly if the patient requires therapeutic paralysis for intubation (recognize if patient is moving extremities and document facial nerve function prior to administering paralytic agents).
   - **Exposure/Environmental Control:** Perform a full physical examination for injury, especially in the non-alert patient, while minimizing hypothermia.

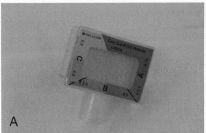 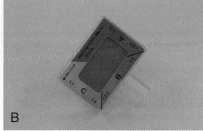

Fig. 69.1 A, Capnograph has turned yellow, indicating return of CO_2. This device attaches to an endotracheal tube and changes color from purple to yellow with CO_2 return. **B.** Capnograph remains purple, indicating no return of CO_2.

2. **What is an AMPLE history?**
   An AMPLE history involves the key elements that can be rapidly obtained by the patient or patient's friends or family when the patient has a limited ability to provide medical history. It consists of: **A**llergies, **M**edications, **P**ast Medical History, **L**ast PO Intake, and the **E**vents leading to the trauma.

3. **What are the methods of verifying a secure airway after intubation or surgical airway procedure?**
   A secured airway must always be verified, including patients who are intubated in the field. The intubation itself should involve direct visualization of the vocal cords. An equal chest rise/fall should be observed. Auscultate for bilateral breath sounds, with consideration of the possibility of right mainstem intubation. Capnography should be rapidly used to assess the proper position; a small plastic insert is placed onto the endotracheal tube and assessed over the duration of several breaths. The return of CO_2 confirms endotracheal positioning and is indicated by a color change from purple to yellow on the capnography insert. Persistent purple coloration indicates no CO_2 return (yellow = mellow, purple = problem) (Fig. 69.1). A chest radiograph can demonstrate the position of the endotracheal tube above the carina but does not necessarily rule out the possibility of esophageal intubation. Bronchoscopic confirmation of endotracheal tube placement is generally not feasible in the trauma bay setting.

4. **What are the indications for chest tube placement?**
   A patient with hypotension and decreased breath sounds in the trauma bay should be presumed to have tension pneumothorax. Decompression should be performed immediately. Needle decompression can rapidly be performed with a 14-gauge needle catheter; recent updates to ATLS recommend needle decompression in the 4th or 5th intercostal space and mid-axillary line for adults (for children, the recommendation is the 2nd intercostal space, mid-clavicular line). Rapid decompression can also be performed with an incision in the anterior axillary 5th intercostal space (generally at the level of the nipple). Entry into the pleural space decompresses the tension pneumothorax; the chest tube can then be placed through this incision (immediate intervention involves the incision; do not wait for a chest tube to be ready if tension pneumothorax is suspected). A chest tube is also placed when hemothorax is suspected on examination or imaging. The initial chest tube output will dictate further management; greater than 1500 cc of blood is an indication for exploratory thoracotomy. Follow-up chest radiography should be performed after chest tube placement. Open chest wounds ("sucking chest wounds") occur where the pleural space/pulmonary circuit directly communicates with the external environment. Large tidal volumes are lost through this open pulmonary wound. Initial management can include "three-sided" occlusive dressing. However, optimal initial management would include chest tube placement on that side of the thorax with a three-sided occlusive dressing to allow decompression and prevent tension pneumothorax.

5. **What are the five locations of blood loss in a trauma patient?**
   - Scalp/street: The scalp and face are highly vascularized areas, and scalp bleeding should promptly be addressed with pressure, sutures, clips, or staples in the significantly injured patient. Prehospital care should include a rapid report that describes any significant blood loss at the scene of the trauma or en route.
   - Chest: Rib fractures (up to 100 mL each), lung laceration, or injury to the great vessels or heart can result in significant thoracic hemorrhage and should be assessed for by examination (observation, palpation, auscultation) and imaging (radiography, ultrasound, computed tomography).
   - Abdomen: Solid organ or mesenteric injury may result in hemoperitoneum and should be assessed for by examination (observation, palpation) and imaging (ultrasound, CT).
   - Pelvis/retroperitoneum: Bleeding may occur from pelvic fractures, vascular injury, or solid organ injury (kidney, pancreas) and can be assessed for by examination, pelvic radiography, and CT.
   - Bones: Blood loss from a pelvic fracture can be as much as 2000 mL; femur fracture, 1000 mL; tibia fracture, 250 to 500 mL; and rib fracture, 100 mL each. Evaluate by physical examination and imaging (radiographs) when injury is suspected.

Table 69.1 Classes of Hemorrhagic Shock

	CLASS I	CLASS II	CLASS III	CLASS IV
Blood loss (mL)	<750	750–1500	1500–2000	>2000
Blood loss (%)	<15	15–30	30–40	>40%
Heart rate	Normal	↑	↑↑	↑↑↑
Blood pressure	Normal	Normal	↓	↓↓
Respiratory rate	Normal	↑	↑↑	↑↑↑

Note that HR and RR are the first to change, rather than a drop in BP.

6. **Define shock.**
   Shock simply means inadequate tissue perfusion. In trauma, the most common cause is *hemorrhagic* shock, which requires immediate hemorrhage control and resuscitation with blood products and/or intravenous fluids. Shock may also result from spinal cord injury (spinal shock or neurogenic shock). Cardiogenic shock may occur due to tension physiology such as tension pneumothorax or cardiac tamponade. Cardiogenic shock from direct myocardial injury is less common in the trauma setting but should be considered for patients with a history of heart disease (i.e., syncopal episode leading to motor vehicle collision), significant anterior chest wall trauma, or sternal fractures. Septic shock should be considered for patients with a significantly delayed presentation such as extremely prolonged extrication or time-consuming transfer from remote locations.

7. **What are the classes of hemorrhagic shock?**
   See Table 69.1. Patients may display normal vital signs despite significant blood loss, as depicted in Table 69.1, warranting thorough evaluation of all trauma patients.

8. **What are the key elements of the neurologic evaluation of a trauma patient?**
   Traumatic brain injury is very common in patients with blunt trauma. The Glasgow Coma Scale is used to rapidly evaluate the eye (4 points), verbal (5 points), and motor responses (6 points). A score ranges from 3 (worst) to 15 (normal) and is used to help classify brain injury (13–15 = minor, 9–12 = moderate, 3–8 = severe). At a minimum, the patient should also be assessed for movement in all four extremities. Stable patients should have motor and sensory evaluations of the extremities during the secondary survey. Based on the identified injuries, further neurologic assessment may be warranted (spine injury, extremity fracture). Imaging (CT brain) in stable patients or immediate intervention with intracranial pressure monitoring by neurosurgery (patients unstable for imaging evaluation) should be considered for all patients with altered trauma.

9. **How are spinal cord injuries assessed?**
   All patients suspected of having spinal cord injury should be properly immobilized. A neurologic exam assesses extremity movement, strength, sensation, and reflexes. A rectal exam is performed to evaluate for tone. Palpation of the entire spinal column for step-offs or tenderness is performed. In the absence of abnormalities on examination, distracting injuries, or intoxication, a gentle assessment of range of motion is then performed. Imaging is warranted for continued suspicion and may include cervical spine radiographs (lateral, anterior-posterior, and odontoid views, including C7 and T1 vertebrae) or computed tomography of the cervical spine (T, L-spine dependent on injury mechanism and exam findings). Magnetic resonance imaging is useful for neurologic deficits not explained by CT imaging and may also be useful for clearing the cervical spine in an obtunded patient who otherwise may suffer from skin breakdown resulting from prolonged preemptive collar placement. MRI is most useful for excluding cervical spine ligamentous injury in the first 24 hours following trauma prior to nonspecific edema development, which MRI can later identify as a false positive.

INITIAL MANAGEMENT OF THE TRAUMA PATIENT

10. **What are the vascular access options for a trauma patient?**
    An ideal vascular access for the trauma patient is a large-bore peripheral intravenous catheter (14- or 16-gauge). This short, large-diameter catheter can allow rapid infusion of blood or fluid but may be difficult to place in an acute setting. Additional options in order of ease of placement and rate of fluid delivery include intraosseous access in the tibia/sternum, saphenous vein cutdown with large-bore peripheral IV placement, and central venous access (femoral, subclavian, or jugular vein).

11. **When is blood transfusion indicated in a trauma patient?**
    A trauma patient who displays hemodynamic instability (HR > 100, SBP < 90) despite a fluid challenge (1 L crystalloid) and is suspected to have ongoing hemorrhage should receive uncrossed, O-negative packed red blood cells, while patient-specific type and crossmatch are performed.

12. **What is the "bloody vicious cycle"?**
Coagulopathy, acidosis, and hypothermia all contribute to each other, resulting in ongoing bleeding that cannot be controlled surgically and is uniformly fatal if not reversed. Aggressive patient and fluid warming and correction of coagulopathy with blood product resuscitation are warranted and may necessitate quick, basic surgery ("damage control surgery" to halt surgical hemorrhage and prevent ongoing contamination) to allow for more optimal resuscitation, including correction of temperature, acidosis, and coagulopathy, to continue in the intensive care unit setting.

13. **What is a massive transfusion protocol?**
Massive transfusion protocols are designed to facilitate transfusion of an appropriate ratio of blood products, including packed red cells, fresh frozen plasma, platelets, and cryoprecipitate. Such protocols facilitate rapid preparation from the blood bank and help ensure appropriate ratios of product are given. Some programs are investigating a return to whole blood transfusion rather than blood product resuscitation by components.

IMAGING OF THE TRAUMA PATIENT

14. **What are the key aspects of the chest radiograph for the trauma patient?**
Chest radiography in a trauma patient allows for rapid assessment for airway deviation, subcutaneous emphysema, pneumothorax, hemothorax, rib fractures, and mediastinal widening, which may be indicative of great vessel injury. It can also assess the positioning of an endotracheal tube, central venous catheter, or nasogastric tube.

15. **What is the FAST?**
Focused abdominal sonography for trauma (FAST) is a rapid bedside test that assesses for fluid (presumed to be blood in the setting of trauma) in various spaces. When performed and repeated during evaluation, it is a sensitive indicator of abdominal bleeding. Prior surgery (adhesions), ascites, body habitus, and user error are pitfalls. It entails four views:
   1. Pericardial view assesses for cardiac activity and blood in pericardial space
   2. Spleen-renal view assesses for blood loss in left upper quadrant
   3. Morrison's pouch is the most dependent portion of the abdomen, right upper quadrant
   4. Pelvis view assesses for blood in perivesicular space/pelvis/lower abdomen
      An extended version of the FAST, referred to as eFAST, can be used to rapidly assess for the presence of pneumothorax.

16. **When is CT angiography of the neck performed?**
CT angiography (CTA) of the neck is used to evaluate for blunt carotid or vertebral artery injury and is obtained when suggestive signs, symptoms, or head and neck radiographic findings are present. CT angiography of the neck is indicated for patients with injuries including cervical seat belt sign, blunt anterior neck trauma, displaced midface fracture, basilar skull fractures involving the carotid canal, diffuse axonal injury, near hanging injury with anoxia, cervical vertebral body or transverse foramen fracture, any cervical spine fracture involving C1 to C3, any ligamentous injury to the cervical spine, or a bruit in a young patient (aged <50 years). Mechanisms for high-energy transfer across the cervical spine, including facial fractures with associated upper thoracic or clavicle fracture or patients with scapular fractures, should be considered for CTA of the neck. Any neck injury resulting from direct force that causes significant swelling, pain, or altered mental status should also be evaluated with CTA of the neck. Hard signs concerning for vascular injury (pulsatile bleeding, expanding neck hematoma, penetrating trauma through the platysma) in surgically accessible zones of the neck should be surgically explored. Inaccessible injuries in Zone I/Zone III of the neck in the stable patient may necessitate CTA imaging.

SPECIAL CONSIDERATIONS IN TRAUMA

17. **What are the key aspects of evaluation of a burn patient?**
The burn patient should be rapidly assessed for associated inhalation injury with a low threshold for airway stabilization (intubation) if suspected. Aggressive fluid resuscitation is vital and should be protocol driven using the Parkland formula or other similar protocols. Urine output monitoring is a good adjunctive resuscitative endpoint. The total burned body surface area should be evaluated. Circumferential burns may require escharotomy to prevent ischemia (extremity) or hypoventilation (chest).

18. **What are the indications for referral of a burn patient to a specialty burn center?**
   1. Partial-thickness burns greater than 10% of total body surface area (TBSA)
   2. Burns involving the face, hands, feet, genitalia, perineum, or major joints
   3. Third-degree burns in any age group
   4. Electrical burns, including lightning injury
   5. Chemical burns
   6. Inhalation injury
   7. Burn injury in patients with preexisting medical disorders that could complicate management, prolong recovery, or affect mortality

8. Any patients with burns and concomitant trauma (such as fractures) in which burn injuries pose the greatest risk of morbidity or mortality. In such cases, if the trauma poses a greater immediate risk, the patient may be initially stabilized in a trauma center before being transferred to a burn unit. Physician judgment will be necessary in such situations and should be in concert with the regional medical control plan and triage protocols.
9. Burned children in hospitals without qualified personnel or equipment for the care of children
10. Burn injury in patients requiring special social, emotional, or long-term rehabilitative intervention

19. **What are the basic elements of triage for a mass casualty event?**
Patients involved in a mass casualty should be rapidly assessed for degree of injury. The ability to walk, airway compromise, respiratory rate, and pulse or capillary refill are signs used in the field to assess severity of injury. Patients with serious but survivable injuries are transported/addressed first; the "walking wounded" require less acute attention, and the patient in extremis should not direct limited resources, attention, or time in the setting of a mass casualty event. Life-saving maneuvers, such as decompression of a tension pneumothorax or direct pressure or tourniquet application of hemorrhage, are carried out in the field.

20. **What considerations are reviewed when "clearing" a polytrauma patient for elective or semi-elective procedures?**
Prior to nonurgent procedures, the multisystem trauma patient should be hemodynamically stable and fully resuscitated (as evidenced by normalized lactate or base deficit). Life-threatening injuries should be stabilized. Injuries undergoing observation must also be considered (such as a splenic laceration, which may bleed with BP lability, or an observed pneumothorax, which can blossom under positive pressure ventilation). Patient position should be considered (unstable fractures are fixated; patient can tolerate supine positioning, such as with severe head injury with increased intracranial pressure). Coagulopathy must be reversed or controlled (some injuries require anticoagulation).

BIBLIOGRAPHY

American College of Surgeons: *Advanced Trauma Life Support*, 10th ed, 2018, American College of Surgeons.
Biffl WL, Cothren CC, Moore EE, et al: Western Trauma Association critical decisions in trauma: screening for and treatment of blunt cerebrovascular injuries, *J Trauma* 67(6):1150–1153, 2009.
Brunicardi F, Andersen D, Billiar T, et al: *Schwartz's Principles of Surgery*, 9th ed, 2010, McGraw Hill.
Feliciano D, Moore E, Mattox K: *Trauma*, 6th ed, 2008, McGraw Hill.

CHAPTER 70

FACIAL TRAUMA

Vincent Eusterman, MD, DDS

KEY POINTS

1. Panfacial fractures require a comprehensive timing and treatment plan for each fracture.
2. Muscle pull can affect a fracture and must be considered to prevent complications.
3. Failure to diagnose and repair a medial canthal tendon injury can lead to functional and cosmetic complications that are difficult to repair secondarily.
4. The quickest way to decompress the eye is by lateral canthotomy with inferior cantholysis.
5. Subcondylar fractures can generally be repaired with an open approach, whereas condylar head and neck fractures are best treated using a closed approach.
6. Bicortical plate screws are used for compression of the mandible, where teeth roots are absent, and monocortical screws are used in the tension areas where roots are present.

Pearls

1. The edentulous mandible has no cross-sectional stability and is too weak to "load share" the fracture site with a small bone plate and requires load-bearing reconstruction.
2. An early clinical finding of optic nerve injury in the traumatized eye is the loss of red color vision.
3. What all Le Fort fractures have in common is that they traverse the pterygomaxillary fissure, interrupting the pterygoid plates and resulting in a mobile palate.
4. A "white-eye blowout fracture" is considered a surgical emergency.
5. The most common sites of mandible fracture are the angle and condyle.
6. The greater wing of the sphenoid supports the zygoma via the sphenozygomatic (SZ) suture and is an excellent reference for displaced zygomaxillary complex fracture repair.
7. A tripod fracture is actually a tetrapod when you add the sphenozygomatic articulation.
8. A transcaruncular approach to the medial orbit enters behind the posterior lacrimal crest where Horner's muscle attaches.

QUESTIONS

1. **What important elements of the physical exam are considered in facial trauma?**
   1. Airway, breathing, and circulation (ATLS)
   2. Disability: cervical spine and brain injury (ATLS)
   3. Cranial nerves: motor (CN VII) and sensory (CNs V_1, V_2, V_3)
   4. Eyes: vision (CN II), pupils, movement (CNs IV, VI) fields, pressure, globe injury, globe position
   5. Ears: hearing, hemotympanum, ear canal fracture, temporal bone fracture (CNs VII, VIII)
   6. Bones: calvarium, midface, and mandible for deformity and dysfunction
   7. Throat: occlusion, TMJ function, bleeding, hematoma, airway, speech, and swallow (CNs IX, X)

2. **What type of imaging should be ordered to evaluate facial trauma?**
   High-resolution (fine-cut) axial computed tomography (CT) with coronal and sagittal reconstruction is ideal. Cervical spine imaging should be included in facial fractures caused by high-energy impacts such as motor vehicle accidents (MVAs). Coronal and sagittal reconstructions are helpful in evaluating the orbital floor, frontal sinus outflow tracts, and mandibular condyles. Three-dimensional CT scans are very helpful in surgical planning when multiple fractures are present. *Direct radiographic* signs of facial fractures include nonanatomic linear lucency, cortical defects or suture diastasis, overlapping bone fragments causing "double density," and facial asymmetry. *Indirect radiographic* signs include soft tissue swelling, periorbital or intracranial air, and fluid in the paranasal sinus.

3. **What characteristics of the mechanism of facial trauma are considered important?**
   Facial fracture results when the tolerance of a facial bone is overcome by kinetic energy transfer (KE = ½mv²) from a blunt or penetrating force. Mechanisms have variable energy from low (falling from standing) to high (MVA). Understanding the mechanism of injury can help predict the extent of facial injury and the risk of associated cervical or brain injuries. High-impact and low-impact forces are defined as more or less than 50 times the force

of gravity (G). Facial bones differ in their ability to withstand force: nasal bones can resist 30 G, zygoma 50 G, mandible angle 70 G, frontal glabella 80 G, midline maxilla and mandible 100 G, and supraorbital rim 200 G. The most common facial fracture is that of the nasal bones.

4. **How is the patient with facial trauma evaluated?**
Each patient must be evaluated and treated according to the ATLS guidelines. Once the patient is medically stable, definitive facial fracture assessment and management can proceed. Facial trauma can range from a minimally displaced nasal fracture to a highly comminuted compound panfacial fracture involving the orbit, brain, and cervical spine. Facial trauma evaluation is best performed by dividing the face anatomically into three sections, as each has its own unique characteristics. The **upper third** assesses frontal bone, frontal sinus, and frontal lobe injury. The **middle third** or "midface" contains nasal, nasal-orbital-ethmoid (NOE), orbit, zygomaticomaxillary complex (ZMC), and maxillary structures. The **lower third** includes the mandible and temporomandibular joint.

UPPER THIRD (FRONTAL BONE)

5. **How would you evaluate a suspected frontal sinus injury?**
High-resolution thin-cut computed tomography (CT) is the best method for evaluating anterior and posterior table fractures and outflow tract injury. In addition to the standard axial and coronal images, sagittal reconstructions of the paranasal sinuses can enhance visualization of the frontal outflow tract. Additional findings such as NOE complex fractures and anterior skull base injury near the junction of the posterior table and the cribriform plate strongly suggest injury to the frontal outflow tract.

6. **What are the treatment goals of frontal sinus repair?**
   - Protection of intracranial structures
   - Stopping cerebrospinal fluid (CSF) leak
   - Prevention of posttraumatic infection or mucocele (late complications)
   - Restoration of facial esthetics

7. **How do you treat a frontal sinus fracture of the anterior table?**
Surgical indications for anterior table fractures include deformity or frontal sinus outflow tract impairment. Minimally displaced (1–2 mm) anterior table fractures are not treated. Fractures requiring repair are treated with open reduction and internal fixation. Approaches include direct access through an open laceration or an osteoplastic flap with open reduction and internal fixation of the anterior table with or without obliteration. Involvement of the frontal sinus outflow tract is important to evaluate. If there is damage to the outflow tract that may lead to scarring and obstruction in the future, the patient may form a frontal mucocele. Observation and medical management with future endoscopic surgery for outflow tract repair is also an option.

8. **How would you treat a posterior table frontal sinus fracture?**
Surgical indications for posterior table fracture include displacement of the posterior table greater than one table width, dural injury, CSF rhinorrhea, frontal sinus outflow impairment, or severely comminuted fractures. The risk of dural injury in these cases is high and consultation with a neurosurgeon is recommended for possible dural repair. Mucosal removal and obliteration with abdominal fat or cranialization of the frontal sinus may be considered.

9. **What is an "osteoplastic flap" used for the frontal sinus obliteration procedure?**
The osteoplastic bone flap is vascularized anterior table frontal bone elevated to access the sinus. It is created by a frontal sinus outline marked on the pericranium using a template from a 6-ft Caldwell radiograph. The frontal pericranium is incised and left attached to the anterior table, preserving its vascularity. Osteotomies are performed and the sinus is opened. The mucosa of the sinus is completely removed, the frontal recess is occluded with temporalis fascia or muscle, abdominal fat may be used to fill the sinus, and the bony flap is replaced. Postoperative CT/MR surveillance imaging is used to detect mucocele formation; however, imaging is often difficult to interpret.

10. **What is "frontal sinus cranialization," and how is it accomplished?**
Cranialization replaces the frontal sinus with the frontal lobe of the brain. It is reserved for severe posterior wall fractures. An anterior pericranial flap is mobilized and preserved. Through a craniotomy the posterior wall of the frontal sinus is removed and the sinus mucosa is stripped away from the remaining bone and outflow tracts plugged. The brain and dura are evaluated by a neurosurgeon for possible debridement and dural closure. The pericranial flap is inserted beneath the brain to separate it from the paranasal sinuses. The brain and dura are permitted to rest against the repaired anterior wall in the area originally occupied by the frontal sinus, which no longer exists.

11. **What are early and late complications of frontal sinus fractures?**
Early complications include wound infection, CSF leak, meningitis, acute sinusitis, deformity, pain, hypesthesia, and brain abscess. *Late* complications include mucocele, mucopyocele, osteomyelitis, cosmetic defect, brain abscess, and headache.

12. **How are CSF leaks in frontal trauma treated?**
    CSF rhinorrhea from fractures of the anterior fossa occurs via the frontal sinus, cribriform plate, ethmoid sinuses, or sphenoid sinuses. Large defects should be repaired early at the time of fracture repair. Small defects can be identified and treated endoscopically. Transient leaks may have stopped due to brain herniation, and delayed treatment could result in meningitis or death.

13. **What are the dangers of raising a coronal flap for facial fracture repair, and how are they avoided?**
    1. Frontal branch of the facial nerve injury can be avoided by incising the superficial layer of the deep temporal fascia at the temporal line of fusion so elevation can be deep to this layer.
    2. Supraorbital and supratrochlear nerve injuries at the supraorbital rims are prevented by removing the inferior lip of the nerve foramen with an osteotome to allow the nerve to move inferiorly.
    3. Laxity of the midface soft tissues occurs if the fascia is not resuspended at the time of closure. Accurate resuspension during closure prevents this.

14. **What endoscopic procedure is used to treat severe chronic frontonasal outflow obstruction?**
    The modified Lothrop procedure (Draf III procedure) may be used to restore severely obstructed frontal outflow pathways after trauma.

MIDDLE THIRD (NOSE, ORBIT, ZYGOMA, MAXILLA)

15. **What key features are evaluated in nasal trauma?**
    Nasal fractures are commonly identified by epistaxis and bony nasal deformity. Often the patient complains of nasal obstruction. The *external examination* should include evaluation of deformity, mobility, step-offs, and telecanthus. The *internal examination* should examine for septal deviation, mucosal tears, or septal hematoma. Clear rhinorrhea may indicate CSF leak. Epistaxis in severe facial trauma may be life-threatening and require surgery or embolization if nasal packing fails.

16. **What are the dangers of a nasal septal hematoma, and how is it treated?**
    A septal hematoma is a collection of blood under the nasal septal perichondrium following trauma. The lack of blood supply to the cartilage can lead to cartilage necrosis or septal abscess and can produce a saddle nose deformity. Urgent treatment includes evacuation of the clot or purulence and adaptation of the mucosa by resorbable sutures or silastic septal splints.

17. **What is the timing for the treatment of nasal bone fractures?**
    Acute nasal fractures are treated best by closed reduction immediately following the fracture (1 to 2 hours) or after swelling has subsided (5 to 10 days). The bones are repositioned and splinted for 7 to 14 days. *Chronic nasal fractures* (>14 days) may be more difficult to treat and often require complete healing (3 to 6 months) followed by formal septorhinoplasty.

18. **What is an NOE fracture?**
    The nasal-orbital-ethmoid (NOE) complex is the confluence of the frontal sinus, ethmoid sinuses, anterior cranial fossa, orbits, frontal bone, and nasal bones. An NOE fracture is a telescoping fracture of the nasal, lacrimal, and ethmoid bones, which occurs from blunt trauma at the nasal bridge. Injury to the bony septal attachment at the cribriform plate can produce a CSF leak and anosmia. NOE fractures involve the attachment of the medial canthal tendons (MCT) and can result in telecanthus. Failure to diagnose and repair an MCT can lead to functional and cosmetic complications that are difficult to repair secondarily. Long-term sequelae of NOE fractures include blindness, telecanthus, enophthalmos, midface retrusion, CSF fistula, anosmia, epiphora, sinusitis, and nasal deformity.

19. **How are medial canthal tendon (MCT) injuries classified?**
    Markowitz classified NOE fractures based on the status of the degree of comminution of the "central fragment" of bone attached to the MCT.
    Type I: fracture lines leave a single, noncomminuted central fragment with MCT attached.
    Type II: the central fragment gets comminuted but the MCT stays attached to its fragments.
    Type III: severe central fragment comminution and the MCT is detached. Types II and III are the most difficult to repair and require transnasal wiring in a posterior-superior direction to minimize medial orbital deformity.

20. **What is a blowout fracture?**
    Orbital blowout fractures result from the hydraulic compression of the orbital contents into the paranasal sinuses. This usually occurs through the thin portion of the orbital floor (0.5 mm) and less frequently through the thin lamina papyracea (0.25 mm), which is supported by the honeycombed ethmoid sinuses. The *pure* form is purely hydraulic without rim injury; the *impure* form is caused by rim deformation and fracture extension posteriorly, creating the blowout.

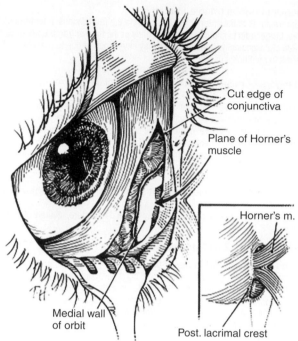

Fig. 70.1 Transcaruncular approach. An incision is made through the caruncle to the bone behind the posterior lacrimal crest where Horner's muscle is attached. The periosteum is incised vertically and the medial extraperiosteal space is entered for fracture repair.

21. **What are the surgical indications for a blowout fracture of the floor?**
    Surgery is indicated for (1) enophthalmos greater than 2 millimeters, (2) double vision on primary or inferior gaze, (3) entrapment of extraocular muscles on forced duction testing, or (4) fracture of more than 50% of the orbital floor on CT imaging.

22. **What is a "white-eyed blowout fracture"? Why is it treated emergently?**
    This is a trapdoor or greenstick fracture of the orbital floor, most commonly seen in children. The orbital floor opens under hydraulic pressure from the compressed globe, forcing the orbital fat and muscle into the maxillary sinus. The elastic bony floor immediately closes on these contents and traps them tightly. Under these circumstances, the sclera remains white without hemorrhage. The child is often nauseated and has severe pain. Careful examination of the irritated child may be difficult, and CT scanning of the orbit should be considered in the diagnosis. Urgent surgery is required to preserve the entrapped ischemic inferior rectus muscle.

23. **What are the surgical approaches to repair orbit wall fractures?**
    Orbital floor fractures are generally approached through a transconjunctival lower lid incision. *Medial wall fractures* are accessed through a transconjunctival or transcaruncular incision and may be treated via an endonasal endoscopic approach through the ethmoid sinuses or, rarely, by an external ethmoidectomy (Lynch) incision. *Lateral wall fractures* are approached through an upper lid skin crease (blepharoplasty) incision or infrabrow incision or through an extended lower lid transconjunctival incision with a lateral canthotomy. *Orbital roof* approaches include upper lid (blepharoplasty), trans-brow, and coronal incisions and, rarely, external ethmoidectomy (Lynch) incisions.

24. **Describe the transcaruncular approach to the medial orbit. Why is it used?**
    The caruncle is divided to access a plane between Horner's muscle and the medial orbital septum to expose the medial extraperiosteal space. Advantages include rapid entry into the orbit, less damage to the skin and muscle layers, better cosmetic results, and less manipulation of the medial canthal tendon and lacrimal sac (Fig. 70.1).

25. **What are common complications of orbital fracture repair?**
    - **Diplopia:** double vision from paresis of an extraocular muscle (usually due to the initial injury) or fibrosis of an extraocular muscle causing restriction
    - **Enophthalmos:** posterior displacement of the eye within the orbit from changes in orbit volume in the setting of fat atrophy or wall malposition

- **Entropion:** inversion of the eyelid toward the globe
- **Ectropion:** eversion of the lid margin away from the globe
- **Proptosis:** forward displacement of the eye due to overcorrection of a blowout fracture
- **Hypoglobus:** downward displacement of the eye in the orbit
- **Telecanthus:** intercanthal distance is larger than the width of the eye
- **Dacryocystitis:** inflammation of the lacrimal sac related to nasolacrimal duct obstruction
- **Orbital cellulitis:** infections in the orbit or from orbital implants

26. **What is the quickest way to decompress the eye with increased intraocular pressure?**
Orbital compartment syndrome (OCS) is an ocular emergency requiring prompt diagnosis and treatment to prevent blindness due to ischemia of the optic nerve and retina. Orbital pressure can be relieved with emergent *lateral canthotomy with inferior cantholysis*. Absolute indications for lateral canthotomy include retrobulbar hemorrhage, resulting in acute loss of visual acuity, increased IOP, and proptosis. In the unconscious or uncooperative patient, an IOP greater than 40 mmHg is an indication for lateral canthotomy (normal IOP is 10 to 21 mm Hg).

27. **What is the first indication that the optic nerve is injured following orbital trauma?**
Traumatic optic neuropathy (TON) is a condition of acute injury to the optic nerve due to direct or indirect trauma. TON is thought to result from shearing injury to the intracanalicular portion of the optic nerve, which can cause axonal injury or disturb the blood supply of the optic nerve. The optic nerve may swell in the optic canal after trauma, resulting in increased luminal pressure and secondary ischemic injury. Patients with TON may have decreased central visual acuity, decreased color vision, an afferent pupillary defect, or visual field deficits. An early clinical finding of optic nerve injury in the traumatized eye is *loss of red color vision*. Treatment is with high-dose corticosteroids or surgical decompression.

28. **What is the difference between a forced duction test and a traction test?**
The *forced duction test* is an upward tug on the anesthetized sclera to test for inferior rectus muscular entrapment after blowout fracture. The *traction test* is the grasping of the lower eyelid and pulling laterally against its medial attachment to determine if there is abnormal laxity indicating a disruption of the medial canthal tendon following NOE fracture.

29. **What is a zygomatic arch fracture, and how is it treated?**
A zygomatic arch fracture is usually a medially displaced deformity in the zygomatic arch from an external blow. The defect can be seen and palpated; the indented bone can impinge on the coronoid process of the mandible and cause pain with jaw movement. Treatment involves fracture reduction often without fixation through a (1) *direct cutaneous approach* using a hook or suture, (2) a *Gilles approach* – an incision behind the hairline over the temporalis muscle to reach the fracture, or (3) a *transoral approach* through a gingivobuccal sulcus incision. Comminuted arch fractures may require a coronal flap and ORIF.

30. **What is a "tripod" fracture?**
The zygoma is the cheek bone or malar bone and forms the lateral orbital wall. It articulates with the temporal bone posteriorly (ZT), frontal bone above (ZF), maxilla below (ZM), and sphenoid bone (SZ) inside the orbit. A tripod or malar fracture is known as a zygomaticomaxillary complex (ZMC) fracture. The often forgotten fourth suture, the spheno-zygomatic (SZ), is at the lateral orbital wall, and, because of the stability of the greater wing of the sphenoid, it can be used to reorient the zygoma in severely displaced ZMC fractures. Technically the ZMC fracture a "tetrapod" rather than a tripod fracture.

31. **What are the midfacial buttresses, and why are they important in fracture treatment?**
The midface is reinforced by strong vertical and weaker horizontal buttresses. Three bilateral vertical buttresses resist the forces of mastication; the *medial buttresses* (nasomaxillary) extend from the nasomaxillary region to the frontal bone. The *lateral buttresses* (zygomaticomaxillary) extend from the molar region superiorly to the zygomaticomaxillary complex along the lateral orbital rim to the frontal bone. The *posterior buttresses* (pterygomaxillary) are from the pterygoid plates to the skull base. The medial and lateral vertical buttresses are accessible for repair, while pterygoid sites are not. Four horizontal buttresses are bridging supports between the vertical buttresses and consist of the palate, a central facial buttress from malar to malar interrupted by the piriform aperture, the frontal bar, and the anterior-posterior zygomatic arch.

32. **How are midface fractures classified?**
In 1901 French military surgeon René Le Fort published a classification of midface fractures that is still in use today. All three fracture types traverse the pterygomaxillary fissure to interrupt the pterygoid plates (Fig. 70.2). **Le Fort I fracture** is a horizontal fracture above the maxillary alveolus that produces a floating palate. The fracture usually involves the nasal aperture and extends above the apices of the teeth, causing the hard palate to move separately from the maxilla. **Le Fort II fracture** is a pyramidal fracture that usually involves the inferior orbital rim. It extends from the nasion through the lacrimal bones and inferior orbital floor and rim through or near the inferior

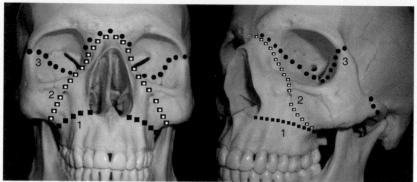

Fig. 70.2 Le Fort fractures. Le Fort I fracture (1) is a horizontal fracture above the maxillary alveolus. Le Fort II fracture (2) is pyramidal and usually includes the infraorbital rim. Le Fort III fracture (3) includes the zygoma and orbit and is considered a craniofacial dissociation when present bilaterally.

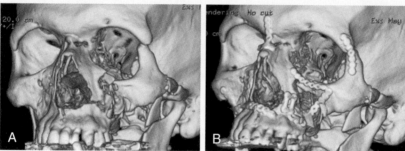

Fig. 70.3 A, Preoperative 3DCT of a patient with a right Le Fort II, left Le Fort I-II-III, and a palate fracture and left coronoid fracture. **B,** Postoperative 3DCT showing the nose and zygoma repositioned and fixed to the skull base. The maxillary buttresses were repaired in relation to **both** the upper stabilized segments and the mandibular occlusion. Note the untreated coronoid fracture in correct position following zygoma repositioning.

orbital foramen and inferiorly through the anterior wall of the maxillary sinus. **Le Fort III fracture** is a transverse fracture that separates the face from the skull, which is known as craniofacial dissociation. It includes fractures through the zygomatic bone, nasofrontal and frontomaxillary sutures, and orbit. The thick greater wing of the sphenoid bone usually prevents the continuation of the fracture into the optic canal, thus preserving vision. Le Fort fractures often present in "mixed combinations" and should be reported as such (Fig. 70.3).

33. **How are midface fractures treated?**
    The goal of midface fracture repair is to restore "form and function." It must be performed in concert with the nose, orbit, zygoma, and maxilla in relation to the mandible. In treating the patient in Fig. 70.3 the upper portions of the midface were treated by stabilizing the nose and ZF suture fractures first with titanium plates. The maxilla was then aligned with the mandible, and the remaining right Le Fort II and left Le Fort I-II-III fractures could be repaired in an accurate and functional way to restore the patient's occlusion and facial form.

34. **What is a "panfacial fracture," and how are panfacial fractures treated?**
    Panfacial fractures are fractures involving the upper, middle, and lower face. Treatment is challenging and requires an individualized treatment plan that utilizes specific principles for each individual fracture. Reconstruction should be performed in the order of stable to unstable (see Fig. 70.3). The mobile zygomatic bone and nasal bones are secured in their correct anatomic position to solid cranial bone. Occlusion and facial height are reestablished first by reconstruction of the mandible to the maxilla, which is then secured to the nasal and zygomatic bones and cranium.

35. **What surgical complications occur in midface fracture repair?**
    1. *Inadequate reduction:* malocclusion (maxilla) and facial deformity (zygoma)
    2. *Imprecise reconstruction of the orbit:* globe malposition
    3. *Diplopia:* from globe malposition, residual entrapment, muscle or nerve injury
    4. *Eyelid malposition:* eyelid incision/dissection trauma, orbital septum injury

5. *Reduced vision and blindness:* rare, preoperative vision evaluation required
6. *Scars and hair loss:* irregular coronal incisions, avoid with careful design and preoperative counseling
7. *Numbness:* traumatic versus surgical nerve injury
8. *Nonunion:* chronic implant infection/extrusion, rare in midface fractures
9. *Dental injury:* avoid tooth roots when placing screws, tooth and gum care with arch bar use
10. *CSF leaks:* recognize early and treat to keep the intracranial cavity separate from nose/sinuses

LOWER THIRD (MANDIBLE)

36. **How is the mandible evaluated in a patient with facial trauma?**
Clinical: facial lacerations, swelling, and hematoma in the fracture area. Bimanual palpation of the inferior border may identify swelling, step-off deformity, or tenderness. Lip numbness occurs in mandibular fractures distal to the mandibular foramen.
Oral examination: deviation of the mouth on opening, limited opening from trismus, TMJ pain, coronoid impingement, occlusal changes, and floor of mouth ecchymosis from periosteal or gingival tearing. Occlusal evaluation may show obvious or subtle malocclusion.
Imaging studies are necessary, and CT scan is preferred over a Panorex. Mandibular fractures usually occur in pairs, and parasymphyseal and condyle fractures often occur together.

37. **How are mandibular fractures classified?**
Mandibular fractures are classified according to anatomic region and by an additional descriptor. Each anatomic region has unique characteristics that require specialized treatment considerations. The additional descriptors describe *severity* (greenstick, simple, compound, comminuted), *displacement* by muscle pull (favorable or unfavorable), and *malocclusion* (open bite, cross-bite). Each of these considerations will contribute to the treatment plan.

38. **What are the anatomic regions of the mandible?**
The mandible is divided into horizontal and vertical parts. The *horizontal mandible* has four anatomic regions: the dense basal bone consisting of the symphysis, parasymphysis, body, and less dense alveolar bone that holds the dentition. The *vertical mandible* has four anatomic regions: the angle, ramus, condyle, and coronoid. Fractures can occur in any of these regions but more frequently in the angle and condyle regions (Fig. 70.4).

39. **How are condylar fractures classified, and why are they considered difficult to treat?**
Condyle fractures are classified by three sites: *the head, neck,* and *subcondylar* (see Fig. 70.4). They can be difficult to treat for several reasons. The fracture occurs *under the facial nerve,* which can be injured during the repair and can be *malpositioned* by the pulling of the lateral pterygoid muscle or by traumatic dislocation, and the *bone quality* of the condylar neck is often inadequate for supporting hardware. The *subcondylar* fracture is, at this time, the only site considered for ORIF. The condylar head or neck fracture sites are often treated nonoperatively with physiotherapy. The malocclusion that occurs from condyle fractures creates an "open bite" deformity.

40. **What are the indications for ORIF of a condyle fracture?**
Absolute and relative indications for open surgery are discussed by Zide and Kent (Table 70.1). Unfortunately, there is no consensus on the treatment of condylar fractures in adults. The type of treatment must be chosen on a case-by-case basis and by professional experience. Physiotherapy (early jaw mobilization) is essential to

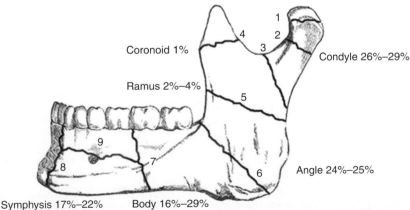

Fig. 70.4 Common mandibular fracture sites: (1) condylar head, (2) condylar neck, (3) subcondylar, (4) coronoid, (5) ramus, (6) angle, (7) body, (8) symphysis (symphysis and parasymphysis), and (9) alveolar.

Table 70.1 Indications for Open Reduction and Internal Fixation (ORIF) of a Condyle Fracture

Absolute Indications

1. Displacement of the condyle into the middle cranial fossa or EAC
2. Inability to obtain adequate occlusion
3. Lateral extracapsular dislocation
4. Contaminated open joint wound

Relative Indications

1. Bilateral condylar fractures in an edentulous patient when splints are unavailable or impossible because of alveolar ridge atrophy
2. Bilateral or unilateral condylar fractures when splinting is not recommended because of concomitant medical conditions or when physiotherapy is not possible
3. Bilateral fractures associated with comminuted midface fractures
4. Bilateral subcondylar fractures with associated (a) retrognathia or prognathia, (b) open bite with periodontal problems or lack of posterior support, (c) loss of multiple teeth and later need for reconstruction, (d) unstable occlusion due to orthodontics, (e) unilateral condylar fracture with unstable fracture base

avoid ankylosis of the TMJ. The three treatments advocated for adults with condylar process fractures include (1) a period of maxillomandibular fixation (MMF) followed by physiotherapy, (2) physiotherapy without a period of MMF, and (3) open reduction with or without internal fixation. ORIF of pediatric condylar or subcondylar fractures is rarely indicated. Instead, nonoperative management with observation, exercises, maxillomandibular fixation, training elastics, and bite-opening splints produce good outcomes with minimal complications.

41. **Why is the mandibular angle subject to high fracture rates?**
    The mandibular angle has a thinner cross-sectional area relative to the neighboring segments of the mandible and the presence of third molars, which weaken the region. The thin bone and tooth socket create a pathologic fracture site by weakening the junction between the vertical and horizontal segments. Unfavorable angle fractures are subject to displacement by pulling from the masseter and medial pterygoid muscles. Mandibular angle fractures pose a unique challenge for surgeons because they have the highest reported postoperative complication rate in any mandibular region.

42. **How is "tension and compression" related to mandibular healing?**
    During chewing, a functional load creates *tension* that separates the superior border of the mandible (Fig. 70.5). This opens the fracture site and allows bacteria and food to enter and produce poor results. *Compression* occurs on the inferior border at the same time and closes the fracture. During repair it is important to place a tension plate on the superior border to reduce movement and separation, which reduces the risks of nonunion and infection.

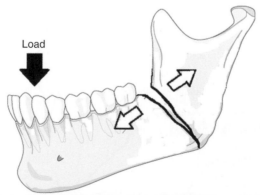

Fig. 70.5 Under chewing load, a mandibular angle fracture opens at the superior border *(open arrows)*. This is considered the "tension" or distracting site, which can be held together with a lightweight mini-plate. "Compression" or closure occurs on the inferior border during loading and needs no plate to keep the fracture reduced. Some surgeons feel that additional help on the inferior border may be necessary.

43. **How is dental occlusion classified?**
    Angle classified three types of occlusion, which should be considered when restoring the bite after mandibular fracture. *Class I* is "normal"; the mesiobuccal cusp (MBC) of the permanent maxillary first molar occludes in the buccal groove (BG) of the permanent mandibular first molar. In retrognathic occlusion the mandible is set back; this *Class II* is a posterior mandible, so the upper MBC is now in front of or mesial to the lower BG. In prognathic occlusion the mandible is protrusive; this *Class III* is an anterior mandible in which the upper MBC is behind (distal to) the lower BG.

44. **What are the indications for closed versus open reduction of mandible fractures?**
    Closed reduction and fixation are considered for nondisplaced favorable fractures, pediatric fractures, grossly comminuted fractures, coronoid fractures, and adult condyle fractures. This is accomplished by maxillomandibular fixation (MMF) using rich arch bars, ivy loops, Risdon wires, dental splints, and dentures. *Open reduction* and fixation are considered for displaced unfavorable fractures, atrophic edentulous mandible fractures, complex facial fractures, and condylar fractures that cannot be treated with closed techniques. This is done by exposing and reducing the fracture and fixing with wires, lag screws, or plates and screws.

45. **Why are edentulous mandible fractures treated differently?**
    Mandibular bone atrophy with loss of teeth and alveolar bone resorption results in a smaller fragile mandible. This remaining bone is "basal bone," which is dense cortical bone that has decreased osteogenesis and reduced blood supply and depends on the periosteum for nourishment. *Closed treatment* using Gunning splints, dentures, and external pin fixation is performed to preserve the blood supply in a noncontaminated environment to promote fracture healing. *Open treatment* requires the placement of heavy load-bearing reconstructive plates using bicortical screws. Edentulous bone has no cross-sectional stability and is too weak to "load-share" the fracture with a small bone plate and monocortical screws. Failure to recognize this important concept when treating edentulous mandibles can lead to serious complications.

46. **How are pediatric mandibular fractures different from adult fractures?**
    Pediatric mandible fractures are more difficult to treat than adult fractures. The teeth are conical in shape and have short roots that are not amenable to MMF. Tooth buds and growth centers can be damaged during the fracture treatment. Children aged 6 years and younger are generally treated with closed reduction techniques to avoid injury to the developing teeth. Children aged 12 years and older should have their permanent teeth in place and can be treated with ORIF using mini-plates. Mandibular growth occurs because of elongation in the condylar region, remodeling, and growth in the ramus and body. Injuries in the condylar region during fracture repair may lead to facial asymmetry.

CONTROVERSIES

47. **Frontal sinus posterior table fracture management.**
    Management of posterior wall frontal sinus fractures is the most controversial. The issue is to assess whether the fragments are displaced. Fine-cut CT scans are helpful in determining whether the fracture is linear or displaced. Linear fractures require no treatment. Nondisplaced fractures with CSF leaks may be observed for 5 to 7 days. According to the current treatment algorithm, frontal sinus exploration is indicated if the wall is displaced. The result of the exploration can result in doing nothing, performing a simple posterior table repair, performing a complete mucosal drill-out and abdominal fat obliteration, or performing a frontal sinus cranialization procedure. Frequently, CT scans do not identify dural tears or herniating frontal lobes, which are often seen when exploring displaced posterior wall fractures.

48. **Outflow obstruction and frontal sinus obliteration versus sinus-sparing techniques.**
    The question of whether frontal outflow tract obstruction can be successfully preserved in selected patient populations (sinus-preserving) in contrast to sinus obliteration procedures remains a controversial topic. There are no head-to-head comparisons between the two techniques. All agree that the consequences of nasofrontal outflow tract obstruction require treatment.

49. **Use of prophylactic antibiotics in the management of facial fractures.**
    There is considerable variability in the management of patients with facial fractures due to the use of prophylactic antibiotics. According to Mundinger, frequent use of pre- and postoperative antibiotics in upper and midface fractures is not supported by the literature. Prophylactic antibiotic use in higher level of evidence studies for comminuted mandible fractures is supported but postoperative use is not. Well-designed, higher-level studies may better guide clinical antibiotic prescription practices.

BIBLIOGRAPHY

Biller JA, Pletcher SD, Goldberg AN, et al: Complications and the time to repair of mandible fractures, *Laryngoscope* 115(5):769–772, 2005.
Bowerman JE: The superior orbital fissure syndrome complicating fractures of the facial skeleton, *Br J Oral Surg* 7:1–6, 1969.
Castro B, Walcott BP, Redial N, et al: Cerebrospinal fluid fistula prevention and treatment following frontal sinus fractures: a review of initial management and outcomes, *Neurosurg Focus* 32(6).E1, 2012.

Champy M, Loddé JP, Schmitt R, et al: Mandibular osteosynthesis by miniature screwed plates via a buccal approach, *J Maxillofac Surg* 6(1):14–21, 1978.

Daudia A, Biswas D, Jones NS: Risk of meningitis with cerebrospinal fluid rhinorrhea, *Ann Otol Rhinol Laryngol* 116:902–905, 2007.

Ellis E III, Zide MF: Transfacial approaches to the mandible. In: Ellis E III, Zide MF, eds: *Surgical Approaches to the Facial Skeleton*, 2nd ed, 2005, Lippincott Williams & Wilkins, pp 151–189.

Ellis E III, Price C: Treatment protocol for fractures of the atrophic mandible, *J Oral Maxillofac Surg* 66(3):421–435, 2008.

Ellis E III: Management of fractures through the angle of the mandible, *Oral Maxillofac Surg Clin North Am* 21(2):163–174, 2009.

Ellis E III, Throckmorton GS: Treatment of mandibular condylar process fractures: biological considerations, *J Oral Maxillofac Surg* 63:115–134, 2005.

Gillies HD, Kilner TP, Stone D: Fractures of the malar-zygomatic compound: with a description of a new x-ray position, *Br J Surg* 14:651–656, 1927.

Hegab A: Management of mandibular fractures in children with a split acrylic splint: a case series, *Br J Oral Maxillofac Surg* 50(6):e93–e95, 2012.

Holt GR, Brennan JA. AAO Resident Manual of Trauma to the Face: Head, and Neck. Available at http://www.entnet.org/mktplace/upload/ResidentTraumaFINALlowres.pdf.

Kachniarz B, Grant M, Darafshar A: *Orbital Fractures. Facial Trauma Surgery*, 2020, Elsevier, pp 113–1121.

Keen WW: *Surgery: Its Principles and Practice*, 1909, WB Saunders.

Kellman RA: Maxillofacial trauma. *Cummings/Otolaryngology: Head and Neck Surgery*, 6th ed, 2014, Mosby Elsevier, pp 325–350.

Kellman RM, Cienfuegos R: Endoscopic approaches to subcondylar fractures of the mandible, *Facial Plast Surg* 25(1):23–28, 2009.

Liu P, Wu S, Li Z, et al: Surgical strategy for cerebrospinal fluid rhinorrhea repair, *Neurosurgery* 66(6 Suppl):281–286, 2010.

Markowitz BL, Manson PN, Sargent L, et al: Management of the medial canthal tendon in nasoethmoid orbital fractures: the importance of the central fragment in classification and treatment, *Plast Reconstr Surg* 87(5):843–853, 1991.

Mundinger G, Borsuk D, Okhah Z, et al: Antibiotics and facial fractures: evidence-based recommendations compared with experience-based practice, *Craniomaxillofac Trauma Reconstr* 8(1):64–78, 2015.

Perez R, Oeltien JC, Thaller S: A review of mandibular angle fractures, *Craniomaxillofac Trauma Reconstr* 4(2):69–72, 2011.

Scholsem M, Scholtes F, Collignon F, et al: Surgical management of anterior cranial base fractures with cerebrospinal fluid fistulae: a single-institution experience, *Neurosurgery* 62:463–471, 2008.

Sharm S, Vashistha V, Chugh A, et al: Pediatric mandibular fractures: a review, *Int J Clin Pediatr Dent* 2(2):1–5, 2009.

Shetty V, Atchison K, Leathers R, et al: Do the benefits of rigid internal fixation of mandible fractures justify the added costs? Results from a randomized controlled trial, *J Oral Maxillofac Surg* 66(11):2203–2212, 2008.

Shorr N, Baylis HI, Goldberg RA: Transcaruncular approach to the medial orbit and orbital apex, *Ophthalmology* 107:1459–1463, 2000.

Smith B, Regan WF: Blowout fracture of the orbit: mechanism and correction of internal orbital fracture, *Am J Ophthalmol* 44(6):733–739, 1957.

Valerie JL, Muriel ER: Ophthalmic considerations in fronto-ethmoid mucoceles, *J Laryngol Otol* 103:667–669, 1989.

Valiati R, Ibrahim D, Abreu ME, et al: The treatment of condylar fractures: to open or not to open? A critical review of this controversy, *Int J Med Sci* 5(6):313–318, 2008.

Winegar BA, Murillo H, Tantiwongkosi B: Spectrum of critical imaging findings in complex facial skeletal trauma, *Radiographics* 33(1):3–19, 2013.

Winkler AA, Smith TL, Meyer TK, et al: The management of frontal sinus fractures. In: Kountakis SE, Onerci TM, eds: *Rhinologic and Sleep Apnea Surgical Techniques*, 2007, Springer, pp 149–158.

Zide MF, Kent JN: Indications for open reduction of mandibular condyle fractures, *J Oral Maxillofac Surg* 41(2):89–98, 1983.

AERODIGESTIVE ANATOMY AND EMBRYOLOGY WITH RADIOLOGIC CORRELATES

Benjamin J. Rubinstein, MD, Craig Villari, MD and Matthew S. Clary, MD

CHAPTER 71

KEY POINTS

1. Three unpaired cartilages (thyroid, cricoid, and epiglottis) and three sets of paired cartilages (arytenoid, corniculate, and cuneiform) constitute the laryngeal framework.
2. Extrinsic laryngeal muscles reposition the laryngeal framework craniocaudally and anteroposteriorly, especially during swallowing while the intrinsic muscles alter true vocal fold position and tension during phonation and respiration.
3. The true vocal folds are covered in squamous epithelium that overlies a gelatinous matrix, the superficial lamina propria, which allows the viscoelastic vibratory properties necessary for phonation.
4. The larynx is primarily formed from the third, fourth, and sixth branchial arches.

Pearls

1. The hyoid bone is not ossified at birth, but it is the first component of the laryngeal framework to ossify, followed by the thyroid cartilage and then the cricoid cartilage.
2. The cricoarytenoid joints are ball-and-socket joints that allow three-dimensional movement to achieve the complex functions required for the larynx.
3. The posterior cricoarytenoid muscle is the only abductor of the true vocal folds.
4. The cricothyroid muscle is the only intrinsic laryngeal muscle *not* innervated by the recurrent laryngeal nerve and is innervated by the superior laryngeal nerve.
5. The interarytenoid muscle is the only intrinsic laryngeal muscle with bilateral innervation.
6. The internal branch of the superior laryngeal nerve penetrates the thyrohyoid membrane to provide sensory innervation to the supraglottic and superior glottic larynx.

QUESTIONS

ANATOMY

1. **What are the three primary subunits of the larynx?**

   The larynx serves three important functions: airway protection, phonation, and swallowing. The larynx is also the portal to the airway; thus anatomical and functional patency is critical to normal breathing. It is sometimes easier to compartmentalize the larynx to better focus on discussion and study. The larynx is commonly divided into three subsections to aid in the description of pathologic processes: the supraglottis, glottis, and subglottis (Fig. 71.1). These anatomic subunits have different histologic characteristics and harbor different benign laryngeal disease processes.

   The supraglottis extends from the rostral edge of the epiglottis to the middle of the laryngeal ventricle. This subsection includes the laryngeal surface of the epiglottis, false vocal folds (also known as the vestibular folds), aryepiglottic folds, and superior portions of the arytenoid cartilages. The glottis extends superiorly from the mid-ventricle to 1 centimeter below the true vocal folds. This subsection contains the true vocal folds and arytenoid cartilages. The subglottis extends from 1 centimeter below the true vocal folds to the most caudal edge of the cricoid cartilage.

2. **What cartilages compose the larynx?**

   The larynx is composed of three unpaired cartilages and three paired cartilages (Fig. 71.2). Two of the unpaired cartilages, the thyroid and cricoid cartilages, are palpable externally and serve as surgical landmarks. The

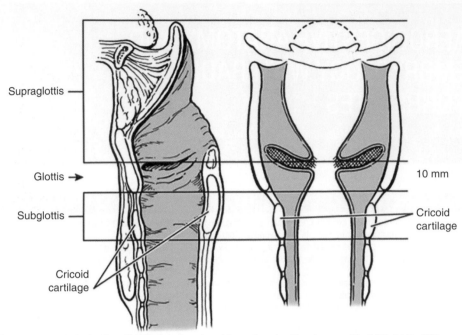

Fig. 71.1 Laryngeal subunits. (From Flint PW, et al.: *Cummings otolaryngology - head & neck surgery,* 6th ed, Philadelphia, 2015, Elsevier, pp. 1601–1633.)[8]

epiglottis and the paired cartilages—the arytenoid, cuneiform, and corniculate cartilages—are internal to the larynx. The cuneiform and corniculate cartilages are sometimes jointly referred to as sesamoid cartilages and serve as structural support to the aryepiglottic folds. The hyoid bone is the most superior aspect of the larynx and serves as an important insertion site for several extrinsic (suprahyoid and infrahyoid) laryngeal muscles. These cartilages can be seen in modified barium swallow studies used to assess dysphagia (Fig. 71.3).

The thyroid cartilage is formed by two alae that fuse at the midline. Each ala contains both superior and inferior cornu, the former tethering to the hyoid via the lateral thyrohyoid ligament, and the latter serves as an articulating joint with the cricoid cartilage. In the midline there is a small notch that helps define the "Adam's apple," which serves as a second connection to the hyoid via the median thyrohyoid ligament.

The cricoid cartilage is the only complete cartilaginous ring of the airway. It has a characteristic three-dimensional shape that is often compared to a signet ring. The ring is oriented such that the narrow portion is anterior in the neck and the larger plate resides posteriorly, offering additional height upon which the arytenoid cartilages sit on its superior surface. The vocal process of the arytenoid cartilage forms the posterior attachment of the vocal folds, which extend to their anterior attachment at the internal midline of the thyroid cartilage.

3. **What muscles are found within the larynx?**
The larynx utilizes two separate groups of muscles, the extrinsic and intrinsic laryngeal muscles, to perform tasks related to phonation, airway protection, and swallowing. The extrinsic musculature connects one structural element of the larynx to another structural element outside of the larynx; conversely, the intrinsic musculature connects one structural element inside the larynx to another.

The extrinsic musculature includes muscles that elevate and depress the laryngeal framework within the neck; while they play a small role in phonation and as accessory muscles of breathing, they are primarily utilized for laryngeal elevation during swallowing. A combination of the activation of the geniohyoid, digastric, mylohyoid, thyrohyoid, or stylohyoid muscles results in laryngeal elevation, while laryngeal depression can be achieved with activation of the strap muscles (sternohyoid, sternothyroid, and omohyoid). The extrinsic musculature has various innervations, including cervical rootlets and cranial nerves V and VII. The final extrinsic muscle group comprises pharyngeal constrictors. The constrictors, all innervated by the pharyngeal plexus, help advance a food bolus into the esophagus. The superior constrictor does not insert on the larynx, but the middle and inferior constrictors do, resulting in elevation and posterior translation with swallows.

Intrinsic musculature is primarily associated with airway protection and phonation. They are all paired muscles except for the interarytenoid muscle (Fig. 71.2). These muscles are classified as adductors or abductors based on the movement of the vocal folds with activation. Adduction results in medial approximation of the vocal folds for phonation, cough, or airway protection. The adductors include the thyroarytenoid, lateral cricoarytenoid,

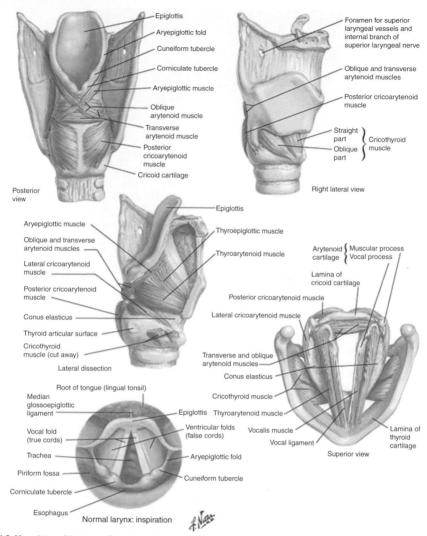

Fig. 71.2 Musculature of the larynx. (From Netter FH: *Atlas of Human Anatomy,* 5th ed, Philadelphia, 2010, Saunders, Plate 78.)[9]

and interarytenoid muscles. Abduction results in lateral excursion of the vocal folds during breathing. The lone abductor is the posterior cricoarytenoid muscle. The cricothyroid muscle is considered an intrinsic laryngeal muscle but it does not directly cause adduction or abduction of the vocal folds. The cricothyroid muscle works to pivot the thyroid cartilage anteriorly along the axis created by the cricothyroid joint, lengthening and tensing the vocal folds to increase pitch.

4. **What type of mucosa is found in the larynx?**
The majority of the mucosa is columnar respiratory epithelium. However, stratified squamous epithelium overlies the vibratory portions of the true vocal fold. The transition points from the respiratory epithelium to the squamous epithelium occur at the superior and inferior arcuate lines; the former is within the laryngeal ventricle, while the latter rests just below the true vocal fold.

This stratified squamous epithelium is thought to be protective against trauma caused by high-frequency collisions of the vocal folds during phonation. Despite this protective quality, the existence of different epithelia and transitions between epithelial types is important for understanding both malignant and benign pathologies. Understanding epithelial types in the larynx can help understand the likely locations for malignancy (squamous

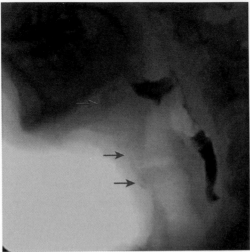

Fig. 71.3 Modified barium swallow showing the hyoid bone (top arrow), thyroid cartilage (middle arrow), and cricoid cartilage (bottom arrow).

cell carcinoma of the glottis) and benign pathology (recurrent respiratory papillomatosis commonly occurs at the transition points between respiratory and squamous epithelia).

5. **What is the laryngeal ventricle?**
   The ventricle is a unique anatomic outpouching between the supraglottic and glottic larynx. The inferior extent is the superior surface of the true vocal folds. The superior limit is not straightforward given the three-dimensional nature of the ventricle. When looking coaxially down the airway the superior extent appears to be the false vocal fold. However, on anatomical dissection one finds that the ventricle extends laterally and superiorly to a cranial extent beyond the false fold. Within this space is the laryngeal saccule, which contains mucus glands that lubricate the vocal folds. Saccular cysts can arise from this location and may be implicated in voice changes or airway obstruction (Fig. 71.4). Alternatively, air-filled dilation of the laryngeal saccule maintaining communication with the ventricle is termed a laryngocele, which also has airway and vocal implications.

6. **What are the quadrangular membrane and the conus elasticus?**
   The quadrangular membrane is a fibroelastic membrane extending from the epiglottis to the false vocal fold, terminating in the ventricular ligament. It roughly comprises the aryepiglottic folds but has no definitive structural integrity. The conus elasticus is also a fibroelastic membrane but it extends from the superior aspect of the cricoid cartilage and spans superiorly to interdigitate with the vocal ligament within the true vocal folds.
   Both the quadrangular membrane and conus elasticus serve as barriers to the spread of malignancy.

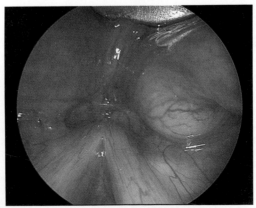

Fig. 71.4 Endoscopic view of the anterior commissure with 70-degree rigid endoscope showing a saccular cyst.

7. **What is the significance of the cricoarytenoid joint? How does the shape of the arytenoid cartilage help to specialize the joint?**

The cricoarytenoid joint is a specialized ball-and-socket joint that is integral in allowing the larynx to perform its vital functions. The joint allows the arytenoids to rotate on a vertical axis while also allowing them the freedom to glide and tip anteromedially.

The arytenoid has a pyramidal shape with the base serving as the socket for the cricoarytenoid joint. The arytenoid has two important appendages known as the vocal and muscular processes. The vocal process serves as the insertion point of the vocal ligament, while the muscular process, as the name implies, serves as the insertion point for several intrinsic laryngeal muscles. The muscles insert in several vectors, allowing the arytenoid to rotate on the cricoarytenoid joint facet, in turn abducting or adducting the vocal fold. This coordinated, highly specialized activation of the laryngeal musculature allows for airway protection and phonation.

8. **What laryngeal muscles are used for respiration?**

Any muscle that helps to adduct or abduct the vocal folds is technically utilized during respiration. For optimal airflow the vocal folds should be in an abducted position for respiration. Therefore the most important muscle is the posterior cricoarytenoid muscle, the lone abductor of the vocal folds, which is innervated by the recurrent laryngeal nerve (RLN). The infrahyoid strap muscles elevate the clavicles and upper ribs and serve as accessory muscles for breathing.

9. **What muscles are used for phonation?**

In contrast to respiration, optimal phonation occurs when the vocal folds are adducted in the midline. The muscles responsible for this motion are the thyroarytenoid, interarytenoid, and lateral cricoarytenoid muscles. These muscles are primarily innervated by the RLN.

The laryngeal framework can also pivot along the cricothyroid joint. This movement allows for tensing of the vocal ligament as it is stretched between the vocal process of the arytenoid cartilage and the insertion of the ligament on the thyroid cartilage. The cricothyroid muscle is responsible for this anterior pivoting, and its activation leads to higher pitched phonation. This muscle is the lone intrinsic muscle innervated by the external branch of the superior laryngeal nerve (SLN).

10. **Can phonation occur through alternative neurolaryngeal pathways?**

The innervation detailed in the previous question is the dominant pathway; however, there are other variations. While most of the intrinsic musculature responsible for adduction of the vocal folds is innervated by the RLN, there is a named anastomosis between the RLN and SLN known as the "nerve of Galen." This anastomosis can lead to some phonatory activation from the SLN and may be important for the maintenance or recovery of strength of the vocal fold following injury to the RLN.

11. **What muscles are used for swallowing?**

Swallowing is an incredibly complex task that involves multiple muscle groups outside the larynx. Swallowing begins with the voluntary transit of a food bolus from the oral cavity to the pharynx. The involuntary pharyngeal and esophageal phases are coordinated by cranial nerves IX, X, and XII. During swallowing, the vocal folds adduct to the midline, creating one level of protection against aspiration. Simultaneously, the extrinsic musculature is activated. This results in laryngeal elevation and epiglottic inversion. Progressive pharyngeal constriction from superior to inferior as well as tongue base contraction helps direct the food bolus toward the upper esophagus, which is now distended due to laryngeal elevation and relaxation of the upper esophageal sphincter (or cricopharyngeus muscle). If food or liquid enters the laryngeal introitus, a cough reflex is stimulated, which is triggered by the sensory branches of the SLN (supraglottic and superior glottic sensation) and RLN (inferior glottic and subglottic sensation).

12. **Do any of the intrinsic laryngeal muscles have bilateral innervation?**

Only one, the interarytenoid muscle, receives bilateral innervation. With denervation of one side of the larynx from an RLN injury, one may see a slight adducting motion of the ipsilateral arytenoid cartilage. This can sometimes be confused with residual ipsilateral innervation but may be due to interarytenoid muscle activation from the contralateral RLN.

13. **What are the layers of the vibratory vocal fold?**

While the vocal fold was once thought to be a solid layer of muscle with an overlying epithelial layer, histologic studies have identified several integral layers, all of which contribute to the unique vibratory function of the vocal folds (Fig. 71.5).

The deepest portion of the vocal fold is the thyroarytenoid muscle and the most superficial portion is the squamous epithelium. Between them is a tri-layered level known as the lamina propria. The intermediate and deep layers fuse together and integrate to form the vocal ligaments. The superficial layer of the lamina propria is a gelatinous matrix that is very important for the unique vibratory qualities necessary for phonation.

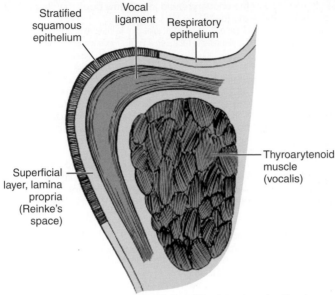

Fig. 71.5 Cross-section of the true vocal fold. (From Flint PW, et al.: Cummings otolaryngology - head & neck surgery, 5th ed, Philadelphia, 2010, Mosby, p. 860.)[10]

EMBRYOLOGY

1. **How does the larynx form in utero?**

    The larynx begins to form during the fourth week of gestation with the emergence of the laryngotracheal groove. This groove begins just caudal to the fourth branchial arch and forms the beginning of the unified upper aerodigestive tract. As the groove deepens, it begins to separate from the primitive esophagus in the coronal plane with the formation of the esophagotracheal septum. Lung buds will eventually descend from the resultant laryngotracheal diverticulum, while the most cranial aspect is destined to form the larynx.

    The larynx forms with contributions from the third, fourth, and sixth branchial arches, as detailed in Table 71.1, with a few exceptions. The hyoid bone forms with contributions from both the second and third branchial arches. The epiglottis originates from the hypobranchial eminence with contributions from both the third and fourth branchial arches.

    Understanding the branchial origins of these structures also provides insight into laryngeal sensory innervation. As the SLN is derived from the same branchial arch as the epiglottis and thyroid cartilages, it follows that the supraglottis and superior aspect of the glottis contain sensory innervation from the SLN. A similar relationship is found with the RLN carrying sensory innervation from the inferior glottis and subglottis.

Table 71.1 Branchial Arch Contributions to the Larynx

BRANCHIAL ARCH	ASSOCIATED NERVE	CARTILAGE/OSSEOUS DERIVATION	MUSCLE DERIVATION
Third	Cranial nerve IX	Greater cornu of hyoid* Epiglottis*	None in larynx
Fourth	Superior laryngeal nerve	Thyroid cartilage Cuneiform cartilage Epiglottis*	Cricopharyngeus Cricothyroid muscle
Sixth	Recurrent laryngeal nerve	Cricoid cartilage Arytenoid cartilages Corniculate cartilages	Intrinsic musculature of larynx

*Indicates structure originates from multiple branchial arches.

The laryngeal framework begins to form around week 5 of gestation and continues through week 9. Early within that time frame the epithelium of the larynx fuses and obliterates the previously present lumen. This lumen must re-form to allow for proper tracheal and lung development; it does so between weeks 7 and 10 of gestation. The laryngeal ventricles form as the lumen recanalizes but manages to leave the tissue, which ultimately becomes the false and true vocal folds.

2. **What in vivo pathologies exist because of derangements of laryngeal embryologic formations?**
Two relatively common pathologies can occur secondary to abnormal embryonic development. Laryngeal webbing occurs with failure to recanalize the lumen of the airway, usually around the 10th week of gestation. Laryngeal clefts form because of incomplete cleavage of the laryngotracheal diverticulum from the primitive esophagus. As the esophagotracheal septum forms in the cranial direction, progression may stall. The earlier the stall occurs during embryologic development, the more severe the laryngeal cleft.

Branchial cleft abnormalities can also involve the hypopharynx. Both third and fourth branchial cleft cysts can originate in the pyriform sinus and, in select cases, cautery of the orifice within the sinus or excision can be curative.

3. **Are any portions of the laryngeal framework ossified at birth?**
No. The hyoid is the earliest structural aspect of the larynx to ossify, occurring around the child's second birthday. The thyroid cartilage begins to ossify in the teenage years and the cricoid cartilage starts to ossify in the third or fourth decade of life. Complete ossification may not occur in any portion of the laryngeal framework but almost always occurs in the hyoid. This lack of ossification may serve as a protective mechanism against laryngeal fractures during childhood.

BIBLIOGRAPHY

Armstrong WB, Vokes DE, Verma SP: Malignant tumors of the larynx. In Flint PW, et al, eds: *Cummings Otolaryngology: Head and Neck Surgery*, 6th ed, 2015, Elsevier.
Bastian RW: Benign vocal fold mucosal disorders. In: Flint PW, et al, eds: *Cummings Otolaryngology: Head and Neck Surgery*, 5th ed, 2010, Mosby Elsevier.
Hirano M. Structure and vibratory behavior of the vocal folds. In: Sawashima M, Cooper FS, eds: *Dynamic Aspects of Speech Production*, Columbia Univ Pr, 1977.
Lee KJ: *Essential Otolaryngology*, 9th ed, 2008, McGraw-Hill.
Netter FH: *Atlas of Human Anatomy. Professional Edition*, 5th ed, 2011, Saunders Elsevier.
Pansky B: *Review of Medical Embryology*, 1982, Macmillian.
Rosen C, Blake Simpson C: *Operative Techniques in Laryngology*, 2008, Springer.
Sulica L: Voice: anatomy, physiology, and clinical evaluation. In: Johnson JT, Rosen CA, Baltimore MD, eds: *Bailey's Head & Neck Surgery Otolaryngology*, 5th ed, 2014, Lippincott Williams & Wilkins.
Tucker HM: *The Larynx*, 1993, Thieme.
Woodson GE: Laryngeal and pharyngeal function. In: Cummings CW, Robbins KT, Schuller DE, Richardson MA, Haughey BH, eds: *Cummings Otolaryngology: Head and Neck Surgery*, 4th ed, 2005, Elsevier.

CHAPTER 72

LARYNGOSCOPY, BRONCHOSCOPY, AND ESOPHAGOSCOPY

Todd M. Wine, MD

KEY POINTS

1. Laryngoscopy is integral to otolaryngology and is required for both diagnosis and treatment in the clinic and the operating theater.
2. Rigid bronchoscopy is not only diagnostic but also therapeutic and can be the key tool in an airway emergency.
3. Communication with the anesthesiologist is of utmost importance during laryngoscopy and bronchoscopy to prevent complications.
4. The narrowest part of the pediatric airway is the subglottis, which should be remembered during intubation to avoid iatrogenic injury.
5. Food impaction assessment should be accompanied by esophageal biopsies to rule out eosinophilic esophagitis.
6. Esophageal button battery foreign bodies are true emergencies requiring prompt removal due to the rapid damage that can occur in just 2 to 3 hours.
7. Using a shoulder roll during rigid esophagoscopy can be helpful in achieving a better angle for the esophagoscope to be advanced into the distal esophagus.

Pearls

1. Correct direct laryngoscopy technique greatly enhances visualization of the vocal cords. Always ensure that there are no contraindications to proper neck flexion and head extension (i.e., unstable cervical spine, Down syndrome).
2. Sizing the airway is inaccurate when acute soft tissue edema is present.
3. The proper depth of anesthesia and spontaneous respiration can be assessed in children by observing the abdomen prior to rigid bronchoscopy.

QUESTIONS

1. **What are laryngoscopy, bronchoscopy, and esophagoscopy?**
   Laryngoscopy is an examination of the larynx. This can be performed indirectly using a head torch and mirror and directly using rigid or flexible laryngoscopes. Bronchoscopy is examination of the trachea, bronchi, and its branches performed using either rigid or flexible bronchoscopes. Esophagoscopy is the endoscopic examination of the esophagus, which may also be performed using either flexible or rigid esophagoscopes.

2. **When is office laryngoscopy indicated in adults?**
   Examination of the larynx in adults is part of the complete physical examination of the head and neck and can be performed using indirect or flexible laryngoscopy. In examining the larynx in an adult the supraglottis, oropharynx, and hypopharynx are often also visualized. Examination of the larynx and surrounding anatomic areas is indicated for complaints of dysphonia, chronic cough, globus sensation, chronic throat discomfort or pain, stridor, neck mass, thyroid mass, and obstructive sleep apnea.

3. **When is office laryngoscopy indicated in children?**
   Examination of the larynx in children is indicated for noisy breathing, voice abnormalities, and obstructive sleep apnea status post adenotonsillectomy.

4. **What are different types of laryngoscopy?**
   Direct laryngoscopy is visualization of the larynx achieved by direct line-of-sight. This requires the use of a laryngoscope to achieve a proper view. The patient is usually anesthetized, although some patients may tolerate laryngoscopy performed with the use of local and/or regional blocks. Direct laryngoscopy is performed to allow insertion of an endotracheal tube (ETT), inspect the larynx in its entirety, and properly expose the portion of the larynx that requires biopsy or excision of a mass.

Indirect laryngoscopy visualizes the larynx and involves instruments to achieve an "indirect" view of the larynx. The laryngeal mirror uses indirect light from an external source (usually a lamp located behind the patient) and a mirror to direct light into the larynx, providing illumination and visualization of the structures. Indirect laryngoscopy can be limited by a patient's gag reflex. Other forms of indirect laryngoscopy involve the use of angled telescopes (70- or 90-degree) or flexible laryngoscopes to visualize the larynx. Rigid endoscopic evaluation with an angled telescope can achieve a high-definition view of the larynx.

Flexible laryngoscopy is often performed in the clinic using a flexible fiberoptic endoscope. The nasal cavity can be treated with a topical decongestant/anesthetic mixture to improve visualization and comfort of the examination. Lubrication of the telescope may also aid in comfort. Flexible laryngoscopy can also be used to evaluate swallowing using a procedure termed flexible endoscopic evaluation of swallowing (FEES). This procedure involves visualization of the larynx while feeding the patient various consistencies to determine if there is aspiration or penetration of the food bolus into the larynx.

Videolaryngoscopy involves attaching a camera to an angled rigid endoscope or a flexible endoscope to project the image onto a monitor. Digital recording devices can record the video, allowing the examination procedure to be stored for later visualization or review.

Videolaryngostroboscopy is videolaryngoscopy with the addition of a stroboscope. The stroboscope uses a microphone or electromyography (EMG) activity to detect the fundamental frequency of the vibrating vocal cords. The stroboscope flashes the light source based on the fundamental frequency, creating the appearance of a vocal cord wave in slow motion. This allows assessment of the mucosal wave of the vocal cord, which can help differentiate various pathologies of the vocal cord.

5. **What are laryngoscopes, and how do they differ?**
Laryngoscopes are instruments used to visualize the larynx while the patient is in the supine position. There are multiple types of laryngoscopes, and their designs differ in order to achieve certain goals. Examples of laryngoscopes optimized for specific functions include an anterior commissure scope (which has an anterior flare and shorter interdental dimension, allowing better view of the anterior commissure), bivalved laryngoscopes for approaching supraglottic and hypopharyngeal tumors, and slotted laryngoscopes that allow for easier intubation. Many different types of laryngoscopes attach to a suspension arm so that the surgeon may perform surgical procedures using a two-handed technique.

6. **How is flexible laryngoscopy performed?**
First the patient is counseled on the steps and side effects of this procedure, as there is minor discomfort involved. The nose is topically prepared using a combination of a local anesthetic and topical decongestant. Lubrication can be applied to the scope to allow for added comfort for the patient. The scope is inserted into the nasal cavity and advanced posteriorly, allowing visualization of the nasal cavity and nasopharynx. The scope is directed inferiorly to allow assessment of the oropharynx and then advanced to a position that allows proper assessment of the supraglottis and glottis. Voluntary vocalization and inspiration can confirm normal vocal cord mobility.

7. **What are the proper positions for direct laryngoscopy?**
The proper patient positioning for rigid direct laryngoscopy is the sniffing position with the head extended on the neck and the neck flexed. A shoulder roll is not required for direct laryngoscopy. To obtain adequate anterior exposure it is sometimes necessary to increase neck flexion further by lifting the head off the table.

8. **What makes laryngoscopy difficult?**
Difficult laryngoscopy does not allow visualization of the larynx. The factors contributing to this are usually anatomical factors. Trismus (inability to open the mouth widely), prominent dentition, micrognathia, tumors, infections, and trauma of the oropharynx and supraglottis can make laryngoscopy difficult.

9. **How is the laryngoscopic view of the larynx classified?**
When using an intubating laryngoscope, the view of the glottic opening should be reported. The grade of the view is important for communicating with other medical providers regarding the future care of the patient and for minimizing the risk involved for patients with known difficult laryngeal exposures. A Grade I view occurs when the entirety of the vocal cords can be seen. A Grade II view occurs with a partial view of the true vocal cords. A Grade III view occurs when only the arytenoids are seen. A Grade IV view occurs when no laryngeal structures are visible.

10. **What should be reported while doing direct laryngoscopy that is part of the head and neck examination?**
As otolaryngologists we are trained to examine the larynx in its entirety. This is most important in patients with head and neck cancers. A thorough examination includes visualization of the base of the tongue, vallecula, epiglottis (remarking on the lingual and laryngeal surfaces), supraglottis, glottis, and hypopharynx.

11. **What are the potential complications of direct laryngoscopy?**
Injury to any structure from the lips to the larynx can occur. Care must be taken to avoid pinching the lips between the laryngoscope and the teeth. Teeth can be inadvertently chipped, loosened, fractured, or avulsed. A tooth guard is used to help minimize dental injury. Difficult exposure of the larynx increases the chances of tooth injury. If dental injury is recognized intraoperatively an immediate dental consultation should be sought. Other risks include injury to the vocal cords. Additionally, laryngospasm can occur, which inhibits adequate ventilation, and, if not treated properly, can lead to respiratory arrest.

12. **What is the narrowest portion of the airway in adults and children?**
In adults the narrowest portion of the airway occurs at the glottis, whereas in children the narrowest portion is the subglottis. As such, knowing how to estimate and measure subglottic size is critical when assessing the airway in children.

13. **How is the appropriate ETT estimated?**
In children the appropriate size of the ETT can be estimated by age. In children aged 2 years and above the formula (4 + age)/4 can estimate the appropriate size. It is important to remember that a newborn should be intubated with a 3.5-mm ETT. As an infant approaches 1 year of age a 4.0-mm ETT becomes appropriate. By 2 years of age a 4.5-mm ETT is appropriate. In adulthood most men can accept an 8.0-mm ETT and women can tolerate a 7.5-mm ETT.

14. **How is subglottic airway size measured?**
Subglottic airway size is determined by performing a leak test. Performing a leak test requires insertion of a series of uncuffed ETTs and viewing and/or listening for a leak to occur around the ETTs. This is for determining the degree of narrowing of a firm stenosis of the subglottic airway. Usually the first tube is 0.5 mm smaller than that expected for the patient's age. There should be a free leak around the tube if the airway has an appropriate diameter. Progressively larger tubes are placed until there is no leak of air at 25 cmH$_2$O or less. The largest tube that allows a leak is considered to be the size of the airway. Based on the patient's age and corresponding ETT that fits, the degree of stenosis can be determined using the scale created by Myer and Cotton (Table 72.1).

15. **When is bronchoscopy indicated?**
Bronchoscopy is indicated whenever symptoms suggest that disease or evidence of disease may be present in the tracheobronchial tree. Symptoms determine the goals of the procedure. For infants and children, indications for bronchoscopy are usually related to stridor, chronic aspiration of liquids, suspected foreign body aspiration, and other diseases of the lower airway and lung parenchyma. In adults bronchoscopy is most often performed when there is hemoptysis, concern for neoplasm, and any other prolonged respiratory disease. In both children and adults, rigid bronchoscopy is vital to achieving success in difficult airway situations when direct laryngoscopy fails. The rigid bronchoscope can be used as a tool to bypass sites of obstruction. If rigid bronchoscopy cannot obtain an airway, a surgical airway is needed in the form of emergent tracheotomy or cricothyrotomy.

16. **What are the different types of bronchoscopy?**
Bronchoscopy can be performed using a rigid or flexible bronchoscope. Historically, rigid bronchoscopy is the older of the two techniques and was formerly termed open bronchoscopy. Rigid bronchoscopes are usually equipped

Table 72.1 Percent Subglottic Stenosis by Endotracheal Tube Size

			ENDOTRACHEAL TUBE SIZE (MM)								
			2	2.5	3	3.5	4	4.5	5	5.5	6
Patient age	Premature		40								
			58	30		No obstruction					
	0–3/12		68	48	26						
	3/12–9/12	No detectable lumen	75	59	41	22					
	9/12–2		80	67	53	38	20				
	2		84	74	62	50	35	19			
	4		86	78	68	57	45	32	17		
	6		89	81	73	64	54	43	30	16	
Grade		IV		III			II		I		

Reproduced with permission from Myer CM, O'Connor DM, Cotton RT: Proposed grading system for subglottic stenosis based on endotracheal tube sizes, *Ann Otol Rhinol Laryngol* 103:319–323, 1994.

with ventilation ports, which are known as ventilating bronchoscopes. Compared with a flexible bronchoscope the use of a rigid bronchoscope is potentially more traumatic and usually requires a deeper plane of anesthesia. When coupled with a Hopkins rod telescope, rigid bronchoscopy allows a more high-definition view of the airway compared to flexible bronchoscopy. In addition to this advantage, rigid bronchoscopy allows ventilation (can be used in emergency situations to secure the airway) and a larger working port, which can allow more efficient removal of foreign bodies or mucosal plugs. Flexible bronchoscopy is performed with a flexible endoscope that can be inserted into the airway under light sedation. Thus a primary advantage is the improved assessment of dynamic airway function, allowing better assessment of conditions such as tracheobronchomalacia. Another advantage is the ability to assess smaller and more distal bronchi. *Bronchoalveolar lavage* consists of instilling sterile sodium chloride into a terminal bronchus and suctioning it out to assess the biochemical nature of the distal airways and alveoli. This fluid can be used to assess for the presence of chronic aspiration and to determine the microbiology of the lung. Biopsies and dilations are other procedures that can be performed during both types of bronchoscopy.

17. **What abnormalities can be seen during bronchoscopy?**
Masses of the trachea or bronchi are readily noted during bronchoscopy. Other abnormalities include stenosis, cobble stoning, thick secretions, compression of the airway from an external source, and malacia. In adults stenosis is most likely to be posttraumatic in origin. While the same is true in children, other possible stenoses include congenital subglottic stenosis and long segment tracheal stenosis due to complete tracheal rings.

18. **How do tracheal dimensions vary with age?**
At 0 to 2 years of age the trachea averages 5.4 centimeters in length. By 16 to 18 years of age it has more than doubled in length to 12.2 centimeters. During that time the diameter increases three-fold, while the cross-sectional area increases six-fold.

19. **What are embryologic abnormalities of the trachea?**
Tracheomalacia is the most common intrinsic tracheal anomaly. This may be secondary to weakness of the cartilage or excess laxity of the posterior wall (membranous) of the trachea. Tracheal bronchus occurs when the right upper lobe bronchus originates directly from the trachea and not from the right main stem. Complete tracheal rings can occur at an isolated ring or may include anything up to the entire length of the trachea. Usually there is a long segment of tracheal stenosis and surgical treatment is necessary whenever the narrowing is severe.

20. **What are the various types of vascular compression of the trachea?**
Innominate artery tracheal compression is an anterior vascular compression that can severely limit the size of the airway. It can cause reflex apnea and recurrent respiratory infections. When severe it can be treated with aortopexy or translocation of the innominate artery. Vascular rings are abnormally connecting arteries of the aortic arch system that can compress the trachea and/or esophagus and cause recurrent respiratory symptoms or dysphagia for solids. The two most common types of vascular rings are the double aortic arch and the right aortic arch with aberrant left subclavian artery and left ligamentum arteriosum. A pulmonary artery sling (the left pulmonary artery originates from the right pulmonary artery and crosses the distal trachea) can also compress the trachea and right mainstem bronchus. Of note, 75% of patients with pulmonary artery sling can have complete tracheal rings. Computed tomography angiography and magnetic resonance angiography provide an accurate diagnosis of the anatomy. Surgical treatment involves translocation of the offending vasculature to relieve airway compression.

21. **What are the keys to rigid bronchoscopy removal of airway foreign bodies?**
Being prepared is of the utmost importance in airway foreign body cases. Proper communication must occur between the operating room staff, anesthesiologist, and surgeon at all times to ensure optimal outcomes. Having an appropriately sized rigid bronchoscope and a backup that is one size smaller is essential. The instruments used to retrieve the foreign body (endoscopic peanut grasper, alligator forceps, etc.) must be tested to ensure that they can fit through the age-appropriate bronchoscope.

22. **What are the indications for esophagoscopy?**
Esophagoscopy is indicated to investigate symptoms pertaining to the esophagus. Dysphagia for solids, refractory reflux, food impaction, and foreign bodies are the main indications for esophagoscopy in children. Dysphagia, gastroesophageal reflux disease, hematemesis, and atypical chest pain are indications for esophagoscopy in adults.

23. **What are the different types of esophagoscopy?**
Flexible esophagoscopy is performed with a flexible endoscope that usually has a port for insufflation of air (helps aid visualization via distension), suction, and irrigation. It can be used for biopsy, to cauterize bleeding, to dilate stenosis using a balloon catheter, and for the removal of foreign bodies. Flexible transnasal esophagoscopy is similar to traditional flexible esophagoscopy except that the scope is thinner (to allow transnasal insertion) and can be tolerated by the awake patient. This has been increasingly used in the office setting for adult patients. Rigid esophagoscopy is a rigid hollow tube inserted into the esophagus to visualize the mucosa of the esophagus.

Table 72.2 Grading System for Caustic Injuries of the Esophagus

GRADE	ENDOSCOPIC FINDINGS
0	Normal
1	Edema and hyperemia of mucosa
2a	Friable, hemorrhage, ulcers, erosions, blisters, exudates, membranes
2b	2a + deep or circumferential ulceration
3a	Small, scattered necrosis
3b	Extensive necrosis
4	Perforation

From Zargar SA, Kochhar R, Mehta S, et al: The role of fiberoptic endoscopy in the management of corrosive ingestion and modified endoscopic classification of burns, *Gastrointest Endosc* 37(2):165–169, 1991.

Visualization can occur unaided or with the help of a Hopkins rod telescope, which greatly enhances the view. Similar to flexible esophagoscopy, biopsies, dilation, and foreign body removal can occur using this modality.

24. **What are the potential complications of esophagoscopy?**
    Trauma to the lips, tongue, throat, and esophagus; fracture or avulsed teeth; aspiration pneumonia; hypotension; arrhythmia; pneumothorax bleeding; and esophageal perforation. Esophageal perforation can be particularly dangerous if not promptly recognized and can lead to life-threatening mediastinitis. Symptoms of chest pain and fever should be taken seriously and perforation of the esophagus should be ruled out. If present, prompt treatment is the key to a successful outcome.

25. **When should esophagoscopy be performed after a caustic ingestion?**
    Mucosal damage is most often caused by caustic ingestion and may continue to occur for some time after exposure. Esophagoscopy immediately after ingestion may underestimate the degree of injury. Esophagoscopy after 48 hours may increase the risk of iatrogenic esophageal perforation. Therefore most sources recommend delaying esophagoscopy until 12 to 48 hours after ingestion to allow the most accurate identification of the degree of injury.

26. **What type of necrosis do acidic and alkaline ingestions induce?**
    Acidic caustic ingestion induces coagulation necrosis. Coagulation necrosis may be helpful in that it creates a coagulum, which protects deeper tissues from injury. *Alkaline caustic ingestion causes liquefaction necrosis.* Liquefaction necrosis causes tissue disintegration, which allows deeper penetration through tissues and is therefore usually associated with more extensive esophageal damage.

27. **What is the grading system used to stage esophageal corrosive injuries?**
    Esophageal corrosive injuries are graded on a scale of 0 through IV (Table 72.2). The scale is based on the extent of mucosal damage. In general, patients with grade 0 to IIa lesions can have oral intake, while IIb to IV require total esophageal rest. No complications are usually associated with grade 0 to IIa injuries. Frequent complications are noted for grade IIb to IV lesions, including esophageal strictures and full-thickness necrosis.

28. **How do button batteries cause soft tissue injury?**
    The primary mechanism by which button batteries cause injury is through their ability to conduct an electrolytic current that produces hydroxide. Leakage of alkaline substances can occur in alkaline button batteries but does not occur in newer lithium button batteries. Lithium button batteries are 3V cells and are more dangerous because they can conduct a greater current. Finally, the battery can exert physical pressure and cause mild injury to the adjacent tissue. Button battery ingestion is an emergency that requires immediate removal because severe injury and subsequent mortality can occur with very short exposures.

29. **What needs to be ruled out when food impaction occurs in a child?**
    Food impaction in a child is highly associated with eosinophilic esophagitis. Therefore while treating food impaction, esophageal biopsies should be performed to investigate the possibility of eosinophilic esophagitis.

30. **How is eosinophilic esophagitis diagnosed?**
    Currently the diagnosis requires 15 eosinophils per high-power field in a tissue sample. Furthermore, the patient should still exhibit this severe eosinophilic infiltrate after being treated with a proton pump inhibitor.

31. **Esophageal foreign bodies are most likely to occur at which location in the esophagus?**
    Foreign bodies most often occur in the region immediately distal to the cricopharyngeus. The cricopharyngeus is a strong concentric muscle that can force a foreign body distal to it. The esophagus is often unable to pass it any further.

32. **What is a Zenker's diverticulum?**

This is a pseudo-herniation through a natural weakness in the posterior hypopharyngeal wall, between the oblique and fusiform fibers of the cricopharyngeus or the inferior pharyngeal constrictor and cricopharyngeus, known as the Killian triangle. When small, this pulsion-type diverticulum is asymptomatic. Over time it gradually enlarges and causes progressive dysphagia. Not only do patients complain of food getting stuck but they also complain of regurgitation of food products. The diagnosis is confirmed on barium swallow depicting a posterior herniation from the proximal esophagus.

33. **How is Zenker's diverticulum treated?**

Treatment has historically consisted of open techniques used to resect, suspend, or ligate the diverticulum along with a cricopharyngeal myotomy. Contemporary treatment is an endoscopic Zenker's diverticulectomy. The cricopharyngeal bar is isolated between the blades of a bivalved esophagoscope and the cricopharyngeal bar is divided using an endoscopic stapling device (if the pouch is large enough), laser, LigaSure, or electrocautery.

BIBLIOGRAPHY

Backer CL, Mongé MC, Popescu AR, Eltayeb OM, Rastatter JC, Rigsby CK. Vascular rings. *Semin Pediatr Surg.* 2016 Jun;25(3):165–75. doi: 10.1053/j.sempedsurg.2016.02.009. Epub 2016 Feb 22. PMID: 27301603.

Contini S, Scarpignato C: Caustic injury of the upper gastrointestinal tract. a comprehensive review, *World J Gastroenterol* 19(25):3918–3930, 2013.

Griscom NT, Wohl EB: Dimensions of the growing trachea related to age and gender, *Am J Roentgenol* 146:233–237, 1986.

Griscom NT, Wohl EB, Fenton T: Dimensions of the trachea to age 6 years related to height, *Pediatr Pulmonol* 5:186–190, 1989.

Litovitz T, Whitaker N, Clark L, et al: Emerging battery-ingestion hazard: clinical implications, *Pediatrics* 125(6):1168–1177, 2010.

Myer CM, O'Connor DM, Cotton RT: Proposed grading system for subglottic stenosis based on endotracheal tube sizes, *Ann Otol Rhinol Laryngol* 103(4 Pt 1):319–323, 1994.

Nielsen HU, Trolle W, Rubek N, et al: New technique using Ligasure for endoscopic mucomyotomy of Zenker's diverticulum: diverticulotomy made easier, *Laryngoscope* 124(9):2039–2042, 2014.

Papadopoulou A, Koletzko S, Heuschkel R, et al: Management guidelines of eosinophilic esophagitis in childhood, *J Pediatr Gastroenterol Nutr* 58(1):107–118, 2014.

Umapathi KK, Bokowski JW. Vascular Aortic Arch Ring. 2021 Aug 1. In: *StatPearls* [Internet]. Treasure Island (FL): StatPearls Publishing; 2022 Jan -. PMID: 32809754.

Zargar SA, Kochhar R, Mehta S, et al: The role of fiberoptic endoscopy in the management of corrosive ingestion and modified endoscopic classification of burns, *Gastrointest Endosc* 37(2):165–169, 1991.

CHAPTER 73

HOARSENESS AND DYSPHONIA

Elliana Kirsh DeVore, MD and Thomas L. Carroll, MD

KEY POINTS

1. Acute laryngitis is often associated with a viral upper respiratory tract infection and resolves within 1 to 2 weeks without antibiotic therapy.
2. Laryngopharyngeal reflux (LPR) is an inflammatory condition of the upper aerodigestive tract caused by the backflow of gastroduodenal contents into the larynx and pharynx. Pepsin, bile salts, and other gastroduodenal proteins directly induce mucosal modifications associated with LPR, while vagally mediated changes indirectly influence symptoms.
3. Systemic inflammatory disorders associated with the larynx include sarcoidosis (supraglottic), amyloidosis (glottic), and granulomatosis with polyangiitis (subglottic).

Pearls

1. During phonation the glottis should be in the closed phase for approximately 45% to 50% or more of each vibratory cycle at the most comfortable pitch and loudness. Glottic insufficiency (GI) exists if the closed phase is less than 45% to 50% and the causes of GI should be considered.
2. Vocal nodules, often overdiagnosed, are by definition bilateral and symmetric and occur at the junction of the anterior and middle thirds of the true vocal folds. More likely, when bilateral lesions are seen, a dominant subepithelial lesion (cyst, polyp, fibrous mass) on one vocal fold opposes a reactive lesion on the other side.
3. Recurrent respiratory papillomatosis (RRP) is primarily caused by HPV types 6 and 11.
4. Muscle tension dysphonia is typically associated with compensation for underlying GI and is unusual as a stand-alone primary diagnosis.
5. If the suspected LPR does not respond to acid suppression, specific testing to rule out nonacid reflux is required to exclude the diagnosis. A barrier treatment such as sodium alginate products or anti-reflux surgery can be offered.

QUESTIONS

1. **Describe the function of the larynx.**
   The larynx plays a role in swallowing, aspiration prevention, respiration, Valsalva maneuver, and phonation. The larynx is a complex three-dimensional structure shaped as a triangle anteriorly and transitioning to a circle posteriorly. It consists of numerous cartilages that support both extrinsic and intrinsic muscles, as described below, and may be divided into the supraglottis, glottis, and subglottis (Fig. 73.1).

2. **What is the mechanism of phonation including the physiology of vocal fold vibration?**
   There are three phases to phonation: pulmonary, laryngeal, and supraglottic/oral. The pulmonary phase creates a column of air via inhalation and exhalation. In the laryngeal phase the vocal folds approximate and vibrate as the air rushes past to create sound. Vocal fold vibration begins at the point of "mucosal upheaval" on the inferior lip of the mucosa in the posterior aspect of the membranous true vocal fold (TVF). When the column of air stops, vibration ceases. Changes in vocal fold length and tension via the thyroarytenoid (TA) and cricothyroid muscles affect the frequency of vibration or pitch. The supraglottis, pharynx, and sinonasal cavities act as resonators to amplify frequencies, creating a unique individual voice. Dysfunction in any of these levels can lead to voice changes, which may be interpreted as hoarseness by the patient. Finally, articulation of words is formed by the action of the palate, tongue, lips, and teeth (dysfunction of these structures from neurologic causes is called dysarthria).

3. **What is the difference between hoarseness and dysphonia? What is aphonia?**
   Hoarseness is a nonspecific term for changes in voice quality and is typically associated with a rough or harsh sound. Hoarseness is regarded as a symptom of an underlying pathology and not a diagnosis. Dysphonia, also a symptom, is an all-encompassing term that describes any problem with voice production, including changes in the quality of the sound produced, increases in vocal effort or fatigue, or pain and discomfort with speaking or singing. Aphonia is an inability to produce a voice.

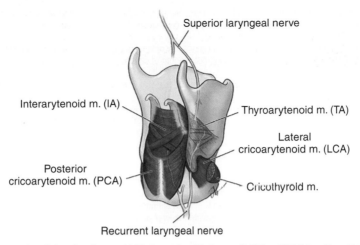

Fig. 73.1 Right posterolateral view of cartilages and intrinsic muscles of the larynx with RLN and SLN (internal branch). (From Rosen CA, Simpson CB: *Operative Techniques in Laryngology*, Berlin, 2008, Springer.)

4. **How is the underlying cause of a patient's dysphonia complaint diagnosed?**
   Clinical history and physical examination, including a complete head and neck examination, are all part of the initial workup to evaluate a dysphonic patient. In addition, voice evaluation by a speech-language pathologist (SLP) including acoustic and aerodynamic measures, laryngeal function studies, and stimulability testing (to determine if a patient is a candidate for voice therapy) is routinely performed in most voice centers before or after visualization of the larynx.

   The larynx can be visualized with a mirror, rigid endoscope, or flexible endoscope in the clinical setting. The mirror examination allows identification of a gross mass in the larynx as well as vocal fold motility; however, it is typically inadequate for detailed evaluation of surface lesions or vibratory anomalies in a dysphonic patient. Videolaryngoscopy allows for better visualization of the laryngeal anatomy including structural pathologies and subtle mucosal changes.

   When the cause of dysphonia is not obvious during static white light endoscopy, laryngovideostroboscopy (LVS) should be performed with either a rigid or flexible laryngoscope. LVS uniquely captures vocal fold vibratory characteristics including phase closure pattern, amplitude of vibration, symmetry of vibration, periodicity of vibration, and other mucosal wave abnormalities if present. With the recent addition of chip-tip camera technology, flexible LVS is becoming a popular modality to complete all portions of the laryngeal examination: structural, neurologic, and videostroboscopic. If possible, the LVS examination should be recorded and saved for future comparisons.

5. **What are pertinent questions in the clinical history of a dysphonic patient? (Include associated laryngeal complaints such as breathing and dysphagia.)**
   - When was the onset of symptoms? What is the duration of symptoms, and is there any progression? Such questions determine whether the process is acute or chronic.
   - Were there any associated events such as an upper respiratory infection; trauma; recent surgery of the head, neck, or chest; an intubation; a period of increased demand or overuse of the voice; or an emotional stressor?
   - How has the quality of voice changed? (Raspy, rough, breathy, weak, tightness, change in pitch.)
   - Is there dysphagia or odynophagia? If present, these symptoms may indicate a problem with the pharynx, esophagus, and/or larynx.
   - Is there a cough? Cough may be associated with LPR, asthma, allergy, infection, or postviral vagal neuropathy. Lung cancer with vocal fold paralysis (secondary to recurrent laryngeal nerve involvement) often presents with dysphonia and cough.
   - Is there hemoptysis? This potentially serious symptom may indicate malignancy.
   - Are symptoms of typical allergy (sneezing, itchy or watery eyes, cat sensitivity), LPR (throat clearing, mucus sensation, cough, globus sensation), or gastroesophageal reflux disease (GERD; heartburn, regurgitation/acid brash, dyspepsia) present?
   - What is the timing of the complaint (i.e., am or pm)? Does the voice get better or worse as the day goes on? Does the voice fatigue with use?
   - What other medical problems exist? Hoarseness may be associated with underlying hypothyroidism, an autoimmune disorder, and medications that cause drying of the laryngeal mucosa.

- What are the occupation and habits of the patient? Singers, teachers, sports coaches, lawyers, or other professional voice users, as well as people who eat a diet contributing to LPR are more likely to suffer from benign causes of dysphonia.
- How are these symptoms affecting the patient's quality of life? Voice health has a significant, multidimensional impact on general health and quality of life, independent of other comorbidities.

6. **Which laryngeal functions are evaluated with the flexible laryngoscopy portion of the examination?**

   Flexible laryngoscopy allows for visualization of the larynx in its physiologic position, and when compared to indirect laryngoscopy it can provide a more comprehensive dynamic voice evaluation in the office setting. Patients are typically decongested and anesthetized with topical medication. The laryngoscope is introduced through a nare and advanced into the oropharynx. The larynx is first observed with the patient breathing quietly, making note of abnormalities in adduction. Next, the patient is asked to produce a sustained "EE" sound and the larynx is evaluated for any lesions, vocal fold abnormality, or atrophy. Continuing the "EE" sound, the patient is asked to slide from low to high pitch and back down. The vocal folds lengthen when moving to a high pitch and shorten when moving to a low pitch. SLN palsies present as abnormalities with vocal fold lengthening maneuvers. The patient then alternates between "EE" and a sniff through the nose. These portions of the examination allow for a better evaluation of vocal fold paralysis. To complete the laryngeal examination, stroboscopy is then performed to evaluate vocal fold motion.

7. **How does stroboscopy generate a slow-motion image of vocal fold vibration?**

   Stroboscopy requires extraction of the frequency of vocal fold vibration via a flat microphone typically held to the patient's neck. The strobe light then shines on the larynx and flashes at specific points in the glottic cycle that are slightly out of phase with the vibration to create the appearance of slow-motion imaging of the vocal folds.

8. **Can you confidently diagnose the etiology of dysphonia without laryngovideostroboscopy?**

   Not really, except in cases of gross abnormality. Even in the case of gross abnormality there are often additional findings that are missed without LVS, such as subtle motion abnormalities or reactive subepithelial lesions of the opposite vocal fold. It is often difficult to reliably assess anything less than gross motion abnormalities of the vocal folds, such as supraglottic hyperfunction, without LVS. LVS improves diagnostic abilities by more than 25% when compared to isolated flexible laryngoscopy and can alter treatment regimens based on these findings.

9. **What are the common causes of dysphonia?**
   - GI with secondary, compensatory muscle tension dysphonia (MTD)
   - Malignant and premalignant exophytic epithelial lesions: leukoplakia (hyperkeratosis, metaplasia, dysplasia) and squamous cell carcinoma. When comparing leukoplakia with erythroplakia, erythroplakia has a higher probability of showing signs of dysplasia or malignancy because it represents a hypervascular lesion (as malignancies often are).
   - Neurologic disorders: spasmodic dysphonia, essential tremor, Parkinson's disease
   - Inflammatory conditions: LPR, vocal process granulomas, Reinke's space edema (polypoid corditis), allergy, irritants, and autoimmune diseases
   - Recurrent respiratory papillomatosis from the lesions themselves or incomplete closure and/or scarring of the vocal folds after intervention leading to GI and secondary MTD
   - Primary MTD: no underlying GI or other pathology is appreciated on LVS but significant supraglottic hyperfunction is present

10. **What is the difference between acute and chronic laryngitis?**

    Acute laryngitis is classically associated with viral upper respiratory tract infection (URTI) and is one of the most common causes of hoarseness. It is self-limiting and resolves with the URTI symptoms within 1 to 2 weeks. Patients typically do not require antibiotics and improve with hydration and voice rest. Chronic laryngitis is general inflammation of the larynx lasting longer than 4 weeks and is often caused by smoking, steroid inhalers such as Advair, fungal infections, or LPR. The voice usually improves if the irritating factors are removed or treated. This may involve smoking cessation, medical or surgical reflux management, antifungal medications, and voice rest.

11. **What is GI?**

    Glottic insufficiency is the inappropriate escape of air during phonation that leads to incomplete or complete but short-phase closure patterns (approximately 40% to 45% or less of each vibratory cycle in the closed position), as seen on LVS. GI may be gross or subtle and secondary to vocal fold scarring, atrophy, paresis, or paralysis. Therapeutic goals seek to augment the affected vocal fold(s) to allow for complete, long-phase closure during phonation (approximately 45% to 50% or more of the vibratory cycle in the closed phase). The presence of benign lesions of the vocal folds often leads to GI.

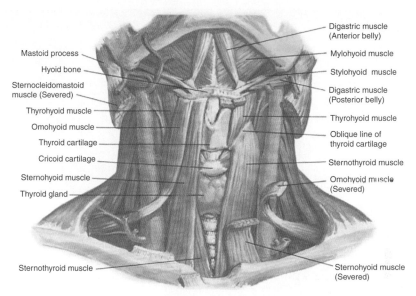

Mastoid process

Hyoid bone

Sternocleidomastoid muscle (Severed)

Thyrohyoid muscle

Omohyoid muscle

Thyroid cartilage

Cricoid cartilage

Sternohyoid muscle

Thyroid gland

Digastric muscle (Anterior belly)

Mylohyoid muscle

Stylohyoid muscle

Digastric muscle (Posterior belly)

Thyrohyoid muscle

Oblique line of thyroid cartilage

Sternothyroid muscle

Omohyoid muscle (Severed)

Sternothyroid muscle

Sternohyoid muscle (Severed)

Fig. 73.2 Anterior view of extrinsic laryngeal musculature. (From Netter FH: *Atlas of Human Anatomy*, 5th ed, Philadelphia, 2010, Saunders.)

12. **What are the different treatments for GI?**
    - Voice therapy (often tried first for many causes of dysphonia)
      Injection augmentation: office-based injections versus operating room (OR) injections. Different substances may be injected into the vocal folds, including autologous fat, human acellular dermis, hyaluronic acid gel, carboxymethylcellulose gel, and calcium hydroxyapatite gel.
      Medialization laryngoplasty with insertion of an implant lateral to the vocal fold composed of a synthetic material such as Silastic or Gore-Tex®.

13. **What is muscle tension dysphonia?**
    Muscle tension dysphonia (MTD) is a pathologic condition in which excessive tension in the extrinsic laryngeal muscles (Fig. 73.2) results in (primary MTD) or from (secondary MTD) an abnormality in the physiology/function of the phonatory mechanism involving the intrinsic laryngeal muscles and/or vocal fold mucosa. Supraglottic laryngeal tissues are often hyperfunctional in cases of MTD.

14. **What is the difference between primary and secondary MTD?**
    Primary MTD is dysphonia in the absence of organic vocal fold pathology and is associated with excessive supraglottic hyperfunction, often in the setting of atypical or abnormal TVF movements during phonation. Secondary MTD occurs in the setting of, and as compensation for, the underlying GI.

15. **What is spasmodic dysphonia (SD)?**
    SD is a focal dystonia affecting the laryngeal muscles during speech. There are two types of SD. **Adductor SD** is characterized by hyperactivity and muscle spasms of the adductor musculature, resulting in a strangled voice quality and breaks during voiced vowels. **Abductor SD** is characterized by dystonia of the abductor muscles, resulting in breathy voice quality and voice breaks during voiceless consonants such as P and F. Symptoms of SD typically improve with singing or the use of minor sedatives such as benzodiazepines. It may worsen with fatigue or physical and emotional stress. The treatment of choice for SD is periodic percutaneous botulinum toxin injection into the affected muscle groups under laryngeal electromyographic or endoscopic guidance.

16. **What are systemic diseases associated with hoarseness?**
    - Neurologic:
      - Hypofunctional disorders: characterized by weak voice, hoarseness, and dysphagia. Examples include Parkinson's disease, motor neuron diseases (amyotrophic lateral sclerosis or ALS, primary lateral sclerosis, postpolio syndrome), neuromuscular junction disorders (myasthenia gravis, Eaton-Lambert disease), and multiple sclerosis.
      - Hyperfunctional disorders: commonly have irregular loudness or pitch and straining of the voice; examples include dystonia, essential tremor, and pseudobulbar palsy.

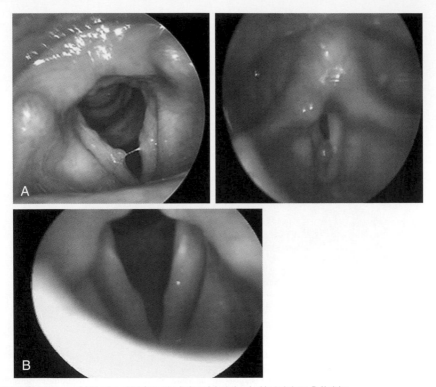

Fig. 73.3 A, Right true vocal fold polyp with left reactive lesion: abducted and adducted views. **B**, Nodules.

- Inflammatory:
  - Rheumatoid arthritis: cricoarytenoid joint involvement with ankylosis and submucosal vocal fold nodules.
  - Sarcoidosis: supraglottic (epiglottis most commonly affected) nodular and "turban-like" thickening.
  - Amyloidosis: laryngeal amyloid deposition most commonly near the glottic level in true and false vocal folds.
  - Granulomatosis with polyangiitis (formerly called Wegener granulomatosis): classically manifests as subglottic stenosis but may also show glottic changes.

17. **Which benign vocal fold lesions might cause hoarseness?**
    - **Polyps:** usually unilateral, broad-based, or pedunculated, found at the junction of the anterior and middle thirds of the membranous TVFs with an opposing reactive lesion (fibrous callous on the opposite TVF). They can be hemorrhagic due to acute trauma (Fig. 73.3A).
    - **Nodules:** always bilateral and symmetric; found at the junction of the anterior and middle thirds of the membranous TVFs (Fig. 73.3B).
    - **Cysts:** fluid-filled (mucus retention cysts) or cellular (epidermoid cysts); found within the superficial lamina propria with an opposing reactive lesion.
    - **Fibrous masses:** often firm, unilateral, broad-based lesions; found at the junction of the anterior and middle thirds of the membranous TVF with an opposing reactive lesion.
    - **Varices and ectasias:** abnormal, enlarged, or tortuous blood vessels; found primarily on the superior aspect of the middle of the membranous TVFs. The common pathology identified in singers with intermittent acute dysphonia.
    - **Granulomas:** fleshy masses due to either trauma such as intubation or persistent contact pressure from glottis insufficiency and secondary MTD in the setting of LPR; classically found on the vocal process of the arytenoids but may appear higher on the arytenoid mucosa or, most commonly in cases of intubation or surgical trauma, on the membranous TVF.
    - **Polypoid corditis/Reinke's edema:** swelling of the superficial lamina propria, associated with smokers and hypothyroidism.
    - **Recurrent respiratory papillomatosis:** exophytic epithelial lesions caused by HPV (typically types 6 and 11 but 16 and 18 are also seen); located anywhere in the larynx, favoring the TVF. Malignant transformation is observed in 1% to 2% of cases.

18. **How are nodules different from other benign vocal fold lesions, and how are they differentiated?**
Nodules are small and discrete lesions located in the membranous portion of the vocal fold, one-third of the distance from the anterior commissure. Vocal nodules are easily identified because they are paired and *symmetric*. Vigilance should be employed during LVS to identify a unilateral dominant phonotraumatic lesion (polyp, cyst, or fibrous mass) with an opposing reactive lesion rather than assuming the diagnosis of nodules, as the treatment may warrant surgical intervention. Polyps are exophytic and asymmetric and appear soft and smooth, often coexisting with a reactive lesion of the opposite vocal fold. Vocal fold cysts are mucous retention or epidermoid cysts located in the superficial layer of the lamina propria, usually at the middle third of the vocal fold in the medial and superior aspect, and are also found in coordination with a reactive lesion of the opposing vocal fold. Fibrous masses are often firm and broad, significantly limiting the mucosal wave, and are seen in the presence of a reactive lesion of the opposing TVF. Vocal process granulomas (VPGs) are not actually found on the membranous vocal fold as compared with the other benign lesions presented; VPGs form on the high-pressure contact area of the vocal processes of the arytenoid cartilage. They have a pathognomonic appearance and typically do not require removal/biopsy but rather regress and become asymptomatic with voice therapy and acid reflux suppressive medications.

19. **How do you treat benign vocal fold lesions?**
For benign, overuse/phonotraumatic lesions such as nodules, polyps, and cysts, the patient typically undergoes a course of voice therapy and rests the voice whenever possible. If voice therapy is not successful or the lesion is too large to have any potential for success, surgical excision of the lesion followed by voice therapy is offered (see below for technique). For RRP, KTP laser excision has emerged as an effective method to preserve voice and avoid injury to the vibratory layer. Other methods to remove RRP include cold knife excision, CO_2 laser excision, and microdebrider excision. KTP laser is also used successfully in the treatment of TVF ectasias and Reinke's edema. Reinke's edema, when excessive, often requires surgical excision.

20. **What is voice therapy, and what is the role of voice therapy in the treatment of dysphonia?**
Voice therapy consists of vocal and breathing techniques that retrain the patient to produce the best sound with the least injury. It is designed to relieve or "unload" the larynx of hyperfunctional behaviors and instills new muscle memory techniques (akin to a baseball pitcher recovering from an arm injury). It is performed over 4 to 6 weeks by an SLP or voice pathologist who specializes in voice therapy. It is offered as first-line therapy for anyone with benign laryngeal pathology who is deemed a candidate for voice therapy by a voice pathologist.

21. **What are the surgical treatments for benign phonotraumatic vocal fold lesions?**
    - Microsuspension laryngoscopy (MSL or suspension microlaryngoscopy) with excision of the offending lesion via the medial microflap technique. The incision for the microflap can be made using cold steel or a CO_2 laser. Dissection using microinstruments then ensues. In some instances the lesion is densely adherent to the overlying epithelium (typical with fibrous mass) or pedunculated (some polyps) and a microflap cannot be separated from the benign lesion. In these cases the epithelium is removed with the lesion (Fig. 73.4).
    - Office-based or operative steroid injections for scars, nodules, or fibrous masses.
    - Office-based or operative KTP laser photoangiolysis for vascular lesions (ectasias or hemorrhagic polyps) or deep fibrous masses that are adherent to the epithelium and would result in a significant TVF defect if excised.

22. **What is LPR disease?**
Laryngopharyngeal reflux disease is an inflammatory condition of the upper aerodigestive tract caused by the backflow of gastroduodenal contents into the larynx and pharynx. Pepsin, bile salts, and other gastroduodenal proteins directly induce mucosal modifications associated with LPR such as vocal fold and laryngeal inflammation. LPR differs from GERD because it affects a different target end organ, the laryngopharynx as opposed to the esophagus, and often involves different presenting symptoms and treatment. LPR is often "silent" because patients do not have typical GERD symptoms such as heartburn or feelings of regurgitation.

23. **How do you diagnose and treat laryngopharyngeal reflux?**
Patients with LPR-induced laryngitis present with symptoms of chronic hoarseness, chronic cough, throat irritation, frequent throat clearing, a mucus sensation in the throat, and globus sensation (a feeling of a lump in the throat and often increased effort with swallowing). All of these symptoms are attributed to LPR but they overlap dramatically with other laryngeal pathologies that lead to GI and secondary MTD. Updated clinical guidelines recommend against prescribing acid-blocking medications to treat isolated dysphonia based on symptoms alone without visualization of the larynx. However, after LVS has been performed and no other pathology is identified a presumed diagnosis of LPR may be applicable and empiric acid suppression and/or alginate trials may be offered. Most patients respond to diet and lifestyle changes along with acid suppression in the form of high-dose, twice-daily proton pump inhibitors because this removes the acid cofactor. Because the nonacidic components of reflux, primarily pepsin, have been demonstrated to be active even at neutral pH, not all patients respond to acid-suppressive medications. Alginate suspensions and chewable tablets are becoming more common in the treatment of LPR, as our understanding of LPR broadens. LPR is not an acid-only problem and pepsin from the

PRE / POST

0 degree   30 degree   70 degree

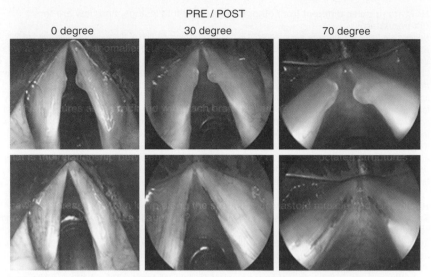

Fig. 73.4 MSL view pre/post microflap excision of right TVF polyp and left reactive lesion with three different telescopic views.

stomach likely plays a larger role in the pathology of the disease. Without dietary changes to avoid acidic foods, dietary acids likely reactivate pepsin that remains in the throat despite medical acid suppression. As with GERD, patients with LPR may benefit from sleeping with the head of the bed elevated; avoiding tomato-based, spicy, or fatty fried foods; and waiting 3 to 4 hours after eating before going to bed.

BIBLIOGRAPHY

Altman KW, Atkinson C, Lazarus C: Current and emerging concepts in muscle tension dysphonia: a 30-month review, *J Voice* 19(2): 261–267, 2005.

Belafsky PC, Postma GN, Reulbach TR, et al: Muscle tension dysphonia as a sign of underlying glottic insufficiency, *Otolaryngol Head Neck Surg* 127:448–450, 2002.

Borges LF, Chan WW, Carroll TL: Dual pH probes without proximal esophageal and pharyngeal impedance may be deficient in diagnosing LPR, *J Voice* 33(5):697–703, 2019.

Carroll TL, Gartner-Schmidt J, Statham MM, et al: Vocal process granuloma and glottal insufficiency: an overlooked etiology? *Laryngoscope* 120(1):114–120, 2010.

Chang JI, Bevans SE, Schwartz SR: Evidence-based practice management of hoarseness/dysphonia, *Otolaryngol Clin North Am* 45:1109–1126, 2012.

Damrose EJ, Berke GS: Advances in the management of glottic insufficiency, *Curr Opin Otolaryngol Head Neck Surg* 11:480–484, 2003.

Davids K, Klein AM, Johns MM: Current dysphonia trends in patients over the age of 65: is vocal atrophy becoming more prevalent? *Laryngoscope* 122:332–335, 2012.

DeVore EK, Carroll TL, Rosner B, Shin JJ: Can voice disorders matter as much as life-threatening comorbidities to patients' general health? *Laryngoscope* 130(10):2405–2411, 2020. doi: 10.1002/lary.28417.

Flint PW, Haughey BH, Lund VJ, et al: *Cummings Otolaryngology: Head and Neck Surgery*, 5th ed, 2010, Mosby Elsevier, pp 805–893.

Francis DO, Smith LJ: Hoarseness guidelines redux: toward improved treatment of patients with dysphonia, *Otolaryngol Clin North Am* 52(4):597–605, 2019.

Lechien JR, Akst LM, Hamdan AL, et al: Evaluation and management of laryngopharyngeal reflux disease: state of the art review, *Otolaryngol Head Neck Surg* 160(5):762–782, 2019.

Lechien JR, Rodriguez Ruiz A, Dequanter D, et al: Validity and reliability of the reflux sign assessment, *Ann Otol Rhinol Laryngol.* 2020;129(4):313–325.

Mau T: Diagnostic evaluation and management of hoarseness, *Med Clin North Am* 94:945–960, 2010.

Mehta DD, Deliyski DD, Hillman RE: Commentary on why laryngeal stroboscopy really works: clarifying misconceptions surrounding Talbot's law and the persistence of vision, *J Speech Lang Hear Res* 53:1263–1267, 2010.

Naunheim MR, Carroll TL: Benign vocal fold lesions: update on nomenclature, cause, diagnosis, and treatment, *Curr Opin Otolaryngol Head Neck Surg* 25(6):453–458, 2017.

Rosen CA, Lombard LE, Murry T: Acoustic, aerodynamic, and videostroboscopic features of bilateral vocal fold lesions, *Ann Otol Rhinol Laryngol* 109:823–828, 2000.

Tae K, Jin BJ, Ji YB, Jeong JH, Cho SH, Lee SH: The role of laryngopharyngeal reflux as a risk factor in laryngeal cancer: a preliminary report, *Clin Exp Otorhinolaryngol* 4(2):101–104, 2011.

CHAPTER 74

VOICE DISORDERS AND VOICE THERAPY

Juliana Litts, MA, CCC-SLP

KEY POINTS

1. Most voice disorders have more than one etiologic factor, and medical, surgical, and behavioral therapies may be warranted individually or in combination at any time.
2. Treatment outcomes for voice disorders are driven by patient perception of limitations related to voice. Treatment goals will be different for each patient depending on their personal voice needs.
3. A multidisciplinary team for treating voice disorders may include otolaryngologists (ENTs), gastroenterologists, neurologists, allergists, speech-language pathologists (SLPs), physical therapists, massage therapists, psychologists, acupuncturists, and singing/vocal coaches.
4. Important components of a voice evaluation include a detailed case history, auditory perceptional observation of patient voicing and respiratory behaviors, and direct visualization of the laryngeal anatomy.

Pearls

1. ENTs have the responsibility to provide medical diagnoses and determine treatment plans that can include behavioral, pharmaceutical, or surgical components related to voice complaints. An SLP knowledgeable in the evaluation and treatment of voice disorders can increase the efficacy of voice evaluation and treatment.
2. When surgical management of a voice disorder is necessary for a patient, voice therapy pre- and postsurgery can improve overall outcomes by addressing maladaptive voice behaviors that may delay recovery or result in relapse.

QUESTIONS

1. **Which pathologies/conditions are appropriate for a referral to an SLP?**
   Voice therapy is most successful in treating patients with normal laryngeal anatomy, which typically carries a diagnosis of muscle tension dysphonia or muscle tension aphonia. Voice therapy can also be highly successful at optimizing patients with mild alterations in anatomy such as vocal fold atrophy, vocal fold nodules, vocal fold polyps, glottic insufficiency, vocal fold scar, vocal fold paralysis, vocal process granuloma, etc.

   Voice therapy can enhance treatment outcomes after medical and/or surgical intervention as it improves the efficiency and coordination of the pulmonary, laryngeal, and resonance systems to decrease extralaryngeal tension and optimize vibration patterns. This promotes improved voice quality and consistency and decreases vocal effort.

   Neurologic voice disorders such as laryngeal tremor and spasmodic dysphonia may benefit from trial voice therapy to reduce laryngeal tension and effort, but treatment with botulinum toxin (Botox) is considered the standard of care for this population. Voice therapy can be used as an adjunct therapy with Botox to reduce compensatory behaviors, with research indicating that these patients may experience significantly better outcomes when compared to patients who received Botox treatment alone, and patients with hypophonia, as seen most commonly in Parkinson's disease (PD), can also be good candidates for voice therapy.

2. **What medical documentation should an SLP complete for an optimal voice assessment?**
   Prior to the initiation of SLP evaluation of voice the patient should be evaluated by an otolaryngologist. Reports and findings including the following are essential to complete an optimal voice assessment: detailed medical and surgical history, current medication list, past and current laryngeal diagnoses, still images or videos of the larynx, radiologic image interpretation of the head and neck (if applicable), and results of any swallowing evaluations (if applicable).

3. **What intake information is collected during an SLP voice evaluation?**
   The main goals of the SLP voice evaluation are to:
   1. Determine the etiologic factors relating to the voice disorder
   2. Determine the severity of the voice disorder
   3. Determine the clinical plan of care and the expected prognosis

Case history, instrumental and physical assessment, acoustic analysis, and perceptual ratings are typically collected during speech-language pathology voice evaluation. SLPs aim to discover behaviors, environmental factors, patterns of occupational and social voice use, and relevant medical and surgical history that impact the patient's voice. The timing and nature of a patient's voice complaints, for example, are extremely valuable pieces of information that help determine the nature of the patient's disorder. Was onset gradual or sudden? Is the problem consistent or intermittent in nature? The patient's vocal hygiene and voice use is also evaluated and discussed.

Physical examination of the head and neck and cranial nerve examination is usually conducted by the referring physician, but can be also performed by the evaluating or treating SLP. SLPs may also conduct an oral mechanism examination such as the Oral Speech Mechanism Screening Examination (OSMSE-3; see chart). This standardized protocol is used to assess the appearance and function of the oral mechanism, including the lips, tongue, jaw, teeth, palate, pharynx, velopharyngeal mechanism, breathing, and diadochokinetic rates. The larynx may also be palpated for the assessment of range of motion.

Assessment of vocal performers requires additional history acquisition and examination. Special attention is given to reported vocal effort, voice production across pitch range, and vocal demands of the patient's performing schedule, among other factors.

4. **Describe the objective measures/evaluation completed during an SLP voice evaluation.**
Rigid laryngoscopy or transnasal flexible laryngoscopy with stroboscopy allows the structure and function of the vocal folds to be assessed, imaged, and digitally recorded. In most states, SLPs with expertise in voice can complete either rigid videostroboscopy or transnasal flexible laryngoscopy with stroboscopy with proper training and physician supervision. The American Academy of Otolaryngology Head and Neck Surgery (AAO-HNS) and American Speech Language and Hearing Association joint position statement outlines the roles of physicians and SLPs in this context. Laryngoscopy can also be an important tool for determining the presence of compensatory vocal behaviors and can be used as a biofeedback tool. Direct observation of vocal folds and vocal fold vibration is an essential component of evaluation as the laryngeal mechanism can be observed and described.

Quantification of other vocal parameters can be performed using advanced equipment to measure the aerodynamic and acoustic properties of voice. As equipment cost and time can be prohibitive for some SLPs, acoustic analysis of voice offers SLPs a noninvasive and low-cost method for obtaining a significant amount of patient data. For example, the fundamental frequency, pitch range, and vocal intensity can be evaluated. Measurements including rates of airflow during phonation, minimum subglottic pressure, and the frequency of breaths while reading the rainbow passage are frequently used during assessment.

5. **Which patient-centered assessments are used during a voice evaluation?**
Throughout a voice evaluation, the SLP listens and forms an impression of the patient's vocal quality, pitch, and vocal intensity (loudness) as a way of describing the patient's voice and setting a baseline for the patient's vocal presentation. The use of digital recording equipment to collect patient speech samples is recommended. Standardized perceptual rating scales such as the Consensus on Auditory Perceptual Evaluation of Voice (CAPE-V) are used to help standardize impressions.

Patients' perceptions of their voice disorder and how it impacts their daily life are important factors that can be quantified using quality of life tools. The Vocal Handicap Index (VHI), Voice Handicap Index-10 (VHI-10), Singing VHI-10 (SVHI-10), and Voice Related Quality of Life Scale (VRQOL) are all subjective quality of life measurements that have been validated for use (Table 74.1).

6. **What are the most common symptoms related to voice disorders?**
The most common symptoms or patient complaints related to voice disorders include changes in pitch, decreased loudness, rough voice quality, breathy voice quality, increased vocal effort, increased vocal fatigue, decreased vocal range, and inconsistency in voice production.

Table 74.1 Voice Handicap Index-10

F1	My voice makes it difficult for people to hear me.	0 1 2 3 4
F2	People have difficulty understanding me in a noisy room.	0 1 2 3 4
F8	My voice difficulties restrict personal and social life.	0 1 2 3 4
F9	I feel left out of conversations because of my voice.	0 1 2 3 4
F10	My voice problem causes me to lose income.	0 1 2 3 4
P5	I feel as though I have to strain to produce voice.	0 1 2 3 4
P6	The clarity of my voice is unpredictable.	0 1 2 3 4
E4	My voice problem upsets me.	0 1 2 3 4
E6	My voice makes me feel handicapped.	0 1 2 3 4
P3	People ask, "What's wrong with your voice?"	0 1 2 3 4

7. **What some common therapeutic approaches to voice therapy?**

All voice therapy should be targeted to improve the efficiency of voice production. There are two common hierarchical methods of voice therapy: resonant voice therapy and flow phonation. These start with a specific target in its simplest form (syllable) and continue to work up to more complicated targets at the word, phrase, and conversational levels. Resonant voice therapy targets awareness of voice sensations in the lips, cheeks, nose, and mouth rather than in the throat, while flow phonation targets awareness of airflow as the dominant feature in voice production. An alternative approach to voice therapy called conversation training therapy is based on motor learning principles, offering voice production targets in conversations that are designed to change the coordination of the voice system to decrease unnecessary segmentation of learning that takes place in the hierarchical approaches. It may be appropriate to use one or more techniques during voice therapy.

8. **Describe common stretches and massage techniques used to decrease laryngeal musculoskeletal tension.**

Stretches of the neck, shoulders, torso, jaw, and tongue and laryngeal massage provide release of extrinsic muscle tension (Table 74.2). Stretches and massages should be completed at least once daily.

9. **What are optimal reflux precautions?**

Gastroesophageal reflux disease (GERD) and laryngopharyngeal reflux (LPR) are commonly observed in patients with laryngeal complaints. Behavioral strategies include, but are not limited to, elevating the head of the bed; avoiding overeating; remaining upright for at least 60 minutes after eating; not exercising after eating; decreasing consumption of caffeine, alcohol, and carbonated drinks; avoiding foods that can trigger acid; weight reduction; avoiding tight clothing; taking medication appropriately; and avoiding excessive drinking of water immediately before bed.

10. **What is vocal hygiene?**

Vocal hygiene refers to the ongoing maintenance of a patient's vocal health. Poor vocal hygiene contributes to vocal pathology, and SLPs aim to educate patients about the benefits of optimal vocal health. The core issues include adequate hydration, elimination of excessive caffeine and alcohol intake, optimal nutrition, elimination and behavioral management of laryngeal irritants such as postnasal drainage and allergies, laryngopharyngeal reflux, and identification and elimination of phonotraumatic behaviors including chronic cough and throat clearing. Adherence to optimal vocal health behaviors contributes greatly to the success of voice therapy.

Table 74.2 Head and Neck Stretches

AREA	DESCRIPTION
Neck	Head side to side
	Head forward and backward (chin up and chin down positions)
	Looking over each shoulder
	Yawn-sigh
Shoulders	Shoulder shrugs
	Shoulder rolls: forward and backward
Torso	Reach up to the ceiling, lean to the sides
	Clasp hands in front of the body and stretch
	Clasp hands behind the body and stretch
Jaw	Massage at masseter muscle and at the TMJ
	Grab jaw and gently pull it down, release tongue
Tongue	Stretch tongue out as far as possible
	Tenderize: gently bite forward and backward on your tongue
Laryngeal massage	Place fingers on thyroid notch
	Feel the top edge of the thyroid cartilage with your thumb and middle finger
	Press fingers inward to feel the thyrohyoid space, feeling the lower border of the hyoid bone
	Gently massage and pull down to unlock tension of the extrinsic musculature

11. **What are common voice therapy goals for a patient with muscle tension dysphonia?**
Behavioral management of muscle tension dysphonia (MTD) seeks to reduce hyperfunctional or hypofunctional vocal production that contributes to laryngeal muscle tension. Common goals for a patient include the implementation of passive and active laryngeal, head, and neck stretches. Management techniques can also include biofeedback; improved airflow with speech at the word, phrase, sentence, and conversational levels; achievement of easy vocal onset; use of resonant voice therapy techniques; and circumlaryngeal massage. Behaviors that contribute to phonotrauma, such as yelling or chronic throat clearing, are discussed and eliminated. The role of stress and its impact on voice is often an important component in examining and discussing patients with MTD. In some cases, referral for the psychosocial management of voice disorders is indicated.

12. **Who should provide voice therapy treatment, and how long is the expected duration of treatment?**
Voice therapy should be provided by a licensed SLP with a background and training in voice rehabilitation. Fewer than 5% of SLPs in the USA report feeling comfortable treating voice disorders. The efficacy of voice therapy significantly improves if provided by a trained SLP. The duration of voice therapy typically lasts approximately 4 to 6 sessions. Therapy is considered complete if the patient has achieved their therapy goals and is no longer limited by their voice or if the patient has failed to continue to progress toward their goals for the following reasons: poor compliance with homework recommendations, insufficient laryngeal anatomy, difficulty in coordinating the laryngeal mechanism into an improved behavior, or lack of internal motivation for changing voice.

13. **Discuss the treatment for paradoxical vocal fold motion (PVFM)/vocal cord dysfunction (VCD).**
The initial treatment for PVFM/VCD involves directing emphasis away from the respiratory system, thereby relaxing the larynx and dissipating the attack. This includes "s breathing," and "f breathing," panting (rapid shallow breathing), and/or yawning to open up the oropharynx. While these maneuvers may be effective for some patients, others find them ineffective.

Pursed lip breathing (PLB) has also been documented as a successful maneuver to dissipate episodes of PVFM/VCD. The patient is first instructed to relax upper body tension and use diaphragmatic breathing. The patient should gently exhale via pursed lips (2–3 seconds), followed by a controlled and silent inhalation (1 second) through the nose. Using PLB allows the building of back pressure to open and relax the airway, reversing the episode of PVFM/VCD. The application of PLB is tailored to the individual and may be used for retraining, pretreating, and moments of attack.

14. **What is an SLP's role with patients with laryngeal cancer?**
An SLP can provide patients who are postsurgical and postradiotherapy with vocal techniques to improve and maintain vocal flexibility, as well as promote vocal hygiene. If a patient undergoes laryngectomy, an SLP is an essential part of the medical team because laryngectomy alters respiration, swallowing, and speech. The SLP can also provide education, recommendations, and training/therapy of postlaryngectomy communication options, including esophageal speech, electrolarynx, and tracheoesophageal voice restoration.

An SLP should also be contacted prior to the treatment of laryngeal cancers for education and counseling when there is concern for postoperative or post-radiation-related dysphagia. Patients typically benefit from ongoing therapy before, during, and after surgery and radiation treatment.

15. **What are hypernasality, hyponasality, and assimilative nasality?**
Hypernasality is an excessive and inappropriate amount of perceived nasal cavity resonance during phonation. Velopharyngeal dysfunction (VPD) and velopharyngeal insufficiency (VPI) are terms used to describe this phenomenon, whether due to impaired motion of the VP mechanism, tissue insufficiency, or both. This includes inappropriate nasal emissions, decreased intraoral pressure, and increased nasal resonance during speaking tasks.

Hyponasality is reduced nasal resonance for /m/, /n/, and "ing" sounds. This is typically a result of an anatomic obstruction including but not limited to large adenoids/tonsils, deviated septum, choanal atresia, nasal cavity turbinate swelling, or allergic rhinitis. Articulation substitutions of /b/, /d/, and /g/ are typically observed.

Assimilative nasality appears when the speaker's vowels or voiced consonants present as nasal when adjacent to nasal consonants. This occurs because the velopharyngeal port opens too soon and remains open inappropriately. This may be due to faulty speech patterns or an exaggerated regional dialect.

16. **What should be completed for a clinical evaluation of nasal resonance disorders?**
Clinicians should listen carefully to voice during spontaneous conversation, vowels in isolation, and speech samples loaded with oral phonemes or nasal phonemes to help the listener distinguish between hyponasality, hypernasality, and assimilative nasality. Another informal screening tool involves having the patient say these two sentences while pinching the nares shut: "My name means money" and "Mary made lemon jam." If the sentence produced sounds "plugged" with both open and occluded nares, the patient has a hyponasal voice quality. If there

is a significant difference between the two sentences, hypernasality may be suspected. Stimulability testing, articulation testing, and oral examination are also included in a patient with a resonance disorder.

17. **What additional laboratory diagnostics should be completed for a thorough nasal resonance disorders evaluation?**

Aerodynamic instrumentation includes pressure transducers and pneumotachometers that measure relative air pressures and airflows emitted simultaneously from the nasal and oral cavities during speech. Acoustic measures may include the use of a nasometer, a noninvasive microcomputer-based system that measures the relative amount of oral to nasal acoustic energy in an individual's speech. Spectrography may also be used as part of acoustic analysis. Visualization via endoscopy or radiologic examination can be used to evaluate the appearance and function of speech mechanisms such as the velopharyngeal mechanism during speech.

18. **What are the treatment options for hypernasality?**

Treatment approaches for a person with a hypernasal voice depend on the organic or functional causes of the underlying hypernasality. If functional causes exist, voice therapy will be initiated with a focus on altering tongue position during speech, change of loudness, auditory feedback, establishing optimal pitch, counseling, opening of the mouth, and respiration training. When a physical inadequacy of the velopharyngeal port is suspected the patient may be referred to an otolaryngologist for surgical options or a prosthodontist to determine the necessity of a palatal lift, obturator, or prosthesis. The SLP shares the results of the patient evaluation and can make recommendations related to the optimal surgical approach or to suggest which dental appliances may work best for the patient.

19. **What are treatment options for hyponasality?**

Appropriate medical evaluation and imaging should precede voice therapy for hyponasality to rule out and manage organic causes such as severe nasopharyngeal obstruction or infection. When indicated, voice therapy for increasing nasal resonance may include auditory feedback, counseling, nasal glide stimulation, and focusing on directing tone into a facial mask during speech.

BIBLIOGRAPHY

American Speech-Language-Hearing Association: The roles of otolaryngologists and speech-language pathologists in the performance and interpretation of strobovideolaryngoscopy [Relevant Paper]. 1998. Available at www.asha.org/policy.

Boone DR, McFarlane SC, Von Berg SL: *The Voice and Voice Therapy*, 7th ed, 2005, Pearson.

Hicks M, Brugman SM, Katial R: Vocal cord dysfunction/paradoxical vocal fold motion, *Prim Care* 35:81, 2008.

Hodges H: Speech therapy for the treatment of functional respiratory disorders. In: Anbar RD, ed: *Functional Respiratory Disorders When Respiratory Symptoms Do Not Respond to Pulmonary Treatment*, 2012, Humana Press, p 251.

Huber J, Stathopoulos E, Ramig L, et al: Respiratory function and variability in individuals with Parkinson disease: pre and post Lee Silverman Voice Treatment (LSVT®), *J Med Speech Lang Pathol* 11:185, 2003.

Rosen CA, Lee AS, Osborne J, et al: Development and validation of the Voice Handicap Index-10, *Laryngoscope* 114(9):1549–1556, 2004.

Sapienza C, Hoffman Ruddy B: *Voice Disorders*, 2nd ed, 2013, Plural.

Stemple JC, Glaze LE, Gerdeman Klaben B: *Clinical Voice Pathology Theory and Management*, 3rd ed, 2000, Singular.

St. Louis KO, Rusello D: *Oral Speech Mechanism Screening Examination*, 3rd ed, 2000, PRO-ED.

Verdolini Abbott K: *Lessac-Madsen Resonant Voice Therapy Clinician Manual*, 2008, Plural.

CHRONIC COUGH

Marie Jetté, PhD, CCC-SLP

KEY POINT

1. The American College of Chest Physicians (ACCP) current guidelines define acute and chronic cough and outline treatment recommendations for these disorders.

Pearl

1. There are no targeted treatments for unexplained or neuropathic chronic cough but limited clinical trial data support benefit from treatment with neuromodulators and speech-language therapy.

QUESTIONS

DEFINITIONS

1. **How does the definition of chronic cough differ from acute cough and subacute cough?**
   The American College of Chest Physicians (ACCP) current guidelines define acute cough as symptoms lasting less than 3 weeks, subacute cough as symptoms lasting 3 to 8 weeks, and chronic cough as symptoms lasting longer than 8 weeks. For children aged ≤14 years, chronic cough is defined as the presence of daily cough of at least 4 weeks in duration.

2. **What is meant by the terms "unexplained cough" and "neuropathic cough"?**
   "Unexplained cough" describes a cough that persists despite a comprehensive diagnostic evaluation, exclusion of common causes, and appropriate therapeutic trials for common causes of cough. The term unexplained cough was chosen over idiopathic cough because it implies that there may be as yet unidentified causes for the cough or that it may be multifactorial. *Cough hypersensitivity syndrome* has been applied to individuals who appear to have common causes of cough and, despite appropriate therapy, have a persistent cough response. The underlying pathophysiology for this remains undefined but has been proposed to follow mechanisms similar to those for chronic pain (lower threshold for stimulation of afferent pain receptors). This has also led to the term neuropathic cough being applied to this group of patients.

3. **What is the burden of illness related to chronic cough?**
   The prevalence of chronic cough in respiratory outpatient practice ranges from 10% to 38%. The prevalence of chronic cough in the general population is estimated to be 9.6%. Cough is also the most common reason for primary care visits in the USA. Approximately US$9 billion is spent annually on over-the-counter (OTC) medications for cough in the USA.

PATHOPHYSIOLOGY OF CHRONIC COUGH

4. **What are the different types of afferent cough receptors?**
   Chemoreceptors react to various stimulants, including water, ammonia, carbon dioxide, sulfur dioxide, cigarette smoke, milk, gastric contents, and capsaicin. Mechanoreceptors respond to pressure (touch), flow, proprioception, and laryngeal muscle contraction. Laryngeal irritant receptors include nociceptive C fibers and G protein-coupled receptors (GPCRs) along with the ion channel receptors, transient receptor, potential vanilloid (TRPV-1) and transient receptor potential ankyrin 1 (TRPA-1). The latter two are ion channels in the membrane (Fig. 75.1).

5. **Where are these cough receptors distributed?**
   There is a network of afferent sensory receptors found in the subepithelial layer throughout the respiratory tract as well as the gastrointestinal tract and cardiovascular system that are capable of triggering cough with appropriate and sufficient stimuli. The larynx, trachea, and lower airways have a rich network of cough reflex afferent nerves that are capable of inducing cough. The main inputs are from the cough receptors themselves, slowly adapting pulmonary stretch receptors (SARs), rapidly adapting pulmonary stretch receptors (RARs), bronchial and pulmonary C-fibers, and Aδ fibers.

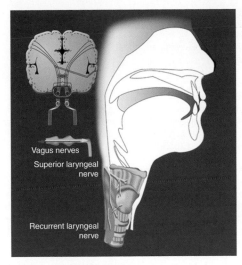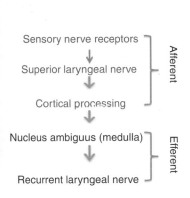

Fig. 75.1 Cough reflex neuronal connections.

6. **Describe the physiology of the cough reflex.**

When an intense stimulus depolarizes the afferent receptor nerve terminal over the threshold, voltage-gated sodium and potassium channels (Kv) are opened and trigger action potentials. Activation of C-fibers can cause mast cell degranulation and release of histamine and bradykinin, leading to airway edema and activation of mechanoreceptors and neuropeptides, resulting in neurogenic inflammation. The afferent input is relayed to the brainstem, where the information can be centrally processed and modulated further before the efferent output leads to the elicitation of a cough. The increased sensitivity of the cough reflex is poorly understood but seems to be driven by a complex interaction between C-fiber receptors, rapidly adapting receptors, and the peripheral and central nervous systems. The nucleus tractus solitarius seems to be a central area for modifying cough through both long-term and short-term neuroplasticity (see Fig. 75.1).

7. **What role does the nose play in the pathophysiology of chronic cough?**

Allergies, infections, and irritants can induce inflammation in the nose, which can lead to symptoms such as sneezing, nasal itching, rhinorrhea, and nasal blockage. These responses are likely mediated by trigeminal sensory nerves. Interestingly, it has been shown that intranasal administration of histamine or capsaicin does not cause coughing but increases the sensitivity to various tussigenic aerosols.

8. **Which neurologic connections between the gastrointestinal tract and the respiratory tract contribute to the cough reflex?**

Vagal afferents from the esophagus and respiratory tract converge in the brainstem. Esophageal afferents may be triggered simply by significant acid secretion into the esophagus, thus triggering a cough response. Previous studies have demonstrated that acid infusion into the esophagus induces bronchoconstriction, presumably through a vagally mediated esophageal-tracheobronchial reflex and dual channel pH monitoring correlated with cough, in terms of both proximal and distal acid reflux. Furthermore, acid infused into the distal esophagus of patients with chronic cough increases the frequency of coughing and cough reflex sensitivity, a phenomenon that can be blocked with topical lidocaine.

ETIOLOGY OF CHRONIC COUGH

9. **What are the common causes of chronic cough?**

Upper airway cough syndrome (previously referred to as postnasal drip) and lower airway conditions, including bronchial asthma, cough variant asthma, eosinophilic bronchitis, atopic cough, and gastroesophageal reflux disease (GERD), are the most common causes (Box 75.1). Atopic cough is defined as a cough that manifests in atopic individuals without bronchial hyperresponsiveness that responds well to antihistamines alone without inhaled steroids, whereas the other lower airway conditions typically require inhaled steroids. These conditions often coexist in various combinations, and failure to address and treat all concurrently may be one of the major impediments to the successful amelioration of chronic cough.

> **Box 75.1** Most Common Causes of Chronic Cough
> - Upper airway cough syndrome
> - Asthma/eosinophilic bronchitis/atopic cough
> - Gastroesophageal reflux disease

10. **What are less common causes of chronic cough?**
Less common causes include chronic bronchitis, chronic infection, interstitial lung disease, angiotensin-converting enzyme (ACE) inhibitors, cardiac diseases including congestive heart failure and mitral valve disorders, and stimulation of hairs in the external auditory canal (Arnold's nerve reflex). Several occupational and environmental exposures have also been associated with chronic cough (Box 75.2).

11. **What distinguishes upper airway cough syndrome from postnasal drip?**
What was previously referred to as chronic postnasal drip has more recently been labeled as upper airway cough syndrome (UACS) in recognition of the fact that posterior nasal drainage may result from several conditions of the sinuses and nasal passages (Box 75.3). Inflammatory signaling and possible neurogenic mechanisms originating in the upper airway may contribute to the development of cough, in addition to the physical and possible chemical irritation of the posterior nasal drainage. While allergic rhinitis is often a culprit, other common causes include chronic rhinosinusitis, nasal polyposis, chronic bacterial overgrowth, fungal disease, anatomic anomalies, and postsurgical changes.

Second, the "unified airway" hypothesis proposes that processes that cause upper airway congestion and postnasal drainage induce inflammation in the lower airways. Such changes may lead to increased sensitivity of the cough receptors in the lower airways, independent of direct stimulation by the postnasal drainage itself. Furthermore, there is evidence that intense irritant exposure to the nose may cause the release of cytokines and various other mediators into the systemic circulation, inducing changes in the lower respiratory tract that may enhance lower airway cough reflex sensitivity.

Findings such as these form the basis for the adoption of the term upper airway cough syndrome in place of postnasal drip, to reinforce that cough may be triggered by immune/inflammatory signaling and neuroplastic

> **Box 75.2** Causes of Upper Airway Cough Syndrome
> - Allergic rhinitis
> - Perennial nonallergic rhinitis
> - Vasomotor rhinitis
> - Nonallergic rhinitis with eosinophilia (NARES)
> - Postinfectious rhinitis
> - Following upper respiratory tract infection
> - Bacterial sinusitis
> - Allergic fungal sinusitis
> - Rhinitis due to anatomic abnormalities
> - Rhinitis due to physical or chemical irritants
> - Occupational rhinitis
> - Rhinitis medicamentosa
> - Rhinitis of pregnancy

> **Box 75.3** Occupational and Environmental Exposures Associated With Chronic Cough
> - Occupational exposures:
>   - Coal and hard rock mining
>   - Tunnel workers
>   - Concrete manufacturing
> - Environmental exposures:
>   - Secondhand smoke
>   - Particulate matter
>   - Irritant gases and fumes
>   - Mold
>   - Perfumes
>   - Mixed pollutants

changes that increase cough receptor sensitivity rather than simply being the result of mechanical and/or irritant receptor triggering by postnasal secretions collecting in the larynx and/or lower respiratory tract.

12. **What is cough variant asthma?**

Cough variant asthma is diagnosed in individuals without wheezing, shortness of breath, or chest tightness who report coughing as their sole symptom when exposed to strong odors, exercise, or other triggers and who have a positive methacholine challenge. Spirometry testing results are typically normal and there may be no bronchodilator response.

13. **What is nonasthmatic eosinophilic bronchitis?**

Individuals with eosinophilic bronchitis report symptoms very similar to asthma and are often initially diagnosed with asthma but exhibit a negative methacholine challenge. Studies of sputum reveal that they have eosinophils and typically respond well to inhaled corticosteroids.

14. **What are the mechanisms by which reflux from the gastrointestinal tract contributes to chronic cough?**

There are several different mechanisms by which gastrointestinal reflux may contribute to chronic cough. This is supported by the observation that PPI therapy alone rarely resolves GERD-related cough. First, there is a convergence of vagal afferents from the esophagus and respiratory tract in the brainstem, as outlined earlier (see Questions 5 and 6). Esophageal dysmotility may lead to esophageal reflux to the larynx that may be aspirated into the lungs or simply irritate the laryngeal mucosa.

Aspiration of gastric contents may or may not be associated with typical symptoms of GERD such as heartburn, regurgitation, water brash, sour taste, chest pain, globus sensation, or pharyngeal symptoms such as dysphonia, hoarseness, and sore throat depending on whether it is predominantly acid or nonacid reflux. Individuals with nonacid reflux often report no significant reflux symptoms but demonstrate signs of aspiration on bronchoscopic lavage with increased lymphocytes or neutrophils and possibly endobronchial signs of squamous metaplasia.

15. **What is the prevalence of cough related to ACE inhibitors?**

Cough induced by ACE inhibitors is estimated to occur in 5% to 35% of users and is reported to be more common in women and nonsmokers. It has also been noted to be more common in patients taking angiotensin-converting enzyme (ACE) inhibitors for congestive heart failure than in those taking them for other cardiovascular diseases such as hypertension. It may cause cough at the first dose or after months of use.

16. **Is there any difference in incidence of chronic cough with ACE inhibitors and angiotensin receptor blockers?**

Studies suggest that the incidence of cough with angiotensin receptor blockers (ARBs) is lower than that with ACE inhibitors, and there is no contraindication to trying ARBs if a patient develops a cough related to ACE inhibitor use. They should be aware of the possibility that the cough may return with ARB use and inform their physician if this occurs.

CLINICAL EVALUATION

17. **Discuss an initial diagnostic approach to chronic cough.**

The ACCP guidelines recommend that if there are signs and symptoms suggestive of upper airway cough syndrome, asthma, nonasthmatic eosinophilic bronchitis, or GERD (which accounts for 80% of all causes of chronic cough), all suspected disorders, should be treated empirically at the same time to determine whether there is a resolution or significant reduction of the cough. Patients who smoke should be encouraged to stop smoking (Fig. 75.2).

If there are any symptoms or physical signs suggestive of cardiopulmonary disease or any suspicion of lung cancer, interstitial lung disease, or bronchiectasis, a chest radiograph should be performed. If there is partial resolution of the cough related to treating any of these entities, the treatment should be continued. It must be emphasized that more than one process may contribute to chronic cough and all must be treated at the same time.

18. **Which symptoms and clinical findings warrant additional medical workup?**

- Hemoptysis
- Smoker with >20 pack/year smoking history
- Smokers older than 45 years with new cough, altered cough, or cough with voice disturbance
- Prominent dyspnea, especially at night
- Substantial sputum production (>1 tbsp/day)
- Hoarseness

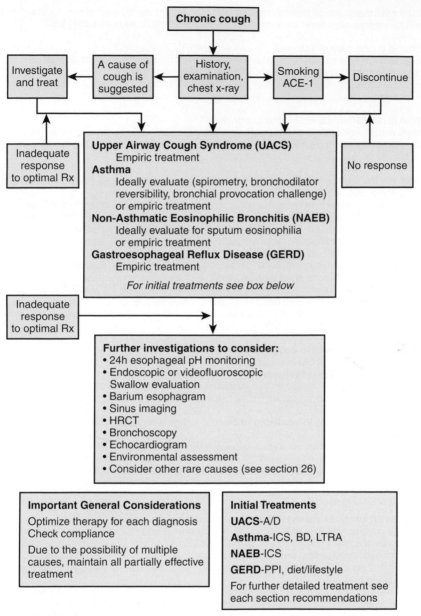

Fig. 75.2 ACCP Guidelines Diagnostic Approach to chronic cough. (Adapted with permission from Irwin RS, Baumann MH, Bolser DC, et al: Diagnosis and management of cough executive summary: ACCP evidence-based clinical practice guidelines, *Chest* 129(1 Suppl):1S–23S, 2006.)

- Systemic symptoms: fever, weight loss
- Complicated reflux symptoms associated with weight loss, anemia, hematemesis or melena, dysphagia, or ondynophagia or failure of empiric treatment for reflux
- Recurrent pneumonia
- Abnormal clinical respiratory examination
- Abnormal chest radiograph

18. **What other tests are useful in evaluation of reflux-associated cough?**
    - Barium esophagram is useful for assessing hiatal hernia, gastroesophageal reflux, and esophago-laryngeal reflux. It is also useful to evaluate other esophageal anomalies.
    - 24-hour esophageal pH/impedance monitoring allows for the evaluation of both acid and nonacid reflux in addition to distal versus proximal events and whether there is any correlation between cough, throat clearing, hoarseness, chest pain, and reflux events. Studies have varied in showing a good correlation between cough events and reflux events. If the cough is triggered solely by acid events in the lower esophagus, there may be a strong correlation between cough events and reflux events. However, if the mechanism is related to laryngopharyngeal reflux with or without aspiration, this may lead to a general increase in sensitivity to a variety of irritant exposures.
    - Esophagogastroduodenoscopy (EGD) is helpful in determining esophageal changes related to reflux or significant damage, indicating Barrett's esophagitis.
    - Esophageal manometry can be useful to assess if there are significant motility issues that may contribute to reflux issues and/or determine whether a patient may be a candidate for gastric fundoplication.

19. **What should be the next step(s) if empiric treatment for the common causes of chronic cough fails?**
    It is imperative that all causes of cough are treated concurrently and optimally. If the cough continues to be present, depending on the clinical history, referral should be made to a specialty cough clinic. Other conditions that might be considered include sleep apnea, eosinophilic bronchitis, tonsillar enlargement, and external ear disease mediated through the auricular branch of the vagus nerve. If the cough remains refractory, further tests should be considered.

    High-resolution computed tomography (CT) scan of the chest can be helpful in ruling out cough caused by things that may be missed by plain chest radiographs such as interstitial lung diseases, bronchiectasis, sarcoidosis, and chronic infections such as atypical mycobacterial infections, lung cancer, aspiration, or mitral valve disease.

    A CT scan of the sinuses can identify anatomic anomalies, polyps, persistent inflammation, and ostial obstruction.

    Skin testing can be used to evaluate significant environmental allergens that may contribute to UACS. Identifying pet, dust mite, cockroach, or mold allergies can lead to remediation that may significantly reduce upper airway congestion and inflammation.

20. **When should bronchoscopy be considered in the evaluation of chronic cough?**
    The current ACCP guidelines suggest that there is not enough evidence for the routine use of bronchoscopy as part of an evaluation of patients with chronic cough. If a thorough pulmonary workup has been performed without identifying a cause, or there is concern for reflux-associated cough or a cough from a chronic low-grade infection such as mycobacteria or mycoplasma, then bronchoscopy may be helpful. Broncheoalveolar lavage (BAL) may show evidence of high neutrophils and/or lymphocytes that have previously been associated with aspiration, and cultures will reveal the presence of noncommensal microbes that may indicate chronic infection/colonization. Biopsies may show changes of squamous metaplasia that are associated with aspiration.

21. **What are useful tests to rule out a cardiac cause of chronic cough?**
    Chest radiographs to look for signs of congestive heart failure and mitral valve calcification are useful, but a CT scan of the chest may be more sensitive in this regard. An echocardiogram is helpful in ruling out mitral valve disease and cardiac wall motion abnormalities.

22. **What are the clinical features of chronic refractory cough?**
    Clinical features include a dry cough that occurs episodically throughout the day. The origin of the cough is the laryngeal region. Triggers include nontussive stimuli that would not normally induce cough, including air conditioning and phonation and low doses of tussive stimuli. Cough is commonly attributed to an initial viral upper respiratory tract infection. Clinically significant dysphonia is observed in 40% of patients with chronic refractory cough.

23. **What is the relationship between cough and paradoxical vocal fold motion disorder?**
    Paradoxical vocal fold motion (PVFM) disorder is an abnormal laryngeal motor pattern with adduction of the vocal folds during inspiration resulting in inspiratory dyspnea, stridor, and laryngeal tension. PVFM disorder can occur concurrently with chronic cough and can be treated using behavioral speech therapy techniques.

THERAPEUTIC APPROACH

24. **What are the treatment options for UACS?**
    First-generation antihistamines such as bromopheniramine, chlorpheniramine, and promethazine have been shown to have central cough suppressive properties, while newer generation nonsedating antihistamines do not

have this property. Decongestants can be combined with first-generation antihistamines and are offered in several combinations. Some studies have suggested that for patients with significant nasal and/or sinus congestion saline nasal rinses can be helpful, although evidence is limited.

25. When should one consider discontinuing ACE inhibitors to determine if they are the cause of the cough?

If there are no signs or symptoms suggestive of more common causes of cough, discontinuation of ACE inhibitors and appropriate replacement therapy should be attempted immediately. A cough caused by ACE inhibitor use will generally subside within 2 to 4 weeks. If there are other factors present that may explain a chronic cough but 4 weeks of empiric treatment fails to lead to substantial resolution, discontinuation of an ACE inhibitor is indicated. If the cough persists despite being off the ACE inhibitor for 4 weeks, it is unlikely to be the cause and it can be re-started. If the cough stops, the ACE inhibitor can be tried again after 2 to 3 months but discontinued permanently if the cough returns.

26. What if substitution of an ACE inhibitor is not an option?

Medication commonly used to suppress cough can be tried, including sodium cromoglycate, theophylline, sulindac, indomethacin, amlodipine, ferrous sulfate, and picotamide.

27. What are medication options for treating unexplained cough?

Persistent cough may be related to cough habituation and neuropathic changes (peripheral and central) created by the cough itself. Central cough suppressants such as dextromethorphan or codeine-containing products are effective for some but there are concerns about the long-term use of narcotics. Benzonatate has been reported to reduce stretch receptor sensitivity in the lungs. Some patients respond to baclofen, transdermal lidocaine patches, or nebulized lidocaine. Peripheral afferent cough suppressants have been proposed to block sensory receptors peripherally and have been shown to suppress cough in randomized controlled trials, but these are not available in the USA (e.g., moguisteine and levodropropizine).

Given the theories that chronic cough is somewhat akin to chronic pain syndrome, it is not surprising that there are recommendations for the use of such agents as tricyclic antidepressants and gabapentin, but data are limited in terms of their efficacy for neuropathic cough.

28. What medical-surgical options are there for treating chronic cough?

Cough that occurs secondary to glottal insufficiency may be subjectively improved with vocal fold injection augmentation either bilaterally or unilaterally. Another option is Botox injection into the bilateral thyroarytenoid muscles. Finally, there is some evidence that nerve block to the SLN using a 50:50 solution of a long-acting particulate steroid and a local anesthetic can reduce subjective cough severity measures.

29. What is the role of behavioral therapy in the treatment of chronic cough?

Behavior modification is typically managed by speech-language pathologists and includes respiratory retraining, laryngeal desensitization, and techniques to suppress and react to cough. Given that chronic cough, paradoxical vocal fold motion disorder, and voice disorders commonly cooccur, therapy should address not only the management of cough but also vocal efficiency and reduction of muscle tension if they are present.

30. How should children with chronic cough be managed?

The management of cough in children should be based on the etiology of the cough. Empirical approaches such as treating UACS due to a sinus condition, GERD, and/or asthma should not be used unless other features consistent with these conditions are present. If an empirical trial is used based on features consistent with a hypothesized diagnosis, the trial should be defined and limited in duration to confirm or refute the potential diagnosis.

BIBLIOGRAPHY

Bascom R, Pipkorn U, Proud D, et al: Major basic protein and eosinophil-derived neurotoxin concentrations in nasal-lavage fluid after antigen challenge: effect of systemic corticosteroids and relationship to eosinophil influx, *J Allergy Clin Immunol* 84(3):338–346, 1989.
Black HR, Bailey J, Zappe D, et al: Valsartan: more than a decade of experience, *Drugs* 69(17):2393–2414, 2009.
Bolser DC: Older-generation antihistamines and cough due to upper airway cough syndrome (UACS): efficacy and mechanism, *Lung* 186(Suppl 1):S74–S77, 2008.
Bolser DC: Pharmacologic management of cough, *Otolaryngol Clin North Am* 43(1):147–155, 2010.
Carr MJ, Undem BJ: Bronchopulmonary afferent nerves, *Respirology* 8(3):291–301, 2003.
Chang AB, Oppenheimer JJ, Weinberger MM, et al: Use of management pathways or algorithms in children with chronic cough: CHEST Guideline and Expert Panel Report, *Chest* 151(4):875–883, 2017. doi: 10.1016/j.chest.2016.12.025.
Chung KF, McGarvey L, Mazzone SB: Chronic cough as a neuropathic disorder, *Lancet Respir Med* 1(5):414–422, 2013.
Chung KF, Pavord ID, Prevalence: pathogenesis, and causes of chronic cough, *Lancet* 371(9621):1364–1374, 2008. doi: 10.1016/S0140-6736(08)60595-4.
Chung KF: Currently available cough suppressants for chronic cough, *Lung* 186(Suppl 1):S82–S87, 2008.
D'Urzo A, Jugovic P: Chronic cough. Three most common causes, *Can Fam Physician* 48:1311–1316, 2002.
Desai D, Brightling C: Cough due to asthma, cough-variant asthma and non-asthmatic eosinophilic bronchitis, *Otolaryngol Clin North Am* 43(1):123–310, 2010.

Dicpinigaitis PV: Angiotensin-converting enzyme inhibitor-induced cough: ACCP evidence-based clinical practice guidelines, *Chest* 129(1 Suppl):169S–173S, 2006.

Dicpinigaitis PV: Cough: an unmet clinical need, *Br J Pharmacol* 163(1):116–124, 2011.

Fujimori K, Suzuki E, Arakawa M: [A case of chronic persistent cough caused by gastroesophageal reflux], *Nihon Kyobu Shikkan Gakkai Zasshi* 31(10):1303–1307, 1993.

Gibson PG, Vertigan AE: Speech pathology for chronic cough: a new approach, *Pulm Pharmacol Ther* 22(2):159–162, 2009.

Ing AJ, Ngu MC, Breslin AB: Pathogenesis of chronic persistent cough associated with gastroesophageal reflux, *Am J Respir Crit Care Med* 149(1):160–167, 1994.

Irwin RS, Baumann MH, Bolser DC, et al: Diagnosis and management of cough executive summary: ACCP evidence-based clinical practice guidelines, *Chest* 129(1 Suppl):1S–23S, 2006.

Irwin RS, French CL, Curley FJ, et al: Chronic cough due to gastroesophageal reflux: clinical, diagnostic, and pathogenetic aspects, *Chest* 104(5):1511–1517, 1993.

Jang DW, Lachanas VA, Segel J, et al: Budesonide nasal irrigations in the postoperative management of chronic rhinosinusitis, *Int Forum Allergy Rhinol* 3(9):708–711, 2013.

Javorkova N, Varechova S, Pecova R, et al: Acidification of the oesophagus acutely increases the cough sensitivity in patients with gastro-oesophageal reflux and chronic cough, *Neurogastroenterol Motil* 20(2):119–124, 2008.

Jervis-Bardy J, Boase S, Psaltis A, et al: A randomized trial of mupirocin sinonasal rinses versus saline in surgically recalcitrant staphylococcal chronic rhinosinusitis, *Laryngoscope* 122(10):2148–2153, 2012.

Jervis-Bardy J, Wormald PJ: Microbiological outcomes following mupirocin nasal washes for symptomatic, *Staphylococcus aureus–*positive chronic rhinosinusitis following endoscopic sinus surgery, *Int Forum Allergy Rhinol* 2(2):111–115, 2012.

Kardos P, Berck H, Fuchs KH, et al: Guidelines of the German Respiratory Society for diagnosis and treatment of adults suffering from acute or chronic cough, *Pneumologie* 64(11):701–711, 2010.

Kohno S, Ishida T, Committee for the Japanese Respiratory Society Guidelines for Management of Cough, et al: The Japanese Respiratory Society guidelines for management of cough, *Respirology* 11(Suppl 4):S135–S186, 2006.

Krouse JH, Altman KW: Rhinogenic laryngitis, cough, and the unified airway, *Otolaryngol Clin North Am* 43(1):111–121, 2010.

Lai K, Chen R, Lin J, et al: A prospective, multicenter survey on causes of chronic cough in China, *Chest* 143(3):613–620, 2013.

Litts JK, Fink DS, Clary MS: The effect of vocal fold augmentation on cough symptoms in the presence of glottic insufficiency, *Laryngoscope* 128(6):1316–1319, 2018. doi: 10.1002/lary.26914.

Magni C, Chellini E, Zanasi A: Cough variant asthma and atopic cough, *Multidiscip Respir Med* 5(2):99–103, 2010.

Malacco E, Santonastaso M, Vari NA, et al: Comparison of valsartan 160 mg with lisinopril 20 mg, given as monotherapy or in combination with a diuretic, for the treatment of hypertension: the Blood Pressure Reduction and Tolerability of Valsartan in Comparison with Lisinopril (PREVAIL) study, *Clin Ther* 26(6):855–865, 2004.

Mazzone SB, Undem BJ: Cough sensors. V. Pharmacological modulation of cough sensors, *Handb Exp Pharmacol* 187:99–127, 2009.

McGarvey LP: Does idiopathic cough exist? *Lung* 186(Suppl 1):S78–S81, 2008.

Mitchell JE, Campbell AP, New NE, et al: Expression and characterization of the intracellular vanilloid receptor (TRPV1) in bronchi from patients with chronic cough, *Exp Lung Res* 31(3):295–306, 2005.

Morice AH, McGarvey L, Pavord I, et al: Recommendations for the management of cough in adults, *Thorax* 61(Suppl 1):i1–i24, 2006.

Morice AH: Chronic cough hypersensitivity syndrome, *Cough* 9(1):14, 2013.

Pavord ID, Chung KF: Management of chronic cough, *Lancet* 371(9621):1375–1384, 2008.

Prakash UB: Uncommon causes of cough: ACCP evidence-based clinical practice guidelines, *Chest* 129(1 Suppl):206S–219S, 2006.

Pratter MR: Chronic upper airway cough syndrome secondary to rhinosinus diseases (previously referred to as postnasal drip syndrome): ACCP evidence-based clinical practice guidelines, *Chest* 129(1 Suppl):63S–71S, 2006.

Pratter MR: Overview of common causes of chronic cough: ACCP evidence-based clinical practice guidelines, *Chest* 129(1 Suppl): 59S–62S, 2006.

Ryan NM, Gibson PG: Characterization of laryngeal dysfunction in chronic persistent cough, *Laryngoscope* 119(4):640–645, 2009.

Sasieta HC, Iyer VN, Orbelo DM, et al: Bilateral thyroarytenoid botulinum toxin type A injection for the treatment of refractory chronic cough, *JAMA Otolaryngol Head Neck Surg* 142(9):881–888, 2016. doi: 10.1001/jamaoto.2016.0972.

Schappert SM: National Ambulatory Medical Care Survey: 1992 summary, *Adv Data* 253:1–20, 1994.

Simpson CB, Tibbetts KM, Loochtan MJ, Dominguez LM: Treatment of chronic neurogenic cough with in-office superior laryngeal nerve block, *Laryngoscope* 128(8):1898–1903, 2018. doi: 10.1002/lary.27201.

Snidvongs K, Pratt E, Chin D, et al: Corticosteroid nasal irrigations after endoscopic sinus surgery in the management of chronic rhinosinusitis, *Int Forum Allergy Rhinol* 2(5):415–421, 2012.

Song WJ, Chang YS, Faruqi S, et al: Defining chronic cough: a systematic review of the epidemiological literature, *Allergy Asthma Immunol Res* 8(2):146–155, 2016. doi: 10.4168/aair.2016.8.2.146.

Tarlo SM: Cough: occupational and environmental considerations: ACCP evidence-based clinical practice guidelines, *Chest* 129(1 Suppl):186S–196S, 2006.

Undem BJ, Carr MJ: Targeting primary afferent nerves for novel antitussive therapy, *Chest* 137(1):177–184, 2010.

van den Berg JW, de Nier LM, Kaper NM, et al: Limited evidence: higher efficacy of nasal saline irrigation over nasal saline spray in chronic rhinosinusitis—an update and reanalysis of the evidence base, *Otolaryngol Head Neck Surg* 150(1):16–21, 2014.

Widdicombe J, Tatar M, Fontana G, et al: Workshop: tuning the "cough center," *Pulm Pharmacol Ther* 24(3):344–352, 2011.

CHAPTER 76

DYSPHAGIA AND ASPIRATION

Elizabeth Cuadrado, MS, CCC-SLP, BCS-S

KEY POINTS

1. As many as 15 million people suffer from some level of dysphagia during their lifetime, with 1 million receiving a new diagnosis of dysphagia every year.
2. More than 60,000 Americans die from complications associated with dysphagia, most commonly aspiration pneumonia. Aspiration pneumonia is one of the leading causes of death among the elderly.
3. The average cost of managing a patient with a feeding tube is reported to be more than $31,000 per patient per year. PEG tubes increase the length of hospital stay and increase patient expenses.
4. A variety of conditions, both acute and chronic, can influence the safety and efficiency of the swallow response, resulting in dysphagia.
5. Dysphagia profoundly affects patients and often leads to depression due to changes in lifestyle and overall decreased quality of life.

Pearls
1. Which cranial nerves are involved in swallowing?
   There are six cranial nerves that contribute to both swallowing and speech, including the following:
   a. CN V: Trigeminal nerve
   b. CN VII: Facial nerve
   c. CN IX: Glossopharyngeal nerve
   d. CN X: Vagus nerve
   e. CN XI: Spinal Accessory nerve
   f. CN XII: Hypoglossal nerve
2. Keeping a cuff inflated on a tracheostomy tube does not mechanically prevent aspiration; it merely contains aspirated material at the level of the cuff, which will leak further into the airway upon cuff deflation unless subglottic suction is in place.
3. The less viscous the food material (e.g., liquids), the more likely it is to be aspirated. This is why the 3-oz water test has been successful in identifying aspiration risk.

QUESTIONS

1. **How do you define normal swallowing?**
   Normal swallowing is divided into phases: (a) the pre-oral anticipatory phase, (b) the oral preparatory phase, (c) the oral transport phase, (d) the pharyngeal phase, and (e) the esophageal phase.
   - Pre-oral anticipatory phase: This phase begins with seeing, smelling, and tasting food. When these senses are triggered, we produce saliva that contains enzymes that start the process of digestion when food is manipulated in the mouth.
   - Oral preparatory phase: After food enters the oral cavity, it mixes with saliva and is manipulated by the tongue, lips, cheeks, palate, and jaw via mashing and rotary chewing motion. The masticated food is formed into a cohesive bolus by the tongue in preparation for swallowing.
   - Oral transport phase: The transport phase of a swallow involves propelling the bolus back between the tongue and palate until the bolus reaches the anterior tonsillar pillars. At this point, a swallow response is initiated and the oral phase of swallow is concluded. The normal oral phase lasts approximately 1 second, even with differing food consistencies, ages, or sex of the individuals.
   - Pharyngeal phase: The pharyngeal phase of a swallow is initiated after the swallow response is triggered. The pharyngeal phase of a swallow involves four main neuromotor components: (a) velopharyngeal closure to prevent oral contents from entering the nasal cavity; (b) sequential contraction of the superior, medial, and inferior pharyngeal constrictors to assist propulsion of the bolus through the pharynx and assist with epiglottic deflection; (c) laryngeal closure via approximation of the true vocal folds and false vocal folds, approximation of the arytenoids to the base of the epiglottis, and epiglottic deflection to prevent aspiration; and (d) opening of the pharyngoesophageal segment (PES), otherwise known as the upper esophageal sphincter. PES opening occurs as a result of three mechanisms: the superiorly directed mechanical tension from laryngeal elevation, signals from the vagus nerve to relax the muscular segment, and the contact pressure exerted by the bolus on the PES.

- Esophageal phase: The esophageal phase of a swallow occurs when the bolus passes through the PES. The bolus is then carried through the esophagus via peristaltic movements of the esophagus to the lower esophageal sphincter, which relaxes to allow material to pass into the stomach.

2. **Define dysphagia.**

Dysphagia is the symptom of difficulty in swallowing that can occur within any phase or combination of phases of swallowing as described above.

3. **What are the most common causes of dysphagia?**

Dysphagia is most commonly caused by neurologic pathology and/or structural trauma. Neurologic pathologies include diseases affecting the cerebral cortex and brainstem, cranial nerves, and/or muscles of swallowing. Cerebral vascular accident (CVA) is the most common cause of dysphagia, followed by neurogenic diseases and head and neck cancers. If only a single cerebral hemisphere is affected by CVA, swallowing may be preserved because the brainstem still receives input from the noninjured hemisphere.

Dysphagia can occur during any phase of swallowing. In the oral preparatory phase, swallowing is controlled by both the cortex and brainstem and is voluntary (i.e., not a reflex). Dysfunction within the oral phase can lead to frequent spillage from the lips, inability to chew, and collection of food residue in the cheeks. These deficits result from decreased lip closure, decreased buccal tension, and decreased strength and/or coordination in the tongue and muscles during mastication. The pharyngeal phase of swallowing is an involuntary phase that is controlled by the brainstem. Pharyngeal phase impairments can include a delayed swallow reflex, decreased velopharyngeal closure resulting in pharyngonasal backflow, insufficient laryngeal closure, insufficient pharyngeal propulsion, and insufficient opening of the upper esophageal sphincter. Esophageal phase impairments include ineffective motility and failure of the lower esophageal sphincter to relax.

4. **How is dysphagia typically diagnosed?**

There are three techniques widely used to diagnose oropharyngeal dysphagia: (a) bedside swallow evaluation, also known as a clinical evaluation; (b) fluoroscopic examination called a modified barium swallow (MBS); and (c) fiberoptic endoscopic evaluation of swallowing (FEES). Esophageal phase dysphagia is commonly assessed via esophagram, manometry, and endoscopy. Bedside tests are noninstrumental assessments and are minimally invasive. This assessment involves merging clinical history, observation, and therapeutic trials to assess the risk factors of dysphagia. The Bedside evaluation has low sensitivity and interrater reliability. In addition, the bedside evaluation is poor in detecting silent aspiration. Modified barium swallow studies (MBSS) allow for an indirect view of the function. The MBS studies can also used to assess the effectiveness of compensatory strategies, which can decrease the presence of airway penetration or aspiration. Fiber-optic endoscopy is used to assess the pharyngeal phase without the use of radiation (Fig. 76.1).

5. **How do you define penetration and aspiration?**

The difference between laryngeal penetration and laryngeal aspiration is based on anatomical boundaries. Laryngeal penetration is defined as misdirected material at or above the level of the true vocal folds. If penetration into the laryngeal vestibule occurs during swallowing but clears with no residue once swallowing is complete, it is known as "transient" penetration. Aspiration is defined as material that passes below the level of the true vocal folds and enters the trachea. "Silent" aspiration is used to describe material that drops below the level of the true vocal cords, without any perception of the event (e.g., coughing, throat clearing, etc.).

6. **What are the steps involved in a bedside swallowing evaluation?**

A bedside swallow evaluation is a noninstrumental assessment. The purpose is to uncover any risk factors for dysphagia, signs of dysphagia, potential mechanisms, and treatment options and to determine if and what instrumental assessments are indicated. Speech-language pathologists (SLPs) look for signs or symptoms of possible oral or pharyngeal dysphagia when someone is eating or drinking. A thorough examination will include a comprehensive chart review, oral motor assessment, assessment of vocal quality, strength of cough, and administration of various food and liquid consistencies to monitor for signs of oral or pharyngeal deficits. If additional information is needed to define function and develop a corresponding treatment plan, an SLP will often perform an instrumental evaluation that allows visualization of swallow function, usually an MBS study or FEES.

For a patient with a tracheostomy tube, a bedside swallowing evaluation will begin by determining why the tracheostomy was placed. Some reasons for tracheostomy can render the beside swallow evaluation unreliable. For example, signs of pharyngeal dysphagia can be undiscernible in a tracheostomized individual with a large and obstructing laryngeal mass. If a bedside evaluation is indicated, it is best to check for cuff deflation and assess finger occlusion to determine the patient's ability to move air around the tracheostomy tube and into the upper airway. If no difficulty is observed, the SLP proceeds with the clinical assessment, including food and liquid trials, if indicated. Signs of aspiration can be further assessed via endotracheal suctioning by trained personnel. Historically, food and liquid trials were dyed blue to make signs of aspiration more apparent. In some cases, a Passy Muir valve (PMV) can improve swallow comfort and safety by increasing subglottic pressure and enabling a more effective cough response to clear the upper airway. If a tracheostomized individual is at high risk of silent aspiration – for example, a stroke patient, an instrumental assessment is often best.

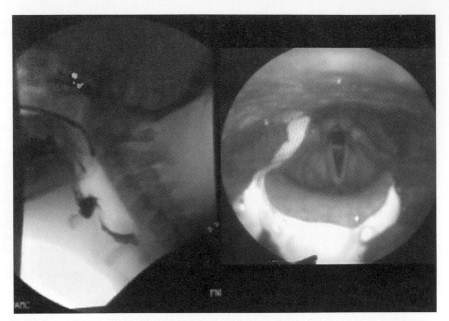

Fig. 76.1 Comparison of MBS and FEES examinations for aspiration/penetration.

7. **What do signs and symptoms of penetration/aspiration look like at the bedside?**
Indicators of penetration/aspiration include coughing upon a swallow, wheezing after intake, choking, chest congestion, tachypnea, noisy or wet breathing, wet vocal quality, throat clearing after a swallow, and rapid sequential swallows to clear a single bolus. Delayed signs of aspiration include infiltrates on a chest x-ray located in gravity-dependent locations, suctioning of postprandial material from the airway, coughing up food particles, and fever.

8. **What is a blue dye test and what is the purpose of its use?**
The modified Evan's blue dye test (MEBDT) is a technique less commonly used today to assess for evidence of aspiration in the tracheostomized patient. Blue dye is placed in food and liquids provided to the patient during a bedside assessment. The patient is deeply suctioned to determine if any blue material has entered the airway. If nothing is recovered during the procedure and assessment, the SLP will wait 24 hours for evidence of delayed aspiration before allowing oral intake and notify both nursing and respiratory therapy that an MEBDT has been provided. The sensitivity and specificity of the MEBDT in predicting oropharyngeal dysphagia vary widely owing to inconsistent protocols and patient populations. A positive test merely shows evidence of aspiration, which requires additional instrumental testing to define the dysfunction. Because fiberoptic endoscopic evaluation of swallowing is more readily available at the bedside and provides more comprehensive information about structure and function, the MEBDT is not used as often.

9. **What portion from an "oral mechanism exam" provides the most insight into a person's risk for aspiration?**
The goal of an oral mechanism examination is to provide information regarding structures, structural relationships, and movement function of the tongue and lips and to identify sensory function within the immediate extra- and intraoral structures. Studies have shown that incomplete lingual range of motion will make a person more likely to aspirate than those with complete lingual range of motion, regardless of complete labial closure and intact facial symmetry. Identifying oral motor weaknesses will heighten awareness during the bedside swallowing assessment.

10. **How do tracheostomy tubes and one-way speaking valves impact a patient's risk for aspiration?**
In patients with a tracheostomy, aspiration and pneumonia have a high incidence (50% to 87%). However, this incidence does not necessarily indicate a causality. It is important to keep in mind why the tracheostomy was needed in the first place. For example, a condition that necessitates a tracheostomy may increase the risk of aspiration, regardless of the tracheostomy; for example, ALS. Many studies have examined the incidence of aspiration with open and closed tracheostomy tubes and found that with the use of finger occlusion or an obturator, the incidence of aspiration was significantly reduced in comparison with those with an open tracheostomy tube. Similarly, the use of one-way valves to occlude the tracheostomy tube has been found to significantly reduce the incidence

and severity of aspiration of thin liquids. One reason for the reduction in aspiration is that the one-way valve increases subglottic air pressure and activation of mechanoreceptors, which are often lost when the tracheostomy tube has been open for a prolonged period. Additionally, improved sensation may also increase the patient's ability to expel material from the throat by coughing and/or throat clearing.

11. **FEES vs. MBS – which test is "better?"**
The answer to this question depends on the patient and which phases of swallowing the clinician believes are involved. Both evaluations provide a visualization of the swallowing mechanism. The FEES exam provides a transverse view, while the MBS studies reveals a sagittal and coronal view. The FEES exam will provide better visualization of secretion management, vocal fold movement, location, and amount of residue. The MBS studies provides better visualization of airway protection and esophageal function. FEES equipment is easily brought to the patient's bedside. This is especially advantageous for patients who have positioning challenges or who might not easily be transported to a radiology suite due to medical acuity or size; however, some individuals may not tolerate nasoendoscopy. MBS studies may be more comfortable for patients; however, they might alter their eating behaviors due to the taste of barium. Furthermore due to the risks associated with radiation exposure, the duration of an MBS study is typically capped at 5 to 6 minutes for adults. Therefore it is challenging to assess the effects of fatigue during MBS studies.

12. **What is the Penetration Aspiration Scale, and why is it so widely used during MBS?**
The Penetration Aspiration Scale (PAS) is an eight-point scale that was developed to provide an objective and consistent way to describe the depth of laryngeal infiltration observed during an MBS study or FEES. A PAS score is assigned to each swallow captured and thus can illustrate a pattern of laryngeal protection as scores are compared between different consistencies. It is widely used because of its favorable intra- and interrater reliability and the ability to easily track outcomes according to changes made on the PAS (Table 76.1).

13. **What is the 3-oz water swallow test, and is it effective in determining risk for aspiration?**
The 3-oz water swallow test is a screening tool that is used to identify patients who are at risk for clinically significant aspiration and who will require a more objective swallow evaluation. Individuals are asked to drink 3 oz of water without interruption. If they show signs of airway infiltration via cough or wet-hoarse vocal quality during the test or for 1 minute afterward, they are considered to have failed. In the initial validation study, the 3-oz water swallow test was able to identify 80% of patients who aspirated on subsequent modified barium swallow examination. A later investigation of 3000 hospital patients with diverse medical histories revealed a sensitivity for predicting aspiration on FEES of 96.5% and a specificity of 48.7% and a false positive rate of 51.3%. Because of the high false positive rate, failure suggests the need for additional testing. A passed test is consistent with safe intake of thin liquid 97.9% of the time.

14. **What is the incidence of dysphagia following intubation?**
Historical studies have reported the incidence of postextubation dysphagia ranging from 3% to 62%. This variability may be related to both study design and the multiple factors that contribute to dysphagia following extubation, including trauma, altered sensation, disuse atrophy, and altered mentation. More recently, postextubation dysphagia was observed in 18.3% of emergency ICU admissions. The literature has shown that pharyngeal muscle atrophy begins 24 hours after intubation. The highest incidence of dysphagia was observed in patients who experienced intubation for longer than 24 hours. Aspiration has been found to be present in 40% or more of medical-surgical and cardiac patients following extubation. Age older than 55 years, medical comorbidities, and a prior history of dysphagia were also found to increase a person's risk of aspiration following intubation.

Table 76.1 Penetration Aspiration Scale	
SCORE	**DESCRIPTION**
1	Material does not enter the airway
2	Material enters the airway, remains above the vocal cords, and is ejected from the airway
3	Material enters the airway, remains above the vocal cords, and is not ejected from the airway
4	Material enters the airway, contacts the vocal cords, and is ejected from the airway
5	Material enters the airway, contacts the vocal cords, and is not ejected from the airway
6	Material enters the airway, passes below the vocal cords, and is ejected into the larynx or out of the airway
7	Material enters the airway, passes below the vocal cords, and is not ejected from the trachea despite effort
8	Material enters the airway, passes below the vocal cords, and no effort is made to eject

15. **Why are infiltrates seen in the RLL more indicative of an aspiration pneumonia?**
Aspirated material is drawn to gravity-dependent portions of the respiratory system, especially since most patients are sitting in an upright position when eating and drinking. The right main stem bronchus is more vertically positioned in most adults than the left, hence the attribution of right lower or middle lobe pneumonias to aspiration and dysphagia.

16. **How do speech-language pathologists (SLPs) treat dysphagia?**
Depending on the patient's diagnosis, the treatment plan will differ and focus on either the oral, pharyngeal, or esophageal phases of swallowing or a combination thereof. Therapy objectives may include ameliorating the deficit; for example, strengthening a muscle group to repair function or compensating for a deficit. Below is an outline of the area of dysfunction and the corresponding treatment methods that can be used to assist in improving dysphagia.
   - Oral preparatory phase:
     - Labial weakness results in anterior spillage of material from the oral cavity. Compensatory strategies focus on reducing anterior spillage, such as using a pincer grasp to assist in closing the weaker labial side and/or presenting all utensils to the stronger side. Strengthening exercises can also be performed. The use of neuromuscular electrical stimulation (NMES) has been controversial and has been shown to cause dyskinesia in facial muscles. Therefore this is not commonly used.
     - Lingual weakness results in poor bolus formation and presents with difficulty in the anterior-posterior movement of a food bolus and "pocketing of food." Isometric tongue exercises can be used to improve muscle strength. External aids, such as mirrors, can provide visual feedback for the pocketed material and anterior spillage. A syringe or modified spoon and education regarding the use of finger sweep or lingual sweep of the cheek to remove any pocketed material are used to assist with anterior-posterior transport. Thermal stimulation techniques can also be used to assist in increasing sensation to the oral cavity, and head tilt positions can assist in moving material to the stronger side of the oral cavity.
   - Pharyngeal phase:
     - Treatment of delayed pharyngeal initiation of the swallow includes thermal stimulation, sour bolus trials, verbal cueing, successive approximations in bolus size, and use of visual feedback via endoscopy.
     - Dysfunction of intrinsic and extrinsic pharyngeal musculature results in poor pharyngeal constriction and an inability to effectively move material through the pharynx. The Mendelson maneuver can be used to provide an isometric hold of the pharynx during contraction to build strength and prolong hyolaryngeal elevation, keeping the pharyngoesophageal segment open longer. Head turning to the weaker side will capitalize on the function of the stronger side to adequately move material through the pharynx. A systematic increase in bolus viscosity combined with fast and effortful swallowing is outlined in the McNeil Dysphagia Therapy Program, which has been shown to increase pharyngeal efficiency.
     - Decreased tongue base retraction will also result in poor transit of material through the pharynx by decreasing epiglottic tilt and increasing pooling in the vallecular space. Swallowing maneuvers, such as the supraglottic swallow, adduct the vocal cords and increase the patient's ability to protect their airway. The Masako maneuver assists in providing isolated exercise to the tongue base to increase strength.
     - Poor laryngeal elevation and excursion will reduce a person's ability to anteriorly displace their trachea to adequately protect the airway. Several therapies exist to help laryngeal motion, including the Shaker exercise, Mendelson maneuver, biofeedback, and effortful swallow. Postural changes will also help to increase a patient's ability to protect the airway, such as chin tuck and head turn positions.

17. **What is neuromuscular electrical stimulation (NMES), more specifically Vital Stim®?**
Vital Stim® is a noninvasive, external electrical stimulation that has been approved by the U.S. Food and Drug Administration (FDA) for the treatment of dysphagia. Different electrode placements target specific areas of muscle dysfunction. Depending on the signs and symptoms seen during MBS, appropriate placement is determined to improve functional swallowing outcomes. See the Controversies section for more information regarding NMES.

18. **Why is it easier for persons with oral-pharyngeal dysphagia to swallow liquids with thicker viscosity?**
One of the most common causes of dysphagia is the delayed initiation of the pharyngeal swallow. A common treatment measure for patients is to thicken their liquids. This compensatory measure allows slower oral-pharyngeal transit time, while creating a more cohesive bolus that is easier to transport through both the oral and pharyngeal cavities. The more viscous the liquid, the slower the transit, allowing patients with delayed pharyngeal swallowing enough time to safely move material through the pharynx and into the esophagus. Thickened liquids should be used cautiously because of their potential effects on hydration, quality of life, blood sugar, and digestion.

19. **What is the Frazier water protocol, and who is appropriate for this?**
The Frazier water protocol (FWP) is a method of minimizing negative sequelae associated with the aspiration of water. Rather than abstain from regular liquids – that is, thin liquids – individuals with dysphagia are encouraged

to drink water according to the structured protocol. Unlike soda or coffee, water has a neutral pH level. Therefore it is well tolerated by the lungs and is quickly absorbed into the bloodstream. The keys to this protocol are good oral hygiene to reduce the bacterial load in the mouth, thus reducing the risk of bacterial exposure to the lungs, and consuming water only between meals. Patients who are NPO due to aspiration, or who benefit from a modified diet, and have good oral care are the best candidates for the FWP. Benefits include reducing the risk of dehydration and pneumonia, improving compliance with swallowing precautions, and improving quality of life.

20. Are there medications that are more likely to cause dysphagia?

Medication-induced dysphagia is far more common than that reported in the medical literature. When dysphagia occurs as a side effect of medication, it is usually caused by a decrease in muscle function, coordination, and/or sensation needed for swallowing. Additionally, medications that cause dry mouth (xerostomia) can interfere with swallowing by impairing the ability to transport food in the mouth. A list of such medications is provided in Table 76.2.

The therapeutic effects of medications can also contribute to dysphagia. When used over a long period of time and in high doses, some medications can cause muscle deterioration, resulting in dysphagia. A list of such medications is shown in Table 76.3.

Table 76.2 Medication-Induced Dysphagia	
Anticholinergic or antimuscarinic	Atropine (Atropar)
	Oxybutynin (Ditropan)
	Tolterodine (Detrol)
Neuromuscular blocking agents	Atracurium (Tracrium)
	Cisatracurium (Nimbex)
	Tubocurarine (Tubarine)
Medications that cause xerostomia	Trycyclic antidepressants
	Antihistamines
	Diuretics
Local anesthetics	Benzocaine (Americaine, Dermoplast)
	Lidocaine (Xylocaine)
Antipsychotic/neuroleptic medications	Haloperidol (Haldol)
	Chlorpromazine (Thorazine)
	Loxapine (Loxitane)

From Balzer KM: Drug-induced dysphagia, *Int J MS Care* 2(1):40–50, 2000.

Table 76.3 Medical Treatments That Can Cause Dysphagia	
Antineoplastics and immunosuppressants	Azathioprine (Imuran)
	Carmustine
	Cyclosporine
	Daunorubicin
High-dose corticosteroids	Dexamethasone (Decadron)
	Prednisolone (Delta Cortef)
	Prednisone (Deltasone)
Antiepileptics, benzodiazepines, narcotics, skeletal muscle relaxants	Gabapentin (Neurontin)
	Phenytoin (Dilantin)
	Carbamazepine (Tegretol)
	Alprazolam (Xanax)
	Clonazepam (Klonopin)
	Diazepam (Valium)
	Baclofen (Lioresal)
	Cyclobenzaprine (Flexeril)

From Balzer KM: Drug-induced dysphagia, *Int J MS Care* 2(1):40–50, 2000.

21. **How does breathing pattern impact swallowing function?**
There are four patterns of breathing that can occur upon initiation and completion of the swallow: EX/EX (expiration-swallow-expiration), EX/IN (expiration-swallow-inspiration), IN/EX (inspiration-swallow-expiration), and IN/IN (inspiration-swallow-inspiration). EX/EX appears to be the most common respiratory pattern in adults with normal swallowing. However, in adults over the age of 65 years and in chronic diseases such as chronic obstructive pulmonary disease (COPD) this respiratory pattern appears to change to EX/IN and can increase the risk of aspiration by drawing any pharyngeal residue into the airway upon immediate inhalation after swallowing. The inspiration-swallow-inspiration breathing pattern is the least frequent respiratory pattern. Interestingly, it has been found to be the dominant respiratory pattern in patients receiving head and neck cancer treatments, placing them at a significantly higher risk of aspiration.

22. **What effect does chemoradiation to the head and neck have on swallowing function?**
Swallow dysfunction is prevalent in patients during and after chemoradiotherapy (CRT) for head and neck cancer. Oral intake toward the end of treatment often declines because of side effects. Some patients with PEG tubes cease intake altogether to avoid the discomfort associated with eating. This inactivity has been known to cause atrophy of the swallowing muscles, which prolongs the transition back to eating and drinking once treatment is complete and side effects resolve. Depending on the treatment site, postradiation effects include fibrosis of the oropharyngeal mucosa and blunting of the epiglottic cartilage. Patients may thus have reduced epiglottic retroflexion, delayed initiation of a swallow, reduced tongue base retraction, and uncoordinated timing of the swallow with respiration, all of which can increase the potential for aspiration. Individuals who have been treated with CRT are at higher risk for "silent aspiration" because of altered sensation. This has been reported in 22% to 42% of patients receiving head and neck CRT. Aspiration pneumonia is an important complication of CRT for patients with head and neck cancers.

23. **What treatment methods have been shown to be beneficial in restoring swallowing function after chemoradiation?**
Prophylactic swallowing exercises and continued muscle activation throughout the treatment and posttreatment periods have been shown to reduce the severity of dysphagia and expedite recovery of swallowing once treatment is completed. Those who participate in swallowing exercises before and during treatment were shown to transition back to full oral intake faster than those who did not. For those who receive a feeding tube before or during treatment, frequent intake should be encouraged, even if it is only water. Education by an SLP is imperative in preserving muscle function for swallowing during CRT and cannot be encouraged enough. Late effects of radiation on swallowing can occur 6 to 18 years after CRT and are typically of sudden onset accompanied by cranial nerve neuropathy. Various treatments for LAD include dysphagia Boot Camp, the McNeil Dysphagia Therapy Program, and expiratory muscle strength training.

CONTROVERSIES

24. **Is NMES an appropriate treatment method for dysphagia?**
As NMES is a relatively newer treatment option for dysphagia (it was approved by the FDA in 2002 for dysphagia), research to support its use remains limited; therefore this modality is not covered by some third-party payers including Medicare. One of the largest trials performed (Xia et al. 2011) reported 120 patients with poststroke dysphagia who were randomly assigned to one of three groups: traditional swallowing treatment alone, e-stim alone, or e-stim plus traditional swallowing treatment. The experimental group that added e-stim to traditional treatment made significantly greater improvements in all four outcome measures than the traditional treatment alone group or the e-stim alone group. Another large study involving individuals with head and neck cancer found that traditional exercise outperformed the use of NMES. The benefits of this modality remain to be explored.

25. **Do tracheostomy tubes contribute to dysphagia?**
While some studies assert that a tracheostomy tube does not alter the elevation and anterior excursion of the hyoid bone and larynx, others indicate that tracheostomy tubes cause altered sensory and motor functions that may decrease swallowing efficiency and cause an anchoring effect that limits laryngeal elevation. It is more likely that the need for a tracheotomy along with an individual's comorbidities (e.g., respiratory failure, trauma, stroke, advanced age, reduced functional reserve, and medications used to treat the critically ill) predisposes patients to dysphagia rather than the tracheostomy tube itself.

BIBLIOGRAPHY

Balzer KM: Drug-induced dysphagia, *Int J MS Care* 2(1):40–50, 2000.
Blonsky E, Logemann J, Boshes B, et al: Comparison of speech and swallowing function in patients with tremor disorders and in normal geriatric patients: a cinefluorographic study, *J Gerontol* 30:299–303, 1975.
Buchholz D: Neurologic causes of dysphagia, *Dysphagia* 1:152–156, 1987.
Carter J, Humbert IA: E-stim for dysphagia: yes or no, *Asha Leader*, 2012 Vol.17 (5), p.12–15
DePippo KL, Holas MA, Reding MJ: Validation of the 3 oz water test for aspiration following stroke, *Arch Neurol* 49:1259–1261, 1992.
Gross RD, Mahlmann J, Grayhack J: Physiologic effects of open and closed tracheostomy tube on pharyngeal swallowing, *Ann Otol Rhinol Laryngol* 112:2:143–152, 2003.

Leder SB, Suiter DM, Murray J, et al: Can an oral mechanism exam contribute to the assessment of odds of aspiration? *Dysphagia* 28:370–374, 2013.

Leder SB, Warner HL, Suiter DM, et al: Evaluation of swallow function post-extubation: is it necessary to wait 24 hours? *Ann Oto Rhinol Laryngol* 128(7):619–624, 2019.

Mandelstam P, Lieber A: Cineradiographic evaluation of the esophagus in normal adults, *Gastroenterology* 58:32–38, 1970.

Martin-Harris B, Brodsky MB, Michel Y, et al: Breathing and swallowing dynamics across the adult lifespan, *Arch Otolaryngol Head Neck Surg* 131(9):762–770, 2005.

Pauloski BR: Rehabilitation of dysphagia following head and neck cancer, *Phys Med Rehabil Clin N Am* 19:889–928, 2008.

Suiter DM, Leder SB. Clinical utility of the 3-ounce water swallow test. *Dysphagia.* 23:244–250, 2008.

Xia W, Zheng C, Lei Q, et al: Treatment of post-stroke dysphagia by vital stim therapy coupled with conventional swallowing training, *J Huazhong Univ Sci Technolog Med Sci* 31(1):73–76, 2011.

CHAPTER 77

BENIGN VOCAL FOLD LESIONS AND PHONOMICROSURGERY

Matthew Naunheim, MD, MBA, Sean X. Wang, MD and Matthew S. Clary, MD

KEY POINTS

1. Phonomicrosurgery is usually reserved for patients who have attempted and failed nonsurgical management, except in cases of very large or suspicious appearing vocal fold lesions.
2. Videolaryngostroboscopy should be performed during the evaluation of a vocal fold lesion to assess mucosal vibratory properties and glottic closure.
3. Many vocal fold lesions caused by excessive phonotrauma recur if the underlying vocal behavior is not corrected.

Pearls
1. The primary management of vocal fold nodules is voice therapy.
2. To achieve the best voice outcome after phonomicrosurgery, the depth of dissection should be limited to the superficial lamina propria.

QUESTIONS

1. **What's the definition of phonomicrosurgery?**
   The term "phonosurgery" was introduced in 1963 to describe procedures that alter vocal quality and pitch. As technology and understanding of the delicate vocal fold anatomy advanced, the term "phonomicrosurgery" became popular. It is usually performed using very fine instruments aided by a high-powered microscope to remove the vocal fold lesion and maximize the preservation of normal vocal fold tissue.

2. **What are the indications for phonomicrosurgery?**
   The most common indication for phonomicrosurgery is for the removal of benign laryngeal lesions to restore the normal prephonatory glottic configuration of the larynx. Occasionally, it can be used to resect precancerous and early cancers of the glottis.

3. **How is phonomicrosurgery different from traditional vocal fold stripping with regard to the management of vocal fold lesions?**
   Vocal fold stripping is usually performed by grabbing the lesion with a cup forceps and "tearing" it off the vocal fold. There is no fine control of the depth with vocal fold stripping. Furthermore the lack of precision may result in excessive removal of normal tissue or incomplete resection of diseased tissue. Stripping is no longer considered the standard of care for the majority of vocal fold lesions.

4. **What are the layers of the membranous vocal fold?**
   Stratified squamous epithelium, basement membrane, superficial lamina propria (SLP), vocal ligament (intermediate and deep lamina propria), and vocalis muscle (see Fig. 77.1).

5. **What are the main components of the lamina propria?**
   Fibroblasts constitute the main cellular component of the lamina propria, while glycosaminoglycans and proteoglycans occupy the interstitial spaces within the extracellular matrix.

6. **Why is the SLP often referred to as the Reinke's space?**
   The superficial lamina propria has often been described incorrectly as a potential space. It is approximately 0.5 millimeters in thickness and has a distinct anatomic structure. Thus the eponym of Reinke's space is a misnomer.

7. **What are the components of the SLP?**
   It is composed mostly of extracellular matrix proteins, water, and loosely arranged fibers of collagen and elastin. SLP is mostly gelatinous.

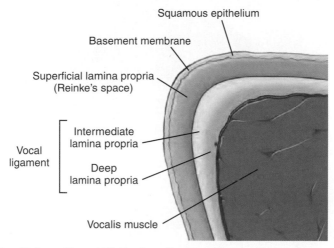

Squamous epithelium

Basement membrane

Superficial lamina propria
(Reinke's space)

Intermediate
lamina propria

Vocal
ligament

Deep
lamina propria

Vocalis muscle

Fig. 77.1 Coronal view of the layers of the vocal fold. (From Rosen CA and Simpson CB: *Operative Techniques in Laryngology,* New York, 2008, Springer, p. 6.)

8. **What are the components of the vocal ligament?**
   It is composed mostly of elastin and collagen. As the vocal ligament transitions from the intermediate to the deep layer of the lamina propria, there is a denser arrangement of collagen. Elastin facilitates tissue stretching, whereas collagen provides connective strength.

9. **What is the body-cover model of the vocal fold?**
   Due to different physical properties, the cover (epithelium and the SLP) vibrates differently from the body (vocal ligament and vocalis muscle). Some authors consider the vocal ligament to be a transitional zone without discrete boundaries between layers. As air passes between the vocal folds from the lung, the cover moves like a wave over the denser vocal ligament and vocalis muscle.

10. **How do laryngeal lesions cause dysphonia?**
    By altering the cover viscosity, interfering with the body-cover relationship, distorting the prephonatory glottic configuration, and changing glottic closure patterns.

11. **What are the principals of phonomicrosurgery?**
    The principals are based on the body-cover model of vocal fold vibration. Given the importance of the interaction between the cover and the body, phonomicrosurgery for most benign lesions has evolved to limit the dissection to the depth and extent of the lesion and to maximize the preservation of normal microarchitecture. The same principle applies for the removal of malignancy; however, the primary goal is to achieve a negative margin. Normal tissue may be sacrificed to ensure cancer extirpation. Additionally, epithelial coverage of the surgical site is a tenet of phonomicrosurgery, when possible. Ideally, microflap techniques should be used to minimize the gap between the epithelial edges, which encourages more rapid healing and is less likely to lead to scarring. Reduction of this epithelial gap may not be possible when the laryngeal lesion involves the epithelium itself (e.g., dysplasia).

12. **What is the plane of dissection for most phonomicrosurgery?**
    In the SLP. Usually, after incising the epithelium of the vocal fold the SLP can be easily entered using a flap elevator. The vocal ligament is dense and appears to be pearly white (see Fig. 77.2).

13. **Can you use lasers to achieve control and precision similar to that of cold steel instruments?**
    Yes. Modern laser technology such as a carbon dioxide (CO_2) laser with an articulating arm can be attached to an operative microscope. With specific software and hardware modifications, the depth and thickness can be precisely controlled (see Fig. 77.3). Other lasers, such as the KTP, can also be used to achieve ablation of tissue while limiting the depth of dissection and thermal injury. The drawback to the use of lasers is the photothermal effect, which causes damage to nearby tissues due to heat. This can be minimized by laryngeal surgeons by optimizing the laser settings.

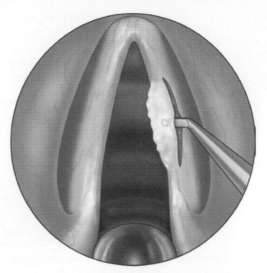

Fig. 77.2 Elevating leukoplakia off the vocal fold using microflap technique. (From Rosen CA and Simpson CB: *Operative Techniques in Laryngology,* New York, 2008, Springer, p. 125.)

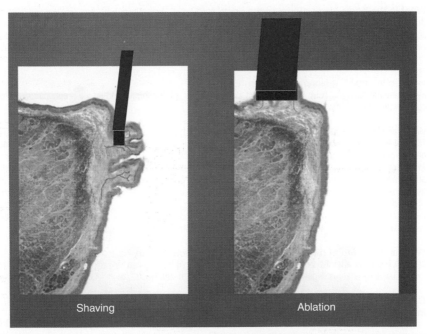

Shaving

Ablation

Fig. 77.3 Microphonosurgery with a CO_2 laser. The left figure demonstrates shaving of respiratory papilloma off the free edge of the vocal fold, seen here in the coronal view. The right figure demonstrates ablating papilloma off the superior surface of the vocal fold. (Courtesy Mark S. Courey, MD.)

14. **Why is laryngostroboscopy a vital part of the preoperative evaluation for phonomicrosurgery?**
    Stroboscopy can assess the vibratory properties and glottic closure pattern of the vocal folds, which cannot be fully seen on laryngoscopy alone. These findings allow the clinician to predict the type and depth of the lesion. Stroboscopy is the only clinically available tool that allows clinicians to assess the pliability and vibratory function of the vocal folds. High-speed photography is another method to evaluate vibratory properties, but it is not readily available for clinical purposes. A detailed description of stroboscopic interpretation can be found in Kitzing (1985).

15. **What are the common benign laryngeal lesions treated with phonomicrosurgery?**
    Vocal fold polyps and cysts, polypoid corditis (Reinke's edema), recurrent respiratory papilloma, and benign keratosis. Nodules, while typically nonsurgical, can also be managed in this fashion.

16. **What are vocal fold nodules?**
    These are bilateral and symmetric midmembraneous vocal fold lesions that are usually due to inefficient voice use. Laryngostroboscopy reveals subtle alterations in the normal vibratory properties of the vocal folds in the midmembranous region, and incomplete closure can be seen. Nodules tend to resolve with behavioral modifications and voice therapy. Vocal fold nodules are rarely managed surgically.

17. **What are vocal fold polyps?**
    These lesions are classically exophytic and can be clear or vascularized in appearance. Inefficient and/or excessive voice use may lead to the formation of clear gelatinous polyps. Some phonotraumatic polyps may have aberrant vessels and present as vascularized polyps that are more reddish in appearance. Vascularized polyps may hemorrhage into the vocal fold if there is an acute episode of violent cough or phonotrauma. Polyps can present unilaterally or bilaterally and usually do not lead to significant perturbation of the normal vibratory properties when they are small; however, most polyps do not respond completely to voice therapy, and many require surgical treatment.

18. **What are vocal fold cysts?**
    These lesions can be unilateral or bilateral. The subepithelial type is thought to be the product of an obstructed mucous gland and may cause mild changes in vibratory properties. A deeper intraligamentous (in the vocal ligament) type may cause significant impairment of vocal fold vibration. Keratin-filled cysts are also occasionally observed. Vocal fold cysts usually do not usually respond to voice therapy and eventually require surgery.

19. **What underlying etiologies are shared by some benign lesions such as vocal fold nodules, polyps, and cysts?**
    The development of these vocal fold lesions is often related to the patient's inefficient phonatory pattern, which leads to excessive vocal fold collision and trauma. Sometimes, the traumatic phonatory pattern may be a compensatory behavior due to glottic insufficiency.

20. **What is Reinke's edema or polypoid corditis?**
    Reinke's edema presents as diffuse swelling of one or both vocal folds. As a result of the significant increase in vocal fold mass, the patient speaks with a lower-pitched and rougher voice. The degree of reduction in the mucosal wave correlates with the size of the lesion. In extreme cases, bilateral Reinke's edema can cause obstruction of the glottic airway. This condition is usually associated with tobacco abuse. Patients are often asked to quit smoking before surgical excision is attempted. Smoking cessation does not reverse Reinke's edema but usually helps to halt progression.

21. **What are vocal fold scars or sulcus vocalis?**
    When there is irreversible loss of viscoelasticity to the superficial lamina propria, a scar or sulcus vocalis is formed. These patients normally have a history of high voice use. If tissue loss is significant, the patient may also experience glottic insufficiency. Phonomicrosurgery rarely improves the mucosal wave vibration. Augmenting the vocal fold with an injectable or permanent implant may correct glottic insufficiency, thus providing more vocal projection and volume. Scars and sulci are often used interchangeably as they have similar effects on vibratory parameters and appearance on stroboscopy but, technically, scar refers to abnormal fibrous tissue in the SLP layer, whereas sulcus refers to loss of SLP tissue.

22. **What kind of the precancerous and cancerous lesions can be treated with phonomicrosurgery?**
    Dysplasia, squamous cell carcinoma in situ, and early vocal fold squamous cell carcinoma.

23. **What are the different techniques for endoscopic excision of early glottic cancer?**
Squamous cell carcinoma in situ and superficial early stage squamous cell carcinomas can be removed with a microflap technique staying superficial to the vocal ligament. If the lesion extends into or through the vocal ligament, endoscopic carbon dioxide laser–assisted cordectomy is an excellent treatment modality that rivals radiation therapy in cure rate.

24. **What is the most important predictor of voice outcome following endoscopic vocal fold cordectomy for cancer resection?**
The deeper the excision, the more unpredictable the voice outcome becomes.

25. **What common pathologies can lead to glottic insufficiency?**
Vocal fold paralysis, paresis, and vocal fold atrophy related to aging or neurologic disease.

26. **Why is preoperative voice therapy important in the management of many benign laryngeal lesions?**
Voice therapy can ameliorate inefficient phonatory patterns, so the patient is less likely to cause further trauma to the vocal folds postoperatively. Furthermore some patients may be satisfied with their voice after therapy and no longer need surgery. Last, for benign laryngeal lesions, phonomicrosurgery is an elective procedure, and one or two sessions of voice therapy can solidify the patient-physician relationship as well as the patient-therapist relationship.

27. **What are the potential complications of phonomicrosurgery discussed with the patient preoperatively?**
Since the larynx is part of the airway, there is always a risk of airway obstruction during and after the procedure. Making an incision in the vocal fold may cause scar formation, thus worsening the patient's voice. A rigid laryngoscope provides the surgeon with exposure of the vocal folds, and the laryngoscope rests on the teeth and tongue; thus dental injury, lip laceration/abrasion, and taste changes can all occur. Lesions that are due to voice abuse may recur if the patient maintains the same vocal behavior.

28. **What equipment is usually needed to perform phonomicrosurgery?**
A specialized laryngoscope is used to expose the larynx. As a general rule, the surgeon should use the largest laryngoscope that the patient can safely tolerate. A suspension system is used to place the laryngoscope in a fixed position. A high-powered operative microscope is used to provide a magnified binocular view of the vocal folds. A 0-degree and/or 70-degree telescope can be used to take operative photographs and closely examine the lesion. The main microlaryngeal instruments are small suctions to remove blood and mucous, sickle knife to make incisions, flap elevators to dissect the lesion, forceps to grab and retract the lesion, and scissors to extend the incision. Lasers can also be used.

29. **What is the typical duration of voice rest after phonomicrosurgery?**
Patients may be placed on complete voice rest for 0 to 14 days and gradually increase their vocal use while working closely with the surgeon and the speech-language pathologist. Some patients may not return to unrestricted voice use until 30 to 60 days postoperatively, especially professional singers and patients with large lesions. The appropriate amount of prescribed voice rest or conservation is under constant debate. Ultimately, postoperative care should be individually tailored based on the type and size of the lesion, the degree of tissue deficiency, the patient's current voice use pattern and projected vocal requirement, and the clinician's experience.

BIBLIOGRAPHY

Goor KM, Peeters AJ, Mahieu HF, et al: Cordectomy by CO2 laser or radiotherapy for small T1a glottic carcinomas: costs, local control, survival, quality of life, and voice quality, *Head Neck* 29(2):128–136, 2007.

Kitzing P: Stroboscopy – a pertinent laryngological examination, *J Otolaryngol* 14(3):151–157, 1985.

Mitchell JR, Kojima T, Wu H, Garrett CG, Rousseau B: Biochemical basis of vocal fold mobilization after microflap surgery in a rabbit model, *Laryngoscope* 124(2):487–493, 2014. doi: 10.1002/lary.24263.

Mortuaire G, Francois J, Wiel E, et al: Local recurrence after CO2 laser cordectomy for early glottic carcinoma, *Laryngoscope* 116(1):101–105, 2006.

Rosen CA: Benign vocal fold lesions and phonomicrosurgery. In: Bailey BJ, Johnson JT, eds: *Head and Neck Surgery – Otolaryngology*, 4th ed, 2006, Lippincott Williams and Wilkins.

Rosen CA, Gartner-Schmidt J, Hathaway B, et al: A nomenclature paradigm for benign midmembranous vocal fold lesions, *Laryngoscope* 122(6):1335–1341, 2012.

Rosen CA, Simpson CB: *Operative Techniques in Laryngology*, 2008, Springer.

Sataloff RT, Hawkshaw MJ, Divi V, et al: Voice surgery, *Otolaryngol Clin North Am* 40(5):1151–1183, 2007.

CHAPTER 78

VOCAL FOLD PARALYSIS

Elliana Kirsh DeVore, MD and Thomas L. Carroll, MD

KEY POINTS

1. Understand the embryology and anatomy of the recurrent and superior laryngeal nerves (RLN and SLN). Unilateral or bilateral injury to one or both of these nerves can lead to a range of dysfunctions in voice, swallowing, and the ability to cough.
2. A comprehensive history focusing on recent surgeries, intubations, or viral illnesses is critical in determining the etiology of vocal fold paralysis. A complete head and neck examination to evaluate other cranial neuropathies or masses is also required. In the setting of unexplained unilateral vocal fold paralysis, a computed tomography (CT) scan of the neck from the skull base through the aortic arch with contrast is typically obtained to evaluate the entire course of the RLN (Box 78.1).
3. In adults, unilateral vocal fold paralysis typically presents with hoarseness, dysphagia, and dyspnea with speaking but not dyspnea with exercise. Bilateral vocal fold paralysis typically presents with dyspnea on exertion and inspiratory stridor. Voice and swallowing may be normal in patients with bilateral paralysis. Bilateral RLN paralysis can be life-threatening and may present as an acute airway emergency (Table 78.1).
4. It is rare for a vocal fold paresis to recover after 6 months from the date of insult. Laryngeal electromyography (LEMG) is often helpful in determining the prognosis for recovery before 6 months have passed from the date of injury. Temporary vocal fold augmentation is used to bridge the gap before paralysis is deemed permanent by time or LEMG criteria.
5. Treatment for unilateral vocal fold paralysis augments and medializes the immobile vocal fold to allow the mobile, opposite vocal fold to meet it and restore glottic competence. Treatment for bilateral vocal fold paralysis is aimed at enlarging the airway, often at the expense of voice, by removing normal vocal fold tissue or lateralizing one of the paralyzed folds.

Pearls
1. The position of the affected true vocal fold (TVF) does not correlate with the level or extent of injury to the vagus nerve or RLN branch. Not all branches of the nerve may recover and the position of the paralyzed or immobile vocal fold may vary over time.
2. Laryngeal EMG is a tool used to measure motor unit recruitment. When the muscle is denervated, fibrillation potentials and positive waves are seen, whereas polyphasic motor units are seen when reinnervation occurs.
3. Augmenting unilateral TVF immobility does not eliminate the risk of aspiration when there is also a sensory deficit from an affected SLN. However, improving the patient's ability to cough more effectively may be sufficient to protect the lungs and tolerate aspiration.
4. Early augmentation with temporary injection in symptomatic patients with unilateral TVF immobility offers better long-term outcomes and a decreased need for permanent augmentation.
5. In bilateral complete vocal fold immobility, tracheostomy may initially be required, but many of these patients can later be decannulated after surgery to enlarge the glottic airway.

QUESTIONS

1. **Describe the anatomy of the vocal folds as part of the larynx.**
   The larynx is divided into the supraglottis, glottis, and subglottis (Fig. 78.2A). The glottis comprises paired true vocal folds (TVFs). The supraglottis encompasses all tissues of the larynx above the TVFs. The laryngeal ventricles extend laterally and superiorly, under the false vocal folds, and end blindly in the laryngeal saccule. The subglottis begins approximately 1 centimeter below the rima glottis (the area where the TVFs meet during phonation), extending to the inferior border of the cricoid cartilage. TVFs are involved in phonation, whereas false vocal folds are typically not. The false vocal folds are formed of mucosa overlying the superior aspect of the thyroarytenoid muscle and other connective tissues. The TVFs are covered by stratified squamous epithelium, differentiating them from the ciliated pseudostratified columnar epithelium of the remainder of the respiratory tract. The superficial lamina propria (Reinke's space) is deep to the squamous epithelium of the TVFs, which together comprise the vocal cover that affords vibration during phonation. The intermediate and deep lamina propria are deeper, forming

461

Box 78.1 Key Historical Questions in a Patient Presenting With Vocal Fold Paralysis

- Symptom frequency, associations, relieving/exacerbating factors, onset, duration
- Avoiding communication because of the effort required?
- Decreased ability to complete everyday tasks/work?
- Decreased participation in strenuous sports/activities?
- Conversion to a relatively sedentary lifestyle? (more common in bilateral paralysis)
- History of aspiration pneumonia/swallowing difficulty?
- Previous neurologic, head and neck, carotid, or cardiothoracic surgery?
- History of alcohol and tobacco use?
- Is it difficult to project the voice?
- History of endotracheal intubation?

Table 78.1 Signs and Symptoms of Vocal Fold Paralysis

Unilateral	• Dysphonia (hoarseness, breathy speech, soft voice) • Dyspnea and fatigue with speaking (but lack of stridor or dyspnea on exertion) • Episodic coughing with thin liquids/dysphagia • Recurrent aspiration pneumonia • Nasopharyngeal regurgitation if high vagal injury • Signs of other cranial nerve involvement; e.g., tongue paralysis or loss of gag • Signs of thoracic malignancy (cough, dyspnea, hemoptysis, etc.)
Bilateral	• Normal voice is possible • Dyspnea on exertion • Stridor with or without activity • Acute airway compromise/stridor postoperatively • Worsening of symptoms after upper respiratory infection

---

the vocal ligament. The vocal ligament sits on top of the vocalis muscle (the medial portion of the thyroarytenoid muscle) and is the superior extent of the conus elasticus, a fibrous tissue condensation extending up from the cricoid cartilage.

2. **Other than phonation, what are the functions of the vocal folds?**
Although phonation is an important function, it is not the primary role of the true and false vocal folds. Protection of the lower airway during swallowing is the most crucial function of the larynx, and the vocal folds are imperative to this. In addition, the TVFs provide the ability to cough and clear the airway and allow increased intraabdominal pressure to build during a Valsalva maneuver.

3. **Describe the innervation of the larynx.**
The larynx is innervated by various sensory and motor branches of the vagus nerve (CN X). After the vagus nerve exits the skull base, it gives off branches, including the superior laryngeal nerve (SLN). The SLN divides into the internal and external branches. The internal branch carries sensory information from the laryngeal mucosa above the TVFs. The external branch innervates the cricothyroid muscle, which contracts to bring the thyroid cartilage closer to the cricoid cartilage, thus lengthening the TVFs and allowing pitch elevation of the voice. After giving off the superior laryngeal nerve, the vagus descends within the carotid sheath, along with the internal carotid artery and internal jugular vein (posterolateral to the internal carotid artery and posteromedial to the internal jugular vein). As the vagus enters the thoracic cavity, it sends a branch cephalad, which is the recurrent laryngeal nerve (RLN). The right RLN splits from the right vagus nerve at the cervicothoracic junction, passing posterior to the right subclavian artery and ascending posterior to the common carotid along the tracheoesophageal groove. One percent of right RLNs arise at the level of the thyroid gland and can be more readily injured during thyroidectomy. The left RLN extends from the vagus nerve at the aortic arch, wrapping posteriorly underneath the ligamentum arteriosum and ascending cephalad in the tracheoesophageal groove. The RLNs enter the larynx near the cricothyroid joint and then split into the anterior and posterior branches. The RLN innervates all of the intrinsic muscles of the larynx (thyroarytenoid [TA], lateral cricoarytenoid [LCA], interarytenoid [IA], and posterior cricoarytenoid [PCA]), except for the cricothyroid muscle. It also supplies sensory innervation to the mucosa of the TVFs and below.

4. **If innervation to the larynx is injured, what can happen?**
It should be understood that innervation of the larynx is more complex than described above. There are anastomoses of the motor and sensory system, as well as between the right and left sides. When the RLN and/or SLN sustain an injury, repair and reinnervation are often incomplete and variable among the smaller terminal branches.

Because the RLN carries adductor (TA, LCA, and IA) and abductor (PCA) fibers, damage to the nerve severe enough to cause Wallerian degeneration results in "cross-wiring" or synkinetic reinnervation and lack of purposeful motion to the affected muscles. Synkinetic TVFs will have good tone and often a normal interference pattern on LEMG, whereas completely denervated TVFs will atrophy.

5. **Describe the embryology pertinent to the RLN.**
The larynx develops from the branchial arch. The supraglottis and superior laryngeal nerve arise from the fourth arch. The cricoid cartilage and recurrent laryngeal nerve arise from the sixth arch. On the right, the sixth segmental artery disappears completely, and the fourth arch artery remains as the subclavian artery. This explains why the right recurrent laryngeal nerve passes under only the right subclavian vessels and has a shorter distance to travel back to the larynx. In contrast, on the left side, the sixth arch artery persists as the ductus arteriosus, which later fibroses to become the ligamentum arteriosum. This remnant necessitates a longer course for the left recurrent laryngeal nerve, forcing it to descend into the chest before returning to the larynx. The effect of this embryologic development on the course of the RLN explains why intrathoracic processes can result in unilateral vocal fold paralysis (Table 78.2).

6. **What is the difference between vocal fold immobility, vocal fold paralysis, and vocal fold paresis?**
It is important to use the correct terminology when evaluating vocal folds that do not move, as it refers to the etiology of their dysfunction. *Immobility* is a general term that does not indicate a cause; it refers to the lack of movement of the vocal folds from any cause, neurologic or mechanical. In addition, any nonmobile vocal fold that has yet to be designated as one with permanent motion impairment is called *immobile* rather than paralyzed. In contrast, *paralysis* of the vocal folds specifically refers to lack of movement (or immobility) from a permanent neurologic cause. If a vocal fold has a partial motion abnormality that is yet to be designated as permanent (i.e., a patient who presents with a new-onset partial vocal TVF motion abnormality) it is called *hypomobile*; it is only given the diagnosis of a TVF *paresis* when it is 6 months or older with no other mechanical explanation and is therefore from a permanent neurologic cause.

7. **Describe the findings on laryngoscopy and stroboscopy seen in vocal fold paralysis.**
In a complete unilateral paralysis, the fold will neither abduct nor adduct and will sit in a neutral position somewhere between adducted and abducted. The position of the immobile or paralyzed TVF does not necessarily distinguish between vagus and RLN injuries. As reinnervation occurs in RLN injury, not all minor branches of the nerve may recover and the position of the affected vocal fold often changes over time. The healthy, opposite vocal fold will have full abduction and adduction capability and will try to cross the midline to meet the paralyzed fold (Fig. 78.1). The arytenoid cartilage on the side of denervation most often falls anteriorly into the airway, but the appearance of the arytenoid does not provide any definitive information on the neurologic status of the affected RLN. On stroboscopy, one may see a transglottic gap without significant vibration or a complete (but dominantly open) closure pattern with asymmetry depending on the position of the immobile TVF. Denervation atrophy after a few weeks or months may lead to greater vibratory amplitude or edge bowing. There is typically supraglottic hyperfunction (secondary muscle tension) due to the compensatory effort by the surrounding intrinsic laryngeal muscles, which may even cause pain/discomfort.

Table 78.2 Causes of Vocal Fold Paralysis/Immobility

Idiopathic (postviral neuropathy)	Tumors of the head and neck
Thyroid or parathyroid surgery	Laryngeal ventricle or piriform sinus mass
Skull base surgery	Intrathoracic, mediastinal neoplasm
Vagal neoplasm	Thoracic/cervical trauma
Anterior cervical fusion surgery	Aortic aneurysm
Carotid surgery	Left atrial dilation ("Ortner syndrome")
Traumatic intubation/extubation	Brainstem infarction (bulbar palsy) (rare)
Arytenoid dislocation	Wallenberg syndrome
Cricothyroid joint fixation	Multiple sclerosis
Rheumatoid arthritis	ALS
Osteomyelitis of skull base	Poliomyelitis
Tuberculosis	Lupus
Chronic alcohol abuse	Granulomatous disease (e.g., sarcoidosis)
Fibrosis from radiation to head and neck	Diabetic polyneuropathy
Endotracheal tube cuff injury to RLN	Polyarteritis nodosum
Thoracic surgery	
Surgery of/near aortic arch	

PHONATION INSPIRATION

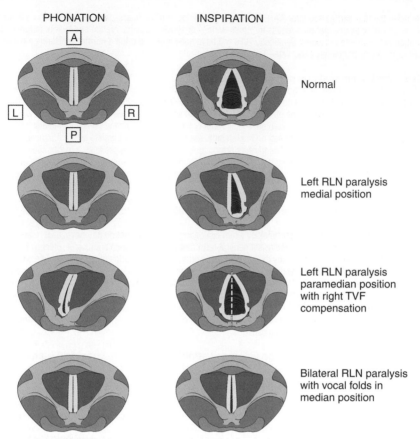

Normal

Left RLN paralysis
medial position

Left RLN paralysis
paramedian position
with right TVF
compensation

Bilateral RLN paralysis
with vocal folds in
median position

Fig. 78.1 Vocal cord paralysis diagrams.

In bilateral vocal fold paralysis, it is important to differentiate between patients with bilateral midline TVFs and those with TVFs that remain paramedian with a glottic gap. When the folds are immobile in the midline, patients typically experience a normal voice but significant airway compromise and respiratory distress. In contrast, when the TVFs lie in a paramedian position, the patient will not routinely have airway compromise but the voice will be severely affected with a transglottic gap on stroboscopy.

8. **What is a glottic gap/glottic insufficiency?**
A glottic gap refers to a pathologic space between the true vocal folds during phonation. It is possible to see this grossly in the setting of severe atrophy or vocal fold paralysis or immobility. Often, laryngovideostroboscopy (laryngoscopy modality that uses a strobe light to provide better visualization of the movement and closure pattern of the vocal folds) is needed to identify a subtler glottic gap due to small benign lesions, paresis/hypomobility, early atrophy, or scarring. Glottic insufficiency is the pathologic and excess loss of air from the vocal folds due to a glottic gap resulting from multiple conditions. Glottic insufficiency is typically the cause of secondary muscle tension dysphonia that presents on examination as hyperfunctional behaviors of the supraglottic structures that are attempting to compensate for the glottic insufficiency. In females a posterior glottic gap is often physiologic and normal.

9. **What is the role of laryngeal electromyography in evaluating vocal fold paralysis?**
Laryngeal electromyography (LEMG) is a test to help characterize the innervation status of an immobile vocal fold. It uses the body's own electricity to demonstrate whether or not the RLN is sending signals to the muscle's motor units or if the muscle is just firing on its own without any input. LEMG can determine if an immobile TVF is from a neurologic cause or a mechanical cause, such as cricoarytenoid joint dislocation, with the latter demonstrating normal LEMG activity. If the muscle is normally innervated, multiple action potentials from many motor units will overlap into a normal *interference pattern*, and there is no spontaneous/random electrical activity. Alternatively, if the muscle is denervated, fibrillation potentials and positive waves are spontaneously observed. During the

time when reinnervation occurs or after incomplete reinnervation, polyphasic motor units are present. LEMG may indicate the potential for return of neuromuscular activity months before a clinical exam shows vocal fold motion. Synkinesis or other poor prognostic findings, such as persistent positive waves/fibrillation potentials after serial LEMGs a few months apart, help the physician recommend early permanent augmentation.

10. **Which other tests should be included in the workup of unexplained unilateral TVF immobility or paralysis?**
    In patients with new-onset unilateral TVF paralysis that cannot be explained by a recent surgery, intubation, trauma, or known pathology, it is important to consider extrinsic causes, specifically masses compressing the recurrent laryngeal nerve anywhere along its course. A CT scan with contrast from the skull base through the aortic arch is the best initial test, as chest x-ray is rarely helpful. If the CT is negative and the history and neurologic examination suggest multiple cranial neuropathies, magnetic resonance imaging (MRI) of the brain and brainstem is indicated. If there is associated stridor that cannot be explained by laryngoscopy, tracheobronchoscopy should be performed. Of note, while the importance of imaging for patients with complete vocal fold paralysis is well established, its routine use in cases of paresis has not demonstrated high clinical yield.

11. **What are the potential sequelae of unilateral true vocal fold immobility?**
    Aspiration pneumonia is a potentially fatal sequela of unilateral true vocal fold immobility, observed in up to 50% of patients with symptomatic dysphagia. Early injection augmentation is offered preventatively in acute TVF immobility in an effort to improve swallow function and "pulmonary toilet" (the ability to cough and clear secretions). Augmenting unilateral TVF immobility by no means guarantees improvement in dysphagia or prevention of aspiration pneumonia, as it may be related to a sensory deficit from SLN dysfunction. However, improving the patient's ability to cough more effectively may be enough to protect the lungs from small aspirations and will also improve voice. In addition to aspiration pneumonia, patients with unilateral true vocal fold paralysis often suffer from severe dysphonia, associated with decrements in voice and health-related quality of life.

12. **What are the potential sequelae of bilateral true vocal fold paralysis?**
    Airway compromise is the primary concern in bilateral TVF paralysis. Most patients do not tolerate the insult if it occurs acutely. Patients who have long-standing bilateral paralysis (or who had a gradual onset) may have stridor at rest or with exercise but function to a satisfactory level when they are otherwise healthy. However, as in the setting of an acute upper respiratory infection, even a small amount of edema in an already narrow glottis can significantly decrease the cross-sectional area of the airway and lead to a life-threatening situation.

13. **What are the treatment options for new-onset unilateral vocal fold immobility?**
    When underlying causes have been ruled out or are concurrently being treated, the first step in managing unilateral TVF immobility in a *symptomatic* patient is temporary injection augmentation of the affected TVF. This can be performed in the office, at the bedside, or in the operating room with a material that typically lasts 2 to 6 months. Early augmentation has been shown to improve long-term voice outcomes and decrease the need for permanent augmentation (the reason for this phenomenon is incompletely understood). Treatment with nimodipine (a calcium channel blocker) may also be considered, as it may improve vocal fold tone and motion recovery by reducing cellular apoptosis and promoting axonal regeneration after neuronal injury.

    LEMG is performed as early as 3 weeks from the time of injury and can be repeated 2 months later, affording prognostic information. Various factors, such as patient age, occupation, comorbid conditions, and preferences, play a role in management. Watchful waiting is satisfactory for many people who can swallow and communicate sufficiently.

14. **What are the treatment options for a long-standing unilateral vocal fold paralysis?**
    Treatment options include injection laryngoplasty, medialization laryngoplasty with or without arytenoid adduction, and RLN reinnervation.

    Injection laryngoplasty, deep into the TA muscle, is accomplished via a percutaneous or peroral route in the office or via suspension laryngoscopy in the operating room. The materials available for long-term (>6 months) augmentation include calcium hydroxylapatite, micronized dermis, hyaluronic acid, and autologous fat (fat is considered the only permanent injectable by many and is almost exclusively performed in the OR because of its harvesting). Injection laryngoplasty can be very effective for a small glottic gap when the paralyzed vocal fold is a midline or paramedian. Early augmentation improves voice outcomes and voice-related quality of life and may reduce the likelihood of requiring open laryngeal framework surgery in the future. However, for larger glottic gaps, injection is often less than satisfactory and medialization laryngoplasty is a more effective treatment (Fig. 78.2A).

    Medialization laryngoplasty, or laryngeal framework surgery, involves the placement of a carved silastic block, Gore-Tex® strip, or prefabricated implant within the paraglottic space, pushing the affected TVF medially (see Fig. 78.2B). An adjunctive treatment to medialization laryngoplasty includes arytenoid adduction with or without arytenopexy. The arytenoid cartilage is repositioned by anchoring sutures in a more physiologic position for phonation. This is employed when there is a large posterior glottic gap or mismatch of the height of the vocal processes of the arytenoid cartilages (Fig. 78.2B). Laryngeal framework surgery provides a permanent solution

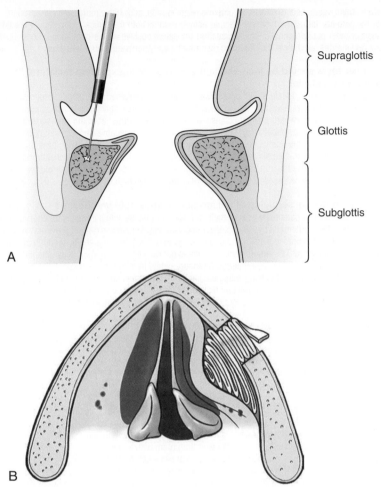

Fig. 78.2 A, Coronal section of the larynx, demonstrating depth of needle placement and location deep in the thyroarytenoid muscle for injection laryngoplasty. **B,** Axial section glottis showing Gore-Tex® medialization. (Adapted from Rosen CA, Simpson CB: *Operative Techniques in Laryngology,* Berlin, 2008, Springer.)

to glottic insufficiency and therefore has been considered the gold standard in the treatment of unilateral vocal fold paralysis. Important considerations include patient education and screening, including evaluation of medical comorbidities (e.g., chronic cough, orthopnea), and counseling to ensure the patient is able to lie awake, supine on the operating room table for up to 3 hours. Patients should be counseled regarding the risks of the procedure, including the potential need for revision surgery, bleeding, infection, implant extrusion, and perioperative airway compromise.

Reinnervation procedures are performed to reestablish the tone of the intrinsic muscles of the larynx. Due to the complex innervation of laryngeal structures, RLN/SLN reinnervation procedures do not reproduce physiologic motion of the TVF and often require augmentation to improve voice during the period of nerve regrowth. Nonetheless, several promising surgical techniques have been developed for selective reinnervation, with positive results in terms of maintaining muscle bulk and promoting voice rehabilitation while avoiding future inflammatory reactions to foreign material, especially in pediatric patients.

15. **What are the treatment options for acute bilateral vocal fold immobility?**
    Patients with bilateral incomplete paralysis can experience partial or even full recovery, and LEMG is employed in this setting to improve prognosis. Treatment options aim to both preserve and protect the patient's airway while awaiting one or both sides to recover motion. Suture lateralization of one vocal fold or tracheostomy is typically used to overcome the acute insult. Theoretically, both of these treatments are reversible and may be removed with nerve recovery or after progressive surgeries to enlarge the airway, as described below.

16. **What are the treatment options for permanent bilateral TVF paralysis?**
    While some patients with acute bilateral TVF paralysis present immediately, others may experience worsening airway symptoms over several weeks as a result of aberrant reinnervation or synkinesis. For cases of permanent bilateral TVF paralysis where the airway is affected and the voice is normal, unilateral or bilateral cordotomy with medial or total arytenoidectomies can be performed. This is typically accomplished in a serially, progressively destructive fashion until a balance between the airway and voice loss is acceptable. These destructive procedures often lead to a breathier voice but provide enough airway improvement to avoid or remove a tracheotomy tube. Alternatively, lateralization procedures of either the vocal fold itself or the arytenoid (arytenoid abduction) can be performed to improve voice quality.
    Emerging treatments for bilateral vocal fold paralysis include laryngeal pacing, botulinum toxin injections, gene therapy, and stem cell therapy; however, more data regarding the safety and efficacy of these interventions are needed before they may be offered to patients.

17. **What is the long-term prognosis in patients with vocal fold paralysis?**
    In cases of unilateral vocal fold paralysis, the outcomes are generally good. With augmentation procedures, most patients can achieve a functional voice with the exception of certain scenarios, such as singing or loudly projecting one's voice. Many experience improvements in voice and general health-related quality of life as a result of treatment. The risk of aspiration remains due to alterations in sensation, leading to an inability to reliably protect the airway. This is especially true when the etiology is a high vagal insult that includes an SLN injury. Augmentation of the affected TVF does not guarantee swallowing improvement, although it often helps to improve the strength of the patient's cough. In the setting of a complete, unilateral RLN injury without SLN involvement, many patients swallow effortlessly because of preserved sensation.
    In bilateral complete vocal fold paralysis, tracheostomy may be initially required, but with surgeries to enlarge the airway at the glottic level many patients with bilateral TVF paralysis can eventually be decannulated. When the voice is affected by paramedian bilateral paralyzed TVFs, medialization and injection augmentation can be used to close the glottic gap, but tracheotomy is often necessary. For patients with persistent and significant dysphagia, a gastrostomy tube may be considered.

BIBLIOGRAPHY

Araki K, Suzuki H, Uno K, Tomifuji M, Shiotani A: Gene therapy for recurrent laryngeal nerve injury, *Genes (Basel)* 9(7):316, 2018.

Arviso LC, Johns MM, Mathison CC, et al: Long-term outcomes of injection laryngoplasty in patients with potentially recoverable vocal fold paralysis, *Laryngoscope* 120:2237–2240, 2010.

Badia PI, Hillel AT, Shah MD, Johns MM III, Klein AM: Computed tomography has low yield in the evaluation of idiopathic unilateral true vocal fold paresis, *Laryngoscope* 123(1):204–207, 2013.

Bakhsh Z, Crevier-Buchman L: Stroboscopic assessment of unilateral vocal fold paralysis: a systematic review, *Eur Arch Otorhinolaryngol* 276(9):2377–2387, 2019.

Butskiy O, Mistry B, Chadha NK: Surgical interventions for pediatric unilateral vocal cord paralysis: a systematic review, *JAMA Otolaryngol Head Neck Surg* 141(7):654–660, 2015.

Carroll TL, Rosen CA: Trial vocal fold injection, *J Voice* 24(4):494–498, 2010.

Costello D: Change to earlier surgical interventions: contemporary management of unilateral vocal fold paralysis, *Curr Opin Otolaryngol Head Neck Surg* 23(3):181–184, 2015.

Friedman AD, Burns JA, Heaton JT, et al: Early versus late injection medialization for unilateral vocal cord paralysis, *Laryngoscope* 120:2042–2046, 2010.

Ivey CM: Vocal fold paresis, *Otolaryngol Clin North Am* 52(4):637–648, 2019.

Li Y, Garrett G, Zealear D: Current treatment options for bilateral vocal fold paralysis: a state-of-the-art review, *Clin Exp Otorhinolaryngol* 10(3):203–212, 2017.

Lichtenberger G: Reversible lateralization of the paralyzed vocal cord without tracheostomy, *Ann Otol Rhinol Laryngol* 111(1):21–26, 2002.

Lin RJ, Klein-Fedyshin M, Rosen CA: Nimodipine improves vocal fold and facial motion recovery after injury: a systematic review and meta-analysis, *Laryngoscope* 129(4):943–951, 2019.

Morris L, Afifi S: *Tracheostomies: The Complete Guide*, 2010, Springer.

Mueller AH, Pototschnig C: Recurrent laryngeal nerve stimulator, *Otolaryngol Clin North Am* 53(1):145–156, 2020.

Oertli D, Udelsman R: *Surgery of the Thyroid and Parathyroid Gland*, 2007, Springer.

Ossoff RH, Shapshay SM, Woodson GE, et al: *The Larynx*, 2003, Lippincott Williams & Wilkins.

Pei YC, Fang TJ, Hsin LJ, Li HY, Wong AM: Early hyaluronate injection improves quality of life but not neural recovery in unilateral vocal fold paralysis: an open-label randomized controlled study, *Restor Neurol Neurosci* 33(2):121–130, 2015.

Rosen CA, Simpson CB: *Operative Techniques in Laryngology*, 2008, Springer.

Statham MM, Rosen CA, Nandedkar SD, et al: Quantitative laryngeal electromyography: turns and amplitude analysis, *Laryngoscope* 120:2036–2041, 2010.

Vaccha B, Cunnane MB, Mallur P, et al: Losing your voice: etiology and imaging features of vocal fold paralysis, *J Clin Imaging Sci* 3:15, 2013.

Walton C, Carding P, Conway E, Flanagan K, Blackshaw H: Voice outcome measures for adult patients with unilateral vocal fold paralysis: a systematic review, *Laryngoscope* 129(1):187–197, 2019.

Zhou D, Jafri M, Husain I: identifying the prevalence of dysphagia among patients diagnosed with unilateral vocal fold immobility, *Otolaryngol Head Neck Surg* 160(6):955–964, 2019.

CHAPTER 79

INTUBATION AND TRACHEOTOMY

Daniel S. Fink, MD

KEY POINTS

1. A general rule for determining the size of the endotracheal tube (ET) in children is **4 + (age in years/4)** for a cuffed tube and **3.5 + (age in years/4)** for an uncuffed tube. It is generally safer to choose a smaller ET tube if the two tube sizes are debated.
2. Tracheostomy does not prevent chronic aspiration.
3. Inspiratory stridor with muffled voice and usually a lack of cough are symptoms of epiglottitis, a possible airway emergency. If the patient is stable, a lateral neck x-ray may demonstrate a "thumb sign," indicating a swollen epiglottis.
4. Biphasic stridor with barking cough is consistent with subglottitis, or "croup." An AP neck x-ray may demonstrate a "steeple sign," indicating subglottic narrowing.
5. Significant bleeding from a tracheostomy should be taken seriously and investigated to rule out trachea-innominate fistula, a surgical emergency that carries a mortality rate of 73%.

Pearls
1. A vertical incision can be used in newborns to decrease the risk of subglottic stenosis.
2. The trachea is the anatomic location in the head and neck with the highest rate of cocaine absorption.
3. A cuff pressure of 34 cm H_2O compromises capillary blood flow to the tracheal mucosa and causes pressure necrosis.
4. What are the steps in the management of an airway fire?
   - Turn off the oxygen flow
   - Douse fire with saline
   - Remove damaged tube
   - Reintubate as atraumatically as possible
   - Administer IV steroids and antibiotics
   - Perform bronchoscopy before leaving the OR to remove any charred tissue or other debris and evaluate the extent of airway injury
   - Delayed extubation with repeat endoscopic airway examinations

---

QUESTIONS

1. **What are common airway grading systems to consider prior to intubation?**
   Friedman Palate Position (Fig. 79.1):
   I   Visualization of entire uvula and tonsils/tonsillar pillars
   II Visualization of the uvula but not tonsils
   III Visualization of the soft palate but not uvula
   IV Visualization of hard palate only
   Similarly, the Mallampati Score (more commonly used in anesthesiology):
   Class I Soft palate, uvula, fauces, pillars visible
   Class II Soft palate, uvula, fauces visible
   Class III Soft palate, base of uvula visible
   Class IV No soft palate visible
   The higher the score, the more difficult exposure of the larynx may be during intubation.

2. **What does the size of the endotracheal tube refer to?**
   The number refers to the inner diameter of the endotracheal tube. Thus a 5.0 ET tube will have an inner diameter of 5 millimeters, a 5.5 ET tube will have an inner diameter of 5.5 millimeters, and so on. The outer diameter of the ET tube can vary according to the material, manufacturer, and type of tube.

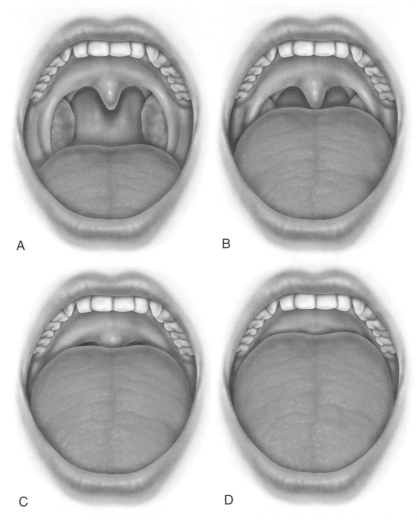

Fig. 79.1 Friedman Palate Position. **A,** I – Visualization of entire uvula and tonsils/tonsillar pillars. **B,** II – Visualization of the uvula but not tonsils. **C,** III – Visualization of the soft palate but not uvula. **D,** IV – Visualization of hard palate only. (From Friedman M, Hani I, Bass L: Clinical staging for sleep disordered breathing. *Otolaryngol Head Neck Surg* 127:13–21, 2002.)

3. **How can you quickly estimate the properly sized endotracheal (ET) tube for children?**
   - Cuffed tube = age 4 years + 3 years
   - Uncuffed tube = age 4 years + 4 years
     This is generally accurate for children aged 1 through 12 years.

4. **How are ET tube sizes chosen for other patients?**
   See Table 79.1.
     As a general rule, between two ET tube sizes, it is safer to put in a slightly smaller ET tube rather than one that is too large and difficult to pass. If ventilation is difficult with a small tube, some ventilation can be administered to stabilize the patient, and a tube exchanger can be used to change the ET tube, with a very low risk of losing the airway.

Table 79.1 Suggested ET Tube Size According to Age

AGE	ENDOTRACHEAL TUBE SIZE (MM)
Neonate	2.5–3.0
Infant, 1–6 months	3.0–3.5
Infant, 6–12 months	3.5–4.0
Toddler	4.0–5.0
Adult female	6.0–7.0
Adult male	7.0–8.0

5. **What is the common airway classification measured during intubation?**
   Cormack-Lehane Classification grades the view of the larynx during direct laryngoscopy:
   Grade I Visualization of the entire glottis
   Grade II Partial view of the glottis; may see only arytenoids
   Grade III Visualization of the epiglottis only; none of the glottis is seen
   Grade IV Not even the epiglottis is visible

6. **What are the typical sounds of obstruction at different levels of the airway?**
   - Trachea – usually expiratory, occasionally inspiratory
   - Subglottis – biphasic stridor, barking cough, hoarse voice
   - Glottis – biphasic or inspiratory stridor, hoarse voice
   - Supraglottic – inspiratory stridor, muffled voice, inability to feed, no cough
   - Oropharynx/nasopharynx – stertor, muffled voice, or hyponasal voice

7. **What are some conservative interventions for upper airway obstruction?**
   Chin lift with jaw thrust, oropharyngeal airway, and *nasopharyngeal airway* are anatomical manipulations that can help alleviate upper airway obstruction. The first two are generally used for unconscious patients. The latter is best used for patients with oral obstruction (i.e., trauma, Ludwig's angina) or in neonates with nasal obstruction who are obligate nasal breathers. *Heliox* can be used to deliver oxygen in cases of airway obstruction. Heliox is a mixture of helium and oxygen and is a lower-density gas compared to room air or pure oxygen. This allows a higher flow rate, which reduces turbulent flow past an obstruction and delivers more oxygen distally to the lungs. This reduced turbulent flow also decreases the pressure gradient needed to move air across an obstruction, thus reducing airway resistance and breathing. Typical concentrations are 21%:79% oxygen to helium. Helium is inert, insoluble in human tissues, and noncombustible. Heliox is used as a temporizing measure while planning to perform a more definitive airway stabilization.

8. **What other noninvasive interventions can improve upper airway obstruction?**
   - *Racemic epinephrine* – administered via nebulizer to cause vasoconstriction and reduce mucosal edema. Racemic epinephrine has been shown to help treat croup and postextubation stridor from laryngeal edema. Racemic epinephrine is not as effective for epiglottitis, and the practice of trying to administer it can be dangerous because agitation for these patients can cause acute obstruction by the swollen epiglottis.
   - *IV steroids* – glucocorticoids, such as dexamethasone, are used to reduce airway inflammation and edema. This is thought to occur through reduced capillary dilation, decreased plasma extravasation, and inflammatory mediator release. They are also indicated for croup and laryngeal edema and are often used for other causes of upper airway obstruction (i.e., abscess or other infectious edema, including epiglottitis and angioedema). IV steroids act gradually, unlike racemic epinephrine, which acts fairly rapidly.

9. **What are the indications for fiber-optic intubation (FOI)?**
   - History of difficult intubation requiring FOI
   - Micrognathia or other craniofacial anomalies
   - Cervical spine issues (fused disks and unstable C-spines)
   - Facial trauma
   - Upper airway obstruction (glottic level or above)
   - Necessity for awake intubation (cannot mask ventilate)
   - Trismus

10. **What are the most common indications for tracheostomy?**
    - Emergent upper airway obstruction or inability to intubate
    - Prolonged intubation/ventilatory support
    - Glottic/supraglottic obstruction (including tumor, infection, trauma, surgical changes)
    - Pulmonary toilet
    - Chronic aspiration (relative indication)
    - Severe sleep apnea not controlled by CPAP or less-invasive surgery

11. **What is the difference between tracheostomy and tracheotomy?**
    Tracheotomy is a procedure that cuts an opening into the trachea. Tracheostomy is technically a term for a more permanent tract that is formed from the trachea to the skin. In reality, a tracheotomy is typically performed, which naturally becomes a tracheostomy as the tract from the skin to airway matures. However, a tracheostomy can be performed at the time of tracheotomy by suturing the skin to the trachea, thus allowing a more stable airway in case of accidental decannulation. These terms are often used interchangeably.

12. **What are the surgical landmarks for tracheotomy?**
    Using a surgical marking pen, the thyroid notch, cricoid cartilage, and sternal notch should be marked.

13. **On what area on the trachea should the tracheotomy be made?**
    Between the second and third tracheal rings. Above this, the tube may erode or fracture the cricoid cartilage, which can lead to subglottic stenosis. Below this, there is a risk to mediastinal structures such as the innominate artery.

14. **What are the basic steps of a tracheotomy?**
    1. The procedure starts with positioning the patient in a supine position with the neck extended. A shoulder roll is very effective in maximizing this extension.
    2. Next, the proper landmarks are marked and the neck is injected with a mixture of lidocaine and epinephrine.
    3. The tracheostomy tube cuff is tested with inflation of the balloon, completely deflated, and then lubricated for ease of insertion. During insertion, the balloon can tear, and the lubricant minimizes trauma to the balloon.
    4. An incision is made in the skin in either a vertical or horizontal direction, depending on the surgeon's preference and patient age. This incision is centered over the second to third tracheal rings, which can be approximated by incising two fingerbreadths above the sternal notch. Incision is carried through the skin, subcutaneous fat, and platysma. Anterior jugular veins may be encountered during this portion of the dissection.
    5. Next, the strap muscles are encountered and divided vertically along the midline raphe to reveal the pretracheal fascia and the thyroid isthmus inferiorly. By staying in the midline with the dissection, bleeding and inadvertent injury to other structures will be minimized.
    6. The thyroid isthmus is retracted either inferiorly or superiorly, depending on its mobility. If it lacks mobility, the isthmus is transected to expose the trachea.
    7. At this point, the anesthesia team should be notified. The anterior surface of the trachea is cleared of its fascial and soft tissue attachments, and any bleeding is attended to to ensure a clear vision of the trachea prior to incision.
    8. Incision into the trachea is made. In adults this is usually a horizontal incision between the second and third rings. In pediatric cases the tracheal incision is vertical through the second and third rings because of the smaller diameter of the trachea. The incisions are made with cold steel to avoid the risk of airway fire using electrocautery. The stoma can be "matured" with either a square section of tracheal cartilage removed ("tracheal window") or a Björk flap (described later in this chapter). The skin edges may also be tacked down to the trachea.
    9. The ET tube is slowly removed by anesthesia under direct visualization by the surgery team. Once it has moved past the opening in the trachea, the tracheostomy tube is inserted using the obturator. The ET tube remains in place until the tracheostomy tube location is confirmed and the tube is fixed in place.

15. **What are the proper steps and precautions after the tracheostomy tube has been placed into the airway?**
    One hand should be kept on the tube AT ALL TIMES. The obturator should be removed, and the inner cannula is inserted into the tracheostomy tube. The cuff should be inflated. Next, the anesthesia circuit is immediately connected and ventilation should be administered. Several items should immediately be assessed: (1) CO_2 return, (2) chest rise, (3) the connection to the tracheostomy tube is checked for condensation, (4) integrity of the balloon is confirmed, and (5) passage of a flexible suction catheter through the tracheostomy tube confirms patency. The anesthesiologist may listen for equal breath sounds. The tube is then sutured and a trach collar is applied.

16. **What is a cricothyroidotomy?**
    In contrast to the tracheotomy procedure described above, a cricothyroidotomy is an emergency procedure for establishing an airway in a life-threatening situation. Many believe that this procedure is easier and quicker than

tracheotomy for the vast majority of medical personnel. There are several kits and techniques that can be used for percutaneous or open cricothyroidotomy, but they typically begin with proper positioning with neck extension and palpation of the cricothyroid membrane between the inferior border of the thyroid cartilage and the superior border of the cricoid. The membrane is approximately 1 cm in height, depending on the neck position. Next, a vertical incision is made through the overlying skin. The cricothyroid membrane is then palpated again and visualized, and a horizontal incision is made in the airway. Following the visualization of air bubbling from the wound, the wound is retracted open (using a tracheal hook, Trousseau dilator, or curved hemostat, etc.), and the tube can be placed with direct visualization of the airway. Some kits involve placing a needle percutaneously, followed by guidewire passage and dilation using the Seldinger technique.

17. **Tracheotomy versus cricothyroidotomy?**
For a planned procedure, tracheotomy is preferred because it provides a long-term and stable airway. A cricothyroidotomy should be converted to a tracheotomy as soon as possible to prevent erosion of the cricoid cartilage or tracheal stenosis.

There is some debate regarding emergent procedures. Some ENT surgeons are comfortable performing tracheotomies so they feel that they should do this in an emergent situation as well. Others feel that a cricothyrotomy is quicker, with less blood loss, and is generally a more reliable landmark in patients with anatomic differences (i.e., short and/or obese necks).

Infants and young children do not have a cricothyroid membrane; thus tracheotomy is required in these populations.

18. **What are the most important intraoperative complications of tracheotomy?**
Complications can be avoided with appropriate communication between the anesthesiologist and operating room staff. For example, airway fire is one of the most devastating complications. This can result from the use of electrocautery during tracheotomy if the FiO_2 concentration is too high. It is imperative to request that the anesthesiologist turn down the FiO_2 several minutes before there is any chance of inadvertently cutting into the trachea using electrocautery. Prior to this point, a high FiO_2 may be needed to properly preoxygenate the patient for extubation and placement of the tracheostomy tube. The ET tube should be slowly removed under direct visualization by the surgeon through the tracheotomy incision. If possible, the anesthesiologist may also watch over the surgical drape barrier. There should be constant communication between the surgeon and the anesthesiologist during this period.

Additional perioperative complications include subcutaneous emphysema, pneumothorax, and pneumomediastinum. Subcutaneous emphysema is thought to occur when air is forced through an incision into the tissue planes of the neck. The mechanisms of pneumothorax or pneumomediastinum are poorly understood. Pneumomediastinum is thought to occur when subcutaneous emphysema is forced further into the chest through negative intrathoracic pressure or a cough that forces air into the deep tissue planes of the neck and mediastinum. One theory for the formation of a pneumothorax is through direct injury to the pleural apices when operating low in the neck. Another is progressive pneumomediastinum causing pleural injury, followed by air tracking into the thoracic cavity.

19. **What is the first intervention for subcutaneous emphysema in a postoperative tracheotomy patient?**
Cutting sutures and inflating the cuff (if not already performed) is the first step. This is followed by a stat chest x-ray and further investigation into the cause.

20. **What are other life-threatening postoperative complications of tracheotomy?**
- Bleeding and/or tracheo-innominate fistula
- Mucus plugging
- Accidental decannulation
- False passage during tracheostomy tube placement

21. **What is a tracheo-innominate (TI) fistula?**
A TI fistula occurs from erosion of the tracheotomy tube through the tracheal wall into the innominate (brachiocephalic) artery. This is an emergency requiring immediate intervention. The fistula typically comes from pressure necrosis from the inflated cuff or the distal tip of the tracheostomy tube. Contributing factors include an overinflated cuff, poor wound healing, and a poorly fitting tube. Fistula formation usually occurs at approximately 2 weeks postoperatively but has been described as early as 2 days. The mortality rate is approximately 73%. Classically, a "sentinel bleed" is described hours or even days prior, wherein there is a brief and intense period of bleeding that spontaneously resolves. This is important to identify, and a CTA may be used to evaluate a stable patient.

22. **How do you handle an urgent bleed in a patient with a tracheotomy?**
If there is a large amount of bleeding from in or around the stoma, the first step is to inflate or overinflate the cuff. If the tube is cuffless, or the patient is coughing up blood through the tube despite overinflation, it should be

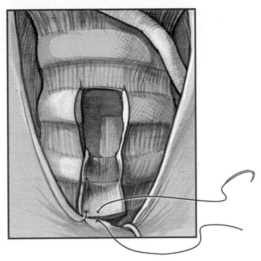

Fig. 79.2 Björk flap. (From Scurry WC Jr., McGinn JD: Operative tracheotomy, *Oper Tech Otolayngol Head Neck Surg* 18(2):85–89, 2007.)

replaced with a cuffed 6.0 ET tube. The cuff should be placed distal to the bleeding site and inflated. Finally, if a TI fistula is suspected, an index finger should be placed through the tracheotomy in an attempt to apply pressure anteriorly against the innominate artery such that it is compressed against the sternum. The patient should be taken immediately to the OR.

23. **What is a Björk flap?**
A Björk flap is created by utilizing a section of the tracheal cartilage that is normally removed during tracheotomy. Superior and lateral cuts are made into the cartilage, but the inferior portion of the cartilage is left intact, leaving an inferiorly based cartilage flap. This flap is then sutured to the muscle/fascial layers and skin of the stoma, such that it serves as the "floor" of the stomal tract. This assists in maintaining a patent stoma in the case of accidental decannulation. The Björk flap creates a tracheostomy that is less likely to spontaneously close upon decannulation (a tracheocutaneous fistula); therefore it is generally used in patients who will undergo a long-term tracheostomy (Fig. 79.2).

24. **What is the basic postoperative care for a tracheotomy?**
Some practitioners prefer to obtain a postoperative chest x-ray to ensure that there is no pneumothorax. However, recent literature has demonstrated that this is generally low yield in patients without signs or symptoms of complications such as pneumothorax. Patients are typically admitted to the surgical ICU for airway monitoring.
    A standard protocol for tracheotomy care is necessary to avoid frequent postoperative complications. The suctioning should be very frequent early on, and it can even be necessary every 15 minutes for the first few hours. As secretions change and lessen, they are needed less frequently. The nurse and respiratory staff should instill saline lavage with suctioning to avoid any mucus plugging, and humidified air is administered to avoid crusting and plugging issues as the innate humidification system of the upper airway has been bypassed because of the tracheotomy.

CONTROVERSIES

25. **When is a cuffed tracheotomy tube indicated? Do they help prevent aspiration?**
A cuffed tube is used when positive airway pressure is required for ventilation. This includes complete ventilatory support and BiPAP/CPAP. Cuffed tubes can also help *slow* aspiration in patients not controlling their secretions. Otherwise, cuffs should always be left deflated. This allows phonation and reduces the risk of pressure-induced injury to the tracheal mucosa.
    Tracheotomy is generally not indicated for aspiration. Cuffed tracheotomy tubes may be helpful in dealing with pulmonary toilet/suctioning of the aspirating patient or decreasing secretions from entering the lungs in patients with sensory or muscle problems of the upper airway. However, cuffed tubes do not prevent chronic aspiration. In fact, tracheotomies can increase the risk of aspiration by preventing proper hyolaryngeal elevation during swallowing.

26. **What are the advantages of an open versus percutaneous tracheotomy?**

Open tracheotomy is a surgical procedure that occurs in the OR. It involves an open wound, with the advantage of better visualization of the trachea prior to entering the airway. It also allows for the identification and control of structures such as small and large blood vessels or the thyroid gland, which theoretically may allow for fewer minor and major complications during the procedure, as well as less postoperative bleeding. However, several large-scale studies have examined the safety of bedside percutaneous tracheostomy in an ICU setting, usually using the dilatational/Seldinger method. The vast majority of these studies have suggested that they are as safe as OR procedures and have similar long-term complications, even in obese patients. Proponents argue that these procedures are faster and far more cost-efficient than open tracheotomies. Critics, however, argue that there is a lack of prospective data and that potentially complicated airways require open procedures. Some critics feel that a potentially catastrophic complication such as transecting a high-riding innominate artery during a percutaneous tracheotomy carries adequate risk for avoiding such procedures. Additionally, in forcing somewhat blunt objects through the skin and trachea, tracheal rings can be crushed, causing long-term tracheal stenosis and/or tracheomalacia.

BIBLIOGRAPHY

Ball JAS, Rhodes A, Grounds RM: A review of the use of helium in the treatment of acute respiratory failure, *Clin Intensive Care* 12:105–113, 2001.

Benjamin BR: Prolonged intubation injuries of the larynx: endoscopic diagnosis, classification, and treatment, *Ann Otol Rhinol Laryngol Suppl* 160:1–15, 1993.

Dennis BM, Eckert MJ, Gunter OL, et al: Safety of bedside percutaneous tracheostomy in the critically ill: evaluation of more than 3000 procedures, *J Am Coll Surg* 216(4):858–865, 2013.

Depuydt S, Nauwynck M, Bourgeois M, et al: Acute epiglottitis in children: a review following an atypical case, *Acta Anaesth Belg* 54:237–241, 2003.

Durbin CG Jr: Tracheostomy: why, when, and how? *Respir Care* 55(8):1056–1068, 2010.

Fernandez R, Tizon AI, Gonzalez J, et al: Intensive care unit discharge to the ward with a tracheostomy cannula as a risk factor for mortality: a prospective, multicenter propensity analysis, *Crit Care Med* 39(10):2240–2245, 2011.

Friedman M, Hani I, Bass L: Clinical staging for sleep disordered breathing, *Otolaryngol Head Neck Surg* 127:13–21, 2002.

Goldenberg D, Gov EG, Golz A, et al: Tracheotomy complications: a retrospective study of 1130 cases, *Otolaryngol Head Neck Surg* 123:495–500, 2000.

Kairys SW, Olmstead EM, O'Conner GT: Steroid treatment of laryngotracheitis: a meta-analysis of the evidence from randomized trials, *Pediatrics* 83:683–693, 1989.

Lalwani AK: *Current Diagnosis & Treatment in Otolaryngology: Head & Neck Surgery*, 2008, McGraw-Hill Medical.

CHAPTER 80

LARYNGEAL AND ESOPHAGEAL TRAUMA

Saied Ghadersohi, MD, Ryota Kashiwazaki, MD and Jeremy D. Prager, MD, MBA

KEY POINTS

1. Laryngeal fractures are uncommon injuries that may be associated with life-threatening airway compromise.
2. The first and most important step in the management of laryngeal trauma is to verify and secure a safe airway.
3. Esophagoscopy should be performed in any patient going to the operating room to rule out concomitant injury.
4. The most common cause of internal laryngeal trauma is endotracheal intubation, especially in the setting of prolonged intubation.
5. Arytenoid dislocations are rare and may present similarly to unilateral vocal cord paralysis.

Pearls

1. An experienced physician should manage the airway, and endotracheal intubation should only be performed under adequate visualization and when the larynx and trachea are in known continuity.
2. Intubating a patient blindly may convert a stable airway to an unstable airway.
3. Avoiding prolonged intubation is the most effective way to prevent internal laryngeal trauma.
4. Choosing the smallest endotracheal tube that will provide adequate ventilation will help to minimize mucosal trauma.
5. Laryngeal trauma should be included in the differential diagnosis when evaluating a patient with vocal cord paralysis.

QUESTIONS

EXTERNAL LARYNGEAL TRAUMA

1. **What is the incidence of external laryngeal trauma?**
   External laryngeal trauma is rare, with an estimated incidence of 1 in 137,000 inpatient admissions and 1 in 30,000 emergency room visits. Laryngeal injuries in the pediatric patient are even more uncommon and account for <0.5% of trauma admissions compared to 1% of adult trauma admissions. The occurrence of blunt trauma injuries has decreased in the past several decades owing to improved automobile safety. However, the incidence of penetrating trauma has increased due to a rise in violent crimes.

2. **What anatomic features are protective against laryngeal trauma?**
   - **Surrounding structures:** Multiple surrounding structures shield the larynx and provide protection from external trauma. These structures include the mandible superiorly, sternum and clavicles inferiorly, sternocleidomastoid muscles laterally, and vertebrae posteriorly. Anterior soft tissue, including the strap muscles, provides minimal protection from the anteriorly directed force. In pediatric patients, the larynx is located higher in the neck in relation to the mandible and is thus further protected.
   - **Laryngeal mobility:** The larynx is mobile in multiple directions, most prominently in the lateral plane but also in the anterior/posterior and superior/inferior planes. This mobility allows it to be pushed out of the way by external forces.
   - **Tissue pliability:** In adults, ossification of the larynx increases the chances of fracture in the setting of blunt trauma. In children, laryngeal cartilages remain pliable and are consequently more resistant to fracture.

3. **Discuss the etiology of external laryngeal trauma.**
   Blunt trauma occurs as the result of an anterior force compressing the larynx against the fixed vertebral column. These injuries most commonly result from motor vehicle accidents despite the use of seatbelts and airbags and

occur when the hyperextended neck is thrust onto the dashboard or steering wheel during rapid deceleration. Similar crush injuries can occur during sports (i.e., ice hockey or karate), hanging, or strangulation. Another subset of these injuries includes "clothesline" injuries in which a thin horizontal structure (e.g., barbed wire fence) is struck at high speed in the cervical region.

The severity of trauma is variable but is generally proportional to the velocity or kinetic energy the struck object imparts to the surrounding tissues. Additional information regarding the size and shape of the blunt or penetrating object is also helpful. A larger force distributed over a smaller surface area is more likely to result in penetrating trauma than blunt trauma. Fortunately, penetrating injuries are much less common and occur as a result of violent crime and military conflicts, such as stab or bullet wounds.

4. **What are the main symptoms and signs of blunt laryngeal trauma?**
Dyspnea, dysphonia, dysphagia, odynophagia, stridor, hoarseness, pain over the anterior neck, and hemoptysis are common symptoms of laryngeal trauma. The severity of symptoms may not correspond with the extent or rate of progression of the injury and the potential for impending airway obstruction.

Physical examination results may range from asymptomatic to critically ill, with typical findings including tenderness or ecchymosis over the larynx; loss of anatomical landmarks on neck palpitation that may indicate hyoid or laryngeal fracture; subcutaneous emphysema, particularly in the setting of positive pressure ventilation; cyanosis; air escaping from the neck wound; or persistent pneumothorax despite chest tube placement. Note that these patients are often at risk of cervical spine and vascular trauma.

Patients may present with mild symptoms and progress to airway compromise over minutes to hours due to progressive edema, hematoma, or instability of the laryngotracheal framework. Eliciting the time course of symptoms and signs is therefore important in determining management. Observation is recommended if history and physical examination are at all concerning, and the patient may require frequent examination by personnel with experience in neck trauma.

5. **Discuss the management of acute airway compromise following laryngeal trauma.**
The initial step in the management of any trauma patient, including those with laryngeal trauma, follows the advanced trauma life support (ATLS) protocol. The first step in airway management is to determine whether the patient displays signs and symptoms of impending airway compromise such as stridor, dyspnea, respiratory distress, or aphonia. If a patient exhibits signs of airway compromise, a secure airway must be obtained as soon as possible. There are several methods that are appropriate for securing the airway in the setting of laryngeal trauma, including intubation, tracheostomy, and cricothyroidotomy.

Several factors must be considered when choosing which method will be used to secure the airway, including patient stability and injury severity. Airway control should occur in the emergency room or, when possible, the operating room to allow for optimal direct and endoscopic evaluation. For endotracheal intubation to proceed, the larynx and trachea must be clearly intact and in continuity to prevent mucosal trauma, destabilization of laryngeal fractures, laryngotracheal separation, and further respiratory compromise. This can be done by placing an endotracheal tube over an endoscope to allow inspection of the airway and intubation. In addition, consideration should be given to the status of the cervical spine, which may be unknown at that point in the evaluation. Spinal stabilization should be maintained until it is clinically and/or radiographically cleared. It is important to note that intubation should be performed by an experienced physician to help prevent intubation-related trauma (Fig. 80.1).

If the airway is determined to be unstable, awake tracheotomy in the operating room should be performed. Cricothyroidotomy is reserved for patients with a rapidly deteriorating airway, those who do not meet the optimal conditions for intubation, or those in whom tracheostomy is not possible due to patient factors or availability of physicians experienced in the surgical airway. Cricothyroidotomy should subsequently be converted to tracheostomy to prevent the development of subglottic stenosis. Following emergent management of the airway, these patients should undergo endoscopic evaluation of the aerodigestive tract in the operating room.

6. **Discuss important aspects of the evaluation and management of a stable patient with external laryngeal trauma.**
A History:
  1 Mechanism of injury: Be suspicious in the setting of a high-velocity impact directed anteriorly to the neck.
  2 Temporal evolution: Determine if symptoms are getting worse.
B Physical exam:
  1 Head and neck examination: Bony and soft tissue trauma, voice quality, respiratory effort, loss of landmarks, crepitus
  2 Associated injuries: Neurologic, vascular, or spinal injuries
C Flexible laryngoscopy: In a stable patient flexible laryngoscopy is the most important next step to assess the airway and extent of injury. Findings including ecchymosis, hematoma, mucosal tears, exposed muscle and cartilage, and vocal cord mobility should be assessed. Serial examinations may be needed if there is progression of symptoms or concerning findings.
D Imaging: Noncontrast computed tomography of the neck will further assess laryngeal structures and any fractures involving the laryngeal framework.

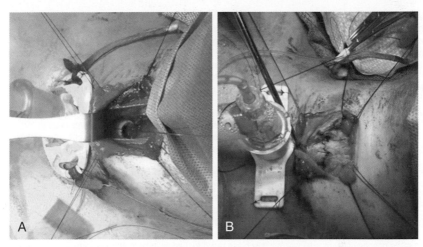

Fig. 80.1 Clothesline injury followed by intubation in the field resulting in complete separation of the larynx and trachea. **A,** The patient was managed by low tracheostomy followed by neck exploration. The airway was separated between the cricoid and the first tracheal ring, which was crushed and fractured. **B,** The second tracheal ring and cricoid were anastomosed.

Definitive management: The extent of injury may then be stratified based on the Schaefer-Fuhrman classification to guide definitive management (Table 80.1).

1 Nonsurgical management:

Appropriate for those with group 1 injuries. This includes a period of observation following injury for 12 to 24 hours, +/- steroids, +/- antibiotics, +/- anti-reflux medications, +/- cool mist, and +/- voice rest. Group 2 patients will also likely benefit from these measures but may need serial fiberoptic examinations to assess the progression of the exam and possible tracheostomy if there is airway compromise.

2 Surgical management:

Patients with group 3 or 4 injuries often require tracheostomy to secure the airway. Endolaryngeal exploration and surgical repair should also be performed with the goal of preserving airway patency and function. Group 5 injuries require tracheostomy placement, which may be very difficult due to the altered anatomy. Often, the distal trachea retracts inferiorly in the neck and potentially into the mediastinum. Re-anastomosis should be performed after securing the airway. Earlier intervention is associated with better voice and airway outcomes, in addition to shorter ICU and overall hospital stays. The surgical approach may require some or all of the following:

A Midline thyrotomy or laryngofissure approach.

B Repair of mucosal lacerations and restoration of mucosal coverage of exposed muscle and cartilage should be attempted.

C Stents are often utilized based on the surgeon's preference or expertise, but in general they should be used when the anterior commissure is significantly disrupted to prevent anterior glottic web formation.

D Repair laryngeal skeletal fractures with wires, sutures, and plating. Plating may be difficult in the more cartilaginous pediatric larynx. Controversy exists regarding plating/repairing all laryngeal framework fractures. Some authors prefer plating even nondisplaced fractures owing to concerns of displacement and voice changes over time.

Table 80.1 Schaefer Fuhrman Classification for Classifying the Severity of Laryngeal Trauma	
Group 1	Minor endolaryngeal hematoma or lacerations, no fractures
Group 2	Edema, hematoma, minor mucosal disruption without exposed cartilage, nondisplaced fractures
Group 3	Massive edema, large mucosal lacerations, exposed cartilage, displaced fractures, vocal cord immobility
Group 4	Same as group 3 but more severe with: Severe mucosal disruption Disruption of the anterior commissure Unstable fracture, two or more fracture lines
Group 5	Complete laryngotracheal separation

7. **What is the preferred imaging modality for the assessment of laryngeal trauma?**
   Chest radiography is often performed as part of the initial trauma evaluation and is helpful in ruling out a pneumo-thorax, tracheal deviation, or pneumomediastinum (suggesting an airway injury). Noncontrast CT is the preferred imaging modality in patients with a stable airway because of its fast acquisition and adequate imaging of the larynx and surrounding structures. A CT angiogram may be considered if vascular injury is suspected.
   It is important to note that airway management should not be delayed for imaging. Imaging is particularly helpful in patients with blunt injury in whom it is difficult to ascertain the severity of the injury.

8. **Which associated injuries should be ruled out in patients with laryngeal trauma?**
   A. Cervical spine injury: Laryngeal fracture can be associated with cervical spine fractures in up to 10% of patients. Based on the National Emergency X-Radiography Utilization Study (NEXUS) criteria, laryngeal trauma qualifies as a "distracting injury," and cervical radiography is indicated to evaluate for the presence of cervical spine injuries. Since a CT scan may be obtained to evaluate the larynx, a cervical spine protocol may be added.
   B. Vascular injury: Usually presents with persistent hemorrhage from an open wound, expanding hematoma in the neck, or a bruit. A CT angiogram can be obtained depending on the location and stability of the patient. Management includes surgical or interventional radiology, depending on the zone of the neck that is involved in the injury.
   C. Pharyngeal/esophageal injuries: Infrequent in penetrating and blunt laryngeal injuries (4% to 6%) but potentially catastrophic with mortality rates approaching 25%. Esophageal injury often results in leakage of saliva or subcutaneous emphysema, which can result in mediastinitis or abscess formation. Management should include esophagoscopy in the first 12 to 24 hours or during airway management to identify any injuries early. Barium or gastrografin esophagram can be considered if there is suspicion of esophageal injury or for follow-up; however, it is not as sensitive as early rigid esophagoscopy. Management can include IV antibiotics, nothing by mouth status for 8 to 10 days, and nasogastric tube placement for feeding or formal transcervical surgical repair of the esophagus.

9. **Propose an algorithm for evaluation and management of external laryngeal trauma.**
   See Fig. 80.2.

10. **What anatomic factors affect laryngeal trauma in the pediatric patient?**
    There are several differences between the pediatric and adult larynx that affect laryngeal trauma in the pediatric population. Some of these factors are protective but some also convey increased risk. First, the larynx lies at the level of C3 in young children and descends gradually until the age of 3 years when it takes on a more adult location at the level of C6. The relatively high location of the pediatric larynx provides some additional protection afforded by the overhanging mandible. Another protective feature of the pediatric larynx is its pliability. Compared with an adult larynx, which is relatively rigid due to ossification, the pediatric larynx remains pliable. The flexibility allows for compression without fracture in the setting of external blunt trauma.
    Conversely, the child's larynx is relatively smaller than the adult airway, which translates to greater potential compromise from edema. Furthermore, the submucosal tissue in a pediatric patient is loosely adherent to the underlying perichondrium when compared with the adult, resulting in the potential for greater soft tissue injury, edema, and hematoma formation. This combination of factors translates to a greater risk of airway compromise in these patients despite the protective factors discussed above.

INTERNAL LARYNGEAL TRAUMA

11. **Discuss the etiology of internal laryngeal trauma.**
    Iatrogenic injury related to endotracheal intubation is the predominant cause of internal laryngeal trauma. The injury can result from the act of intubation or the presence of an endotracheal tube, and risk factors include prolonged intubation, excessive endotracheal tube (ET) size, intubation in the emergency setting, and intubation without neuromuscular blockade. Acute complications include mucosal lacerations, arytenoid dislocation, and tracheal rupture, among others. Trauma related to prolonged intubation is the result of long-standing excessive pressure from the ET or cuff, leading to tissue necrosis, inflammation, and subglottic stenosis from scar formation. Longer duration correlates with greater histologic damage.
    There are several locations that are at risk for injury from prolonged intubation, including the narrowest por-tions of both the adult and pediatric airway: the glottis and subglottis, respectively. In children, intubation injury in the subglottis can result in subglottic stenosis. In adult patients, damage at the level of the glottis generally occurs posteriorly and can result in posterior glottic stenosis and even bilateral vocal cord immobility (Fig. 80.3).

12. **What is the incidence of subglottic stenosis following endotracheal intubation?**
    The incidence in pediatric patients (those most at risk) ranges from approximately 1% to 8%. More recent reports have indicated an incidence between 0% and 2%. Of patients with acquired subglottic stenosis, approximately 90% of cases are due to endotracheal intubation.

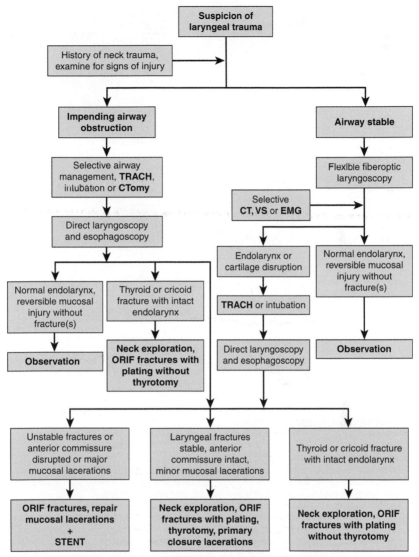

Fig. 80.2 Algorithm for early treatment of acute external laryngeal trauma. CT = computed tomography; CTomy = cricothyroidotomy; EMG = electromyography of the larynx; ORIF = open reduction and internal fixation of laryngeal skeletal fractures; STENT = endolaryngeal stent or lumen keeper; TRACH = tracheotomy; VS = videostroboscopy of larynx. (Used with permission. From Schaefer SD: Management of acute blunt and penetrating external laryngeal trauma. *Laryngoscope* 124(1):233–244, 2014.)

13. **What are other causes of internal laryngeal trauma?**
    Caustic ingestion and inhalation burns are two other causes of internal laryngeal injury. The larynx is involved in 40% of cases of caustic ingestion. Thermal injury of the larynx occurs in 30% of patients with burns. These injuries tend to produce more severe stenosis than postintubation trauma.

14. **What is arytenoid dislocation?**
    Arytenoid dislocation is a rare injury that can occur as a result of external laryngeal trauma with disruption of the laryngeal framework or, more commonly, as a result of upper aerodigestive tract instrumentation (intubation). Dislocation occurs either anteriorly or posteriorly. Anterior dislocation results from anterior displacement of the cartilage during laryngoscope or ET insertion, whereas posterior cartilage displacement can result from forces applied by the ET as it passes through the glottis. Another possibility is extubation with an inflated cuff, which translates posteriorly directed forces on the cartilage.

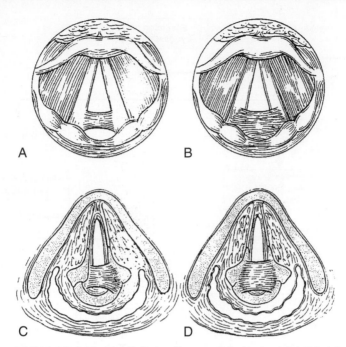

Fig. 80.3 Posterior subglottic stenosis. **A,** Interarytenoid adhesion with a mucosally lined tract posteriorly. **B,** Posterior commissure and interarytenoid scar without a mucosally lined tract posteriorly. **C,** Posterior commissure scar extending into the right cricoarytenoid joint. **D,** Posterior commissure scar extending into both cricoarytenoid joints. (From Zalzal GH, Cotton RT: Glottic and subglottic stenosis. In: Flint PW, Haughey BH, Lund VJ, et al, eds, *Cummings Otolaryngology: Head and Neck Surgery,* 5th ed, Philadelphia, 2010, Mosby Elsevier, p. 2916.)

15. How common is arytenoid dislocation?

Arytenoid dislocation is extremely rare, with an estimated incidence of 0.1% of tracheal intubations.

16. How does an arytenoid dislocation present?

Common presenting symptoms include dysphonia, vocal fatigue, cough, and inability to project the voice due to reduced vocal cord mobility. Some patients may also experience swallow dysfunction. In the acute phase after laryngeal trauma, the patient may also have a sore throat or pain with swallowing.

Flexible fiberoptic laryngoscopy and/or videostroboscopy demonstrate diminished ipsilateral vocal cord movement with abnormal position of the arytenoid cartilage as well as a height discrepancy between the vocal cords (CT scans may also reveal incorrect position of the arytenoid cartilage). Laryngeal electromyography can distinguish vocal cord paralysis from arytenoid dislocation, as paralysis is associated with predictable changes in electrical activity, and arytenoid dislocation should be associated with normal electrical activity in the acute or subacute setting.

17. Describe treatment for arytenoid dislocation.

Early intervention is recommended to prevent joint ankylosis. Microlaryngoscopy with arytenoid repositioning is effective in most patients who undergo this treatment. Voice therapy as an adjunctive treatment is also helpful.

BIBLIOGRAPHY

Ahmed N, Massier C, Tassie J, Whalen J, Chung R: Diagnosis of penetrating injuries of the pharynx and esophagus in the severely injured patient, *J Trauma* 67:152–154, 2009.

Armstrong WB, Detar TR, Stanley RB: Diagnosis and management of external penetrating cervical esophageal injuries, *Ann Otol Rhinol Laryngol* 103:863–871, 1994.

Bent JP III, Silver JR, Porubsky ES: Acute laryngeal trauma: a review of 77 patients, *Otolaryngol Head Neck Surg* 109(3 Pt 1):441–449, 1993.

Esteller-More E, Ibanez J, Matino E, et al: Prognostic factors in laryngotracheal injury following intubation and/or tracheostomy in ICU patients, *Eur Arch Otorhinolaryngol* 262:880, 2005.

Flint PW, Haughey BH, Lund VJ, et al: eds: *Cummings Otolaryngology: Head and Neck Surgery,* 2015, Saunders Elsevier.

Hoffman JR, Mower WR, Wolfson AB, et al: Validity of a set of clinical criteria to rule out injury to the cervical spine in patients with blunt trauma, *N Engl J Med* 343:94, 2000.

Jalisi S, Zoccoli M: Management of laryngeal fractures – a 10-year experience, *J Voice* 25(4):473–479, 2011.

Jewett BS, Shockley WW, Rutledge R: External laryngeal trauma analysis of 392 patients, *Arch Otolaryngol Head Neck Surg* 125(8):877–880, 1999.

Mendelsohn AH, Sidell DR, Berke GS, John MS: Optimal timing of surgical intervention following adult laryngeal trauma, *Laryngoscope* 121(10):2122–2127, 2011.

Nahum AM: Immediate care of blunt laryngeal trauma, *J Trauma* 9(2):112–125, 1969.

Norris BK, Schweinfurth JM: Arytenoid dislocation: an analysis of contemporary literature, *Laryngoscope* 121:142–146, 2011.

Randall DR, Rudmik LR, Ball CG, Bosch JD: External laryngotracheal trauma: Incidence, airway control, and outcomes in a large Canadian center, *Laryngoscope* 124:E123–E133, 2014.

Schaefer SD: The treatment of acute external laryngeal injuries. "State of the art," *Arch Otolaryngol Head Neck Surg* 117(1):35–39, 1991.

Schaefer SD: The acute management of external laryngeal trauma. A 27-year experience, *Arch Otolaryngol Head Neck Surg* 118(6):598–604, 1992.

Schaefer SD: Management of acute blunt and penetrating external laryngeal trauma, *Laryngoscope* 124(1):233–244, 2014. doi: 10.1002/lary.24068.

Walner DL, Loewen MS, Kimura RE: Neonatal subglottic stenosis – incidence and trends, *Laryngoscope* 111(1):48–51, 2001.

Zalzal GH, Cotton RT: Glottic and subglottic stenosis. In: Flint PW, Haughey BH, Lund VJ, et al, eds: *Cummings Otolaryngology: Head and Neck Surgery, 5th ed*, 2010, Mosby Elsevier, p. 2916.

Page numbers followed by *"f"* indicate figures, *"t"* indicate tables, and *"b"* indicate boxes